Geriatric Trauma and Acute Care Surgery

Aurelio Rodriguez
Robert D. Barraco • Rao R. Ivatury
Editors

Geriatric Trauma and Acute Care Surgery

Springer

Editors
Aurelio Rodriguez
University of Maryland School of Medicine
Drexel University College of Medicine
Baltimore, MD
USA

Robert D. Barraco
Lehigh Valley Health Network
USF Morsani College of Medicine - Lehigh Valley
Allentown, PA
USA

Rao R. Ivatury
Virginia Commonwealth University
Richmond, VA
USA

ISBN 978-3-030-09623-6 ISBN 978-3-319-57403-5 (eBook)
https://doi.org/10.1007/978-3-319-57403-5

Softcover re-print of the Hardcover 1st edition 2018

Printed on acid-free paper
This Springer imprint is published by the registered company Springer International Publishing AG part of Springer Nature
The registered company address is: Gewerbestrasse 11, 6330 Cham, Switzerland

Contents

Contributors

Sharline Z. Aboutanos, M.D., F.A.A.P., F.A.C.S. Richmond Plastic Surgeons, Richmond, VA, USA

Daniel T. Altman, M.D. Department of Orthopaedic Surgery, Drexel University College of Medicine, Allegheny General Hospital, Allegheny Health Network, Pittsburgh, PA, USA

Tiffany N. Anderson, M.D. University of Florida Academic Health Center, Gainesville, FL, USA

Robert D. Barraco, M.D., M.P.H., F.A.C.S., F.C.C.P. Lehigh Valley Health Network, Allentown, PA, USA

Justin Boccardo, M.D., F.A.C.S. Department of Vascular Surgery, Bayfront Punta Gorda, Punta Gorda, FL, USA

Kai Bortz, M.S.N., R.N.-B.C., C.M.S.R.N., C.N.L., T.C.R.N Transitional Trauma Unit, Lehigh Valley Health Network, Allentown, PA, USA

Benjamin N. Breyer, M.D. University of California - San Francisco Urology Department, San Francisco General Hospital, San Francisco, CA, USA

Laura S. Buchanan, M.D. R Adams Cowley Shock Trauma Center, University of Maryland Medical Center, Baltimore, MD, USA

Wayne Campbell, M.D. Department of Medicine-Infection Deseases, Union Memorial Hospital, Baltimore, MD, USA

Alexander Chen Medstar Union Memorial Hospital, Baltimore, MD, USA

JoAnn Coleman, D.N.P., A.C.N.P., A.O.C.N. Department of Surgery, Sinai Hospital of Baltimore, Baltimore, MD, USA

Mark Crye, M.D. Department of Cardiovascular and Thoracic Surgery, Allegheny Health Network, Pittsburgh, PA, USA

James Edmond Conway, M.D., Ph.D. Department of Neurosurgery at Sinai Hospital and Baltimore Neurosurgery and Spine Center, Baltimore, MD, USA

Baltimore Neurosurgery and Spine Center, Baltimore, MD, USA

Edward E Cornwell III, M.D., F.A.C.S., F.C.C.M., F.W.A.C.S. Department of Surgery, Howard University Hospital, Washington, DC, USA

Connie DeLa'O, M.D., M.S. Division of Trauma, Acute Care Surgery and Surgical Critical Care, West Virginia University, Morgantown, WV, USA

Mathew A. Van Deusen, M.D. Department of Cardiovascular and Thoracic Surgery, Allegheny Health Network, Pittsburgh, PA, USA

Jose J. Diaz, C.N.S., F.A.C.S., F.C.C.M. R Adams Cowley Shock Trauma Center, University of Maryland Medical Center, Baltimore, MD, USA

Therese M. Duane, M.D., M.B.A. Department of Surgery, John Peter Smith Health Network, Fort Worth, TX, USA

Juan Duchesne, MD, FACS, FCCP, FCCM Trauma and Critical Care, Tulane University, New Orleans, LA, USA

Russell D. Dumire, M.D., F.A.C.S. Conemaugh Memorial Hospital, Johnstown, PA, USA

James K. Dzandu, Ph.D. Department of Trauma, Honorhealth John C. Lincoln Medical Center, Phoenix, AZ, USA

David Elliott, M.D. Médecins Sans Frontières/Doctors Without Borders, Richmond, VA, USA

Paula Ferrada, M.D., F.A.C.S. VCU Surgery Trauma, Critical Care and Emergency Surgery, Richmond, VA, USA

Ellen P. Fitzpatrick, M.D. Department of Orthopaedic Surgery, UC Davis Medical Center, Sacramento, CA, USA

Molly Flanagan, M.D. VCU Surgery Trauma, Critical Care and Emergency Surgery, Richmond, VA, USA

Rajesh R. Gandhi, M.D., Ph.D. Department of Surgery, John Peter Smith Health Network, Fort Worth, TX, USA

Ira Martin Garonzik, M.D. Department of Neurosurgery at Sinai Hospital and Baltimore Neurosurgery and Spine Center, Baltimore, MD, USA

Baltimore Neurosurgery and Spine Center, Baltimore, MD, USA

Amy J. Goldberg, M.D., F.A.C.S. Department of Surgery, Lewis Katz School of Medicine at Temple University, Philadelphia, PA, USA

James M. Haan, M.D. Trauma Services, Trauma Services Via Christi Hospitals, Via Christi Hospitals St. Francis Campus, Wichita, KS, USA

Laura Harmon, M.D. Department of Surgery, R Adams Cowley Shock Trauma Center, University of Maryland, Baltimore, MD, USA

Sharon Henry, M.D. Program in Trauma University of Maryland School of Medicine, University of Maryland Medical Center R A Cowley Shock Trauma Center, Baltimore, MD, USA

David N. Herndon, M.D., F.A.C.S. Department of Surgery, University of Texas Medical Branch (UTMB), Galveston, TX, USA

Department of Surgery, Shriners Hospitals for Children®—Galveston (SHC-G), Galveston, TX, USA

Gabriel Hundeshagen, M.D. Department of Surgery, University of Texas Medical Branch (UTMB), Galveston, TX, USA

Department of Hand, Plastic and Reconstructive Surgery, Burn Trauma Center, BG Trauma Center Ludwigshafen, University of Heidelberg, Ludwigshafen, Germany

Rao R. Ivatury, M.D. Virginia Commonwealth University, Richmond, VA, USA

Janeen Jordan, M.D. University of Florida Academic Health Center, Gainesville, FL, USA

Kimberly Joseph, M.D., F.A.C.S., F.C.C.M. Department of Trauma and Burns, John H. Stroger Hospital of Cook County, Chicago, IL, USA

Bellal Joseph, M.D. Division of Trauma, Department of Surgery, University of Arizona, Tucson, AZ, USA

Jessica Jurkovich, AGACNP-BC, MSN, CCRN Department of Trauma, Critical Care and Acute Care Surgery, Oregon Health Science University, Portland, OR, USA

Stephen Curran Kane, B.S. Baltimore Neurosurgery and Spine Center, Baltimore, MD, USA

Mark Katlic, M.D., M.M.M., F.A.C.S. Department of Surgery, Sinai Hospital of Baltimore, Baltimore, MD, USA

Elizabeth D. Katrancha, DNP, CCNS, RN, CNE, CSN Department of Nursing, University of Pittsburgh, Johnstown, PA, USA

Jessica G. Kingsberg, M.D. Silver State Orthopedics, Las Vegas, NV, USA

Jonathan Levy, M.D. Department of General Surgery, Allegheny Health Network, Pittsburgh, PA, USA

Leah Kohri, B.S.N., C.C.R.N. Multitrauma Critical Care, R Adams Cowley Shock Trauma Center, Baltimore, MD, USA

Rosemary Kozar, M.D., Ph.D. Department of Surgery, R Adams Cowley Shock Trauma Center, University of Maryland School of Medicine, MD, USA

Margaret H. Lauerman, M.D. Program in Trauma University of Maryland School of Medicine, University of Maryland Medical Center R A Cowley Shock Trauma Cente, Baltimore, MD, USA

Anna M. Ledgerwood, M.D. Wayne State University School of Medicine, Detroit, MI, USA

Jong O. Lee, M.D. Department of Surgery, University of Texas Medical Branch (UTMB), Galveston, TX, USA

Victor Ryan Lewis, B.A. Baltimore Neurosurgery and Spine Center, Baltimore, MD, USA

Manuel Lorenzo, M.D. Associates in Surgical Acute Care, Dallas, TX, USA

Charles E. Lucas, M.D., F.A.C.S. Michael and Marian Ilitch Department of Surgery, Wayne State University School of Medicine, Detroit, MI, USA

Arturo R. Maldonado, M.D., Ph.D., F.A.C.S. Bethesda North Trauma Center, Bethesda North Hospital, Cincinnati, OH, USA

Ajai Malhotra, M.D. Acute Care Surgery, University of Vermont College of Medicine, Burlington, VT, USA

Alicia J. Mangram, M.D., F.A.C.S. Department of Trauma, Honorhealth John C. Lincoln Medical Center, Phoenix, AZ, USA

Cathy A. Maxwell, Ph.D., R.N. Vanderbilt University School of Nursing, Nashville, TN, USA

Jack W. McAninch, M.D. University of California - San Francisco Urology Department, San Francisco General Hospital, San Francisco, CA, USA

Jay Menaker, M.D. Division of Surgical/Critical Care, Department of Surgery, Program in Trauma, R Adams Cowley Shock Trauma Center, University of Maryland School of Medicine, Baltimore, MD, USA

Dave Milzman, M.D., F.A.C.E.P. Georgetown University School of Medicine, Washington, DC, USA

Department of Emergency Medicine and Divison of Trauma, Washington Hospital Center, Washington, DC, USA

Study Center for Brain Injury, Washington Hospital Center, Washington, DC, USA

Frederick Moore, M.D. University of Florida Academic Health Center, Gainesville, FL, USA

Benjamin J. Moran, M.D. Department of Surgery, Lewis Katz School of Medicine at Temple University, Philadelphia, PA, USA

Matthew Mowry, R.N., M.S.N., C.E.N. Trauma Performance Improvement Coordinator, Level 1 Adult Trauma Center, Allegheny General Hospital, Pittsburgh, PA, USA

Gregory P. Murphy, M.D. University of California - San Francisco Urology Department, San Francisco General Hospital, San Francisco, CA, USA

Lena M. Napolitano, M.D. Division of Acute Care Surgery (Trauma, Burns, Surgical Critical Care, Emergency Surgery), Department of Surgery, University of Michigan, Ann Arbor, MI, USA

Russell J. Nauta, M.D., F.A.C.S. Harvard Medical School, Boston, MA, USA

Mount Auburn Hospital, Cambridge, MA, USA

Adrian W. Ong, M.D. Department of Surgery, University of Pennsylvania, Philadelphia, PA, USA

Department of Surgery, Reading Health System, Reading, PA, USA

Juan L. Peschiera, M.D. Bethesda North Trauma Center, Bethesda North Hospital, Cincinnati, OH, USA

Elizabeth L. Price, R.N., M.S.N., A.C.N.S.-B.C. Department of Trauma Services, John Peter Smith Health Network, Fort Worth, TX, USA

Ashanthi Ratnasekera, D.O. Crozer Keystone Health System, Chester, PA, USA

Peter Rhee, M.D. Division of Trauma, Department of Surgery, University of Arizona, Tucson, AZ, USA

T. Robert Qaqish, M.Sc., M.D. Department of Surgery, Sinai Hospital of Baltimore, Baltimore, MD, USA

Sarada Rao, M.D. Georgetown University School of Medicine, Washington, DC, USA

Department of Surgery, Eastern Virginia Residency Program, Norfolk, VA, USA

Aurelio Rodriguez, M.D., F.A.C.S. University of Maryland School of Medicine, Drexel University College of Medicine, Baltimore, MD, USA

Peter B. Letarte, M.D., F.A.A.N.S., F.A.C.S. Neurosurgeon, Premier Health, Dayton, OH, USA

Thomas M. Scalea, M.D. Division of Surgical/Critical Care, Department of Surgery, Program in Trauma, R Adams Cowley Shock Trauma Center, University of Maryland School of Medicine, Baltimore, MD, USA

C.W. Schwab, M.D., F.A.C.S., F.R.C.S.(H)glas Division of Traumatology, Surgical Critical Care and Emergency Surgery, Department of Surgery, Perlman School of Medicine, University of Pennsylvania, Philadelphia, PA, USA

Elizabeth Seislove, M.S.N., R.N., A.V.P. Trauma Services, Hospital Corporation of America (HCA), Nashville, TN, USA

Jason Sheaffer, R.N., M.S.N. Blocker Burn Unit, University of Texas Medical Branch at Galveston, Galveston, TX, USA

Vanessa Shifflette, M.D. Associates in Surgical Acute Care, Dallas, TX, USA

Lars Ola Sjoholm, M.D. Department of Surgery, Trauma Program Lewis Katz School of Medicine at Temple University, Philadelphia, USA

Deborah M. Stein Department of Surgery, University of Maryland school of Medicine, R Adams Cowley shock Trauma Center, University of Maryland Medical Center, Baltimore, MD, USA

Joseph F. Sucher, M.D., F.A.C.S. Department of Trauma, Honorhealth Deer Valley Medical Center, Phoenix, AZ, USA

Nicole L. Werner, M.D., M.S. Division of Acute Care Surgery (Trauma, Burns, Surgical Critical Care, Emergency Surgery), Department of Surgery, University of Michigan, Ann Arbor, MI, USA

Edward R. Westrick, M.D. Department of Orthopaedic Surgery, Drexel University College of Medicine, Allegheny General Hospital, Allegheny Health Network, Pittsburgh, PA, USA

Jack Wilberger, M.D., F.A.C.S., F.A.A.N.S. Department of Neurosurgery, Allegheny General Hospital, Drexel University College of Medicine, Pittsburgh, PA, USA

Syed Nabeel Zafar, M.D., M.P.H. Department of Surgery, Howard University Hospital, Washington, DC, USA

Jami Zipf, R.N., B.S.N. Conemaugh Health System, Johnstown, PA, USA

Part I

Introduction

1 Introduction

C.W. Schwab

Our ELDERS—special care for special people …

I became interested in the geriatric injury shortly after leaving the United States Navy. I was 34 years "young" and entered my first academic position in Tidewater, Virginia. Every year we would see a surge of older Americans seriously injured while vacationing or enjoying the milder climate of the eastern shores of Virginia and North Carolina. These elders were "different" and the information, especially in the standard surgical textbooks and the few trauma books of the day, did not mention any other special population except pediatrics. The first paper we published was on flail chest in the elderly, a small retrospective case study. It attempted to point out the dissimilarities of presentation, acute management, natural history, and poor outcomes of blunt high-energy chest trauma in the "old" vs. the young. Throughout my career, I have maintained an intellectual focus on this enlarging part of our practices.

The words elderly, geriatric, and senior conjure a picture of slow, frail, and mental struggle. My own father, born in 1907, lived till age 91 and was independent, physically active, and as "sharp as a tack." Perhaps out of respect for him, I adopted the term "elder" and replaced, where I could, the more frequently used above terms. An "elder" is a person of influence within certain cultures or in a family and community. Many societies and governing bodies use the term "elder" to connote a person of great influence, experience, and wisdom. For the sake of simplicity, I will use the terms geriatric, elderly, and senior interchangeably, but as you read this new textbook keep the image of the "elder" in mind.

"Elderly" is not easy to define for medical purposes as chronologic age does not accurately define one's physiologic age. Nor does age alone give us an ability to predict recovery from injury or a critical medical emergency. An accepted definition for geriatrics is 65 years and older, but the foundations for this reside in government so as to administer such tasks as census tracking or qualifying citizens for social security. Age alone does not explain the health and medical characteristics of our patients. Each patient over 65 years is a blend of genetics, biologic and mechanical aging, medical conditions, and sequelae of any treatments. Each of us "ages" at a different rate as does each organ system.

C.W. Schwab, M.D., F.A.C.S., F.R.C.S.(H)glas
Division of Traumatology, Surgical Critical Care and Emergency Surgery, Department of Surgery, Perlman School of Medicine, University of Pennsylvania, Philadelphia, PA, USA
e-mail: schwabc@uphs.upenn.edu

A. Rodriguez et al. (eds.), *Geriatric Trauma and Acute Care Surgery*,
https://doi.org/10.1007/978-3-319-57403-5_1

Thus, the ability to predict outcomes is complex and requires assessment of the type and severity of injury or insult, physical and mental fitness, and especially the preinjury or illness functional state. In my own experience, the prediction equations for elderly outcomes are *only* guidelines and modestly sensitive. What I have found is that higher pre-event intact cognitive abilities and higher physical fitness reset the chronologically aged person to a younger cohort and predict better outcome.

It's important to grasp the statistics, epidemiology, and impact of the elder populations as it relates to medicine. As we speak, the face of the world's population is changing with the percentage of those living older than 65 years rapidly approaching 17%, while children 7 years and younger falling toward 7%. By 2030, if trends continue, one-fifth of the United States' population will be over the 65-year mark and those living into their 90s will be a large proportion of that 20%.

Globally, this elderly momentum is occurring in most well-developed countries. Thus in the few next decades, caring for our elders will become a *very* large part of all aspects of medical practice, especially emergency, trauma, and intensive care. Trauma centers are seeing an increasing number of older patients as people live longer, and are more active and exposed to increased risk for injury. Falls have become the most common mechanism of injury at most trauma centers and are equal in number to those combined by *all* motor vehicular mechanisms. Pennsylvania, the country's sixth largest state population, has one of the highest proportions of Americans over 65 years. Twelve million people live in the state, and two million in central rural PA, and are well served by a network of trauma centers. Trauma registry data from one busy rural center show the impact of the above on their emergency and trauma practices. From 2012 to 2015, the trauma center evaluated over 4000 trauma patients older than 65; 40% of all trauma patients and 15% of these elders were greater than 80 years of age. Falls were the dominant mechanism and fall from standing was the most common MOI within the "older old" subgroup of patients.

As physicians and nurses, we know that improving care to special populations requires advancing knowledge and standardizing approaches to these patients. Whether that special population is defined by an uncommon procedure (Whipple procedure, high-risk cardiac or CNS surgery, etc.), condition (spinal cord injury, immune suppressed, etc.), or age (pediatrics, geriatrics), outcomes will improve when these two facets inform our practices and therapies. The third impactful element is the team approach to complex medical situations. This team concept has shown its value by integrating disciplines and specialists and expanding the clinical focus across the spectrum of an illness. The care of the "elder" is no different and requires specialists at the medical management and rehabilitation of the emergencies of older patients. Though surgery is a critical factor, leading this team concept is a requirement to assure optimal care of the most vulnerable patients. At our own institution, we have been fortunate to have a vibrant gerontology department. The gerontology service with its team of experts in medicine, nursing, pharmacy, occupational and physical therapy, social service, and hospice is invaluable to help older patients and their families. They have adapted to the demands of the trauma center, become integrated on our teams, and advanced our understanding of older people at every phase. They display a passion for "caring" for seniors as "elders." They bring extraordinary judgment and humanism to the bedside and further help families navigate difficult and uncharted waters. This beneficial linkage to the trauma, emergency, surgical, and critical care services should be a part of a modern hospital and an essential requirement to any accredited trauma center.

It is not surprising that both Drs. Rodriguez and Barraco practice at two of Pennsylvania's busiest trauma centers. Perhaps more than others, they feel the impact of the demographic momentum on a daily basis. Years ago, Dr. Rodriguez promoted the concept of "special care for special people" and organized his hospital's resources to support the elderly trauma patient. His passion and zeal have been contagious. This new textbook embraces the team approach. Drs. Rodriguez, Ivatury, and Barraco are to be complimented for combining medical and nursing experts as authors to advance the understanding of the "elder" with life-threatening emergencies. This unique approach will help to standardize our clinical approach and ultimately improve outcomes.

2 Why This Book and Why Now? A Rationale and Systems Impact for Geriatric Trauma and Acute Care Surgery

Robert D. Barraco, Aurelio Rodriguez, and Rao Ivatury

Present State

As the founding Chair of the Geriatric Trauma Committee of the American Association for the Surgery of Trauma, Dr. Steven Shackford stated that we are in the midst of a Silver Tsunami. The geriatric population in the USA is growing (Fig. 2.1). Census projections have those aged 85 and over exceeding 20 million in the year 2050. This is not only a US problem but also one that is global. According to the World Health Organization report on Global Health and Aging, the world population aged 65 and over will triple from 524 million in 2010 to 1.5 billion in 2050 [1]. Of course, much of this growth will be in developing countries. As experience in Pennsylvania has shown, geriatric trauma volumes continue to rise, yet most of the injured elderly are seen at nontrauma centers (Figs. 2.2 and 2.3). This, coupled with the fact that the geriatrician workforce is not keeping up, is creating a healthcare crisis. In 2007, there was one geriatrician for every 2546 elderly Americans. In 2030, there will be one for every 4254 elderly Americans [2]. Everyone associated with the care of the injured elderly need to become content experts in the area to optimize the team approach to the care of the geriatric trauma patient. Back in 2006, the American Geriatrics Society issued a position statement on interdisciplinary care, espousing its benefits for the patients, families, and caregivers [3]. The John A. Hartford Foundation also supported this concept through its Geriatric Interdisciplinary Team Training Program. That is why this book enters into the prehospital, physician, nursing, and disposition spaces.

The Impact

Many sources as well as several chapters in this book discuss various aspects of the impact on healthcare of this population shift. According to a 2002 article in the International Journal of Epidemiology, much of the impact of the aging population will not come from the growth of the elders but from the slowing of the growth of the working-age population. That will mean fewer people to pay taxes for public programs that support the elders. The ratio of people 16–64 compared to those adults aged 65 and over will decline by 43% [4].

R.D. Barraco, M.D., M.P.H., F.A.C.S., F.C.C.P. (✉)
Lehigh Valley Health Network,
Allentown, PA, USA
e-mail: robert_d.barraco@lvh.com

A. Rodriguez, M.D., F.A.C.S.
Drexel University College of Medicine, University of Maryland School of Medicine, Baltimore, MD, USA
e-mail: arod@zoominternet.net

R. Ivatury, M.D., F.A.C.S., F.C.C.M.
Virginia Commonwealth University,
Richmond, VA, USA
e-mail: raoIvatury@gmail.com

A. Rodriguez et al. (eds.), *Geriatric Trauma and Acute Care Surgery*,
https://doi.org/10.1007/978-3-319-57403-5_2

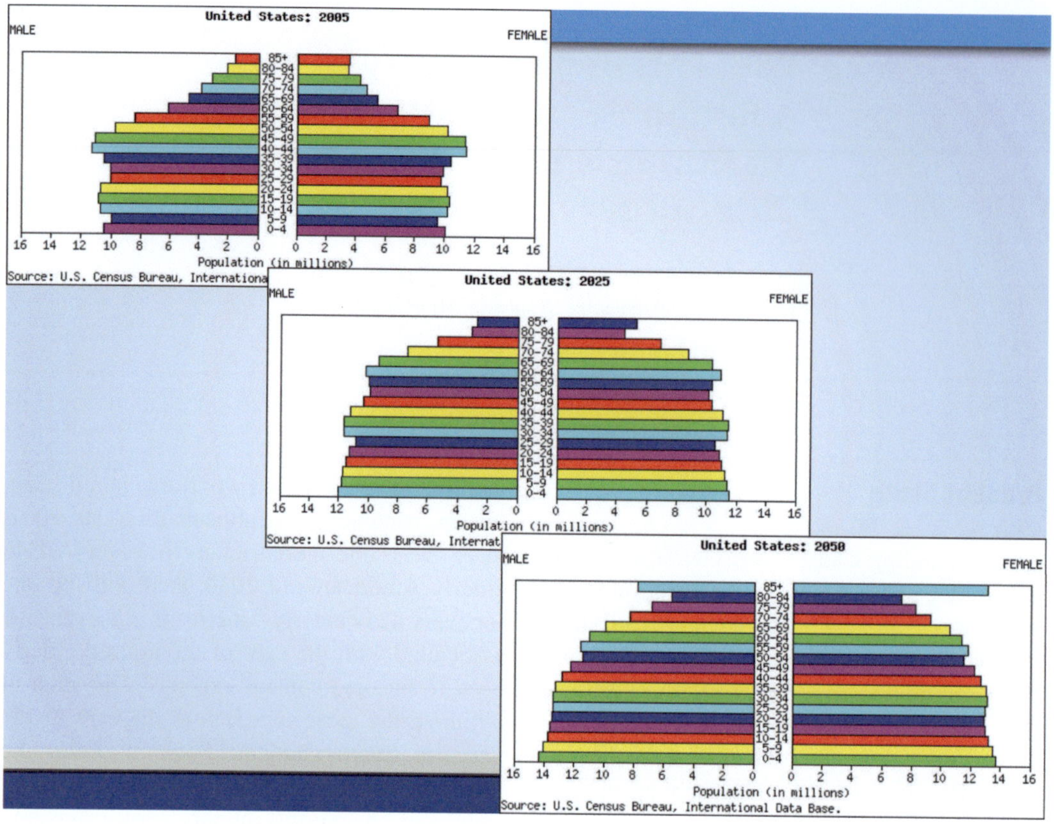

Fig. 2.1 Census projections 2005-2050

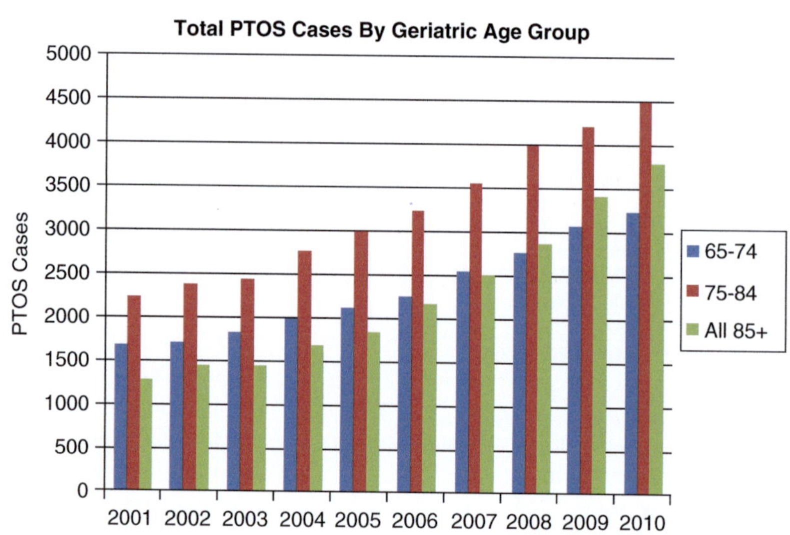

Fig. 2.2 Trauma registry cases age 65 and over in Pennsylvania from 2001–2010

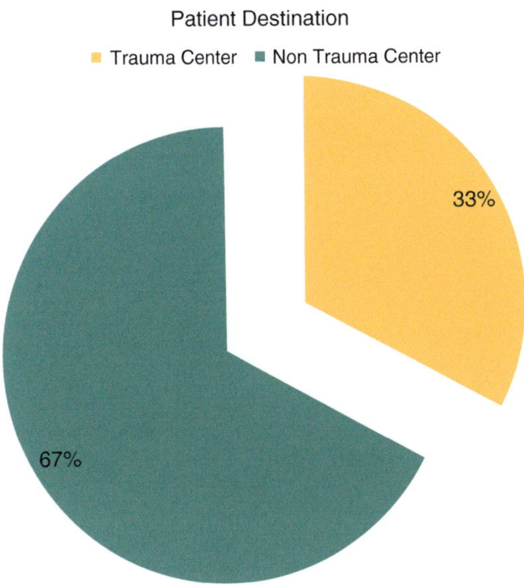

Fig. 2.3 Patient Destination from field age 65 and over in Pennsylvania

Table 2.1 Summary of 2007 AHA report on chronic conditions in those born between 1946 and 1964

More than 6 of every 10 will have more than one chronic condition
Over 21 million or 1 in 3 will be considered obese
Over 14 million or 1 in 4 will have diabetes
Almost 26 million or 1 in 2 will have arthritis
24 million or almost 1 in 2 will suffer a nonfatal fall
423,000 hip fractures per year in 2030

What does this mean for healthcare? Globally, leading causes of death will come from noncommunicable chronic diseases [1]. The focus also will shift in the USA from treatment of acute illness to chronic. There will also be a shift from acute to long-term care and a need for better integration in health systems [4]. According to a 2007 report from the American Hospital Association, those in the USA living with more than one chronic condition will increase sevenfold between 2000 and 2030, from over 5 million to over 37 million. This means the potential for much increased healthcare spending. Those with five or more chronic conditions spend almost six times more per person on healthcare than those with one chronic condition [5]. Table 2.1 summarizes the key findings of the AHA report.

Several chronic conditions will be particularly challenging. Cancer, dementia, obesity, diabetes, hypertension, and hypercholesterolemia as well as falls will top the list. The impact of these conditions will be felt in the care of the injured and acute care surgery patients and in all of healthcare. Cancer cases will increase to 27 million by 2030. 115 million people will have Alzheimer's by the year 2050 worldwide. Obesity will continue to increase, costing Medicare an average of 34% more than those not suffering from obesity. Diabetes among Americans will increase to 46 million in the year 2030. Increases in hypertension will cause increases in cardiovascular disease if prevention is not initiated [6].

Falls are already a major cause of morbidity and mortality in elders. Over one-third of elders fall, resulting in significant injuries in up to 30% [5]. As a result of an increasing number of falls, hip fractures will more than double in 2050. These patients with more chronic conditions will create more challenging and complex care problems for caregivers.

The impact will be felt among providers and hospitals with increases needed in resources. Hospital admissions will more than double and elders will make up over half of all hospital admissions [5]. As a result, this will exacerbate the projected nursing and physician shortages. By 2020, the nursing gap will approach one million nurses [7] and the physician gap will approach 200,000 [8]. In addition to shortages in these areas, there are also shortages in ancillary services such as lab and imaging technologists and pharmacists [5]. As a result of increased arthritis, hip fractures, and other orthopedic trauma, the demand for orthopedic surgeons will outstrip the supply [5].

Systems Response

As was mentioned earlier, interdisciplinary team care needs to be the focus of the future. Hospitals and healthcare systems have already begun such a transition. Crew Resource Management techniques and teamwork tools such as TeamSTEPPS are being taught to healthcare workers. Training of nurses in NICHE (Nurses Improving Care for Healthsystem Elders) programs improves geriatric education of staff and models of care for the patients. Also, several programs have been created and shown early success in the interdisciplinary care of geriatric trauma patients. The G-60 program by Dr. Mangram, one of the authors of the book, will be covered in her chapter [9]. Additional programs by two of the editors of this book, Dr. Rodriguez and his Geriatric Trauma Institute and Dr. Barraco and the Geriatric Trauma Section at Lehigh Valley Health Network, have also shown great promise [10, 11]. The former showed a decreased length of stay and decreased hospital charges of patients admitted to the geriatric trauma service compared to patients admitted to a nontrauma service. The latter showed decreased hospital and ICU length of stay and mortality with implementation of a geriatric interdisciplinary trauma team compared to historical controls.

Combatting the shortages in personnel involves a two-pronged approach. The first is more efficient utilization of facilities and providers. This can involve workflow and patient flow improvements, new technology, and mobile-based access for patients. Lean methodology for process improvement and studying workflow has spread from the business world to healthcare and achieved some significant results. New electronic health records are revolutionizing healthcare. With mobile applications, patients can see results, schedule appointments, message their healthcare team, and even be seen in virtual visits by providers. The second is recruitment and retention of healthcare personnel as well as increasing the pool via increases in medical school and nursing school numbers. Concern for provider wellness, reducing burnout, and allowing frontline staff's increased participation in improving care have been pursued to increase employee satisfaction and thereby patient satisfaction.

The growing chronic and long-term care needs will need special attention in this era of population health and increased utilization data. Complex care teams are being created in some health systems to address the needs of the highest utilizers in order to prevent their admission. Use of wearable technology to monitor patients as outpatients has also begun to help spot potential problems before they require admission. These technologies can help patients stay at home and avoid hospitals or long-term care facilities by making care in the home easier.

Injury prevention needs to play a major role, especially in the area of falls. Examination of medications, including that of anticoagulants, needs to be a part of any initiatives in this area. Studying frailty and interventions to help mitigate its effects are critical. Physical and occupational therapy can play a role here. Exercise programs, vitamin D, and environmental modifications were recommended in the Evidence Based Review from the Eastern Association for the Surgery of Trauma in 2016 [12].

This book will examine many other changes in the systems as well as the care of the geriatric trauma and acute care surgery patient. It is interdisciplinary as geriatric care must be to achieve optimal outcomes. We hope that you will find the following pages useful and within it the impetus for future changes in your practice.

References

1. Suzman R, Beard J. Global health and aging: preface. National Institute on Aging website. www.nia.nih.gov/research/publication/global-health-and-aging/preface. Published October 2011. Updated January 22, 2015. Accessed 1 Aug 2015.
2. Retooling for an aging America: building the health care workforce. Institute of Medicine, Board on Health Care Services, Committee on the Future Health Care Workforce for Older Americans National Academies Press; 2008.
3. Mion L, Odegard PS, Resnick B, Segal-Galan F, Geriatrics Interdisciplinary Advisory Group, American Geriatrics Society. Interdisciplinary care for older adults with complex needs: American Geriatrics Society position statement. J Am Geriatr Soc. 2006;54(5):849.
4. Weiner JW, Tilly J. Population ageing in the United States of America: implications for public programmes. Int J Epidemiol. 2002;31(4):776–81.
5. American Hospital Association. When I'm 64: how boomers will change health care. Chicago, IL; 2007.

6. https://www.nia.nih.gov/research/publication/global-health-and-aging/assessing-costs-aging-and-health-care.
7. FCG projections based on HRSA. What is behind HRSA's projected supply, demand, and shortage of registered nurses; 2004.
8. FCG projections based on HRSA. Physician supply and demand: projections to 2020; 2006.
9. Mangram AJ, Mitchell CD, Shifflette VK, Lorenzo M, Truitt MS, Goel A, Lyons MA, Nichols DJ, Dunn EL. Geriatric trauma service: a one-year experience. J Trauma Acute Care Surg. 2012;72(1):119–22.
10. De La'O CM, Kashuck J, Rodriguez A, et al. The Geriatric Trauma Institute: reducing the increasing burden of seniors trauma care. Am J Surg. 2014;208(6):988–94.
11. Barraco RD. The Geriatric Trauma Team: the cutting edge of elder trauma care. ICU. Winter 2008/2009;8(4).
12. Crandall M, Duncan T, Mallat A, Greene W, Violano P, Christmas AB, Barraco RD. Prevention of fall-related injuries in the elderly. J Trauma. 2016;81(1):196–206.

Part II

General Evaluation, Risk Assessment and Goals of Care (Trauma and Acute Care Surgery)

Check for updates

3 General Evaluation, Risk Management, and Goals of Care

Alicia J. Mangram, Joseph F. Sucher, and James K. Dzandu

Introduction

There is a clear understanding that the geriatric population of the world is growing and with it we are seeing a concomitant increase in geriatric trauma. Over one million Americans aged 65 years and older sustain traumatic injury yearly and at least 46,000 of these patients die. More than 55% of injuries are due to falls, 14% due to motor vehicle collision (MVC), 8% due to asphyxiation, and 10% coded as "unspecified cause" (see Fig. 3.1) [1].

There is substantial evidence that there is a higher morbidity and mortality among the geriatric trauma patients when compared to the adult trauma patients [2–8]. But what defines "geriatric" trauma? In the literature, geriatric trauma age ranges from 55 to 70 years. Advanced Trauma Life Support (ATLS) recommends patients older than 55 years of age be transported to a trauma center. The Eastern Association for the Surgery of Trauma (EAST) guidelines defines elderly as any patient over 65 years of age [9]. Caterino et al. reported an increased mortality in patients aged 70 and older compared to younger adults when stratified by injury severity score (ISS) [10].

At our level 1 trauma center, we define our geriatric patients as greater than 60 years of age. This determination was made after a 2010 review of the National Trauma Data Bank (NTDB) between 1999 and 2008 [11]. In this study, we asked the question "Should age be a factor to change from a level II to a level I trauma activation?" Patients with similar ISS were matched. We found a statistically significant difference in morbidity between those over 60 years of age versus those less than 60 (see Table 3.1). We concluded that the NTDB for elderly patients shows a significant increase in morbidity and mortality with lower levels of injury at 60 years of age. A high index of suspicion is imperative in the management of this age group. Additionally, the importance of under-triage and its adverse impact was emphasized. Increasing the level of trauma response may allow for earlier resuscitation and definitive care, resulting in better outcomes. Based on this initial retrospective review, we created our "G-60" trauma service operationally defined as any trauma patient 60 years of age and older. Over the last 6 years we continue to focus on trying to understand the differences in this population of patients compared to those younger

A.J. Mangram, M.D., F.A.C.S. (✉)
J.K. Dzandu, Ph.D.
Department of Trauma, Honorhealth John C. Lincoln Medical Center, 250 E. Dunlap Avenue, Phoenix, AZ 85020, USA
e-mail: Alicia.mangram@honorhealth.com; alicia.mangram@jcl.com; James.Dzandu@honorhealth.com

J.F. Sucher, M.D., F.A.C.S.
Department of Trauma, Honorhealth Deer Valley Medical Center, 19829 N. 27th Street, Phoenix, AZ 85027, USA
e-mail: joseph.sucherMD@honorhealth.com

A. Rodriguez et al. (eds.), *Geriatric Trauma and Acute Care Surgery*,
https://doi.org/10.1007/978-3-319-57403-5_3

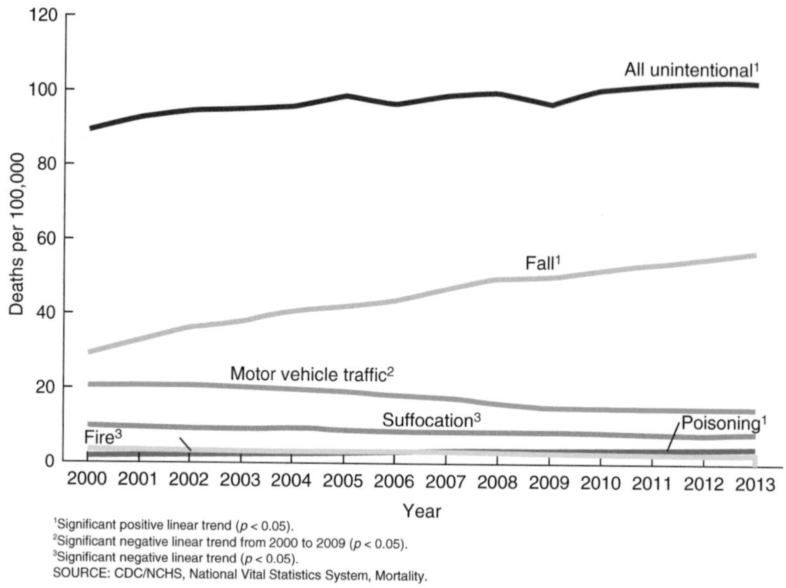

Fig. 3.1 Age-adjusted death rates, by cause of death among adults aged 65 and over: United States 2000–2013 [1]. Data based on information obtained from death certificates of individuals who died from (1) all unintentional injuries, (2) fall, (3) motor vehicle traffic, (4) suffocation, and (5) poisoning. Geographical coverage included 50 states and the District of Columbia from 2000 to 2013. Note the significant positive linear trend for fall deaths per year with clear death risk due to falls (also see [38])

Table 3.1 Review of NTDB 1999–2008 [11]

ISS category	% of morbidity		*p*-Value
	Age 13–60	Age >60	
Minor (0–9)	1.5	5.0	0.001
Major (10–15)	4.8	10.4	0.001
Severe (16–24)	10.9	16.4	0.001
Critical (>24)	27.3	28.0	0.050

than 60 years in an ongoing effort to improve quality of care and patient outcomes.

The difference between the elderly and young adults may seem obvious. We know that the physiologic reserve to injury is different than their younger counterpart [3, 12–18]. As we age we begin to have physiologic changes (Table 3.2) as well as an increase in the number of chronic medical conditions on the rise in patients 65 and older include hypertension, hypercholesterolemia, diabetes mellitus, cancer, mental illness, and back problems. According to a survey from Johns Hopkins, mental illness, diabetes mellitus, heart disease, COPD, congestive heart failure, and kidney disease are listed as the top chronic diseases in the elderly but higher among the lower socioeconomic groups [19]. These chronic conditions begin to rise significantly in the fourth decade of life and affect nearly 9/10 Americans by the eighth decade (see Fig. 3.2) [20]. Many other factors lead to injury in older adults including cognitive impairment, gait imbalance, decreased visual acuity with loss of depth perception, and slowed reaction times [21]. Trauma recidivism is another important component to recognize as a traumatic event places the elderly at threefold risk for future trauma [22–26].

Polypharmacy, or patients' concurrent use of multiple medications, is directly related to the presence of multiple chronic conditions. The polypharmacy bag includes antihypertensives, antiarrhythmics, hypoglycemics, antiplatelets, and anticoagulants. One of the newest of these medication classes is now the most feared by trauma surgeons: the New Oral Anticoagulants (NOACs). These direct thrombin inhibitors and factor Xa inhibitors are not detectable by the standard coagulation assays (PT, aPTT, INR) and the only one with a specific reversal agent at this time is Dabigatran (a direct thrombin inhibitor) [27].

Table 3.2 Physiologic changes in geriatric trauma patients (adapted from UpToDate—Geriatric Trauma) [73]

Organ system	Changes	Implications
Pulmonary	↑ Chest wall rigidity	↓ Respiratory reserve
	↓ Vital capacity	↑ Risk of hypoxia
	↓ Forced expiratory volume	↑ Risk of hypercapnia
	↓ Alveolar surface area	↑ Risk for invasive ventilator support
	↓ Chest wall compliance	↑ Risk for ventilator associated pneumonia
	↓ Oxygen exchange	↑ Risk of rib fractures
Cardiac	↓ Cardiac output	↓ Cardiac reserve
	↓ Sensitivity to catecholamines	↑ Risk for hypotension
	↑ Cardiac and arterial disease	Potential need to raise threshold for what is considered hypotension
	Beta and calcium channel blockers	Vital signs may not reflect severity of injury
	Antiplatelet agents/anticoagulants	↓ Response to shock
		↑ Risk of bleeding complications
Renal	↓ Glomerular filtration rate	↑ Risk of acute renal (nontrauma) injury
	↓ Renal mass	↑ Risk of contrast-induced nephropathy
		↓ Clearance of certain medications
Hepatic	↓ Hepatic function	↓ Clearance of certain medications
Gastrointestinal	↓ Gastric acid	↑ Risk of aspiration pneumonia
	↓ Lower esophageal sphincter tone	↑ Risk of ileus
	↓ Peristalsis	↓ Wound healing
	↓ Nutrition	↑ Wound complications
		↓ Reserve for maintaining lean muscle mass
Immune/endocrine	↓ Immune response	↑ Risk of infection
	↑ Hyperglycemia	↓ Wound healing
		↑ Wound complications
Musculoskeletal/integumentary	↓ Muscle mass	↑ Risk of fracture
	Osteoporosis	↓ Mobility
	Arthritis	↓ Pliability
	Thin skin	↓ Thermoregulation
		↑ Risk for recidivism
		Rapid deconditioning impairing recovery
Neurologic	↓ Autoregulatory capability	↑ Risk of ischemia due to injury from decreased cerebral perfusion
	Brain atrophy	↑ Risk for occult injury
	Dementia	↑ Risk for recidivism

Another challenge is that we are seeing an increase in fall-related injury as a common mechanism compared to the younger adults. This deceptive, relatively low-energy mechanism, has become an increasingly important cause of high morbidity and mortality [7, 28–36]. Recent estimates suggest that more than 2.3 million elderly adults with fall-related injuries are treated in emergency departments each year, at an estimated cost of more than $30.4 billion [37]. Approximately one-third of the population over the age of 65 experiences falls each year, a figure that rises to over 50% among individuals aged 80 and above [35]. In a recent study of "Why Elderly Patients With Ground Level Falls Die Within 30 Days and Beyond," Mangram et al. concluded that this low-energy mechanism is a significant cause of mortality in the first 30 days due to traumatic brain injury, and early identification and aggressive care are paramount [38].

Finally, to add further complexity, triage of the elderly is a difficult challenge. Elderly

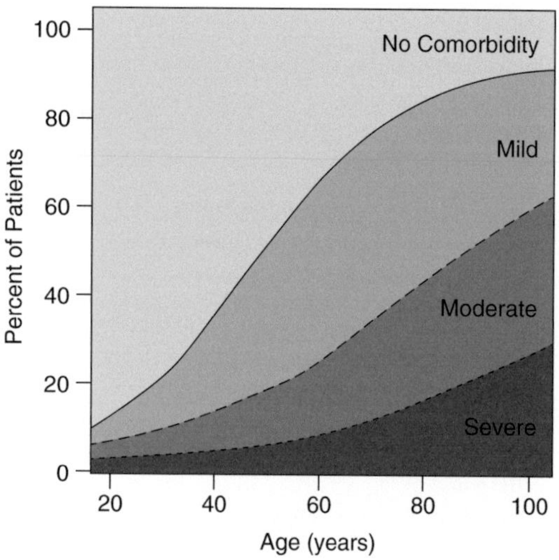

Fig. 3.2 Prevalence of overall comorbidity by severity across the age spectrum [20]

patients' vital signs are unreliable as a marker of shock state [5, 39–41]. Although shock index may have utility in identifying geriatric trauma patients at risk, there is no definitive study to confirm or refute this hypothesis [42, 43]. Interestingly, the elderly tend to present with less acute neurologic impairment in traumatic brain injury as compared to their younger counterparts [44]. Lehmann et al. [45] reviewed the Washington State Trauma Registry from 2000 to 2004 and found that elderly patients were significantly less likely to have trauma team activation than those <65 years old (14% vs. 29%, $p < .01$), despite similar severe injuries (ISS > 15), and more often required urgent craniotomy (10% vs. 6%, $p < .01$). Additionally, under-triaged patients had a fourfold increase in mortality and discharge disability rate compared to their younger cohorts. Again, under-triage is an important issue that has a major adverse impact on morbidity and mortality [45–50]. Consequently the development of geriatric triage criteria and a triage system is important for improving outcomes [46, 49]. Demetriades et al. [51] noted that 63% of severely injured geriatric patients (ISS > 15) and 25% of patients with critical injuries (ISS > 30) did not have any of the standard hemodynamic criteria for trauma team activation.

We should be aware of the fact that many of our elderly trauma patients will present with significant chronic medical conditions and often prescribed multiple medications. Additionally, they may have deceptively low-risk mechanisms of injury without significant perturbations in their neurologic assessment or vital signs. Therefore, it is imperative to maintain a high index of suspicion and be efficient. This may require us to create new criteria for trauma team evaluation.

The initial evaluation and management of trauma patients are exceptionally standardized as a result of the inception of the Advanced Trauma Life Support (ATLS) course originally conceived in 1976 by Dr. James Styner. The original aims of the ATLS courses were to train those doctors who do not manage trauma on a regular basis, such as rural general practitioners, in the initial management of the severely injured patient. The pilot courses were ran in Auburn, Nebraska, in 1977. This course has expanded nationally and internationally under the auspices of the American College of Surgeons Committee on Trauma by 1980 [52]. Injury, however, remains the fourth leading cause of death overall in the United States, the seventh leading cause of death for those aged 65 and older, and is responsible for more years of life lost than any other disease with an occurrence of 124 medical contacts per 1000 population [1]. Because of ATLS, trauma centers and trauma surgeons all speak the same ABCDE language (i.e., Airway, Breathing, Circulation, Disability, and Exposure). But even within this specialized area, we learned that the physiologic response to trauma in infants and the very young is different compared to adults. As a result, specialized pediatric level I centers were developed and became necessary to continue to raise the quality of care.

However, it is only in this last decade that we have really begun to see the impact of the increasing geriatric population on our trauma system. Individuals 65 years and older comprise 13% of the population in 2010 and this is expected to grow and constitute 19.3% of the population by 2030 [53]. Trauma centers are already seeing a disproportionate increase in geriatric trauma patients, as 23.7% of patients in the NTDB were over 65 in 2011 [54]. Thus, the clinically significant question is this: "Should the care given to older trauma patients be distinctive from the care we give to younger trauma patients"? The Eastern Association for the Surgery of Trauma (EAST) practice management guidelines work group on geriatric trauma asked six different questions regarding geriatric trauma care [9]. For example, is advanced age a criterion for trauma center referral and activation? Is an elevated base deficit a surrogate marker for severe injury and the need for intensive care? Ultimately the EAST group concluded, "In the relative absence of data to the contrary, our elderly patients should receive care at centers that have devoted specific resources to attaining excellence in the care of the injured using similar criteria to those used in younger patients". Of note, Zafar et al. [8] performed a retrospective analysis of the NTDB in 2015 on 295 centers with 1.9 million patients and reported that "older patients were 34% less likely to die if they presented to centers treating a high versus low proportion of older trauma (odds ratio, 0.66; 95% confidence interval, 0.54–0.81)." Earlier in 2014, Matsushima et al. [55] retrospectively analyzed the Pennsylvania Trauma Registry data between 2001 and 2010 and noted "Higher rates of in-hospital mortality, major complications, and failure to rescue were associated with lower volumes of geriatric trauma care and paradoxically with higher volumes of trauma care for younger patients. These findings offer the possibility that outcomes may be improved with differentiated pathways of care for geriatric trauma patients.

There is little doubt that the elderly population requires special attention. This special attention is not just limited to the prehospital management and triage, or to the initial evaluation and resuscitation. There needs to be ongoing aggressive treatment and management throughout the continuum of care. Again, the goal is to try to improve outcomes while mitigating the known increased morbidity and mortality risk that we have seen in this population over the years.

General Evaluation and Risk Assessment

The initial evaluation of the G-60 trauma patient evokes the added attention to the high probability of preexisting conditions. Staying with the universal language ABCDE, we will provide additional thoughts and extension to the language.

A = Airway

The premise of ATLS is to treat the greatest threat to life first. Thus traditionally, when the trauma patient arrives we immediately check for a patent airway, often by simply talking with the patient. This holds true for all patients, other than the very young or those with neurologic disability. Known pitfalls taught by ATLS: inability to intubate, occult airway injury, and equipment failure are all true, but in our elderly patients we have to add additional concerns, such as the potential lack of dentition or presence of dentures. For instance, it can be more difficult to create an adequate seal with a bag valve mask (BVM) in the edentulous patient. Placement of an endotracheal tube usually relies on an estimate of depth based on position at the lips. In those patients without teeth, the lips are positioned towards the oral cavity, thus increasing the risk of a right main-stem intubation. Limited neck movement caused by arthritic changes may also present difficulties in securing an airway [56]. The presence of ill-fitting dentures predisposes this group to the potential of airway obstruction. Finally, geriatric patients are at increased risk for depressed gag and cough reflexes, predisposing them to aspiration.

B = Breathing

There are numerous chronic diseases and physiologic changes in the pulmonary system and chest wall that predispose the elderly to increased risk of hypoxia, hypercapnia, and respiratory distress. The elderly can have increased work of breathing due to decreased chest wall compliance and/or chronic obstructive pulmonary disease (COPD). Exacerbating this can be decreased thoracic muscle mass, reducing the ability to maintain maximal minute ventilation. Further, in the elderly, residual volume (RV) and functional residual capacity (FRC) increase, while forced expiratory volume in 1 s (FEV1) and inspiratory and expiratory functional reserve volumes are reduced. This, combined with decreased compensatory response to hypoxia, increased coronary artery disease, cerebral vascular disease, and peripheral vascular disease (e.g., carotid artery disease), increases the elderly patient's risk for ischemic complications [57]. Therefore, all elderly patients should be placed on supplemental oxygen regardless of their oxygen saturation while undergoing the initial trauma evaluation.

Consideration for all pharmacologic agents may require changes in dosing and agents used. The increased fat to lean muscle mass, decreased hepatic clearance, and decreased renal function, all alter the pharmacokinetics of many agents. Benzodiazepines used for sedation may require decreased dosing, and narcotic administration may require increases in the interval of delivery. The baroreceptor response to hypotension can be reduced in the elderly, and myocardial muscle and smooth muscle contractility can be impaired. Therefore, etomidate has been suggested as the drug of choice for induction in the elderly, as it causes less hemodynamic depression than propofol or high-dose benzodiazepines. Finally, neuromuscular blockade (NMB) agents may have an increased time to effect and a prolonged effect owing to decreased cardiac output and decreased metabolism [56]. Careful assessment of duration of NMB is necessary so adequate sedation can be provided.

Owing to osteoporosis and chest wall rigidity, this population is at risk for rib fractures, which is an independent risk factor of mortality. Bulger et al. [58] reported that blunt thoracic trauma patients ≥65 years old had twice the mortality and thoracic morbidity than their younger patients with similar injuries. Other injuries to the lungs, such as pulmonary contusion, hemothorax, and pneumothorax, can also have significant impact on morbidity and mortality. Therefore, early and aggressive management in the intensive care unit includes blunt chest wall treatment protocols that aggressively reduce pain without narcotics (e.g., percutaneous intercostal nerve blocks, thoracic epidural catheter placement, IV acetaminophen), intensive care-level pulmonary therapy, judicious use of crystalloid fluid to reduce the risk of pulmonary edema, and early rib fixation for those patients who fail medical management or who are at high risk for pulmonary complications [59, 59–62]. Our group has described rib fixation with muscle-sparing minimally invasive thoracotomy (MSMIT), showing improved pulmonary function by postoperative day 5 [63].

C = Circulation

Cardiac function and smooth muscle contractility can be impaired in the elderly, predisposing them to hypotension even in the face of relatively limited hypovolemia. However, hypotension is relative for any patient, as the incidence of hypertension is 70.3% in patients over 65 years of age [64]. Oyetunji et al. [65] reviewed the NTDB records between 2001 and 2006 for 700 trauma centers and reported that the optimal cutoff for the definition of hypotension in elderly patients may be 117 mmHg (versus the conventional value of SBP <90 mmHg). Given the knowledge that vital signs alone are poor predictor of shock, and may be even more so in the geriatric trauma population, has led others to consider further testing with venous lactate levels. In 2013 Salottolo et al. [43] reported that venous lactate levels better predicted mortality (OR = 2.62) vs. initial vital signs or shock index (OR = 1.71 and OR = 1.18, respectively). Of note, this study used SBP <90 mmHg to describe shock.

As discussed previously, G-60 trauma patients have an increased incidence of polypharmacy, which may include numerous medications that decrease the ability to respond to shock state. Beta-blockers are the primary culprit of this polypharmacy phenomenon. Often discussed but easily overlooked in the controlled chaos of acute trauma is the fact that these agents may prevent the normal compensatory tachycardia required to maintain perfusion in hypovolemic states, thus lulling the provider into a false sense of security. Also, diuretics can lead not only to volume depletion, but also to electrolyte depletion. This can further exacerbate preexisting cardiac arrhythmias and create labile hemodynamics.

The topic often comes up regarding invasive hemodynamic monitoring with pulmonary artery catheters (PACs) in hemorrhagic shock, and the elderly seem to be a special group of patients that some believe benefit from utilization of this diagnostic adjunct. Although much has been written concerning the benefits of PAC monitoring, most of this was during a time of massive crystalloid resuscitation in an effort to push "supranormal" oxygen delivery [17, 66]. The translation of this innovative concept into practice, however, did not result in increased oxygen utilization or improved outcomes. Ultimately, it is our considered opinion that PACs should be reserved for use in those patients who are not responding to standard hemorrhagic shock resuscitation principles. It is a very rare occurrence to require more than the standard central venous pressure monitoring coupled with continuous arterial blood pressure monitoring using a minimally invasive indirect cardiac output systems. Additional information may be gained by echocardiography that can provide information on structure and function of the myocardium as well as some estimate of filling status. Adverse changes in the structure and function of several organs and organ systems have been shown to be associated with aging (Table 3.2).

D = Disability

Which came first, the trauma or the neurologic deficit? The question is moot in the initial evaluation. No matter what the etiology, maintaining the universal ABCDE language optimizes patient safety, efficient evaluation, and rapid care. This is what is paramount in all patients, but especially in the geriatric population because neurologic insult is a leading cause of mortality. Of course, this group comes with the potential for preexisting chronic neurologic diseases such as dementia, Parkinson's, or previous cerebral vascular accident to name a few. Additionally, age-related changes of cerebral atrophy increase the risk of subarachnoid and subdural hemorrhage and atherosclerotic disease predisposes this group to ischemic stroke due to blunt cervical injury or shock. As noted previously, geriatric patients can present with a higher GCS than their younger counterparts with similar traumatic brain injury (TBI) [44]. Cervical spine injury is common in ground-level falls. Given the high incidence of osteoporosis and arthritic changes in the spine, even falls from bed are known to lead to significant cervical spine injury [67]. Therefore, despite even a low mechanism of injury, liberal use of CT and MRI imaging is warranted [30].

E = Exposure

Complete examination requires optimal exposure, not only in an effort to identify acute injuries, but also to ensure chronic conditions are identified. As noted previously, diabetes and peripheral vascular disease are common chronic conditions of the elderly. Add to this decreased mobility, and neuropathic conditions along with changes in the skin and underlying soft tissue due to aging. All this is a setup for the elderly to have decreased soft-tissue integrity and increased incidence of skin and soft-tissue wounds, both acute and chronic. If not identified and addressed, these wounds may become a serious, life-threatening event for the patient during the hospitalization for what otherwise may have been an isolated injury.

Other skin changes of aging, such as thinning of the skin, changes in the microvascular circulation, and decreased subcutaneous tissue, predispose the elderly to poor response to temperature extremes. Elderly patients are at increased risk for both hypothermia and hyperthermia, and early definitive measures should be taken to ensure that the patient has adequate treatment to maintain normothermia.

F = Frailty

We now propose to expand our trauma ABCDE language at this point to include the assessment of frailty. As noted earlier age, ISS, or vital signs alone are not independent predictors of outcome. Those patients aged >80 years that present with shock and ISS >25 have a mortality rate that exceeds 80% [68]. However we need to focus on the greater majority of the patients at risk. The leading cause of trauma in the elderly is falls and with this mechanism of injury age alone does not predict outcome. As such, we perceive 60 is the new 40, 70 is the new 50, and 80 is the new 60. But that's not to say that all 80-year-olds are robust and without chronic illness, as it is true that many 50-year-olds are not "healthy." To account for this wide variation in health status, tools have been developed to assess frailty across the spectrum of ages. "Frailty can be defined as a phenotype of multi-system impairment and expanding vulnerability which is associated with a higher risk of adverse health outcomes that are not entirely explained by aging" [3]. There are other definitions of frailty, just as there are multiple tools to assess frailty. Joseph et al. published two articles using a 50-point questionnaire to assess frailty [69, 70]. These studies identified frail individuals as higher risk for "unfavorable" discharge disposition (other than home or rehabilitation center) and increased risk for inpatient complications. In 2014, Joseph et al. [71] published their third study, now utilizing the Trauma-Specific Frailty Index (TSFI), an abbreviated tool using 15 variables derived from the original two studies. This prospective study from 2011 to 2013 evaluated 200 patients aged 65 and older at their level I trauma center. The mean age was 77 years, 72% were male, 82% were white, and the median ISS was 15. Thirty percent (30%) of patients had an unfavorable discharge disposition. A TSFI score had a 1.5-fold increase in likelihood of unfavorable discharge disposition.

In the same year, Mangram et al. [72] published their results using the Vulnerable Elderly Survey-13 (VES-13) tool created in 2000 to assess for vulnerable elderly in the community. A simple-to-use tool, it relies on patient or family self-reporting of 13 variables to gauge frailty. Mangram et al. prospectively evaluated 322 patients aged 60 and older from 2012 to 2014 at a level I trauma center. The mean age was 77, 62% female, 83% white, and the mean ISS 9.9, of which fifty-five percent (55.4%) of patients were vulnerable. Of the vulnerable, 73% were female and only 23% of vulnerable patients had a favorable discharge (discharge to home). They concluded that VES-13 predicted that vulnerable patients were four times more likely to have an unfavorable discharge disposition (discharge to other than home).

These studies evaluating frailty over age are immensely important in recognizing the enormous impact frailty has in this population. It may help to institute targeted interventions for these patients. It may also aid in having frank discussions with family as to the prognosis of these patients.

Goals of Care

The G-60 trauma patient group has unique challenges as it relates to goals of care. Preexisting conditions, polypharmacy, changes in physiology, and frailty set the elderly apart from their younger counterparts. The preinjury functional state often dictates the parameters within which we work. Patients with an "acceptable" preinjury functional state should have the goal of care to restore health and optimize functional recovery. For others who may present in a moribund preinjury state, the goal of care may be limited to palliation. Therefore, there is a wide spectrum of goals and considerations that is limited mainly by the unalterable preinjury functional status. Additionally, there are commonly held perceptions by the patient and/or the family that the elderly are "too old" to have surgery, or that they are "too weak" to recover from the traumatic insult. Concurrently, surgeons and anesthesiologists alike may have their own predisposed biases that make them less comfortable with treatment of the elderly. These societal perceptions and professional biases can lead to under-triage, delay of care, and/or less aggressive interventions in the elderly that may lead to worse outcomes. Therefore, we submit to the readers that care for the elderly should be definitive in its goal and aggressive in its expedience. The following two articles highlight how optimizing triage, and implementation of a geriatric trauma team with evidence-based care, decreases complications and improves mortality.

In 2012 we published our 1-year experience that directly addressed these issues through the implementation of care specifically for the G-60 patient. After creation of a goal-directed geriatric trauma service in a level I trauma center we performed a retrospective review of 673 geriatric trauma patients [14]. The control group (G-60) consisted of trauma patients during the first year after implementation of the G-60 service compared to an age-matched cohort from the year prior to implementation. We observed a decrease in adverse outcomes among the G-60 group in all categories: average emergency department length of stay, average emergency department to operating room time, average surgical intensive care unit LOS, and average hospital LOS (see Table 3.3). A 3.8% mortality rate was found in the G-60 group compared with a 5.7% mortality rate in the control group. Our analysis also showed a rate of 0% pneumonia, 1.3% respiratory failure, and 1.5% urinary tract infection in the G-60 group, while the control group had a rate of 1.8% pneumonia, 6.8% respiratory failure, and 3.9% urinary tract infection (see Table 3.4).

In the same year, 2012, Bradburn et al. [53] published their findings on the implementation of a "high-risk" geriatric protocol (GP) in a level II trauma center. They defined the geriatric trauma patient as age 65 years and greater. High-risk geriatric patients were placed on an aggressive treatment pathway that included rapid and thorough evaluation, addition of a geriatric consultation, and rapid definitive care. With this protocol, they showed a reduction in mortality (OR 0.63, $p = 0.046$) as compared to a retrospective cohort prior to implementation of the high-risk geriatric protocol. High-risk patients were identified by mechanisms of injury, significant medical comorbid conditions, presence of anticoagulants, altered mental status, need for blood or plasma transfusion, need for emergency surgery, base deficit ≥6 mmol/L, and/or lactic acid ≥2.4 mmol/L. The latter markers of base deficit and elevated lactic acid being very important, as elderly patients may present with normal vital signs, but in fact have occult end-organ perfusion deficits. In 2003, Jacobs noted a 66% increase in mortality in those patients 55 years and older with a base deficit ≥6 mmol/L [13]. Again, these studies highlight the importance of optimizing triage, early identification of shock, and aggressive care pathways for G-60 trauma patients.

In conclusion, empirical evidence that people are living longer and have multiple comorbidities requires that we change our systems of care and become better prepared. We have reviewed the universal language of trauma, ABCDE, and due to the rising tide of elderly we have added "F" for the assessment of frailty. Evidence-based strategies to drive identification of high-risk patients and implement definitive and aggressive care to meet the unmet needs of this rapidly expanding group of patients should be the ultimate goal. As it is unlikely that there will be resources to create stand-alone geriatric trauma centers, we submit that the focus should be on a multidisciplinary team approach, mirroring the successes we have in the ICU, and expanding it across the continuum of care. Finally, regardless of preinjury functional status, aggressive care-even aggressive palliative care-is key to optimizing outcomes for the geriatric trauma patient.

Table 3.3 Time efficiency goals [14]

Results	Control (n = 280)	G-60 (n = 393)	p-Value
ED LOS (H)	6.1	4.2	0.0001
Time to OR (H)	52.9	37.6	0.0103
ICU LOS (D)	5.2	3.0	0.0002
Hospital LOS (D)	7.0	4.8	0.0002

Table 3.4 Morbidity and mortality [14]

Morbidity	Control (n = 280)	G-60 (n = 393)	p-Value
UTI	11 (3.9%)	6 (1.5%)	0.05
Respiratory failure	19 (6.8%)	5 (1.3%)	0.0001
Congestive heart failure	4 (1.4%)	0	0.05
Acute renal failure	4 (1.4%)	0	0.05
Pneumonia	5 (1.7%)	1 (0.2%)	0.0078
DVT	0	1 (0.2%)	0.398
PE	2 (0.07%)	0	0.0934
Decubitus ulcer	1 (0.03%)	0	0.2358
Mortality	16 (5.7%)	15 (3.8%)	0.2

References

1. Kramarow E, Chen Li-Hui, Hedegaard H, Warner M. Deaths from unintentional injury among adults aged 65 and over: United States, 2000–2013 [Internet]. National Vital Statistics System: Centers for Disease Control; 2015. p. 1–8. Report No. 199. http://www.cdc.gov/nchs/data/databriefs/db199.pdf.
2. Hashmi A, Ibrahim-Zada I, Rhee P, Aziz H, Fain MJ, Friese RS, et al. Predictors of mortality in geriatric trauma patients: a systematic review and meta-analysis. J Trauma Acute Care Surg. 2014;76(3):894–901.

3. Joyce MF, Gupta A, Azocar RJ. Acute trauma and multiple injuries in the elderly population. Curr Opin Anaesthesiol. 2015;28(2):145–50.
4. MacKenzie EJ, Morris JA, Smith GS, Fahey M. Acute hospital costs of trauma in the United States: implications for regionalized systems of care. J Trauma. 1990;30(9):1096–101. discussion 1101–3
5. Perdue PW, Watts DD, Kaufmann CR, Trask AL. Differences in mortality between elderly and younger adult trauma patients: geriatric status increases risk of delayed death. J Trauma. 1998;45(4):805–10.
6. Taylor MD, Tracy JK, Meyer W, Pasquale M, Napolitano LM. Trauma in the elderly: intensive care unit resource use and outcome. J Trauma. 2002;53(3):407–14.
7. Wang H, Coppola M, Robinson RD, Scribner JT, Vithalani V, de Moor CE, et al. Geriatric trauma patients with cervical spine fractures due to ground level fall: five years experience in a level one trauma center. J Clin Med Res. 2013;5(2):75–83.
8. Zafar SN, Obirieze A, Schneider EB, Hashmi ZG, Scott VK, Greene WR, et al. Outcomes of trauma care at centers treating a higher proportion of older patients: the case for geriatric trauma centers. J Trauma Acute Care Surg. 2015;78(4):852–9.
9. Calland JF, Ingraham AM, Martin N, Marshall GT, Schulman CI, Stapleton T, et al. Evaluation and management of geriatric trauma: an Eastern Association for the Surgery of Trauma practice management guideline. J Trauma Acute Care Surg. 2012;73:S345–50.
10. Caterino JM, Valasek T, Werman HA. Identification of an age cutoff for increased mortality in patients with elderly trauma. Am J Emerg Med. 2010;28(2):151–8.
11. Shifflette VK, Lorenzo M, Mangram AJ, Truitt MS, Amos JD, Dunn EL. Should age be a factor to change from a level II to a level I trauma activation? J Trauma. 2010;69(1):88–92.
12. Schwab CW, Kauder DR. Trauma in the geriatric patient. Arch Surg. 1992;127(6):701–6.
13. Jacobs DG. Special considerations in geriatric injury. Curr Opin Crit Care. 2003;9(6):535–9.
14. Mangram AJ, Mitchell CD, Shifflette VK, Lorenzo M, Truitt MS, Goel A, et al. Geriatric trauma service: a one-year experience. J Trauma Acute Care Surg. 2012;72(1):119–22.
15. Scalea TM, Simon HM, Duncan AO, Atweh NA, Sclafani SJ, Phillips TF, et al. Geriatric blunt multiple trauma: improved survival with early invasive monitoring. J Trauma. 1990;30(2):129–34; discussion 134–6.
16. Demetriades D, Karaiskakis M, Velmahos G, Alo K, Newton E, Murray J, et al. Effect on outcome of early intensive management of geriatric trauma patients. Br J Surg. 2002;89(10):1319–22.
17. McKinley BA, Marvin RG, Cocanour CS, Marquez A, Ware DN, Moore FA. Blunt trauma resuscitation: the old can respond. Arch Surg. 2000;135(6):688–93; discussion 694–5.
18. McMahon DJ, Schwab CW, Kauder D. Comorbidity and the elderly trauma patient. World J Surg. 1996;20(8):1113–9; discussion 1119–20.
19. Chronic condition among Older Americans [Internet]. American Association of Retired Persons; 2016 [cited 2016 Jun 17]. http://assets.aarp.org/rgcenter/health/beyond_50_hcr_conditions.pdf.
20. Piccirillo JF, Vlahiotis A, Barrett LB, Flood KL, Spitznagel EL, Steyerberg EW. The changing prevalence of comorbidity across the age spectrum. Crit Rev Oncol Hematol. 2008;67(2):124–32.
21. Bonne S, Schuerer DJE. Trauma in the older adult. Clin Geriatr Med. 2013;29(1):137–50.
22. McGwin G, May AK, Melton SM, Reiff DA, Rue LW. Recurrent trauma in elderly patients. Arch Surg. 2001;136(2):197–203.
23. Rittenhouse K, Harnish C, Gross B, Rogers A, Miller JA, Chandler R, et al. An analysis of geriatric recidivism in the era of accountable care organizations. J Trauma Acute Care Surg. 2015;78(2):409–14.
24. Allan BJ, Davis JS, Pandya RK, Jouria J, Habib F, Namias N, et al. Exploring trauma recidivism in an elderly cohort. J Surg Res. 2013;184(1):582–5.
25. Smith RS, Fry WR, Morabito DJ, Organ CH. Recidivism in an urban trauma center. Arch Surg. 1992;127(6):668–70.
26. Reiner DS, Pastena JA, Swan KG, Lindenthal JJ, Tischler CD. Trauma recidivism. Am Surg. 1990;56(9):556–60.
27. Connors JM. Antidote for factor Xa anticoagulants. N Engl J Med. 2015;373(25):2471–2.
28. Spaite DW, Criss EA, Valenzuela TD, Meislin HW, Ross J. Geriatric injury: an analysis of prehospital demographics, mechanisms, and patterns. Ann Emerg Med. 1990;19(12):1418–21.
29. Tornetta P, Mostafavi H, Riina J, Turen C, Reimer B, Levine R, et al. Morbidity and mortality in elderly trauma patients. J Trauma. 1999;46(4):702–6.
30. Sterling DA, O'Connor JA, Bonadies J. Geriatric falls: injury severity is high and disproportionate to mechanism. J Trauma. 2001;50(1):116–9.
31. Spaniolas K, Cheng JD, Gestring ML, Sangosanya A, Stassen NA, Bankey PE. Ground level falls are associated with significant mortality in elderly patients. J Trauma. 2010;69(4):821–5.
32. Cook A, Cade A, King B, Berne J, Fernandez L, Norwood S. Ground-level falls: 9-year cumulative experience in a regionalized trauma system. Proc (Bayl Univ Med Cent). 2012;25(1):6–12.
33. Ayoung-Chee P, McIntyre L, Ebel BE, Mack CD, McCormick W, Maier RV. Long-term outcomes of ground-level falls in the elderly. J Trauma Acute Care Surg. 2014;76(2):498–503.
34. Parker S, Afsharpad A. Ground-level geriatric falls: a not-so-minor mechanism of injury. Case Rep Orthop [Internet]. 2014 [cited 2015 May 6]. http://www.ncbi.nlm.nih.gov/pmc/articles/PMC4241333/.
35. Rau C-S, Lin T-S, Wu S-C, Yang JC-S, Hsu S-Y, Cho T-Y, et al. Geriatric hospitalizations in fall-related

injuries. Scand J Trauma Resusc Emerg Med [Internet]. 2014;22:63. [cited 2015 May 6]. http://www.ncbi.nlm.nih.gov/pmc/articles/PMC4232632/.
36. Tchalla AE, Dufour AB, Travison TG, Habtemariam D, Iloputaife I, Manor B, et al. Patterns, predictors, and outcomes of falls trajectories in older adults: the MOBILIZE Boston Study with 5 years of follow-up. PLoS One [Internet]. 2014;9(9):e106363. [cited 2015 May 7]. http://www.ncbi.nlm.nih.gov/pmc/articles/PMC4153626/.
37. Joseph B, Pandit V, Khalil M, Kulvatunyou N, Zangbar B, Friese RS, et al. Managing older adults with ground-level falls admitted to a trauma service: the effect of frailty. J Am Geriatr Soc. 2015;63(4):745–9.
38. Mangram A, Dzandu J, Harootunian G, Zhou N, Sohn J, Corneille M, et al. Why elderly patients with ground level falls die within 30 days and beyond? J Gerontol Geriatr Res. 2016;5(2):1–7.
39. Martin JT, Alkhoury F, O'Connor JA, Kyriakides TC, Bonadies JA. Normal vital signs belie occult hypoperfusion in geriatric trauma patients. Am Surg. 2010;76(1):65–9.
40. Heffernan DS, Thakkar RK, Monaghan SF, Ravindran R, Adams CA, Kozloff MS, et al. Normal presenting vital signs are unreliable in geriatric blunt trauma victims. J Trauma. 2010;69(4):813–20.
41. Osler T, Hales K, Baack B, Bear K, Hsi K, Pathak D, et al. Trauma in the elderly. Am J Surg. 1988;156(6):537–43.
42. Pandit V, Rhee P, Hashmi A, Kulvatunyou N, Tang A, Khalil M, et al. Shock index predicts mortality in geriatric trauma patients: an analysis of the National Trauma Data Bank. J Trauma Acute Care Surg. 2014;76(4):1111–5.
43. Salottolo KM, Mains CW, Offner PJ, Bourg PW, Bar-Or D. A retrospective analysis of geriatric trauma patients: venous lactate is a better predictor of mortality than traditional vital signs. Scand J Trauma Resusc Emerg Med. 2013;21:7.
44. Salottolo K, Levy AS, Slone DS, Mains CW, Bar-Or D. The effect of age on Glasgow Coma Scale score in patients with traumatic brain injury. JAMA Surg. 2014;149(7):727–34.
45. Lehmann R, Beekley A, Casey L, Salim A, Martin M. The impact of advanced age on trauma triage decisions and outcomes: a statewide analysis. Am J Surg. 2009;197(5):571–4; discussion 574–5.
46. Ichwan B, Darbha S, Shah MN, Thompson L, Evans DC, Boulger CT, et al. Geriatric-specific triage criteria are more sensitive than standard adult criteria in identifying need for trauma center care in injured older adults. Ann Emerg Med. 2015;65(1):92–100.e3.
47. Staudenmayer KL, Hsia RY, Mann NC, Spain DA, Newgard CD. Triage of elderly trauma patients: a population-based perspective. J Am Coll Surg [Internet]. 2013;217(4):569–76. [cited 2016 Jun 16]. http://www.ncbi.nlm.nih.gov/pmc/articles/PMC3839622/.
48. Rogers A, Rogers F, Bradburn E, Krasne M, Lee J, Wu D, et al. Old and undertriaged: a lethal combination. Am Surg. 2012;78(6):711–5.
49. Werman HA, Erskine T, Caterino J, Riebe JF, Valasek T. Members of the Trauma Committee of the State of Ohio EMS Board. Development of statewide geriatric patients trauma triage criteria. Prehosp Disaster Med. 2011;26(3):170–9.
50. Chang DC, Bass RR, Cornwell EE, Mackenzie EJ. Undertriage of elderly trauma patients to state-designated trauma centers. Arch Surg. 2008;143(8):776–81; discussion 782.
51. Demetriades D, Sava J, Alo K, Newton E, Velmahos GC, Murray JA, et al. Old age as a criterion for trauma team activation. J Trauma. 2001;51(4):754–6; discussion 756–7.
52. Carmont M. The Advanced Trauma Life Support course: a history of its development and review of related literature. Postgrad Med J. 2005;81(952):87–91.
53. Bradburn E, Rogers FB, Krasne M, Rogers A, Horst MA, Beelen MJ, et al. High-risk geriatric protocol: improving mortality in the elderly. J Trauma Acute Care Surg. 2012;73(2):435–40.
54. Goodmanson NW, Rosengart MR, Barnato AE, Sperry JL, Peitzman AB, Marshall GT. Defining geriatric trauma: when does age make a difference? Surgery. 2012;152(4):668–75.
55. Matsushima K, Schaefer EW, Won EJ, Armen SB, Indeck MC, Soybel DI. Positive and negative volume-outcome relationships in the geriatric trauma population. JAMA Surg. 2014;149(4):319.
56. Murray D, Dodds C. Perioperative care of the elderly. Contin Educ Anaesth Crit Care Pain. 2004;4(6):193–6.
57. Cook DJ, Rooke GA. Priorities in perioperative geriatrics. Anesth Analg. 2003;96(6):1823–36.
58. Bulger EM, Arneson MA, Mock CN, Jurkovich GJ. Rib fractures in the elderly. J Trauma. 2000;48(6):1040–6. discussion 1046–7
59. Truitt MS, Murry J, Amos J, Lorenzo M, Mangram A, Dunn E, et al. Continuous intercostal nerve blockade for rib fractures: ready for primetime? J Trauma Inj Infect Crit Care. 2011;71(6):1548–52.
60. Truitt MS, Mooty RC, Amos J, Lorenzo M, Mangram A, Dunn E. Out with the old, in with the new: a novel approach to treating pain associated with rib fractures. World J Surg. 2010;34(10):2359–62.
61. Holcomb JB, McMullin NR, Kozar RA, Lygas MH, Moore FA. Morbidity from rib fractures increases after age 45. J Am Coll Surg. 2003;196(4):549–55.
62. Todd SR, McNally MM, Holcomb JB, Kozar RA, Kao LS, Gonzalez EA, et al. A multidisciplinary clinical pathway decreases rib fracture–associated infectious morbidity and mortality in high-risk trauma patients. Am J Surg. 2006;192(6):806–11.
63. Ali-Osman FR, Mangram AJ, Shirah GR, Hollingworth AK, Sucher JF, Oguntodu OF, Dzandu JK. Rib fixation with minimally invasive muscle sparing thoracotomy. Quickshot Abstract Number 48, presented at 68th Annual Meeting of the Southwestern Surgical Congress; 2016 Coronado, CA.

64. Keenan NL, Rosendorf KA. Prevalence of hypertension and controlled hypertension – United States, 2005–2008. Morb Mortal Wkly Rep. 2011;60(01):94–7.
65. Oyetunji TA, Chang DC, Crompton JG, Greene WR, Efron DT, Haut ER, et al. Redefining hypotension in the elderly: normotension is not reassuring. Arch Surg. 2011;146(7):865–9.
66. McKinley BA, Sucher JF, Todd SR, Gonzalez EA, Kozar RA, Sailors RM, et al. Central venous pressure versus pulmonary artery catheter-directed shock resuscitation. Shock. 2009;32(5):463–70.
67. Wang H, Coppola M, Robinson RD, Scribner JT, Vithalani V, de Moore CE et al. Geriatric trauma patients with cervical spine fractures due to ground level fall: five years experience in a level one trauma center [Internet]. 2013 [cited 2015 May 6]. http://www.ncbi.nlm.nih.gov/pmc/articles/PMC3601504/pdf/jocmr-05-75.pdf.
68. DeMaria EJ, Kenney PR, Merriam MA, Casanova LA, Gann DS. Survival after trauma in geriatric patients. Ann Surg. 1987;206(6):738–43.
69. Joseph B, Pandit V, Rhee P, Aziz H, Sadoun M, Wynne J, et al. Predicting hospital discharge disposition in geriatric trauma patients: is frailty the answer? J Trauma Acute Care Surg. 2014;76(1):196–200.
70. Joseph B, Pandit V, Zangbar B, Kulvatunyou N, Hashmi A, Green DJ, et al. Superiority of frailty over age in predicting outcomes among geriatric trauma patients: a prospective analysis. JAMA Surg. 2014;149(8):766–72.
71. Joseph B, Pandit V, Zangbar B, Kulvatunyou N, Tang A, O'Keeffe T, et al. Validating trauma-specific frailty index for geriatric trauma patients: a prospective analysis. J Am Coll Surg. 2014;219(1):10–7.e1.
72. Mangram AJ, Corneille MG, Moyer MM, Stienstra A, Collins M, Chaliki S, et al. Pre-injury VES-13 score at admission predicts discharge disposition for geriatric trauma patients. Ann Gerontol Geriatr Res. 2014;1(2):1–4.
73. Colwell Christopher. Physiologic changes in geriatric trauma patients [Internet]. UpToDate; 2015 [cited 2016 Jun 21]. http://www.uptodate.com/contents/geriatric-trauma-initial-evaluation-and-management.

Part III

Trauma: Prehospital Care (Fluids, Immobilization and Transport, Triage, OOH DNR and POLST)

4 Prehospital Care

Juan Duchesne and Connie DeLa'O

Background

Traumatic injury in the geriatric population is increasing in prevalence and is associated with higher mortality and complication rates compared with younger patients. An appreciation for the decreased physical reserve, presence of various co-morbid diseases, and increased risk of elderly-specific complications, such as delirium that are more common in elderly patients, has prompted development of elderly-specific care protocols within the multi-disciplinary trauma service model.

The 2008 Report on Older Americans issued by the Federal Interagency Forum on Aging-Related Statistics continues to emphasize that the US population is becoming older. Although no surprise to EMS providers who encounter this population on a daily basis, the 2008 report points out that the US population of 65 and older is now greater than 37 million, accounting for more than 12% of the total population. This statistic takes on new meaning when you consider that this segment of the population has grown from 3 to 37 million in the 1900s alone. Furthermore, with the baby boomer generation retiring, it's expected to reach 71.5 million by 2030.

A closer look at these statistics also reveals that the geriatric population of 85 and older will reach close to ten million in the same time period. These statistics are important for proper trauma triage by EMS agencies because the rising geriatric population, along with an increased level of independence in this age group, will place an increased demand on EMS and trauma systems [1]. Because of this, it is of relevance to better understand the proper prehospital resuscitation strategies of this generation.

Triage and Physiological Reserve

Recent reports indicate that our geriatric population is under-triaged when they experience a traumatic injury. According to a study by Ferrera et al. in 2000, 94% of the reported mechanisms of injury (MOI) in the geriatric population were due to falls, motor vehicle crashes, and pedestrian-related accidents (Table 4.1) [3]. It's interesting to note that 55% of the hospitalizations for trauma are due to low-energy mechanism falls.

Traditionally, the geriatric patients with trauma have been triaged in a similar fashion and by the same guidelines as our adult population. However, several studies have revealed that these two populations have different survival rates from similar

J. Duchesne, MD, FACS, FCCP, FCCM (✉)
Trauma and Critical Care, Tulane University, New Orleans, LA, USA
e-mail: jduchesn@tulane.edu

C. DeLa'O, M.D., M.S.
Division of Trauma, Acute Care Surgery and Surgical Critical Care, West Virginia University, Morgantown, WV, USA
e-mail: Connie.delao@hsc.wvu.edu

A. Rodriguez et al. (eds.), *Geriatric Trauma and Acute Care Surgery*,
https://doi.org/10.1007/978-3-319-57403-5_4

Table 4.1 Physiologic aging and clinical correlates

Physiologic change
Altered temperature controls from hypothalamus dysfunction
Decreased sweating and skin changes, loss of skin collagen/elastin
Lean body mass replaced by fat
Fluid volume changes
Altered thirst GI disorders
Diuretic use
Cardiovascular
Decreased contractility coronary artery disease conduction system abnormalities reduced postural reflexes
CNS
Decreased brain mass adherent dura
Neuronal transmitter decrease
Reduced hearing, sight, smell
Gait instability, sluggish reflexes declining immune function

Modified from Evans R. Physiology of aging. In: Sanders AB, editor. Emergency care of the elder patient. St. Louis: Beverly Cracom; 1996. p. 11–27 [2]

trauma. Thus, the first critical intervention in the care of our elderly trauma patients is to not under-triage them [4, 5].

Refined Geriatric Triage

The Trauma Committee of the State of Ohio performs periodic reviews of their statewide trauma registry [6]. In 2007, a focused review of the geriatric trauma population unveiled a startling trend: Patients older than 72 years of age, regardless of the severity of their injuries, had increased mortality. When reviewing single and multiple body regions injured, the geriatric patients died at a higher rate than the nonelderly adult population—3.9–2.6% and 8.42–6.25%, respectively.

Another concerning piece of information from this report was a subset analysis that indicated traumatized geriatric patients died at a significantly higher rate than the adult population (15.89% vs. 1.99%) when they were admitted to a non-ICU setting in a nontrauma center hospital. In addition, the death rate of geriatric patients compared against adult patients at trauma centers was significantly different (81.51–91.19%). These two data sets seem to support the theory that all too often the geriatric population is under-triaged to nontrauma centers.

Based on this important information the following Geriatric Trauma Triage Guidelines emerged:

1. Patients 70 years of age or older should be considered geriatric for the purposes of the triage guidelines.
2. Geriatric trauma patients should be triaged for evaluation in a trauma center for the following indications:
   (a) Glasgow Coma Score <15 with suspected traumatic brain injury (TBI)
   (b) Falls with evidence of traumatic brain injury (even from a standing position)
   (c) Systolic blood pressure <100 mmHg
   (d) Geriatric pedestrian struck by motor vehicle
   (e) Known or suspected proximal long-bone fracture sustained in a motor vehicle crash (MVC)
   (f) Multiple body regions injured

Based on their data the geriatric patient suffering from TBI with a GCS <15 had the same mortality rate as an adult with a GCS = 10. This data is helpful but has some limitations. The baseline GCS on many of our geriatric patients may not be 15. Utilizing the number without clinical correlation may actually lead to over-triage of these geriatric trauma patients.

So, the geriatric patient, with an obvious head injury, and a GCS less than 15, should be triaged to a trauma center. These criteria apply to patients who fell from a standing height. These falls have been traditionally viewed as a minor MOI, even in the geriatric population, yet data has demonstrated differently.

We must also consider the occurrence of spinal cord injuries in this population. Because geriatric bone structure is much more brittle than in adults, a seemingly minor fall can more easily lead to spinal column fractures and potentially spinal cord injuries. Thus, we must elevate our index of suspicion regarding the trauma suffered in our geriatric patients from simple falls [7].

According to the Ohio report, the Ohio trauma registry is not specifically able to identify injury qualifiers [6]. But one MOI was able to be analyzed. The report showed that geriatric patients struck by an automobile suffered more than double the mortality rate than the adult population—16.63% to 7.45%, respectively. Because an auto-pedestrian accident can involve a high amount of force and the geriatric patient is susceptible to more severe injuries with less force, the report recommends following this guideline to appropriately triage these patients to a trauma center.

The report also provided data on the outcome of geriatric trauma patients that incur long-bone (humerus or femur) fractures from MVCs. The increased odds of mortality for the geriatric patient from this type of injury correlates with the decreased severity of MOI needed to cause fatal injuries in this group.

Evaluating Clinical Signs

The traditional clinical marker for shock has been a systolic blood pressure (SBP) less than 90 mmHg. As referenced earlier, elasticity of the vascular system decreases with age, resulting in a steadily trending higher baseline. Therefore, shock (often detected by decreased SBP) can be masked by a higher baseline SBP in the geriatric population.

The Ohio report analyzed the mortality of the geriatric patients as related to SBP and found that the mortality of a geriatric patient with a SBP <100 mmHg is equal to the SBP of 90 mmHg in the adult population. Therefore the recommendation for triage of geriatric patients to a trauma center should be triggered by a SBP = 100 mmHg [6].

Different Physiologic Response

In many geriatric patients, their physiologic capacity to compensate for the traumatic insult is significantly impaired [8, 9]. This occurs as a result of normal aging processes further compounded by the effects of chronic illness [10–13]. Every system in the body is affected by aging, most important of which are the pulmonary and cardiovascular systems. The pulmonary system is impacted by decreases in functional capacity and lung elasticity as a person ages. This negatively impacts tidal volume, which is required for proper ventilation. Compound this with overlying chronic obstructive pulmonary disease (COPD) and the patient's ability to compensate during stress can be severely impaired [14]. Therefore, seemingly minor injuries, such as rib fractures, can cause significant respiratory compromise.

Also, the cardiovascular system, which is important to maintain tissue perfusion, particularly in a shock state, is drastically affected by aging [15]. Inelasticity of the arteries, poorly functioning heart valves, decreased cardiac function (cardiac output), and decreased sensitivity to the catecholamine response of fight or flight all impact the patient's ability to mount a response to injury and shock. This can be further compounded by baseline coronary artery disease, previous myocardial infarction, and congestive heart failure (CHF) [16]. It's, therefore, critical that elderly patients with an underlying medical condition be closely monitored when suffering a traumatic injury.

The aging of other important body systems can also have an impact on elderly trauma patients. Cerebral atrophy causes shrinkage of the brain, which creates tension on the cerebral veins and, in turn, can tear more easily and cause subdural hematomas. Decreased renal function can impact the patient's ability to survive a protracted recovery period. Decreased immune system response can prevent the ability to fight infection [11].

Further, the elderly patient's ability to physiologically compensate for the stress of trauma is not only reduced by the normal aging process and chronic disease, but compromised by the medications typically taken by this population. Some key medications to be concerned about include the blood thinner Coumadin (warfarin) and the antiplatelet agents, such as aspirin and Plavix (clopidogrel), which can lead to significant bleeding complications.

Beta-blockers and calcium channel blockers can reduce cardiac output when it may be needed most—during acute traumatic stress.

Diuretics, such as Lasix (furosemide), can make these patients relatively volume depleted (dehydrated), which can then compromise their ability to mount a response to lowered blood pressure. All of these compounding factors set the geriatric patient up for a poor outcome from a traumatic insult, even a seemingly insignificant trauma.

Beyond the physiologic response problem in this population, there's speculation that hospitals not structured to treat the geriatric trauma patient may actually contribute to the increased morbidity and mortality of this disease process. Fallon et al. advocate the concept that a resource-based, multidisciplinary approach to these patients supports better outcomes [17]. This level of care can best be provided by an appropriately certified trauma center. Outcomes may be further improved with the addition of a geriatric trauma team as a consulting service.

Primary and Secondary Surveys Address Need for Resuscitation

In a patient who appears to be terminally ill, inquiry regarding preexisting advance directives (living will, DNR) should be made to reduce the likelihood of an unwanted resuscitation (further detail will be discuss later in this chapter) If the answer is not immediately available, rescuers should proceed in favor of resuscitation.

Attention to airway, breathing, and circulation forms the basic approach to emergency care at any age. Special considerations follow:

Special Considerations for Airway Breathing

- Loose dentures should be removed if they obstruct airway or impair formation of a tight seal when bag-valve-mask is needed. Place an oral/nasal airway if patient is unconscious.
- When using bag-valve-mask to support breathing, deliver lower tidal volumes (e.g., 500–600 cc) 7–8 cc/kg. This avoids gastric distention which may impair ventilation or promote vomiting.
- Limited mobility of the C-spine, spinal curvature, and bony prominences require extra care and padding in the application of cervical collars and backboard immobilization.

Special Considerations for Circulation

- Correct hand placement for chest compression is paramount, as rib fractures are common with compression in the frail older patient.
- RAPID identification and defibrillation of pulse less ventricular tachycardia or fibrillation guarantee the best chance for survival. Avoid placing paddles or pads over palpable pacemakers or internally implanted defibrillators.
- Hypotension may reflect problems with the volume (dehydration, bleeding, sepsis), pump (depressed left ventricular function from CHF), or heart rate (too fast or too slow). In the absence of overt CHF, a fluid bolus or balanced blood component transfusion is indicated in the presence of severe hemorrhage.

Special Considerations for Disability and Exposure

- Use the AVPU (alert, voice, pain, none) system to describe responsiveness, and assess orientation to person, place, and time. Consider the *Cincinnati Stroke Scale*, a simple tool to screen for acute stroke (Kothari) [18]. Other stroke scales can be used as per your individual system. Any NEW facial asymmetry (ask patient to smile), change in speech, or upper extremity drift when arms are extended and eyes closed is suggestive of stroke. Follow your system guidelines for stroke scales [19].
- Head-to-toe assessment via history, inspection, and palpation in trauma is essential to identify all injuries. Splint obvious fractures to reduce pain. Attention to thermal adjustment (fans, sprays, ice vs. blankets) during transport for patients with altered mental status due to heatstroke or hypothermia is warranted depending upon available resources and local regulations.
- Diabetes is common in the older patient; exclude treat hypoglycemia in all patients with acute change in mental status or behavior.

- Acknowledge and treat severe pain with low doses of parenteral narcotics as per regional guidelines. Splinting injured extremities significantly reduces pain.

Special Considerations for Immobilization and Transport

Immobilization and transport require special considerations in the geriatric trauma patient. Pre-existing conditions are important factors to consider prior to preparing a patient for transport to definitive care and may lengthen the initial assessment. In preparing to transport the advanced-age patient, knowledge of pre-existing conditions resulting in reduced mobility or altered anatomy is imperative, as are potential complications that may be encountered.

- With an increasing incidence of osteoporosis and osteoarthritis in the geriatric population, range of motion can be a significant limiting factor and render the patients at increased risk of fractures, even in the setting of minor trauma. Kyphosis, spondylosis, canal stenosis, and other physical deformities are not an uncommon occurrence in this population. A neutral position for normal anatomy may be impossible in the geriatric patient who has degenerative changes altering the anatomy. Standard cervical immobilization may be anatomically impossible. Forcing such patients into a neutral position can lead to further injury. Vickery discussed the extensive potential complications of spinal board immobilization in a review of the literature [20]. Creative immobilization may be required for safe transport. The use of pillows, blankets, and other items which are readily available can be helpful in creative packaging for transport of such patients.
- Abnormal spinal curvature can also lead to impairments in ventilation. As the thoracic cage becomes stiffer and more reliant on the diaphragm, sensitivity to intra-abdominal pressures may provoke respiratory difficulty. Impairment of sphincter tone, diminished ability to clear secretions, impaired ciliary mechanisms, and presence of dental prostheses increase the risk for aspiration. Normal aging and changing of bone structure over time can cause difficulty in creating a seal on bag-valve-mask ventilation. These anatomical factors, coupled with age-related respiratory functional changes, can lead to rapid respiratory decline.
- Geriatric skin is thin and fragile and fat pads are thinner. Hence, pressure sores can arise rapidly, especially in the occipital, scapular, and lumbosacral regions, as bony prominences rest directly on the board. Localized mechanical pressure can lead to impaired blood supply, tissue hypoxia, and ultimately tissue death. The use of immobilization boards may cause tissue injuries much sooner than in the younger patient. Additional padding should be used on pressure points to prevent rapid breakdown. The use of adhesive tapes can also cause significant tissue trauma from avulsion of fragile skin [21].
- Impairment in temperature control is common in the older patients. Hypothermia easily ensues with rapid heat loss in exposed patients. Hypothermia is particularly common in trauma with prolonged extrication and environmental exposures. Warmed fluids, warming blankets, and increased ambient temperatures should all be employed to help prevent additional temperature loss.

Advance Directives and End-of-Life Treatment Decisions

An understanding of the various forms of advance directives and how they may differ from do-not-resuscitate or -intubate orders is critical for the prehospital setting. Patient autonomy remains a focal point for geriatric trauma patients and the creation of advanced directives has continued to preserve patient autonomy. Advance Directives (ADs) are legal documents which allow a patient or their surrogate to direct the care of the patient to health care providers. In 1976, in an effort to promote and preserve patient autonomy, the advance directive became a document created to detail the end-of-life wishes of a patient and guide end-of-life care when a patient may be unable to express their wishes personally (Brown) [22]. In the United States, this was further supported with the creation of the Patient Self-Determination Act, which required institutions to provide patients information regarding formulation of advance directives (Omnibus) [23]. European support for patient autonomy is also well documented (Council, French Parliament) [24, 25].

With a focus on patient autonomy, promotion of advance directive use became increasingly common. The prevalence of patients with advanced directives certainly has increased since its inception. In Silviera's 2010 study reviewing geriatric deaths, they found that in American subjects, 42.5% of the patients needed decision making about medical treatment before death. Of this cohort, 67.6% already had an advance directive already in place with requests for limited care (Silviera) [26]. This study suggests that patient comfort with the topic has increased, but no universal standard for topics covered in advance directives exists within most health care systems and a wide range of issues may be addressed. The global movement of patient autonomy and end-of-life treatment decisions has affected prehospital care as well.

Types of Advance Directives and End-of-Life Treatment Plans

In an advance directive, a patient provides instructions specific to lifesaving measures. The goal of the directive is not limited to restricting care measures but ensuring that the patient's personal preferences are maintained. The directive may instruct providers against proceeding with certain interventions. Such interventions may include intubation, cardiac compression, or use of vasopressor medications. The directive may have specific parameters for implementation of treatment plans. A common parameter includes in the event of a terminal diagnosis, to proceed or not proceed with interventions deemed aggressive by the patient. This may also include a request to have or not have artificial means of nutrition provided in such circumstances. Advance directives may include a living will, durable power of attorney for health care, or both. The benefit of advance directives is that it not only defines a patient's care goals but also allows for discussion of end-of-life planning and decision making before the time arises.

Living Will

A living will is a type of advance directive document which details the wishes of the patient in regard to life-sustaining treatment. This is a legal written document and does not go into effect unless the patient is terminal, in a coma, or on life support. While an advance directive may provide guidelines, a living will in the United States is a legal document.

Durable Power of Attorney

A durable power of attorney (DPOA) for health care is a type of advance directive document which details and names a surrogate decision maker in the event the patient is unable to express their wishes personally. It is a legally binding document. The person who is assigned as the surrogate decision maker may be referenced as a health care proxy, health care agent, health care surrogate, or patient advocate depending on the laws in place. The duration of the DPOA may be unlimited or limited to a specific time, such as a deployment, and is detailed in the document. A terminal illness is not required for a DPOA to take effect.

Physician Orders for Life-Sustaining Treatment (POLST)

This document was created in order to address what were viewed as deficiencies in the advance directives and code status orders already in place and specifically designed for patients likely to die within a year. The form includes instructions for the use of emergency medical services, hospitalizations, use of intensive care, as well as other orders including resuscitative orders. The form's goals are to provide end-of-life care preferences which are then translated into acknowledged medical orders and are completed by a physician (Schmidt) [27]. These forms are orders which can be followed by prehospital personnel and are universally valid regardless of the setting and not limited to do-not-resuscitate or -intubate (Bomba) [28]. The goal of a POLST is to include a complete scope of treatment plan in a formal medical order. Some states maintain a registry of such orders that are readily accessible by hospital and prehospital staff.

Common Treatments Addressed in Advance Directives and End-of-Life Care Plans

- *Resuscitation*: This may include the utilization of cardiopulmonary resuscitation, defibrillation use, or use of vasopressors to elevate blood pressure.
- *Vasopressor Support*: This may include medications which are utilized to augment blood pressure and cardiac function within a failing system.
- *Ventilatory Support*: This may include mechanical ventilation which provides a mechanical device to assist or replace spontaneous respiration. Noninvasive support measures may include continuous positive airway pressure (CPAP) or bilevel positive airway pressure (BIPAP).
- *Extracorporeal Support Devices*: This may include hemodialysis, continuous renal replacement therapy, use of PA catheters or cardiac support devices, extracorporeal membrane oxygenation (ECMO), extracorporeal life support, cardiopulmonary bypass, etc.
- *Nutritional Support*: Tube feeds, parenteral nutrition, or intravenous fluids to supply the body with nutrients and fluids when a patient is unable to take them in: Limitations on nutritional support may include its use for a limited time, no use of supplemental nutrition per tube, or restrictions to temporary feeding devices only, in effect, disallowing a permanent feeding tube.
- **Antibiotic/Antiviral Use**: The use of these medications to treat infections may alter how aggressive the treatment plan is near the end of life.
- **Organ/Tissue Donation**: A driver's license may have organ/tissue donation wishes already designated. In an advance directive, specifics for donation can be provided. In some cases, life-sustaining procedures will be temporarily required until donation is completed.
- **Comfort Measures/Care Only**: This is often referenced as allowing for a natural death. The goal of this treatment focuses on comfort to the patient. This may include use of medications for symptomatic control of pain, secretions, anxiety, or other end-of-life comfort needs. Instructions to not transfer a patient to a hospital facility for life-sustaining treatment may also be included in this directive.
- **Limited Additional Interventions**: This may allow interventions in addition to those considered comfort care or measures alone. Basic medical treatment may be considered to include medications, antibiotics, intravenous fluids, and less invasive airway measures but generally declines intensive care transfer.
- **Full Medical Treatment**: This allows for all medical treatments without specific limitations. It also allows for transfer to a hospital or intensive care unit and utilization of invasive treatments unless otherwise specified.

Controversies in Advance Directives

Advance directives often have terminology which is considered vague, requiring interpretation by a surrogate or health care provider. They may address only a portion of the potentially required treatment plan. Cardiopulmonary resuscitation is most commonly addressed, yet the directive for intubation is often unknown (Lahn) [29]. Additionally, directives for the treatment period prior to an arrest are often not addressed. The use of BIPAP or CPAP may circumvent the need for intubation. This critical decision-making point may prevent a potential arrest from occurring. Additionally, if a patient has a DNI order but no known directive regarding cardiopulmonary resuscitation, should a prehospital provider then provide CPR but not intubate the patient? A clinical dilemma may exist which requires interpretation. Ultimately, clinical judgment should dictate treatment plan when clear directives are not provided.

A health care proxy may override previously stated preferences. Seghal et al. found this often related to specific circumstances requiring an override of preferences, for example, a temporary hold on DNR/I for the purpose of surgery [30]. However, a living will is a legal document and therefore should be upheld. In circumstances that are not clear, hospital ethics committee involvement should be considered.

Do-not-resuscitate (DNR) and do-not-intubate (DNI) orders are not the same as an advance directive, though they may be included in an AD. A DNR or DNI is an order which a physician makes within the medical record. An advance directive often addresses the desire for cardiopulmonary resuscitation or intubation but is not limited to these orders.

In the prehospital setting, an advanced directive may not be readily available to a prehospital provider. Multiple studies have documented the lack of availability of advance directives despite legislative promotion of their creation (Lahn, Weinick) [29, 31]. It is not uncommon that the patient is transferred from a skilled nursing facility to a hospital for evaluation and advance directives are not known for the patient. In the era of electronic medical records, these documents are more readily available in multiple hospital settings; however, this may not be readily available to the prehospital providers. If able, the patient should be asked if they have an advance directive, and if not, what their wishes are. When in doubt, clinical judgment should supercede.

Conclusion

The number of patients over age 65 requiring EMS assistance is growing every year. By the year 2020, these patients will make up the majority of runs serviced by prehospital providers. It is critical for every prehospital provider to have the specialized knowledge to optimize care for this group of patients. It is time to reassess how we triage our geriatric trauma patients. We must maintain a high index of suspicion for serious injury in this population. States should review, validate, and present geriatric trauma triage criteria to guide EMS providers in their decision about what is the best triage and resuscitation guidelines for the eldest patients in order to give them the best chance of survival.

References

1. Strange GR, Chen EH. Use of emergency departments by elder patients: five-year follow up study. Acad Emerg Med. 1998;5(12):1157–62.
2. Evans R. Physiology of aging. In: Sanders AB, editor. Emergency care of the elder patient. St. Louis: Beverly Cracom; 1996. p. 11–27.
3. Ferrera PC, Bartfield JM, D'Andrea CC. Outcomes of admitted geriatric trauma victims. Am J Emerg Med. 2000;18(5):575–80.
4. Phillips S, Rond PC 3rd, Kelly SM, et al. The failure of triage criteria to identify geriatric patients with trauma: results from the Florida trauma triage study. J Trauma. 1996;40(2):278–83.
5. Sterling DA, O'Connor JA, Bonadies J. Geriatric falls: injury severity is high and disproportionate to mechanism. J Trauma. 2001;50(1):116–9.
6. State of Ohio State Board of Emergency Medical Services Trauma Committee: Geriatric trauma task force report and recommendations. www.ems.ohio.gov/datacenter/Geriatric%20Trauma%20Triage%20Study.pdf.
7. Hoffman JR, Mower WR, et al. Validity of a set of clinical criteria to rule out injury to the cervical spine in patients with blunt trauma. N Engl J Med. 2000;343:94–9.
8. Evans D. Alzheimer's disease in a community population of older persons. Higher than previously reported. JAMA. 1989;262(18):2551–6.
9. Kiel DP, Eichorn A, et al. The outcomes of patients newly admitted to nursing homes after hip fractures. Am J Public Health. 1994;84(8):1281–6.
10. Scalea TM, Kohl L. Geriatric trauma. In: Feliciano DV, Moore EE, Mattox KL, editors. Trauma. Norwalk, CT: Appleton-Lange; 1996. p. 899–915.
11. Gleason PP, Meehan TP, et al. Associations between initial antimicrobial therapy and medical outcomes for hospitalized elderly patients with pneumonia. Arch Intern Med. 1999;159:2562–72.

12. Telfer S, Fenyo G, et al. Acute abdominal pain in patients over 50 years of age. Scand J Gastroenterol. 1988;23(Suppl 144):47–50.
13. Deehan DJ, Heys SD, et al. Mesenteric ischemia: prognostic factors and influence of delay on outcome. J R Coif Surg Edinb. 1995;40:112–5.
14. Wenzel V, Idris AH, et al. Respiratory system compliance decreases after cardiopulmonary resuscitation and stomach inflation: impact of large and small tidal volumes on calculated peak airway pressure. Resuscitation. 1998;38:113–8.
15. Thiemann DR, Coresh J, et al. Lack of benefit for intravenous thrombolysis in patients with MI who are older than 75 years. Circulation. 2000;101:2239–46.
16. Kennedy RD, Caird FI. Physiology of the aging heart. Cardiovasc Clin. 1981;12:1–8.
17. Fallon WF Jr, Rader E, Zyzanski S, et al. Geriatric outcomes are improved by a geriatric trauma consultation service. J Trauma. 2006;61(5):1040–6.
18. Kothari R, Pancioli A, et al. Cincinnati Prehospital Stroke Scale: reproducibility and validity. Ann Emerg Med. 1999;33:373–8.
19. The National Institute of Neurological Disorders and Stroke RT-PA Stroke Study Group. Tissue plasminogen activator for acute ischemic stroke. N Engl J Med. 1995;333:1581–7.
20. Vickery D. The use of the spinal board after the prehospital phase of trauma management. Emerg Med J. 2001;18(1):51–4.
21. Pudelek B. Geriatric trauma: special needs for a special population. AACN Clin Issues. 2002;13(1):61–72.
22. Brown BA. The history of advance directives: a literature review. J Gerontol Nurs. 2003;29:4–14.
23. Omnibus Budget Reconciliation Act of 1990, Pub Law No. 101-508. 1990.
24. Council of the European Union. Council conclusions on common values and principles in European Union Health Systems. Official Journal of the European Union, June 22, 2006. http://eur-lex.europa.eu/LexUriServ/LexUriServ.do?uri=OJ:C:2006:146:0001:0003:EN:PDF. Accessed 28 Mar 2016.
25. French Parliament. Law No. 2002-303 of 4 March 2002 on patients' rights and the quality of the health system. http://www.legifrance.gouv.fr/affichCodeArticle.do;jsessionid=AB85CDED5DA6C2F01D482487F7BC0C7E.tpdjo07v_2?cidTexte=LEGITEXT000006072665&idArticle=LEGIARTI000006685759&dateTexte=20100225&categorieLien=id. Accessed 28 Mar 2017.
26. Silveira MJ, Kim SY, Langa KM. Advance directives and outcomes of surrogate decision making before death. N Engl J Med. 2010;362(13):1211–8.
27. Schmidt TA, Zive D, Frommes EK, Cook J, et al. Physician orders for life-sustaining treatment (POLST): lessons learned from analysis of the Oregon POLST Registry. Resuscitation. 2014;85(4):480–5.
28. Bomba PA, Kemp M, Black JS. Polst: an improvement over traditional advance directives. Cleve Clin J Med. 2012;79:457–64.
29. Lahn B, Friedman P, Bijur M, et al. Advanced directed in skilled nursing facility residents transferred to emergency departments. Acad Emerg Med. 2001;8:1158–62.
30. Sehgal A, Galbraith A, Chesney M, Schoenfeld P, Charles G, Lo B. How strictly do dialysis patients want their advance directives followed? JAMA. 1992;267:59–63.
31. Weinick RM, Wilcox ER, Park RT, et al. Use of advanced directives for nursing home residents in the emergency department. Am J Hosp Palliat Care. 2008;25:179–83.

Part IV

Emergency Medicine

5 The Role of the Emergency Physician for Injured Geriatric Patient Care in the ED

Dave Milzman and Sarada Rao

Introduction

The rapidly aging population is now shifting the focus of healthcare. As the population lives longer, a greater percentage of individuals are living longer, more active, and subsequently at more of a risk to suffer from a traumatic injury. This means that more older persons are at risk to fall down and fracture a hip and suffer from a subdural hematoma and more at risk to be struck in a crosswalk and suffer from multiple trauma. Injuries in the geriatric population presenting to the emergency department (ED) are undergoing a change in presentations and complexity. Geriatric trauma is increasing both in absolute number and proportion of annual trauma admissions, with admissions in level I and II trauma centers up from 23% in 2003 to 30% in 2009 [1]. The geriatric trauma patient is three to five times more likely to die from trauma than a younger patient who sustains a similar mechanism of injury [2, 3].

As the number of elderly patients continues to grow, the healthcare system will need to embrace the challenges of caring for older adults [4]. Certainly there exists some major differences in mechanisms of injurious forces suffered by older patients compared to 18–25-year-old counterparts, as well as patient tolerance for injury with resultant trauma. Blunt trauma is overwhelmingly the predominant mechanism of injury for geriatric patients. Enhanced care means increased vigilance for recognizing preinjury health issues and risks for increased morbidities and mortalities in these patients. It is therefore imperative that emergency physicians are able to be prepared to care for these individuals who oftentimes have complex medical conditions, arrive with atypical presentations that can obscure the diagnostic process, and require special needs during their visit. Rapid early intervention for medical complexities is important as older populations tend to have worse outcomes than their younger counterparts [2, 5]. This chapter explores these evolving management models within the context of contemporary emergency care for geriatric adults.

Historically, the traditional emergency care model has been used in the diagnostic process in the care for geriatric patient. This model focuses

D. Milzman, M.D., F.A.C.E.P. (✉)
Georgetown University School of Medicine, Washington, DC, USA

Department of Emergency Medicine and Divison of Trauma, Washington Hospital Center, Washington, DC, USA

Study Center for Brain Injury, Washington Hospital Center, Washington, DC, USA
e-mail: milzman@georgetown.edu

S. Rao, M.D.
Georgetown University School of Medicine, Washington, DC, USA

Department of Surgery, Eastern Virginia Residency Program, Norfolk, VA, USA

A. Rodriguez et al. (eds.), *Geriatric Trauma and Acute Care Surgery*,
https://doi.org/10.1007/978-3-319-57403-5_5

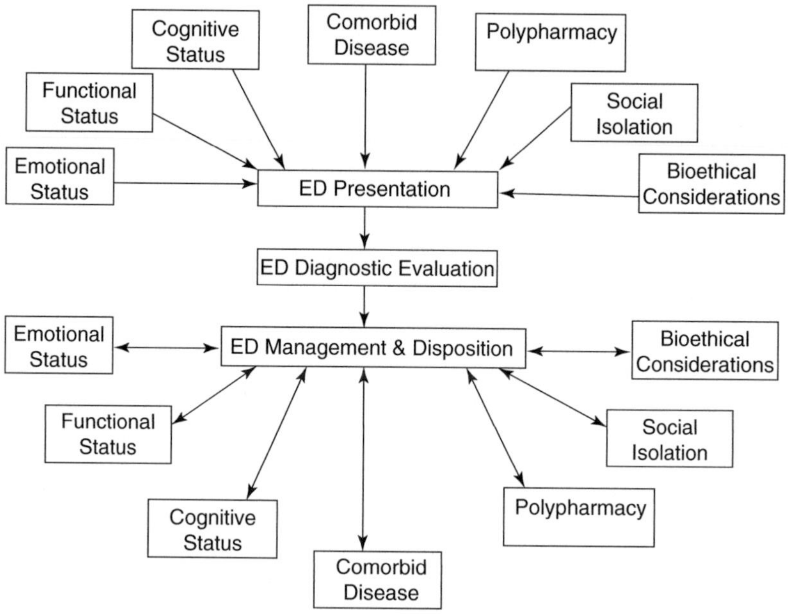

Fig. 5.1 Geriatric ED model of care [1]. There are differences from standard EM care models where many more factors impact both patient presentation and especially disposition (with permission from The Clinics Elsevier Publications, Pending approval)

on a linear and therapeutic medical decision making. While this can be useful in younger individual who comes into the emergency room, it is ineffective for an older emergency or trauma patient. The geriatric emergency care model is multifactorial and incorporates essential elements of older adult well-being including social isolation, transportation limitations, fixed incomes, cognitive status, and functional disability (Fig. 5.1) [1, 6].

Role of the ED Doctor in the Prehospital and Hospital Triage

The role of the emergency physician in prehospital care of the acutely injured patient has changed markedly in the past decade with increased role and responsibility as surgeon coverage in trauma has also changed. The idea that only a surgeon can adequately assess an injured patient is over. Now in this age of mostly nonoperative management of nonorthopedic injuries, the emergency department assessment has proven most valuable in optimal resource allocation with apparently similar outcomes. The initial evaluation of trauma starts with discussing triage with prehospital providers. Emergency physicians have always served as leaders in EMS care and their expertise in triage is well documented [7, 8].

Emergency physicians are the first line of care for the majority of patients presenting to the hospital. Even when sent from an office for medical clearance; the judgement for patient stability is attained through ED screening. Decisions on trauma center activation also rest with a discussion between the emergency medical services (EMS) and emergency physician in order to decide whether a patient is triaged to trauma or can be sent to the emergency department.

The current American College of Surgeons' Committee on Trauma guidelines recommend that all injured patients aged 55 years and older should be considered for transfer to a trauma center as a special consideration [9]. There is little current support in the literature for age, alone, to upgrade trauma patients and this semi-arbitrary number needs to be amended. The triage rule, to send all patients with advanced age, has not been found statistically correct [10, 11]. The problem with this data is that it is not independent of other factors such as preexisting disease, medication (especially those affecting platelets and coagulation), and decreased mental capacity and level of self-care. The ability to ascertain such information, prehospital, at the scene or en route, is most difficult. The reliability of such information, from an injured patient or rarely bystander/family member, is not a reasonable expectation.

More recent research has failed to find that enhanced consideration of age 55 years of age results in reduced mortality with an unacceptable rate of over-triage to trauma centers [10, 12]. Age alone, as secondary triage criteria, needs reconsideration without physiologic or serious mechanism of injury findings. There are trauma attendings that believe that over-triage rates approaching 30–35% are acceptable to prevent increased death or disability and that it must be increased for geriatric trauma patients [13]. Trauma team activation must account for a lack of a clear history of events and understanding of the injury mechanism. Early over-triage often occurs because injury mechanism or initial assessment appears to warrant trauma center evaluation. It is well understood that older patients have lower physiologic reserve and delay in injury detection is linked to worse outcomes [14, 15].

Use of prehospital predictors such as Revised Trauma Score function poorly for geriatric patients and yet not enough treating emergency physicians and trauma surgeons recognize this fact. New reports using systolic blood pressure criteria in the National Trauma Triage Protocol for geriatric trauma "110 (SBP in mmHG) is the new 90" are vital to improving care of geriatric patients [16]. These added "considerations" require more time and thought on part of EMS. More widespread teaching of early shock markers in geriatric patients is needed. These include narrowing of the pulse pressure, higher "normal" resting heart rates and blood pressures, and less physiologic reserve as well as less tolerance of the usual 2.0 L of IV fluid bolus resuscitation in patients with increased rates of renal and cardiac dysfunction [16]. Shock Index (SI) is an accurate and specific predictor of morbidity and mortality in geriatric trauma patients. It is not part of usual triage at this time but has been found superior to heart rate and systolic blood pressure for predicting mortality in geriatric trauma patients. A value (SI = HR/SBP) greater than or equal to 1 should be transferred to a Level 1 trauma center [17].

Additionally rapid neurological assessment with Glasgow Coma Score (GCS) also requires some modification for prehospital decision making in geriatric patients. Changing the EMS trauma triage cutoff for elders from GCS 13 to GCS 14 results in improved sensitivity for clinically relevant outcomes. In injured elders, with GCS 14 have greater odds of mortality and TBI than younger adults with GCS 13 [18].

EP are best positioned to retrain or at least reorient prehospital providers. They must make quick determinations in the department if geriatric patients at greatest risk for occult injuries need early enhanced care approach; that can only be received from a trauma team activation. Geriatric patients often with minor mechanisms may require ED upgrade for higher risk injuries such as hip and pelvic fractures and likely TBI.

Information of prescription drug use is not known prehospital. Therefore, patients at increased risk from medication with antiplatelet or anticoagulants suffer delayed intervention. Preexisting disease states often require trauma center triage and the ED is better equipped and experienced to serve as a better arbiter to decide on trauma team activation with enhanced rapid diagnosis and treatment of such injury.

It is extremely common for EMS to under-triage geriatric injuries, usually nonvertical fall from standing and low-speed vehicular crash which account for majority of geriatric trauma mechanisms [12, 19–21]. Due to preexisting injuries, lower bone densities, and greater rates of anticoagulant and antiplatelet medications more injuries result from low-force trauma [22]. Accurately describing injuries in geriatric patients rarely is fully available prehospital. An abundance of evidence describes that injured geriatric patients are less likely to be appropriately triaged for initial care at trauma centers despite the fact that the risk for adverse, postinjury outcome is more likely due to limits of patient comorbidities, and cardiovascular reserve as well as "general frailty" [12, 20, 21].

The study of the Maryland system found that among over 26,000 patients, under-triage was found increased among geriatric patients (>65 years) compared to younger patients 50% versus 17.8%, $p < 0.001$, respectively [20]. There clearly is a discoverable bias against elderly receiving transport to higher trauma center level. The reason includes EMS provider bias, due to beliefs they possess for poorer geriatric patients outcomes [23]. Too often decisions are made that older patients fail to survive many complex injuries and may be under-triaged. However, the opposite is actually true, where the majority of geriatric trauma victims return to independent living [24].

Diagnostic and Therapeutic Decision Making in the ED for Geriatric Trauma

Care of the whole patient, especially the chronically ill, geriatric patient, is likely outside the norm for most trauma attendings and their trauma team. The ED is more used to such complicated, multisystem medical failures. The determination of what caused the trauma and obtaining pre-event status is valuable and can alter treatment decisions. This precipitating medical event in older trauma patients will complicate assessment, response to treatment, and outcome. This problem in geriatric trauma requires treating physicians to assess initially for traumatic injury but also be well aware of possible medical conditions that may also need treatment that caused or at least contributed to the traumatic injury. Hypoglycemia, stroke, or seizure while driving may mimic a TBI and needed intervention delayed [24].

Does a fall and hip fracture require a trauma center evaluation? An intertrochanteric fracture from a fall alone is an ISS of 9 and if there is another abrasion or injury we now are pushing double digits in a patient likely with significant comorbidities and older age, would rapid evaluation and earlier operative clearance and resuscitation improve outcome? This question has been addressed by having designated geriatric teams care for such patients routinely in the ED. There are many evidence-based reports of success and improved care with shorter hospital days and fewer complications when the patients were admitted in the past, under orthopedic teams with medical consults [25, 26]. Geriatricians routinely oversee the medical management for the patient and provide operative risk assessment and surgical clearance. Then the designated orthopedic surgery team can focus solely on the perioperative and postoperative care of the prosthetic and healing. The improved care comes from better medical workup of ongoing causation of the trauma, not just repairing a specific injury, which likely fails to address a larger ongoing medical problem [27].

The role of the treating physician in a trauma center has been shown to be optimized when the most experienced physicians are present. The great problem is not that a board-certified EP cannot be adequately trained to care for an injured geriatric patient and achieve similar outcomes as a surgeon. The concern is that in the setting of overcrowded EDs there is inadequate triage, time, and personnel to assure that geriatric patients are both assessed and treated in a manner that reduces delays in detection and maximizes early and appropriate resuscitative efforts, and relief of suffering. The current state of ED overcrowding appears to clearly point toward figuring out enhanced geriatric medical in trauma centers, due to lack of adequate timely intervention in the ED. For acutely injured patients. there is not good data to prove this assertion currently. However; this finding appears to be so obvious that waiting for randomized, controlled trials may not be necessary. ED triage of geriatric trauma only works in efficient, not overcrowded, ED where the lag from triage to physician assessing critical and emergent patients is minimal.

In the latest edition of Optimized Care of the Injured patient, the role of attending physician is clearly described as "having the best and the brightest medical professionals available to treat injured patients" [28]. The guidelines state the responsibility for board-eligible or board-certified general surgeons and emergency medicine physicians to be "available 24 h a day in facilities providing the highest level of care and cannot abdicate that responsibility to a resident in training"[8, 10, 28]. In addition, the attending requires significant trauma experience more than simply Advanced Trauma Life Support certification. ATLS was designed not for a leader in trauma care, but as a minimum standard for care of trauma patients in setting of limited resources.

The need for an experienced trauma leader is most apparent in dealing with complicated geriatric patients where occult injury is not usually apparent, history seldom is clear, and most often the mechanism of injury is underwhelming. Minor fall from standing can produce significant traumatic brain injuries such as subdural hematoma and hip fractures, whereas a younger patient may not even seek care for a similar fall. Early on, altered mental status, headache, and minor neuro changes that may be symptoms of TBI can be masked by prior CVA, dementia, medication, or prior chronic complaints. Almost none of the ACS COT triage criteria will adequately predict most injuries in geriatric patients [9, 28]. The usual is anything but usual in geriatric trauma patient care. Under-triage occurs too frequently in this population due to minor-appearing mechanisms expecting same outcomes as with younger, healthier patients with many fewer pre-existing disease states. Most providers fail to consider the frailty and medication use of geriatric patients. Also, there is failrly widespread use of antiplatelet and anticoagulant therapy in geriatric patients compared to younger matched set, as well as a lesser ability to withstand minor mechanism without suffering fracture, is well documented [29, 30].

Recent findings in ED and trauma ordering of head CT, using the ACEP guidelines instead of Canadian head CT decision rules, show great increases in nontherapeutic uses of brain CT [31]. Actual positive findings are small, less than 5% of all scans, and those with occult findings requiring neurosurgical intervention are less than 1% of all geriatric brain CT obtained. This is not stating that traumatic lesion does not occur in geriatric patients; geriatric brain injury is increased compared to nonelderly and occurs despite less severe mechanisms [32, 33]. Since most geriatric head injuries happen from falls from a standing mechanism, usual trauma team activation by mechanism is not met. However, resultant injury rates occur with significant TBI resulting greater than 10% of time (brain AIS >2) [29, 30]. Furthermore, initial GCS on these patients is not sufficiently low <13, to achieve trauma team activation, or patients are assumed chronically altered and end up in the ED [18].

There are no matched prospective evaluations of isolated geriatric head trauma treated in ED compared to trauma center evaluation. The use of nonstandardized scores like the CRASH CT found that elderly patients with TBI deserve tailored assessment and care by providers familiar with the issues that make their clinical course unique [33]. The increased rates of preexisting disease, higher rates of anticoagulants, and complicating comorbidities all make it essential for rapid evaluation and diagnosis of these patients to optimize their outcomes. Too often delayed detection will lead to lower success for neurosurgical intervention. Trauma center care results in obtaining brain CT faster and more often than comparable ED evaluations of geriatric fall patients.

The older patient is a truly changing dynamic; age is no longer the major determinant as well as general health. In past studies, increasing age was directly correlated with preexisting disease states [34]. However, the younger patient with renal disease has increased mortality independent of age and ISS. Similarly, once a patient has more than two PED, they have 18% increased mortality controlling for injury compared to those without PED, independent of age [34, 35]. In the new view of trauma patients, a healthy 65-year-old should do better than a hypertensive, diabetic, obese 38-year-old patient. We are currently lacking good studies for at what age, even a healthy, disease-free geriatric patient starts to note increased mortality compared to an also healthy younger patient. Knowledge of a patient's usual heart rate and blood pressure, or at least a good approximation, is most important. When in doubt, use usual markers such as lactate, and shock index and pulse pressure which can rapidly assist the treating physician as to early presence of hypoperfused shock state.

The role of the emergency physician can be critical in the early resuscitation of the elderly trauma patient and unfortunately in the busy ED fails to provide sufficient early intervention that a trauma center could improve upon. The critical immediate postinjury assessment and resuscitation period is too often full of delays in exact injury identification and inadequate and long course in adequate fluid response.

The early need for invasive monitoring, especially in the geriatric patient, is an important question that had been well studied in the late 1980s by Scalea et al. with improvements in outcome demonstrated with early invasive monitoring with pulmonary artery catheters [36]. This major improvement came at the same time that the PA catheter was being blamed for increased mortality in the medical ICU population; that makes Scalea's study even more important [37]. Recently, the rapid and heavily invasive approach to sepsis treatment has been demonstrated as adding little improvement in patient outcome in large multicenter studies from North America, the United Kingdom, and Australia (respectively) PROCESS, PROMISE, and ARISE [38–41]. All found the usual ED care of the sickest sepsis patients was equal to advanced, more invasive care, even in geriatric patients [42].

It is clear that repeat evaluation using standard resuscitation methods performed as well as invasively monitored patients have improved outcomes. Sepsis is not exactly the same mechanism as trauma, but the resuscitation timing is not so different. Most important is bedside assessment and continuous reassessment until the patient has demonstrated improvement and stability not only in vital signs but also in biomarkers. The availability of a senior physician at the bedside is the key difference in trauma center handling of the geriatric patient and a focused exam in the ED. The usual consultation the next day as is routine for geriatricians with orthopedic cases is not adequate for trauma. Only the emergency physician and trauma surgeon are available on an immediate basis 24/7 to provide not only consultation but also immediate assessment and intervention.

Pitfalls of the Emergency Department

The emergency physician often has too many other responsibilities during a shift to focus solely on resuscitation of single patients for prolonged time periods. It is a failure of the ED, limited by overcrowding with patients, which reduces availability for the physician at the bedside to provide necessary patient care adn resuscitation in a timely manner.

In geriatric patients, a key question in resuscitative decision is the timing of transfusion of blood products versus early crystalloid for traumatic shock. In the emergency department the great majority of geriatric patients receive IV fluids, mainly crystalloid. This is done not to assure renal perfusion and maintain normal pulse pressure, but instead to treat standard vital signs: tachycardia, and hypotension. In geriatric patients, all too often overlooked or overcompensated for is the concern of decreased cardiac output, and the risk of decreasing pulmonary oxygenation and increasing lung water from fluid overload.

However, most recent data favors judicious fluid resuscitation favoring keeping patients slightly dryer, but meeting needed improvement in pressure and biomarkers [28]. If resuscitation forgoes invasive monitoring of central pressures and oxygenation, frequent repeat marker analysis is necessary to confirm lack of occult shock state. It is relatively rare to get back to the excellence of the late 1980s and early 1990s when traumatologists like Scalea were resuscitating geriatric patients with PA catheters with continuous ScvO2 to detect acute changes in perfusion [37]. These interventions like the Early Goal Directed Protocols, outlined so well with Rivers in 2000 [38], are rarely employed now, nearly two decades later, as evidence-based medicine retrospective analysis has failed to support such important interventions in their entirety.

The most recent sepsis research into protocols found that "usual care" in the ED has improved greatly [39–41]. The problem remains, however, that are we really comparing similar patients? In stage II and III traumatic shock, patients, especially geriatric patients, benefit greatly from excessive intervention and monitoring in the trauma bay compared to the ED. Even trauma centers have gone away from invasive monitoring and more expectant care. This style of resuscitation may reduce some morbidity of over-resuscitation but will not allow for optimal care of some of the most severely injured geriatric patients.

The lack of recognition of decreased baseline mental capacities directly impacts excessive workup and causes increased hospital length of stays. Cognitive impairments including dementia (in many forms) have been found in over one-quarter of geriatric ED patients, although less than one-third of these patients actually had documentation. Delays in emergency department patient assessments have become more routine now than at any time in the past 30 years. Misunderstanding of even falls from standing in the elderly on ED triage nurse and even with physician-assisted triage will result in delayed assessment and significant delay in some brain trauma and orthopedic injuries. Only the careful and thorough rapid trauma team evaluation allows for such improved outcome in injured geriatric patients.

The acceptable rate of radiographic and lab evaluation is not always that much different from that obtained in the ED with the huge caveat that it is done in much more rapid and organized manner. Trauma team activation allows for a better "team" assessment of injured patients, especially geriatric, and without the time delay that could be more than 2–4 h and set the patient up for increased morbidity and mortality form delay in diagnosis, proper consultation with specialist, and delivery of therapeutic operative care.

This is not to say that the ED always underperforms. It is, however; most likely that a large percentage of geriatric patients brought to the ED after suffering a traumatic injury are misunderstood due to appearances and underestimation of injury mechanism. Usual mechanisms of injury in geriatric patients include low falls, not vertical falls, from height, lower vehicular speeds, and fewer blunt assault and penetrating traumatic injuries, which make ED personnel to mistreat injured elderly patients.

Difficulties to Determine Final Destination of the Patient

There are two main decisions to be made on patient arrival by EMS: whether to keep the patient in ED or upgrade to trauma team activation. Often, difficulty in properly assigning geriatric patient destination is very institution dependent. The key determinant should always be patient stability. In any case, an unstable patient, with any possible trauma, should undergo trauma activation. The exception would be if medical causation is clearly identifiable as cause of the traumatic event, and those patients can stay in ED if an emergency attending physician is immediately available to care for the patient.

Since many geriatric patients present following relatively minor mechanisms but with semisignificant derangement of initial presentation, there is a great variability in triaged destination. Reviewing mechanisms in geriatric trauma is an important clue to optimal destination of the patient for care. If there is a high-speed vehicular crash with an alert patient, trauma activation is most appropriate as long as no obvious arrhythmia, or correctable mental status abnormality. Causes of high-speeed MVCs such as diabetes (medication-induced hypoglycemia), seizure, stroke or cardiac arrhythmia causing syncoope; all could be important to treat than soley ruling out the traumatic injury. Fall from standing, down steps, or other minor mechanical mishap during what should be normal ambulation likely is better treated in the emergency department.

An ideal scenario is to have a geriatric patient evaluated where nursing and support staff is most comfortable with the disease process. For example, oversight of medical emergencies that include monitoring for arrhythmias as well as neurologic or respiratory issues that involve noninvasive ventilatory support is better managed in the emergency department whereas injuries that involve open fractures, traumatic brain injury, complex wounds, and surgical abdomens are much better taken care of through trauma activation. The clear key is speed to determine diagnosis and comfort level with treatment intervention. Administering large amounts of blood products in ventilated patients goes best in trauma whereas insulin or amiodarone drips are better managed in the emergency department. A list of suggested causative mechanisms and hospital disposition focuses on optimal outcome based on perceived timely intervention.

The greatest impact on outcome, excluding severity of injury and underlying preinjury general health, is time to treatment of a medical cause of trauma. Rapid assessment utilizing whole-body scan radiograph, FAST, and identifying perfusion deficit in geriatric trauma is much more important in this population as they have reduced clinical reserves to withstand even short periods of shock. Proper triage prehospital would be optimal, but current geriatric guidelines are limited and difficult for even the best prehospital provider to accurately discern. Age alone is a poor predictor. An important example would be a 48-year-old (nongeriatric patient) on dialysis with history of liver disease and prior TED on a newer anticoagulant who suffered a trip and fall compared to a healthy 64-year-old biking. Limitations on handling medically complex patients have clearly been identified in trauma centers where consultation to nonsurgeons is limited and not planned. Having the emergency physician take lead on such cases clearly can improve speed, knowledge, and care of the patient.

Again, there is limited data to confirm this mostly anecdotal finding. Multicenter investigations to determine the optimal destination of contnued patient resuscitation are needed. It also remains unclear where geriatric postoperative patients or nonoperative observation patients can best be monitored. Most medical wards are not adept at usual surgical monitoring and surgical wards may not be as comfortable with medical patient care. The treating team needs to be actively directing care, so the ultimate placement should rest with the physician providing the greatest ongoing care.

During the assessment phase in the ED elderly patients routinely receive less analgesia than nonelderly patients [43]. They are under-resuscitated due to overestimation of nontolerance of fluid administration and delays in definitive care due to ED delay in diagnosis and proper consultation, with many specialty evaluations (surgical) waiting until the following day. There are also issues with delays in initiating proper diet in geriatric patients and in ensuring that diet placed in front of them actually gets consumed. Few studies exist that document the impact of advanced nutritional assessment, but of the existing studies that demonstrate poor nutrition, mortality is increased in geriatric pneumonia patients who lack adequate diet at 72 postadmit [44].

Would comfort care measures be better attained on a trauma service than admitted geriatric trauma in the ED. There are currently insufficient studies that compare similar patients with significant outcome markers. The determinants of a reduced mortality are multifactorial and difficult to unbundle from inherent patient physiologic and protoplasm issues compared to rapidity and thoroughness of interventions as well as accuracy.

Significance and Repercussions, in the Outcome, Related to the ED Patient Stay Before Final Decisions Are Made

Does a trauma team activation for a geriatric fall patient with rapid imaging of brain and a total body scan for possible associated fractures improve the usual ED care? The new 'usual' wait to be seen in the E.D. needs to be compared for morbidity and mortality. However, improvements will likely not be discernible by measuring mortality differences due to low death rates and morbidity change will also be difficult to determine for comparison will not be easy to match to controls. Length of stays may be shorter in the ED with a simple return to home, whereas detecting additional injury can result in longer stays. This more accurate placement, to rehabilitation sites; However, will cause delays in proper SNF placement [45]. To avoid anecdotal conclusions, multisite studies must be designed to see if the idea of geriatric trauma centers will improve care, reduce morbidities, and reduce longer term disability.

Geriatric trauma centers and even geriatric ED sections require a closer evaluation. Among acute injuries, patients older than 55 and certainly over 65 years are less likely to be involved in usual traumatic injuries due to much reduced exposure to causative mechanisms [46]. Falls, vehicular crash, and some interpersonal violence are the leading presenting mechanisms to trauma centers and ED for geriatric injuries. In pediatric trauma care there is a clear advantage to having the trauma team evaluate patients and lead to reduced delays in intervention and improved outcomes. Before creation of the trauma team, relevant specialists were individually called to the ED for patient evaluation. When a formal trauma response team was organized, time required for ED treatment of severe trauma was decreased, and consequently survival was better than predicted compared with the reference major trauma outcome study population [47]. The need for geriatric trauma center with enhanced designation and a better integrated surgical-medical cooperative team format would allow for enhanced integration of care in most expedient manner [47, 48]. Delays will exist in all complicated patients, but identifying early and initiating protocol-driven diagnostics can reduce delays in identifying medically sick and needy trauma patients.

Conclusion

In years to come, the proportion of older patients presenting to the emergency department is expected to increase exponentially. These patients are at greater risk for adverse outcomes than younger patients. The currently used disease-oriented models do not sufficiently consider the complexity of older ED patients. In order to address these emerging issues and provide better care for the growing, aging population care, future emergency medicine management models will need to incorporate appropriately trained personnel, reliable streams of communication between prehospital trauma services and emergency department as well as inpatient services, well-developed and comprehensive protocols, and lastly a geriatric-friendly infrastructure. The implementation and wide use of such age-centered approaches will help to further improve the quality of care for acutely injured geriatric patient.

The emergency physician is uniquely prepared and capable to assist the trauma team in both assessment and concern for preexisting illness concerns as well as limited tolerance for "usual" resuscitation protocols. The medical side of trauma care is not foreign to trauma surgeons. However, the focus may be alternatively delayed. Trauma team activation for geriatric patients requires a true "team" approach with the surgeon needing to recognize early if the presenting injury is actually secondary to the causative medical condition that may be responsible for the injury. In that case, early consultation with the emergency physician can be vitally important in optimizing outcome. There is limited, existing evidence-based practice detailing who is really most capable of providing care to injured elderly patients.

Prehospital Geriatric Patient Assessment

Criteria for injured Geriatric Patient to be sent to Trauma Center, Not the E.D.

Vital Signs

GCS < 15 with any suspected TBI
SBP ≤ 100 mmHg or any Shock Index (HR/SBP) > 1
HR > 110 or > 90 if patient is on Beta Blocker or other heart rate controlling medication
RR < 10 or > 24 or assisted ventilation to maintain pulse Ox >94%

Mechanism Criteria

Falls (any height) with any evidence of TBI
Any vehicular pedestrian collision,
Any vehicular crash with a long-bone fracture or multiple body regions injured
And all traumatic injury mechanism with the following age and pre-existing disease states
All patients > 70 years
Age > 55 years with more than 2 preexisting conditions
Age > 65 with more than 1 preexisting condition

Preexisting Disease Considerations:

Stroke
Diabetes
Active Coronary Artery Disease, Prior MI
CHF
COPD

Use of Anticoagulant or Clotting Disorder
All Immune Compromised patients (AIDS, Cancer patients on Chemotherapy)
Liver or Renal Failure and Hemodiaslyis patients

For resuscitation, judicious use of fluids initial bolus of 500CC less likely for interosseous infusion success.

References

1. Carpenter CR, Platts-Mills TF. Evolving prehospital, emergency department, and "inpatient" management models for geriatric emergencies. Clin Geriatr Med. 2013;29(1):31–47.
2. Taylor MD, Tracy JK, Meyer W, Pasquale M, Napolitano LM. Trauma in the elderly: intensive care unit resource use and outcome. J Trauma. 2002;53(3):407–14.
3. JM K, Sciadini MF, Sinclair E, O'Toole RV. Geriatric trauma: demographics, injuries, and mortality. J Orthop Trauma. 2012;26(9):e161–5.
4. Centers for Disease Control and Prevention. The state of aging and health in America 2013. Atlanta, GA: Centers for Disease Control and Prevention, US Department of Health and Human Services; 2013.
5. Meldon SW, Reilly M, Drew BL, et al. Trauma in the very elderly: a community-based study of outcomes at trauma and nontrauma centers. J Trauma. 2002;52:79Y84.
6. Sanders AB, Witzke DB, Jones JS, Richmond K, Kidd P. Principles of care and application of the geriatric emergency care model. In: Sanders AB, editor. Emergency care of the elder person. St. Louis, MO: Beverly-Cracom Publications; 1996. p. 59–93.
7. Mohan D, Barnato AE, Rosengart MR, et al. Trauma triage in the emergency departments of nontrauma centers: an analysis of individual physician caseload on triage patterns. J Trauma Acute Care Surg. 2013;74(6):1541–7.
8. Sasser SM, Hunt RC, Faul M, et al. Centers for Disease Control and Prevention. Guidelines for elder triage of injured patients: recommendations of the National Expert Panel on Field Triage, 2011. MMWR Recomm Rep. 2012;61(RR-1):1–20.
9. Committee on Trauma, American College of Surgeons. Collaborative clinical services. In: Rotondo M, Cribari C, Smith S, editors. Resources for optimal care of the injured patient. Chicago: American College of Surgeons; 2014. p. 76–87.
10. Kohn MA, Hammel JM, Bretz SW, Stangby A. Trauma team activation criteria as predictors of patient disposition from the emergency department. Acad Emerg Med. 2004;11(1):1–9.
11. A H, Ibrahim-Zada I, Rhee P, Aziz H, Fain MJ, Friese RS, Joseph B. Predictors of mortality in geriatric trauma patients: a systematic review and meta-analysis. J Trauma Acute Care Surg. 2014;76(3):894–901.
12. Phillips S, Rond PC 3rd, Kelly SM, et al. The failure of triage criteria to identify geriatric patients with trauma: results from the Florida Trauma Triage Study. J Trauma. 1996;40(2):278–83.
13. Gage AM, Traven N, Rivara FP, Jurkovich GJ, Arbabi S. Compliance with Centers for Disease Control and Prevention elder triage guidelines in an established trauma system. J Am Coll Surg. 2012;215(1):148–54.
14. Davis JW, Kaups KL. Base deficit in the elderly: a marker of severe injury and death. J Trauma. 1998;45:873–7.
15. Sterling DA, O'Connor JA, Bonadies J. Geriatric falls: injury severity is high and disproportionate to mechanism. J Trauma. 2001;50:116Y119.
16. JB B, Gestring ML, Forsythe RM, Stassen NA, Billiar TR, Peitzman AB, Sperry JL. Systolic blood pressure criteria in the National Trauma Triage Protocol for geriatric trauma: 110 is the new 90. J Trauma Acute Care Surg. 2015;78(2):352–9.
17. Pandit V, Rhee P, Hashmi A, Kulvatunyou N, Tang A, Khalil M, O'Keeffe T, Green D, Friese RS, Joseph B. Shock index predicts mortality in geriatric trauma patients: an analysis of the National Trauma Data Bank. J Trauma Acute Care Surg. 2014;76(4):1111–5.
18. JM C, Raubenolt A, Cudnik MT. Modification of Glasgow Coma Scale criteria for injured elders. Acad Emerg Med. 2011;18(10):1014–21.
19. Yilmaz S, Karcioglu O, Sener S. The impact of associated diseases on the etiology, course and mortality in geriatric trauma patients. Eur J Emerg Med. 2006;13:295–8.
20. Chang DC, Bass RR, Cornwell EE, et al. Undertriage of elderly trauma patients to state-designated trauma centers. Arch Surg. 2008;143:776–81. discussion 782
21. Scheetz LJ. Effectiveness of prehospital trauma triage guidelines for the identification of major trauma in elderly motor vehicle crash victims. J Emerg Nurs. 2003;29:109.
22. McMillian WD, Rogers FB. Management of prehospital antiplatelet and anticoagulant therapy in traumatic head injury: a review. J Trauma. 2009;66:94.
23. Meldon SW, Reilly M, Drew BL, et al. Trauma in the very elderly: a community-based study of outcomes at trauma and nontrauma centers. J Trauma. 2002;52:79–84.
24. Bonne S, Schuerer DJE. Trauma in the older adult: epidemiology and evolving geriatric trauma principles. Clin Geriatr Med. 2013;29(1):137–50.
25. Vidán M, Serra JA, Moreno C, Riquelme G, Ortiz J. Efficacy of a comprehensive geriatric intervention in older patients hospitalized for hip fracture: a randomized, controlled trial. J Am Geriatr Soc. 2005;53:1476–82.
26. Fisher AA, Davis MW, Rubenach SE, Sivakumaran S, Smith PN. Outcomes for older patients with hip fractures: the impact of orthopedic and geriatric medicine cocare. J Orthop Trauma. 2006;20:172–80.

27. Gowing R, Jain M. Injury patterns and outcomes associated with elderly trauma victims in Kingston, Ontario. Can J Surg. 2007;50(6):437–44.
28. Calland J, Ingraham A, Martin N, et al. Evaluation and management of geriatric trauma: an Eastern Association for the Surgery of Trauma practice management guideline. J Traum Acute Care. 2012;73:S345–50.
29. Sterling DA, O'Connor JA, Bonadies J. Geriatric falls: injury severity is high and disproportionate to mechanism. J Trauma. 2001;50(1):116–9.
30. Cohn B, Keim S, Sanders A. Can anticoagulated patients be discharged home safely from the emergency department after minor head injury? J Emerg Med. 2014;46(3):410–7.
31. Hodgkinson S, Pollit V, Sharpin C. Early management of head injury, summary of updated NICE guidance. BMJ. 2014;348:g104.
32. Sadro C, Sandstrom C, Verma N, et al. Geriatric trauma: a radiologist's guide to imaging trauma patients aged 65 years and older. Radiographics. 2015;35:1263–85.
33. JA S, Wang J, Mills B, et al. The application of the CRASH-CT prognostic model for older adults with traumatic brain injury: a population-based observational cohort study. J Head Trauma Rehabil. 2016;31:E8–E14.
34. Milzman DP, Boulanger BR, Rodriguez A, et al. Pre-existing disease in trauma patients: a predictor of fate independent of age and injury severity score. J Trauma. 1992;32(2):236–43.
35. Ferraris VA, Ferraris SP, Saha SP. The relationship between mortality and preexisting cardiac disease in 5,971 trauma patients. J Trauma. 2010;69(3):645–52.
36. Scalea T, Holman M, Fuortes M, et al. Central venous blood oxygen saturation: an early accurate meansurement of volume during hemorrhage. J Trauma. 1988;28:725.
37. Scalea T, Simon H, Duncan A, et al. Geriatric blunt multiple trauma: improved survivial with early invasive monitoring. J Trauma. 1990;30:129–36.
38. Nguyen HB, Jaehne AK, Jayaprakash N, et al. Early goal-directed therapy in severe sepsis and septic shock: insights and comparisons to ProCESS, ProMISe, and ARISE. Crit Care. 2016;20(1):160–72.
39. Process Investigators, Yealy DM, Kellum JA, Huang DT, Barnato AE, Weissfeld LA, et al. A randomized trial of protocol-based care for early septic shock. N Engl J Med. 2014;370(18):1683–93.
40. ARISE Investigators, Anzics Clinical Trials Group, Peake SL, Delaney A, Bailey M, Bellomo R, Cameron PA, et al. Goal-directed resuscitation for patients with early septic shock. N Engl J Med. 2014;371(16):1496–506.
41. Mouncey PR, Osborn TM, Power GS, Harrison DA, Sadique MZ, Grieve RD, et al. Trial of early, goal-directed resuscitation for septic shock. N Engl J Med. 2015;372(14):1301–11.
42. Angus DC, Barnato AE, Bell D, Bellomo R, Chong CR, Coats TJ, et al. A systematic review and meta-analysis of early goal-directed therapy for septic shock: the ARISE, ProCESS and ProMISe Investigators. Intensive Care Med. 2015;41(9):1549–60.
43. VS MD, Thompson KA, Lewis PR, Sise CB, Sise MJ, Shackford SR. Frailty in trauma: a systematic review of the surgical literature for clinical assessment tools. J Trauma Acute Care Surg. 2016;80(5):824–34.
44. Mangram AJ, Shifflette VK, Mitchell CD, et al. The creation of a geriatric trauma unit "G-60". Am Surg. 2011;77(9):1144–6.
45. Smith JSJ, Martin LF, Young WW, Macioce DP. Do trauma centers improve outcome over non-trauma centers: the evaluation of regional trauma care using discharge abstract data and patient management categories. J Trauma. 1990;30:1533–8.
46. Bouras T, Stranjalis G, Korfias S, et al. Head injury mortality in a geriatric population: differentiating an "edge" age group with better potential for benefit than older poor-prognosis patients. J Neurotrauma. 2007;24:1355–61.
47. Fallon WF Jr, Rader E, Zyzanski S, et al. Geriatric outcomes are improved by a geriatric trauma consultation service. J Trauma. 2006;61(5):1040–6.
48. State of Ohio, State Board of Emergency Medical Services, Trauma Committee. Geriatric Trauma Task Force Report and Recommendations. www.ems.ohio.gov/datacenter/Geriatric%20Trauma%20Triage%20Study.pdf.

Part V

Head Injury

6 Geriatric Concussions

Russell D. Dumire

Overview and Epidemiology

The geriatric population currently constitutes the most rapidly growing segment of the US as well as world population. In addition, this rapidly growing population is enjoying a level of freedom and independence not realized by previous generations due to advances in healthcare as well as rapid growth of social support organizations and assisted living communities. The geriatric population (people aged 65 and older) comprises approximately 12% of the US population. However, as the 77 plus million members of the baby boomer generation continue to age, the number of people over the age of 65 will exceed 71 million by the year 2030 and represent approximately 20% of the US population. The US Census Bureau also projects that between the years 2005 and 2050 the geriatric population will more than double and in the same period of time the number of individuals aged 85 and older is expected to exceed 20 million in the United States alone [18, 68, 69].

Trauma is the seventh leading cause of death in the geriatric population; however [54, 57], deaths associated with traumatic brain injury constitute approximately 30% of this overall mortality. Mortality rates from TBI start to increase at age 30 but the likelihood of death is maximal after age 70 [24]. In general, mild traumatic brain injury rarely results in death but one must remember that the geriatric population is at much greater risk of significant injury when compared to their younger cohorts [28, 40, 59]. This higher incidence in mortality is, in part, due to a combination of increased incidence of preexisting diseases, decreased physiologic reserve, as well as a general lack of knowledge among healthcare providers in regard to the geriatric population [25, 43, 46]. Indeed, similar outcomes following traumatic events can be obtained in the geriatric population as compared to the younger population if the injury or potential injury is identified early and aggressively pursued [51, 62, 63, 67]. A high index of suspicion and keen attention to detail are of critical significance in this patient population. Understanding the physiologic changes associated with aging as well as the confounding issues of the polypharmacy often associated with comorbidities is also an essential component in the evaluation and management of this patient population. Low-energy mechanisms of energy such as ground-level falls should raise the suspicion of the possibility of a more significant injury in general and specifically occult head injury in geriatric population. Early individualized management of the geriatric patient following a mild TBI can provide the best opportunity for their eventual return to the community with an acceptable quality of life [41, 45]. It should be noted that at this time, there exist no evidence-based guidelines

R.D. Dumire, M.D., F.A.C.S.
Conemaugh Memorial Hospital, Johnstown, PA, USA
e-mail: rdumire@conemaugh.org

A. Rodriguez et al. (eds.), *Geriatric Trauma and Acute Care Surgery*,
https://doi.org/10.1007/978-3-319-57403-5_6

in regard to the diagnosis, evaluation, and management of concussion/mild traumatic brain injury (MTBI) in the geriatric population. There even exists a great deal of variation in the definitions of what constitutes geriatric and MTBI.

The diagnosis of mild traumatic brain injury acutely in the geriatric population can be challenging as it is often near impossible to discern whether alterations in mental status were caused by the fall or if their presence was a possible contributing factor leading to the injury itself. When dealing with trauma in the geriatric population, we must keep in mind that the golden hour is made up of platinum minutes especially in our platinum patients. Delays in diagnosis result in increased morbidity and mortality in all age groups including the geriatric population where the potential for injury is too often underappreciated as well as under-triaged resulting in delays in diagnosis as well as initiation of therapy [33, 56, 65].

On an annual basis, 1.4 Americans each year will suffer from a traumatic brain injury, and of these, 50,000 will die, 235,000 will be hospitalized, and over 80,000 patients each year will experience some type of long-term disability which has resulted in an estimated 5.3 million Americans currently living with disabilities resulting from brain injury [18, 21, 35]. In 2006 alone, over $2.8 billion was spent on treating traumatic brain injury in patients 65 years and older. This volume of injury translates to a financial burden of $75–$100 billion per year for the care of patients with traumatic brain injury of which the geriatric population constitutes approximately 30%. When thinking about traumatic brain injury in the geriatric population, one can remember the 30% rule. The geriatric population continues to demonstrate a relatively constant annual incidence of trauma of approximately 30% with 30% of these having an associated traumatic brain injury consuming approximately 30% of the health care resources spent on trauma annually and is associated with 30% fatality rate. As the public has become more aware of both severe and mild traumatic brain injury over the last several years, we can see a decline in the incidence of TBI-related death overall, with the exception of the geriatric population which continues to increase [5, 18, 50].

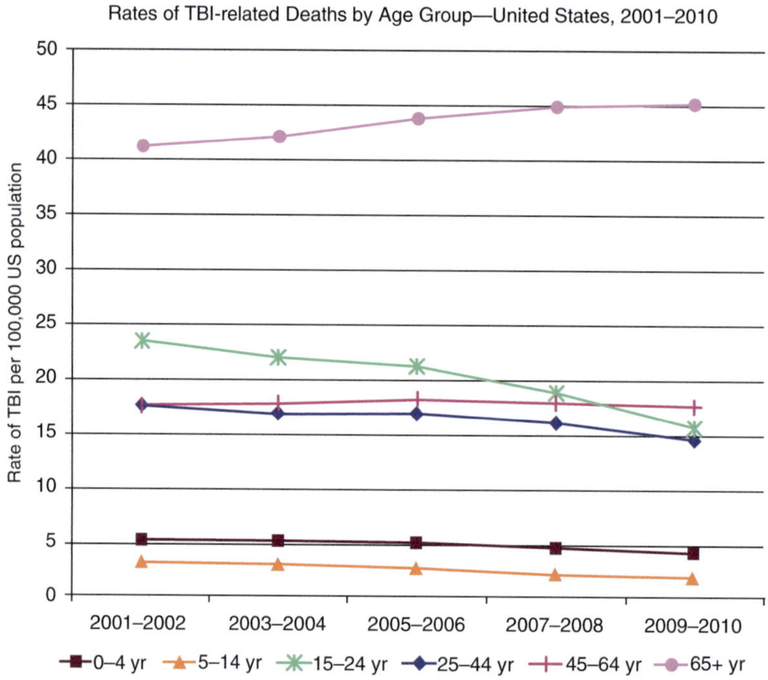

Source: Faul M, Xu L, Wald MM, Coronado VG. Traumatic brain injury in the United States: emergency department visits, hospitalizations, and deaths. Atlanta (GA): Centers for Disease Control and Prevention, National Center for Injury Prevention and Control; 2010.

All traumatic brain injury is not the same and fortunately only 10% of traumatic brain injury cases are classified as severe which is defined as a Glasgow Coma Scale of 8 or less following a traumatic event. Mild traumatic brain injury constitutes approximately 80% of all brain injury and is defined by a Glasgow Coma Score between 13 and 15 following traumatic event. The CDC defines concussion or mild traumatic brain injury (MTBI) as "a complex pathophysiologic process affecting the brain induced by traumatic biomechanical forces secondary to direct or indirect forces to the head. MTBI is caused by a blow or jolt to the head that disrupts the function of the brain. This disturbance of brain function is typically (but not always) associated with normal structural neuroimaging findings (i.e., CT scan, MRI)" [70, 71]. The Eastern Association for the Surgery of Trauma defines MTBI in its 2012 update as "an acute alteration in brain function caused by a blunt external force and is characterized by a Glasgow Coma Scale (GCS) score of 13 to 15, loss of consciousness for 30 minutes or less, and duration of posttraumatic amnesia of 24 hours or less and **if a CT scan of the brain has been performed, its result must be normal**" [16]. A comprehensive review of the existing literature related to concussion and the geriatric population reveals a great deal of variation in both the definition of mild traumatic brain injury and the definition of the geriatric population [13]. Mild TBI results in a constellation of physical, cognitive, emotional, and/or sleep-related symptoms and may or may not involve a loss of consciousness (LOC). Duration of symptoms is highly variable and may last from several minutes to days or weeks. Approximately 15% of people with mild traumatic brain injury still manifest symptoms a year or more after the injury [1]. This fact is particularly concerning in the geriatric population in that many already have coexisting degenerative limitations and are already walking a fine line between independent living and a nursing home. Many times a seemingly trivial injury is the tipping point resulting in institutionalization of a previously independently living geriatric patient. Approximately 50% of patients 65 years of age and older who are admitted after any traumatic event end up in a nursing or skilled facility post-hospital discharge and most never return to independent living [8, 28, 49].

Definitions

The commonly accepted definition of the geriatric population is that population 65 years of age and older; however, many of the earlier studies included patients 55 years of age and older. This review/discussion of geriatric mild traumatic brain injury will include all data sources due to the very limited data available concerning concussions in the geriatric population. For the purposes of this discussion, the currently accepted definition of the geriatric population includes patients 65 years and older and a concussion is defined as a condition meeting the above Eastern Association for the Surgery of Trauma (EAST) definition and no anatomic evidence of injury on neuroimaging studies. The basic defining characteristics of a concussion/MTBI include:

Loss of consciousness for a period of 30 min or less and a Glasgow Coma Score of 13–15

Loss of memory for events immediately before or after the accident with posttraumatic amnesia not greater than 24 h

Any alteration in mental state at the time of the accident (disorientation and/or confusion)

Patients may also demonstrate one or more of the following associated symptoms following a traumatically induced disruption of brain function. These are often referred to as the postconcussion syndrome:

Fatigue
Headaches
Visual disturbances
Memory loss (short-term greater than long-term memory)
Poor attention/concentration
Sleep disturbances
Dizziness/loss of balance
Irritability-emotional disturbances
Feelings of depression
Nausea
Loss of smell
Sensitivity to light and sounds
Mood changes/depression
Disorientation and/or confusion
Slow or impaired thought processes
Suicidal ideation in the elderly population

Using the above definition, the terms mild traumatic brain injury (MTBI) and concussion can be used interchangeably. One should also note that many of these symptoms are also symptoms associated with the aging process and progressive organ dysfunction which further complicates the recognition and diagnosis of mild traumatic brain injury in the geriatric population.

Discussion

The physiologic effects of aging begin in the third decade of life, and although the various organ systems are affected at different rates, the process itself progresses at a relatively constant rate [11, 19]. Although individuals may phenotypically express these changes differently, the decline in organ function including neurologic function continues to progress. This variable rate of decline in organ system function accounts for the difference in physiologic and chronological age and is heavily influenced by comorbidities, medications, and previous injury. Most notably, the geriatric population will manifest an overall decrease in their functional reserve capacity and therefore a less severe mechanism of injury may result in more severe underlying consequences due to preexisting comorbidities, polypharmacy, and its effect on physiologic response to injury as well as diminished functional capacity in all of the major organ systems. The existence of these comorbidities results in a diminished functional capacity but also remember that the medical treatment (polypharmacy) of the comorbidity may also blunt or limit physiologic responses and predispose to injury [39]. For example, diuretics that require the elderly patient to get up at night combined with the antihypertensive which predisposes towards orthostasis in combination with diminished vision and balance can result in a fall. Recent data demonstrates that one in four adults have at least two chronic conditions requiring medical treatment and more than half of older adults have three or more chronic conditions. The average number of medications being taken by a patient 65 years of age and older is 5 with 12–20% being on 9 or more medications [2–4, 39, 55].

Many of the changes associated with aging such as loss of muscle mass, slowing reflexes, and deterioration in the senses of sight and sound are predisposing factors for injury in the geriatric population. Other changes such as bone demineralization predispose to more severe anatomic injury. For instance, between the ages of 20 and 80, the maximal cardiac output is reduced between 30 and 50%. Cardiac output decreases in a linear fashion of approximately 1% per year after the age of 30 in patients with no underlying cardiac disease. This decline is amplified in the presence of underlying cardiac disease. There is also a decline in respiratory function as manifested by a drop in FEV1 of approximately 30 mL per year after the age of 30 and by age 75 the pulmonary capacity is only 40–50% of that at age 30. The result is a lower arterial oxygen content as well as a decreased ability to pump oxygen to the vital organs in times of stress. This lack of overall physiologic reserve may represent an additional reason as to why more geriatric patients present with anatomic injury such as ischemic insults following trauma. However, I can find no evidence-based studies to support this theory.

Anatomically, the brain undergoes progressive atrophy with aging decreasing in size (volume) by approximately 10–12% between the ages of 30 and 70. These anatomic changes are also associated with subtle but progressive changes in cognition, function, as well as memory, which may complicate the process of mental status evaluation in these patients. The cerebral atrophy associated with aging is associated with an increase in CSF which allows for more room to accommodate bleeding and swelling which may delay the onset of clinical symptoms when the patient may actually have a significant underlying brain injury that has yet to clinically manifest itself. This atrophy also predisposes to anatomic traumatic brain injury, in particular subdural hemorrhages, due to the stretching of the dural veins. Geriatric patients experience MTBI more frequently than severe TBI and they have a very high rate of intracranial hemorrhage following mild head injury [24, 36, 53]. Initial review of our Geriatric Trauma Institute (GTI) data also demonstrates that in our population of geriatric patients presenting after a fall and confirmed loss of consciousness, all exhibited anatomic evidence of more severe injury. It is also likely that the diagnosis of a concussion would be overlooked in the geriatric patient with preexisting confusion, disorientation, or dementia that sustained a fall and has no clinical evidence of anatomic injury. This may lead to an underreporting of as well as an underestimation of the overall incidence of concussion in this population. Although this may seem of little consequence, there is current data which suggest that concussions at any age may result in subtle yet persistent deficits and repeated concussions compound these deficits [15, 23, 31, 47]. Prevention of the first concussion in the geriatric population may ultimately be the single most important event in keeping this population viable and independent. The vast majority of geriatric trauma results from ground-level, low-energy falls. Therefore targeting this common etiology is a reasonable starting point.

Mechanism

Falls are, by far, the most common cause of trauma in general in the geriatric population as well as geriatric traumatic brain injury [54, 62, 63]. These falls are almost always ground-level/low-energy falls with most of them occurring at home. The diagnosis of injury is often delayed in this patient population due to a low index of suspicion based upon mechanism of injury as well as the ability of injuries to progress without early clinical findings as a result of the anatomic changes associated with the aging process. This delay in diagnosis undoubtedly contributes to the overall increased morbidity and mortality in this vulnerable patient population. Falls account for approximately 60% of geriatric trauma cases admitted to the hospital and the death rate associated with unintentional falls in the geriatric population continues to rise on an annual basis. Approximately 36% of geriatric patients who fall will require a repeat ED visit or will die within 1 year following the initial fall and 50% of these patients will experience a repeat fall within the next 6–12 months [35]. The history of a single fall is the most important risk factor in predicting subsequent falls in this patient population, and if the fall results in hospitalization, there is a 50% chance that the patient will not return home but rather be placed in a nursing home or other skilled facility [5, 8, 34, 64]. The clinical effects of repetitive MTBI in the geriatric population present a significant issue that has received very little formal investigation and warrants further study. However, there is data that demonstrates a cumulative effect of repeated head injuries. Repeated mild head injuries are associated with persistence of symptoms and diminished performance scores. Age at the time of injury does not influence the incidence of symptoms [1]. These falls are often a result of the physiology of aging due to impaired senses, slowed reflexes, and loss of muscle tone in addition to the polypharmacy present in many geriatric patients due to their comorbidities. Motor vehicle collisions, auto-pedestrian accidents, assaults, elder abuse, and suicide constitute the majority of the remaining etiologies associated with geriatric traumatic brain injury.

Data from the CDC demonstrates that a geriatric patient dies from a fall-related injury approximately every 20 min in the United States today with traumatic brain injury associated approximately 30% of the time [69]. The vast majority of patients sustaining a traumatic brain injury are classified as mild whereas only 10% of patients overall comprise the severe traumatic brain injury group. Traumatic brain injury in the geriatric trauma population accounts for approximately 80,000 emergency department visits per year and, as previously mentioned, the vast majority being classified as mild traumatic brain injury (MTBI). Despite the great preponderance of MTBI across all age groups, there are no nationally accepted standards for the diagnosis and treatment of MTBI. The lack of a standard definition of MTBI makes comparison of studies difficult as many of the older studies included patients with and without anatomic evidence of injury on neuroimaging techniques and a GCS of 13–15 while the more recent studies typically exclude patients with anatomic evidence of injury as well as oftentimes excluding the geriatric population [13]. As the proportion of the world population of geriatric patients increases, so too will the incidence of traumatic events including mild traumatic brain injury. However, there is currently a paucity of data related to all aspects of geriatric mild traumatic brain injury including incidence, diagnosis, and management [49]. Just as the pediatric patient is not a small adult, the geriatric patient is also not just an older adult. Extrapolation of data and results from existing concussion studies is difficult due to the underrepresentation or often exclusion of geriatric patients from their study groups and therefore may not accurately represent the pathophysiology of mild traumatic brain injury in the geriatric population.

Diagnosis and Evaluation

The diagnosis of mild traumatic brain injury in the geriatric population presents unique challenges in that there exists a baseline variation in functional as well as cognitive capacity in this very diverse patient population. In addition, the complete and thorough evaluation of the geriatric patient may be complicated due to multiple comorbidities, polypharmacy, and its effect on the neurological examination as well as the inability to completely evaluate this patient population due to limitations such as the increased incidence of MRI-noncompatible hardware such as pacemakers, nerve stimulators, and other implanted hardware. This prevents the complete evaluation of patients with significant or persistent symptoms and may result in missing an anatomical injury and erroneously classifying the patient as a concussion when in fact they truly have a more severe anatomic traumatic brain injury. It is for this reason we must be cautious when comparing statistics and outcomes between the younger and older populations. In addition, the symptoms of and therefore the diagnosis of concussion are difficult to delineate in the geriatric population due to several confounding factors. In only 50% of the cases can the geriatric patient or their family reliably tell us if there was any associated loss of consciousness or alteration in baseline neurologic function before or after the fall [58]. Many of the commonly associated signs and symptoms of a concussion such as confusion, disorientation, mood swings, and sleep disturbances may be preexisting conditions in this patient population. The signs and symptoms of mild traumatic brain injury are often so subtle that they are often overlooked by family members as well as physicians. In addition, the symptoms may not be present initially and manifest themselves over weeks following the injury and are often overlooked by the patient as well as family members. Upon review of our own institutional data over the last 2 years, there were no instances of a geriatric patient sustaining a ground-level fall resulting in a confirmed loss of consciousness that presented with a GCS of 13–15 which did not have anatomic evidence of injury on CT scan with the exception of those patients who clearly and reliably communicated a disorientation or loss of consciousness prior to the fall. Anecdotally, it appears as if the neurologic disruption resulting from a fall (not present prior to) in this population is almost always associated with an anatomical injury.

Recent studies of geriatric patients with a mild head injury demonstrate that 14% of patients had evidence of lesion on CT; 20% of these lesions required neurosurgical intervention [36]. Routine CT scan of the head is now recommended for all patients aged 65 and older presenting with neurological symptoms and signs or history of head trauma to aid TBI diagnosis [6]. One must also consider the fact that approximately 9–10% of the geriatric population is taking some type of antiplatelet or anticoagulation medication which increases the incidence of associated intracerebral bleeding even with what appears to be minor traumatic events [51, 62]. The signs and symptoms of this slowly progressive bleed may not become apparent for many hours following the event. Unless the evaluating physicians have a high index of suspicion, this injury may be missed until it becomes clinically apparent at which point the patient's prognosis significantly worsens. It is because of this that many local institutional practice guidelines and recommendations are being developed regarding the care of geriatric patients in general across the country. Unfortunately, there still is very little to no data available on a standardized approach to the care of mild traumatic brain injury in the geriatric population. Some applicable recommendations include the following:

1. CT scans should be performed on patients with suspected brain injury if available [16].
2. Patient taking warfarin who presented with a mild traumatic brain injury should have an INR determined as early as possible [16].
3. Patients on antiplatelets or anticoagulation with a presumed to potential mild traumatic brain injury should be triaged to early CT scan even in the absence of clinical symptoms [12].
4. Patients with multiple comorbidities or significant mechanisms of injury should be evaluated at a trauma center [12, 16, 44, 66].
5. Same level or ground-level falls in the geriatric population with any alteration mental status should be evaluated at a trauma center [8, 61, 63].
6. Preestablished triage and treatment protocols in this patient population result in expedited diagnosis of significant injury and result in improved outcomes in the geriatric population [38].
7. Trauma centers with a higher volume of geriatric patients, geriatric specific protocols, and or geriatric services obtain better overall outcomes with lower associated cost [37, 38].

We have many tools available to assist in the diagnosis and management of all patients with TBI or potential TBI. However, when using a tool, one must know the limitations of that tool. Our most valuable tool, the clinical examination by a knowledgeable practitioner, may be limited in the geriatric population due to progressive degenerative changes or blunted physiologic responses due to concurrent medications. The Glasgow Coma Score (GCS), a basic tool in the neurologic assessment of trauma patients, has been proven an inaccurate predictor of acute injury in the geriatric population as well as predictor of long-term outcome, with the exception of an admission GCS of 3 in this population which uniformly is associated with poor outcomes [32]. A classification system that considers the GCS score in addition to the presence or absence of intracranial pathology in the postacute phase of initial evaluation and treatment of the geriatric population which also accounts for the extent and severity of preexisting disease is required to accurately predict outcome in this population [4, 7, 20, 26].

Preventative strategies that reduce the risk of injury need to be developed as well as standardized diagnostic protocols and treatment strategies. This approach offers the best chance of decreasing the incidence of traumatic brain injury in the geriatric population as well as to provide a reliable database to serve as the basis of further research in this area [42]. Particular attention needs to be given to high incidence of polypharmacy in this patient population and it remains the responsibility of the entire spectrum of health care providers to try and streamline the medication lists and minimize any potentially harmful medications using tools such as the Beers and the START/STOPP [48] criteria. Over one-third of adverse drug events leading to emergency room visits involve warfarin, insulin, and digoxin. The Screening Tool of Older Persons Potentially Inappropriate Prescriptions (STOPP) criteria is associated with a more significant decrease in avoidable adverse drug events than the Beers criteria [3]. Reassessment of the need for anticoagulants and antiplatelet on a regular basis is required as functional capacity and fall risk can change quite quickly in this population as well. Home safety evaluations should also be an important aspect of geriatric care as well as aggressive fall prevention programs and exercise programs in order to decrease the risk of falls. Anecdotally, upon reviewing the data from our Geriatric Trauma Institute (GTI), the overwhelming majority of falls in this population occur at home and at night with poor lighting after rising from bed on the way to the bathroom. Many times the reason for getting out of bed is the need to void which is often related to diuretics. Streamlining of medications or adjusting their timing as well as installing floor-level lighting or motion activated lighting in addition to insuring safe flooring could potentially result in a significant reduction in this common mechanism.

Due to the inherent difficulties in the differentiation between MTBI and more severe injuries in the geriatric population, it would be reasonable to obtain a CT scan of the head (CTh) in most if not all geriatric patient with a potential for underlying head injury even if clinically asymptomatic. Although there is little data concerning functional outcomes in MTBI patients 65 and older, there is data supporting better overall functional capacity and outcomes following severe TBI in this patient population with aggressive, early treatment [13, 21, 27, 28, 52, 67]. Failure to obtain a CTh may result in under-triaging more severe injuries and therefore not treating aggressively as well as negatively skew MTBI data in this patient population.

While the diagnosis and management of MTBI remains a complicated issue, the real opportunity in the geriatric patient who has suffered a MTBI may be in the prevention of subsequent injuries. If the geriatric patient is to remain functionally independent, it is imperative that efforts be made to prevent subsequent injuries or possibly even prevent the first event through preventative strategies. A single fall in this patient population should trigger a multidisciplinary approach that includes a home safety evaluation, vision testing, gait and balance assessment, assessment of current medications, and usage in addition to the medical assessment. If the geriatric patient operates a motor vehicle, yearly vision, cognitive, and motor assessments should be considered [29]. These discussions are best initiated by the primary care physician. However, these important and sensitive discussions occur very rarely during a primary care visit [9, 10]. A primary barrier to the initiation of a "driver retirement" process is the perception by the patient of a loss of independence and the lack of resources to the primary care physicians for implementation of supportive services which would help the geriatric patient maintain independence without a need to continue driving once the physiologic consequences of aging make this an unsafe activity for the patient and the public in general. The focus of these discussions should be on maintaining the physical independence of the patient as long as safely possible and how a single motor vehicle collision could significantly compromise this goal.

Exercise programs such as Tai Chi have shown great promise in decreasing the rate of falls [17, 22, 30, 64]. However, one must remember that the "fear of falling" is common in older people and associated with serious physical, psychological, and social isolation. Exercise (planned, structured, repetitive, and purposive physical activity aimed at improving physical fitness) has been shown to reduce the fear of falling by improving strength, gait, and balance which has also been associated with reducing the incidence of falls in general in this high-risk population. Unfortunately, the population most likely to engage in these programs is also the portion of the geriatric population that has already chosen not to remain physically and socially isolated. It is the homebound geriatric population's fear of falling that keeps them from the senior centers and other venues that are most in need and the most difficult to reach. This withdrawal and lack of activity due to their fear predispose them to falling as well as to more serious injuries from the fall [14, 60]. Strategies to reach this population must become part of the community or regional prevention initiative as well.

Summary

The issue of MTBI/concussions in the geriatric population remains an underappreciated and often underdiagnosed entity due to the confounding issues of comorbidities, polypharmacy, and physiologic changes in physical and mental function associated with the natural aging process. The exact incidence remains unknown and the physiologic consequences, both short and long term, have not yet been sufficiently studied due to the lack of a uniform definition of MTBI as well as what defines a geriatric patient. At this point in time, there exists a complete lack of evidence-based recommendations in regard to the diagnosis and management of geriatric MTBI and extrapolation of data from younger cohorts as well as animal studies which does not take into account the physiologic changes associated with aging is inappropriate. As the proportion of our population older than 65 who are either living independently or semi-independently in group or assisted living communities continues to increase, the consequences of these injuries may become more obvious and hopefully, with time, more evidence-based recommendations based on appropriate studies of this population will become available. More importantly, preventative measures which prevent the primary fall/insult and subsequent or repeated injuries may prove to be the optimal strategy to keeping our geriatric patient vibrant and functioning in their communities and families as they enjoy their platinum years in a state of health previously unseen in past generations.

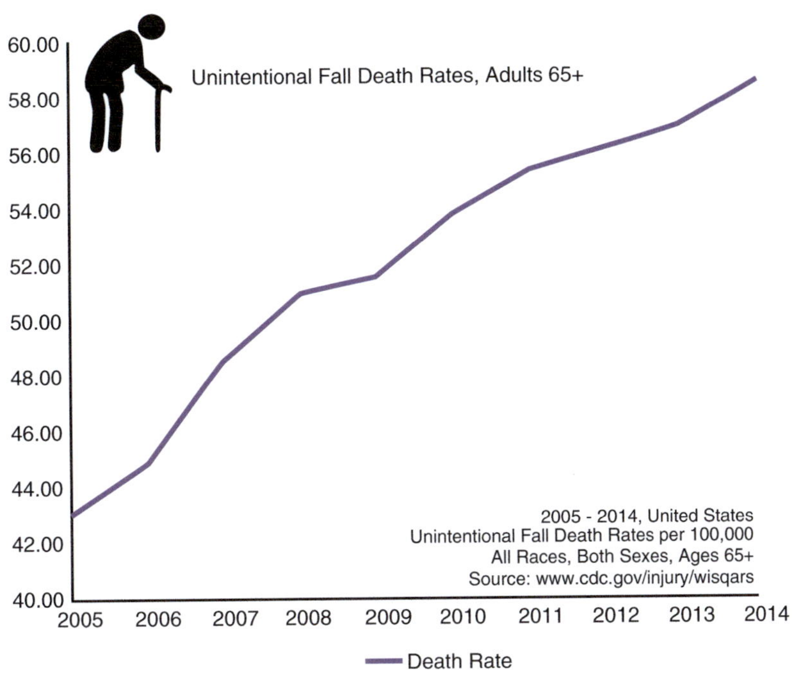

Source: http://www.cdc.gov/homeandrecreationalsafety/falls/adultfalls.htm

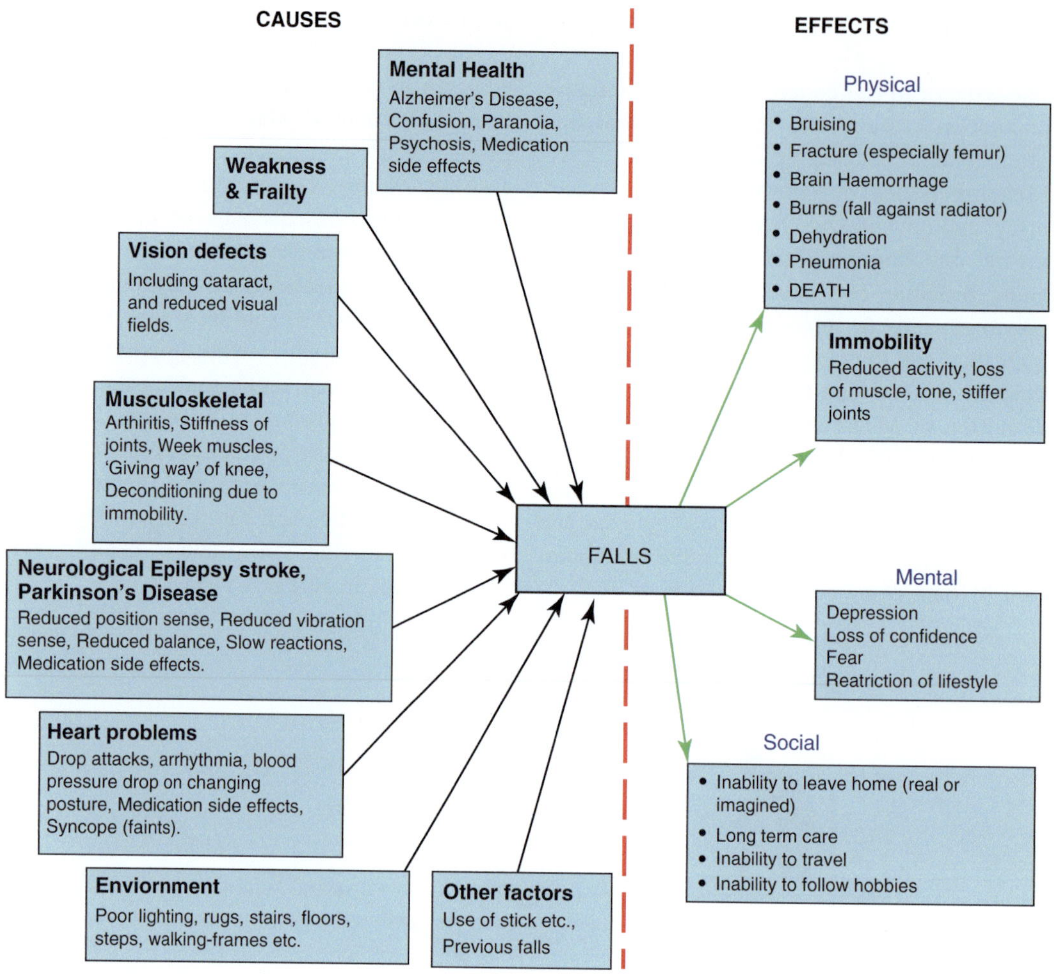

Source: http://www.physio-pedia.com/Falls

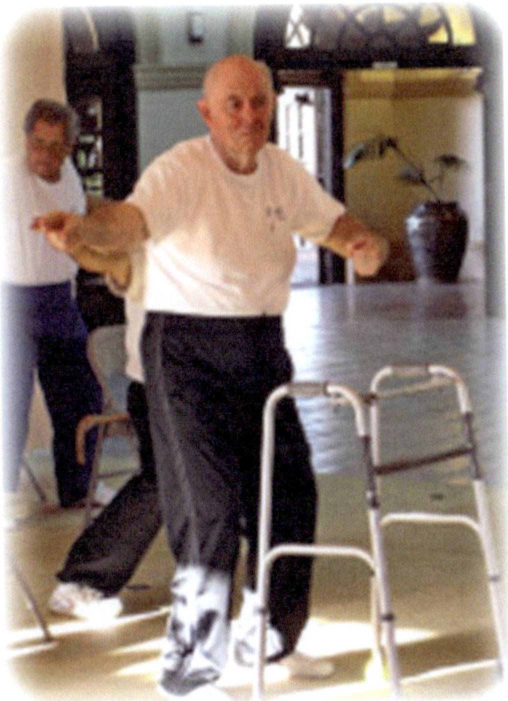

References

1. Albrecht MA, Masters CL, Ames D, Foster J. Impact of mild head injury on neuropsychological performance in healthy older adults: longitudinal assessment in the AIBL cohort. Front Aging Neurosci. 2016;8:1–11.
2. Ambrose AF, Paul G, Hausdorff JM. Risk factors for falls among older adults: a review of the literature. Maturitas. 2013;75(1):51–61.
3. American Geriatrics Society 2015 Beers Criteria Update Expert Panel. American Geriatrics Society 2015 Updated Beers Criteria for potentially inappropriate medication use in older adults. J Am Geriatr Soc. 2015;63(11):2227–46.
4. American Geriatrics Society Expert Panel on the Care of Older Adults with Multimorbidity. Guiding principles for the care of older adults with multimorbidity: an approach for clinicians. J Am Geriatr Soc. 2012;60:E1.
5. Arai H, Ouchi Y, Yokode M, Ito H, Kita T. Members of subcommittee for aging. Toward the realization of a better aged society: messages from gerontology and geriatrics. Geriatr Gerontol Int. 2012;12(1):16–22.
6. Barbosa RR, Jawa R, Watters JM, Knight JC, Kerwin AJ, Winston ES, Barraco RD, Tucker B, Bardes JM, Rowell SE, Eastern Association for the Surgery of Trauma. Evaluation and management of mild traumatic brain injury: an Eastern Association for the Surgery of Trauma practice management guideline. J Trauma Acute Care Surg. 2012;73(5 Suppl 4):S307–14.
7. Barnett K, Mercer SW, Norbury M, et al. Epidemiology of multimorbidity and implications for health care, research, and medical education: a cross-sectional study. Lancet. 2012;380:37.
8. Bergeron E, Clement J, Lavoie A, Ratte S, Bamvita JM, Aumont F, Clas D. A simple fall in the elderly: not so simple. J Trauma. 2006;60(2):268–73.
9. Betz ME, Kanani H, Juarez-Colunga E, Schwartz R. Discussions about driving between older adults and primary care providers. J Am Geriatr Soc. 2016;64(6):1318–23.
10. Betz ME, Jones J, Carr DB. System facilitators and barriers to discussing older driver safety in primary care settings. Inj Prev. 2015;21(4):231–7. https://doi.org/10.1136/injuryprev-2014-041450. Epub 23 Jan 2015.
11. Boss GR, Seegmiller EJ. Age-related physiological changes and their clinical significance. West J Med. 1981;135(6):434–40.
12. Bradburn E, Rogers FB, Krasne M, Rogers A, Horst MA, Beelen MJ, Miller JA. High-risk geriatric protocol: improving mortality in the elderly. J Trauma Acute Care Surg. 2012;73(2):435–40.
13. Carroll LJ, Cassidy JD, Peloso PM, Borg J, von Holst H, Holm L, Paniak C, Pépin M, WHO Collaborating Centre Task Force on Mild Traumatic Brain Injury. Prognosis for mild traumatic brain injury: results of the WHO collaborating centre task force on mild traumatic brain injury. J Rehabil Med. 2004;36(43 Suppl):84–105.
14. Connell BR, Wolf SL. Environmental and behavioral circumstances associated with falls at home among elderly individuals. Arch Phys Med Rehabil. 1997;78(2):179–86.
15. Cowen TD, Meythaler JM, DeVivo MJ, Ivie CS III, Lebow J, Novack TA. Influence of early variables in traumatic brain injury on functional independence measure scores and rehabilitation length of stay and charge. Arch Phys Med Rehabil. 1995;76(9):797–803.
16. Eastern Association for the Surgery of Trauma. The EAST Practice Management Guidelines Work Group [on-line]. Practice Management Guidelines for Geriatric Trauma. 2005. www.east.org/tpg/geriatric.pdf.
17. Gillespie LD, Robertson MC, Lamb SE. Interventions for preventing falls in older people living in the community (Review). The cochrane library. Cochrane Database Syst Rev. 2012;(9):CD007146.
18. Faul, M.; Xu, L.; Wald, MM; Coronado, VG. Services USDoHaH. Traumatic brain injury in the United States: emergency department visits, hospitalizations, and deaths. 2010. Atlanta, GA: Centers for Disease Control and Prevention, National Center for Injury Prevention and Control; 2010.
19. Fried LP, Ferrucci L, Darer J, Williamson JD, Anderson G. Untangling the concepts of disability,

frailty, and comorbidity: implications for improved targeting and care. J Gerontol A Biol Sci Med Sci. 2004;59(3):255–63.

20. Friese RS, Wynne J, Joseph B, Rhee P. Age and mortality after injury: is the association linear? Eur J Trauma Emerg Surg. 2014;40(5):567–72. Epub 21 Feb 2014
21. Frankel JE, Marwitz JH, Cifu DX, et al. A follow-up study of older adults with traumatic brain injury: taking into account decreasing length of stay. Arch Phys Med Rehabil. 2006;87(1):57–62.
22. Gillespie LD, Robertson MC, Gillespie WJ, Sherrington C, Gates S, Clemson LM, Lamb SE. Interventions for preventing falls in older people living in the community. Cohhrane Database Syst Rev. 2012;12:CD005465.
23. Goldstein FC, Levin HS, Goldman WP, et al. Cognitive and neurobehavioral functioning after mild versus moderate traumatic brain injury in older adults. J Int Neuropsychol Soc. 2001;7(3):373–83.
24. Harris C, DiRusso S, Sullivan T, Benzil DL. Mortality risk after head injury increases at 30 years. J Am Coll Surg. 2003;197:711–6.
25. Harvey LA, Close JC. Traumatic brain injury in older adults: characteristics, causes and consequences. Injury. 2012;43(11):1821–6. https://doi.org/10.1016/j.injury.2012.07.188. Epub 11 Aug 2012
26. Hashmi A, Ibrahim-Zada I, Rhee P, et al. Predictors of mortality in geriatric trauma patients: a systematic review and meta-analysis. J Trauma Acute Care Surg. 2014;76(3):894–901.
27. Hollis S, Lecky F, Yates DW, Woodford M. The effect of pre-existing medical conditions and age on mortality after injury. J Trauma. 2006;61(5):1255–60.
28. Hukkelhoven CW, Steyerberg EW, Rampen AJ, et al. Patient age and outcome following severe traumatic brain injury: an analysis of 5,600 patients. J Neurosurg. 2003;99:666–73.
29. Ikpeze T, Elfar JC. The geriatric driver: factors that influence when to stop driving. Geriatr Orthop Surg Rehabil. 2016;7(2):106–9. https://doi.org/10.1177/2151458516644818. Epub 24 Apr 2016
30. Kendrick D, Kumar A, Carpenter H, Zijlstra GA, Skelton DA, Cook JR, Stevens Z, Belcher CM, Haworth D, Gawler SJ, Gage H, Masud T, Bowling A, Pearl M, Morris RW, Iliffe S, Delbaere K. Exercise for reducing fear of falling in older people living in the community. Cochrane Database Syst Rev 2014;(11):CD009848.
31. Klein M, Houx PJ, Jolles J. Long-term persisting cognitive sequelae of traumatic brain injury and the effect of age. J Nerv Ment Dis. 1996;184(8):459–67.
32. Kehoe A, Rennie S, Smith JE. Glasgow Coma Scale is unreliable for the prediction of severe head injury in elderly trauma patients. Emerg Med J. 2015;32(8):613–5. https://doi.org/10.1136/emermed-2013-203488. Epub 3 Oct 2014
33. Kodadek LM, Selvarajah S, Velopulos CG, Haut ER, Haider AH. Undertriage of older trauma patients: is this a national phenomenon? J Surg Res. 2015;199(1):220–9. https://doi.org/10.1016/j.jss.2015.05.017. Epub 18 May 2015
34. LeBlanc J, de Guise E, Gosselin N, Feyz M. Comparison of functional outcome following acute care in young, middle-aged and elderly patients with traumatic brain injury. Brain Inj. 2006;20(8):779–90.
35. Liu SW, Obermeyer Z, Chang Y, Shankar KN. Frequency of ED revisits and death among older adults after a fall. Am J Emerg Med. 2015;33(8):1012–8.
36. Mack LR, Chan SB, Silva JC, Hogan TM. The use of head computed tomography in elderly patients sustaining minor head trauma. J Emerg Med. 2003;24:157–62.
37. MacKenzie EJ, Rivara FP, Jurkovich GJ, et al. A national evaluation of the effect of trauma-center care on mortality. N Engl J Med. 2006;354(4):366–78.
38. Mangram AJ, Mitchell MA, Schifflette V, Lorenzo M, Truitt G. Geriatric trauma service: a one year experience. J Trauma Acute Care Surg. 2012;72(1):119–22.
39. Marcum ZA, Pugh MJ, Amuan ME, Aspinall SL, Handler SM, Ruby CM, Hanlon JT. Prevalence of potentially preventable unplanned hospitalizations caused by therapeutic failures and adverse drug withdrawal events among older veterans. J Gerontol A Biol Sci Med Sci. 2012;67(8):867–74.
40. McGwin G Jr, MacLennan PA, Fife JB, Davis GG, Rue LW. Preexisting conditions and mortality in older trauma patients. J Trauma. 2004;56(6):1291–6.
41. Meldon SW, Reilly M, Drew BL, Mancuso C, Fallon W Jr. Trauma in the very elderly: a community-based study of outcomes at trauma and nontrauma centers. J Trauma. 2002;52(1):79–84.
42. Mercer SW, Smith SM, Wyke S, et al. Multimorbidity in primary care: developing the research agenda. Fam Pract. 2009;26:79.
43. Milzmann DP, Boulanger BR, Rodriguez A, Soderstrom CA, Mitchell KA, Magnant CM. Pre-existing disease in trauma patients: a predictor of fate independent of age and injury severity score. J Trauma. 1992;32(2):236–43.
44. Morris JA, MacKenzie EJ, Edelstein SL. The effect of preexisting conditions on mortality in trauma patients. JAMA. 1990;263(4):1942–6.
45. Morris JA, MacKenzie EJ, Damiano AM, Bass SM. Mortality in trauma patients: the interaction between host factors and severity. J Trauma. 1990;30(12):1476–82.
46. Mosenthal AC, Lavery RF, Addis M, et al. Isolated traumatic brain injury: age is an independent predictor of mortality and early outcome. J Trauma. 2002;52(5):907–11.
47. Mosenthal AC, Livingston DH, Lavery RF, et al. The effect of age on functional outcome in mild traumatic brain injury: 6-month report of a prospective multicenter trial. J Trauma. 2004;56(5):1042–8.
48. O'Mahony D, O'Sullivan S, Byrne S, Gallagher P. STOPP/START criteria for potentially inappropriate prescribing in older people. Age Ageing. 2015;44:213–8.

49. Papa L, Mendes M, Braga C. Mild traumatic brain injury among the geriatric population. Curr Tran Geriatr Gerontol Rep. 2012;1:135–42.
50. Perdue PW, Watts DD, Kaufmann CR, Trask AL. Differences in mortality between elderly and younger adult trauma patients: geriatric status increases risk of delayed death. J Trauma. 1998;45(4):805–10.
51. Pretorius RW, Gataric G, Swedlund SK, Miller JR. Reducing the risk of adverse drug events in older adults. Am Fam Physician. 2013;87(5):331–6. Review
52. Rapoport MJ, Feinstein A. Outcome following traumatic brain injury in the elderly: a critical review. Brain Inj. 2000;14(8):749–61.
53. Reynolds FD, Dietz PA, Higgins D, Whitaker TS. Time to deterioration of the elderly, anticoagulated, minor head injury patient who presents without evidence of neurologic abnormality. J Trauma. 2003;54(3):492–6.
54. Schwab CW, Kauder DR. Trauma in the geriatric patient. Arch Surg. 1992;127(6):701–6.
55. Shanthi GS, Krishnaswamy B. Risk factors for falls in elderly. J Ind Acad Geriatr. 2005;2:57–60.
56. Shimoda K, Maeda T, Tado M, Yoshino A, Katayama Y, Bullock MR. Outcome and surgical management for geriatric traumatic brain injury: analysis of 888 cases registered in the Japan Neurotrauma Data Bank. World Neurosurg. 2014;82(6):1300–6. https://doi.org/10.1016/j.wneu.2014.08.014. Epub 14 Aug 2014
57. Smith DP, Enderson BL, Maull KI. Trauma in the elderly: determinants of outcome. South Med J. 1990;83(2):171–7.
58. Styrke J, Stalnacke BM, Sojka P, Bjornstig U. Traumatic brain injuries in a well-defined population:epidemiological aspects and severity. J Neurotrauma. 2007;24(9):1425–36.
59. Susman M, DiRusso SM, Sullivan T, et al. Traumatic brain injury in the elderly: increased mortality and worse functional outcome at discharge despite lower injury severity. J Trauma. 2002;53(2):219–23.
60. Teno J, Kiel DP, Mor V. Multiple stumbles: a risk factor for falls in community-dwelling elderly. J Am Geriatr Soc. 1990;38(12):1321–5.
61. Thompson HJ, Dikmen S, Temkin N. Prevalence of comorbidity and its association with traumatic brain injury and outcomes in older adults. Res Gerontol Nurs. 2012;5(1):17–24.
62. Thompson HJ, McCormick WC, Kagan SH. Traumatic brain injury in older adults: epidemiology, outcomes, and future implications. J Am Geriatr Soc. 2006;54(10):1590–5.
63. Timmons T, Menaker J. Clin Geriatr. 2010;18(4):20.
64. Tinetti ME. Clinical practice. Preventing falls in elderly persons. N Engl J Med. 2003;348:42–9.
65. Tornetta P 3rd, Mostafavi H, Riina J, et al. Morbidity and mortality in elderly trauma patients. J Trauma. 1999;46(4):702–6.
66. Werman HA, Erskine T, Caterino J, Riebe JF, Valasek T. Members of the Trauma Committee of the State of Ohio EMS Board. Development of statewide geriatric patients trauma triage criteria. Prehosp Disaster Med. 2011;26(3):170–9.
67. Whitmore RG, Thawani JP, Grady MS, Levine JM, Sanborn MR, Stein SC. Is aggressive treatment of traumatic brain injury cost-effective? J Neurosurg. 2012;116(5):1106–13. https://doi.org/10.3171/2012.1.JNS11962. Epub 6 Mar 2012

Websites

68. US Census Bureau, population division. National population projections released 2008 (based on Census 2000). Washington, DC: US Census Bureau, Population Division; 2008. www.census.gov/population/www/projections/2008projections.html
69. Federal Interagency Forum on Aging-Related Statistics. Older Americans 2010. Key indicators of well-being. Federal Interagency forum on aging-related statistics. US Government Printing Office, Washington, DC; 2010. www.agingstats.gov/agingstatsdotnet/Main_Site/Data/2010_Documents/Docs/OA_2010.pdf.
70. Hall MJ, DeFrances CJ, Williams SN, Golosinskiy A, Schwartzman A. Division of Health Care Statistics. National Hospital Discharge Survey: 2007 summary. National Health Statistics reports number 29; 2010. www.cdc.gov/nchs/data/nhsr/nhsr029.pdf.
71. Report to Congress Traumatic Brain Injury in the United States: Epidemiology and Rehabilitation Submitted by the Centers for Disease Control and Prevention National Center for Injury Prevention and Control Division of Unintentional Injury Prevention. www.cdc.gov/traumaticbraininjury/pdf/tbi_report_to_congress_epi_and_rehab-a.pdf.

7 Traumatic Extra-Axial Hemorrhage in the Elderly

Jack Wilberger

Introduction

Traumatic brain injury (TBI) in the elderly (>65 years of age) presents unique medical, surgical, and ethical challenges that require enhanced trauma team and neurosurgical communication and collaboration to ensure optimal treatment decisions and outcome.

This chapter focuses on traumatic extraaxial hemorrhages—ASDH, epidural hematoma (EDH), and chronic subdural hematoma (CSDH)—to elucidate treatment considerations in the context of epidemiology, pathophysiology, impact of comorbid factors, and outcome.

Additional issues of anticoagulation and palliative care of these patients are highlighted.

Epidemiology

The incidence of severe TBI in the elderly has dramatically increased coincident with the ageing population. O'Conner et al., utilizing the National Trauma Data Bank, found a 20–25% increase in trauma center admissions for TBI in those >75 years old compared to the general population between 2007 and 2010 [1].

The US Census Bureau estimates that those >65 comprized 35 million of the population in 2006 and will grow to greater than 86 million by 2050 [2].

Harvey et al. studied the TBI hospitalization rate in elderly patients from 1999 to 2011. Acute subdural hematoma (ASDH) accounted for 43% of hospitalizations. Falls at 82% were the most common cause and increased by 8.4% per year [3].

While those >65 years comprise 10% of all patients suffering from TBI, they result in 50% of all TBI deaths. Those >75 years have the highest TBI hospitalization rate—264/100,000—twice the rate of any other age-related group [4].

Pathophysiology of the Ageing Brain and Body

Treatment decisions in the elderly with TBI should be grounded in an understanding of the physiology of the ageing brain.

After 20 years old the brain loses mass by 0.1% per year and accumulates an increasing amount of harmful aluminum, iron, and free radicals.

There is an approximately 20% decrease in cerebral blood flow which can be further exacerbated by cerebrovascular disease.

There is an age-dependant decrease in neurotransmitters and receptors [5].

J. Wilberger, M.D., F.A.C.S., F.A.A.N.S.
Department of Neurosurgery, Allegheny General Hospital, Drexel University College of Medicine, Suite 302, 420 East North Ave, Pittsburgh, PA 15212, USA
e-mail: jwilberg@wpahs.org

A. Rodriguez et al. (eds.), *Geriatric Trauma and Acute Care Surgery*,
https://doi.org/10.1007/978-3-319-57403-5_7

Ageing also reduces plasticity and repair mechanisms. Although the natural reduction in cell number and plasticity has been studied in the context of memory [6], plasticity plays an important role following traumatic brain injury.

Constitutional issues also affect an individual's proneness and response to a TBI: poor eyesight, impaired balance, muscle deconditioning, medications, bone health, cardiac arrhythmias, postural hypotension, and neuropathy.

Medical Comorbidities

Various studies have shown that those >65 years, still independently living, have a high incidence of medical comorbidities [7] (Fig. 7.1).

Mosenthal et al. found that 70% of those over 65 years had a significant medical comorbidity compared to those younger [8].

The incidence of dementia, depression, and Parkinsonism is likewise higher in fall-related TBI [9].

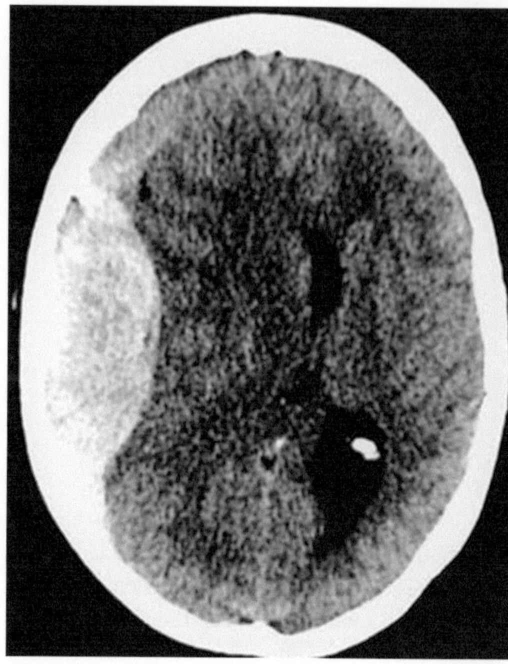

Fig. 7.1 CT scan of a typical chronic subdural hematoma with hypodense fluid layering cortex with midline shift

Acute Epidural Hematoma

Acute epidural hematoma (EDH) is rare—presumably because of the dense adherence of the dura to the skull in this age group (Fig. 7.1). There is a single large publication on this topic. LeRoux and Nadvi undertook a retrospective review of 3249 patients with EDH over a 23-year period. Of those >65 years <1% had an EDH. When such occurred, 56% occurred from assaults, 25% from falls, and 19% from motor vehicle crashes. Approximately one-third of patients had a good outcome while no patient with a Glasgow Coma Score (GCS) <8 or >75 years old had a good outcome [10].

Acute Subdural Hematoma

Acute subdural hematoma (ASDH) is the most common TBI pathology in the elderly. Brain atrophy, associated with "stretched" subdural veins, is the most common explanation. However, cortical arterial bleeding—the hyperacute ASDH—is not uncommon (Fig. 7.2).

This has generally been felt to be a lethal injury in this population.

Hanif et al. studied patients with ASDH who underwent surgical evacuation. Mortality was 50% in those >70 years, compared to 25.6% in those 40–70 years and 26% in those <40 years. Overall poor outcome was 74% in those >70 years, 48% in those 40–70 years, and 30% in those <40 years [11].

In 2012, Leitger et al. studied a cohort of ASDH patients treated between 2002 and 2010, with 44% over age 61. Nonsurgical management was associated with significantly higher mortality. The in-hospital mortality rate was 46.7%. However age-related mortality was highest ($p = 0.008$). [12].

However, very recently, Raj et al. reported on 44 ASDH patients over 75 years of age treated between 2009 and 2012 with a mean follow-up of 4.2 years. Greater than 70% of the patients were

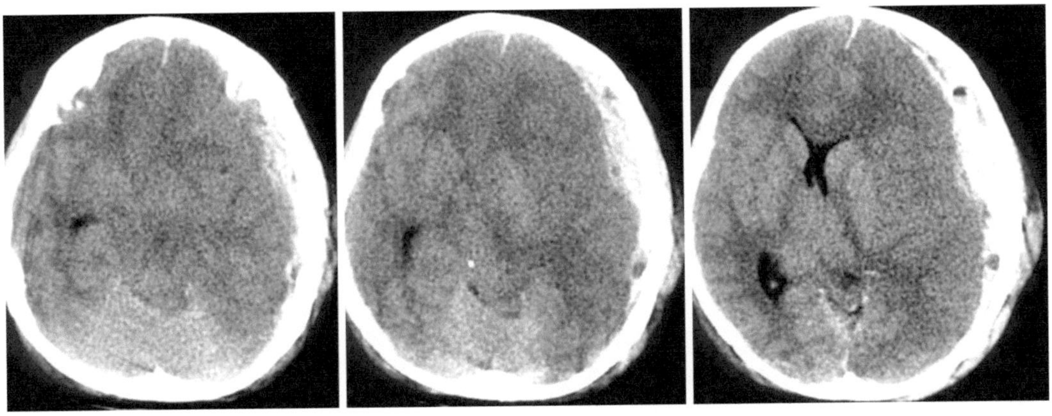

Fig. 7.2 Classic lens-shaped epidural hematoma, with significant midline shift

on anticoagulants and living independently at the time of injury. Such patients had a 1-year mortality of 42% compared to those patients who were not living independently. Of 1-year survivors 77% were still alive. However functional outcomes were not addressed [13].

Chronic Subdural Hematoma

Chronic subdural hematoma (CSDH) is common in the elderly, often precipitated by a seemingly minor trauma to the head. As the brain atrophies with ageing the bridging cortical veins are stretched and vulnerable to rupture with trivial trauma.

Symptoms may be delayed by weeks or months and typically include worsening headaches, altered mental status, focal neurological deficits, and/or seizures.

The peak incidence occurs in the seventh to eighth decades with an estimated incidence of up to 7.35/100,000 in those >70 years [14] (Fig. 7.3).

While multiple surgeries from twist-drill drainage to burr hole drainage to craniotomy have been proposed and debated, the outcome has uniformly been reported as favorable.

While CSDH has traditionally been considered a "benign" entity, easily treated surgical problem, Miranda et al. reported differently.

On review of 209 CSDH cases with at least 1-year follow-up, survival was significantly decreased from expected actuarial survival.

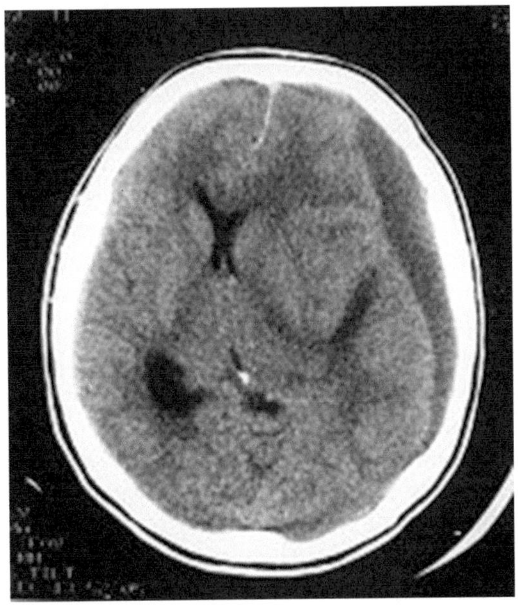

Fig. 7.3 CT scan of a hyperacute subdural hematoma with significant underlying brain injury and edema

There was a marked increase in mortality rate (OR 2.1, $P = 0.0012$) which was not impacted by type of surgery, size of the CSDH, or anticoagulation [15].

Anticoagulation

Various studies have shown that 9–15% of patients >65 years who suffer from a TBI are on antiplatelet or anticoagulation medications [16].

Table 7.1 Reversal strategies for non-Coumadin anticoagulants

Direct thrombin inhibitors	Reversal
Dabigatran	1. Anti-inhibitor coagulant complex (Feiba, activated PCC—25 U/kg)
	2. Alternative Prothrombin complex 4-factor (Kcentra—25-50 U/kg)
Factor Xa inhibitors	
Apixaban	1. Prothrombin complex 4-factor Feiba, activated PCC—25 U/kg)
Rivaroxaban	2. Anti-inhibitor coagulant complex (Feiba, activated PCC—25–50 U/kg)

Antiplatelet medications can be readily reversed by platelet infusions with or without DDAVP.

Coumadin can likewise be reversed by vitamin K and fresh frozen plasma or prothrombin concentrate complex (PCC), the advantage of the latter being a low-volume infusion in those who may well be already cardiovascularly compromised.

However there is increasing use of direct thrombin and factor Xa inhibitors for which the only absolute reversal is hemodialysis.

A number of strategies have been employed to "reverse" these agents with varying success (Table 7.1).

Palliative Care

In general, regardless of pathology, the elderly have a higher mortality rate after TBI. Pennings et al. found an in-hospital mortality rate of 79% compared to those <65 years [17].

Given this situation, the question of does surgery or other aggressive treatment have a role in the management of these patients becomes an ethical issue.

The concept of "risk of unacceptable badness"—such a bad outcome that the patient would not want to experience—becomes important [18].

Unfortunately, many times such decisions have to be made by the healthcare team in the absence of family, advance directives, or a living will.

The responsible physician or team may need to consider not performing a procedure if it is felt there is a significant chance the outcome will be poor and unacceptable to the patient.

References

1. O'Conner KD, Cothbert JP, Whyte J, et al. Traumatic brain injury among older adults at Level I and II trauma centers. J Neurotrauma. 2013;30 (24):2001–13.
2. Flanagan SR, Hubbard MR, Riordan B, Gordan WA. Traumatic brain injury in the elderly: diagnostic and treatment strategies. Clin Geriatr Med. 2006;22(2):449–68.
3. Harvey LA, Close JC. Traumatic brain injuries in older adults: characteristics, causes and consequences. Injury. 2012;43(11):188–92.
4. Stippler M, Holguin E, Nemoto E. Traumatic brain injury in elders. Ann Longterm Care. 2012;20:1309–13.
5. Knight J, Nigam V. Exploring the anatomy and physiology of ageing Part5—the nervous system. Nurs Times. 2008;104:18–9.
6. Morrison JH, Hof PR. Life and death of neurons in the ageing brain. Science. 1997;278(5337):412–9.
7. Hoffman C, Rice D, Hy S. Persons with chronic conditions: their prevalence and cost. JAMA. 1996;276: 1437–9.
8. Mosenthal AC, Livingston DH, Lavery RF, et al. The effect of age on functional outcome in mild traumatic brain injury: 6 month report of a prospective multicenter trial. J Trauma. 2004;56:1042–8.
9. Coronado VG, Roland-Brown V, Thomas KE. The CDC traumatic surveillance system. Characteristics of persons 65 years and older hospitalized with a traumatic brain injury. J Head Trauma Rehabil. 2005;20:215–23.
10. LeRoux AA, Nadvi SS. Acute extradural hematoma in the elderly. Br J Neurosurg. 2007;21(1):16–20.
11. Hanif S, Abudundle O, Ali Z, Pidgeon C. Age related outcome in ASDH following traumatic brain injury. Ir Med J. 2009;102(8):255–7.

12. Leitger J, Mauritz W, Brazinova A, et al. Outcome after severe brain trauma due to acute subdural hematoma. J Neurosurg. 2012;117:324–33.
13. Raj R, Mikkonen ED, Kivisaari R, et al. Mortality in elderly patients operated for an acute subdural hematoma: a surgical case series. World Neurosurg. 2015;10:592–7.
14. Adhiyaman V, Asghar M, Ganeshram KN, Bhoumick BK. Chronic subdural hematoma in the elderly. Postgrad Med J. 2002;78:71–5.
15. Miranda LB, Braxton E, Hobbs J, et al. Chronic subdural hematoma in the elderly: not a benign disease. J Neurosurg. 2001;114:72–6.
16. www.east.org/tpg/geriatric.pdf- 2005.
17. Pennings JL, Bachulis BL, Simons CT, et al. Survival after severe traumatic brain injury in the aged. Arch Surg. 1993;128(7):787–93.
18. Gillett GR, Honeybul S, Ho KM, et al. Neurotrauma and the RUB: where tragedy meets ethics and science. J Med Ethics. 2010;36(12):727–30.

8 Traumatic Subarachnoid Hemorrhage

Jack Wilberger

Introduction

Traumatic subarachnoid hemorrhage (t-SAH) is common across the spectrum of mild moderate and severe traumatic brain injury (TBI).

It not only increases in incidence with advancing age but also adversely impacts outcome.

Indeed, trauma is the most common cause of subarachnoid hemorrhage.

Until recently it was felt that the most common sequela of subarachnoid hemorrhage—vasospasm, and its associated morbidity and mortality—rarely occurred after t-SAH. However, such is not the case. Thus vigilance for the possibility of vasospasm is an important management tenant.

This chapter focuses on the epidemiology, effects of the aging brain and comorbidities, outcomes, and management of t-SAH.

Epidemiology

Prior to computerized tomography (CT), t-SAH was found to be the most common posttraumatic finding at autopsy [1].

With CT up to 60% of patients have been reported to show evidence of t-SAH, with more severe TBI having the highest rates [2, 3].

In a large European study 33% of moderate to severe TBI demonstrated t-SAH on an early CT [4].

Typically, the t-SAH is minor—affecting several cerebral sulci (Fig. 8.1); however it can be quite extensive mimicking aneurysmal subarachnoid hemorrhage (Fig. 8.2).

The amount and location of the blood are important in prognosis.

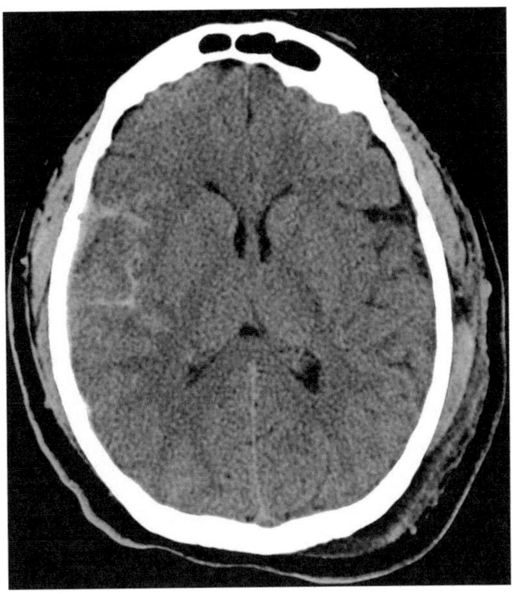

Fig. 8.1 Minimal t-SAH in right frontal cortex

J. Wilberger, M.D., F.A.C.S., F.A.A.N.S.
Department of Neurosurgery, Drexel University College of Medicine, Suite 302, 420 East North Avenue, Pittsburgh, PA 15212, USA
e-mail: jack.wilberger@AHN.org

A. Rodriguez et al. (eds.), *Geriatric Trauma and Acute Care Surgery*,
https://doi.org/10.1007/978-3-319-57403-5_8

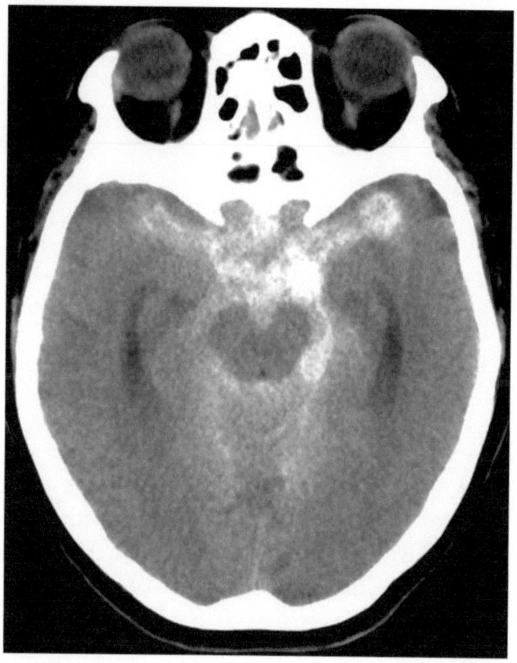

Fig. 8.2 t-SAH mimicking aneurysmal SAH

The Ageing Brain and Medical Comorbidities

Ageing brain volume loss is estimated to be 0.1% per year with an associated 20% decrease in cerebral blood flow. The latter can be further compromised by atherosclerotic changes.

These factors have been implicated in the high incidence of t-SAH with increasing age.

Additionally, of those over 65 years of age still living independently the majority have a very high incidence of medical comorbidities [5].

One of the big concerns however is the rate of utilization (9–15%) of antiplatelet or anticoagulation medications in this population.

While antiplatelets can be reversed by platelet transfusions and/or DDAVP, and Coumadin by fresh frozen plasma or prothrombin complex concentrate, there is increasing use of direct thrombin and factor XA inhibitors for which the only proven reversal is hemodialysis [6].

Interestingly, Maung et al. recently studied the outcomes from traumatic injury comparing patients on warfarin to those on new oral agents (NOA).

In a multivariate regression analysis patients on warfarin (OR 2.215, p = 0.001), but on an NOA (OR 0.871, p = 0.823), was an independent risk factor for mortality.

While there were only a small number of TBI patients included in the study and the type of structural injury was not described, 19.3% on warfarin died compared to 16.7% on an NOA [7].

Thus in these situations careful clinical and CT monitoring is warranted.

Outcomes

Several studies have shown t-SAH to be one of the most independent negative prognostic factors in TBI outcome [8].

With advancing age, the incidence of vegetative outcome or death increases from 50% in those 16–25 years of age to 85% in those over 55. However, a TBI severity factor is clearly implicated—as the lower the GCS the higher the morbidity and mortality [9].

It has been shown that t-SAH increases ICU length of stay, posttraumatic epilepsy, and hydrocephalus and is associated with potentially significant neuropsychological deficits [10, 11].

There are those who will however question whether the t-SAH is not an epiphenomenon and the degree and extent of the primary and secondary brain injury play a more important role in outcome.

Management

In general, with type of t-SAH depicted in Fig. 8.1, and the patient anticoagulated, the anticoagulation is held but not reversed and the patient is monitored clinically on a frequent basis, With no neurological changes a repeat CT in 18–24 h is appropriate.

If the t-SAH is minor and the scan is not worsening or is improving discharge with a follow-up

CT in 2–3 weeks is reasonable. Studies have shown that >90% of these patients do well.

With more extreme t-SAH and poor neurological status (GCS <8), reversal of anticoagulation is appropriate, along with ICP monitoring—assuming that surgical decompression is not indicated.

Particularly concerning in aneurysmal SAH is vasospasm, leading to significant ischemia and associated increased morbidity and mortality.

Such can also occur after t-SAH with an angiographic incidence of 2–4.1% and transcranial Doppler (TCD) incidence of up to 60%—based on increased flow velocities [12]. Vasospasm is typically defined by a mean flow velocity of >120 cm/s.

t-SAH vasospasm appears to occur earlier (3–4 days) than aneurysmal vasospasm (7 days), but has the same time course of 12–14 days [13].

In the Harders study, 27% of patients with minor t-SAH, 25% with moderate t-SAH, and 46% with major t-SAH had increased flow velocity on TCD [4]. It is important to note however that increased TCD flow velocity does not directly translate to clinically significant vasospasm—potentially leading to ischemia and infarction.

An article by Oertel et al., in a study of 299 patients, using TCD and cerebral blood flow studies found that hemodynamically significant vasospasm may occur in the absence of t-SAH, especially in patients with lower GCS scores ($P < 0.001$) [14].

A confounding factor is that while angiographic or TCD evidence of "significant" vasospasm may be frequently found, it may not be clinically significant. Such is obviously difficult to sort out in a severe TBI patient.

Nevertheless, if there is no neurologic improvement in a GCS <8 patient (with t-SAH) without ICP, CT, or MRI—or other potential contributors—subclinical status epilepticus, hyponatremia, etc.—the possibility of vasospasm should be considered.

It is generally recommended that TCD monitoring be begun in these patients within 48 h. If the flow velocities are indeed increasing, then angiography is warranted and intra-arterial therapy should be considered.

A standard treatment for symptomatic aneurysmal SAH has been the use of calcium channel blockers (CCB) such as nimodipine or nicardipine—although currently intra-arterial balloon dilation or infusion of verapamil to dilate constricted vessels is a primary treatment consideration.

There have been six clinical trials of CCB in t-SAH.

A Cochrane review meta-analysis resulted in the following:

Outcome	Odds ratio
Severe disability/persistent vegetative state	0.65
Death	0.59

The results achieved a small statistical significance. However, the various studies were very heterogeneous making it difficult to translate to clinical practice [13].

It is important to note that if a CCB blocker is indeed utilized for documented clinical vasospasm, hypotension is not an insignificant risk and it is well known that such indeed significantly worsens outcome from TBI.

Conclusions

TBI is a very heterogenous disease entity with the potential for multiple structural and metabolic/pathophysiologic derangements that may be changing during the time course of the injury.

It is however important to take into account the role t-SAH may play—more so in severe rather than minor TBI.

As has been elucidated, while t-SAH is associated with worse outcome with advancing age, the exact reason for this remains to be determined.

The vast majority of those with a good GCS and minor t-SAH do well.

Such is unfortunately not the case with a low GCS and extensive t-SAH.

The possibility of clinically significant vasospasm in those with extensive t-SAH and no other explainable reason for their neurologic condition/or deterioration must be kept in mind when treating this population and TCDs should be added to the clinical monitoring and appropriate angiography and interventional therapies be considered when appropriate.

Treatment algorithm—Minor-t-SAH

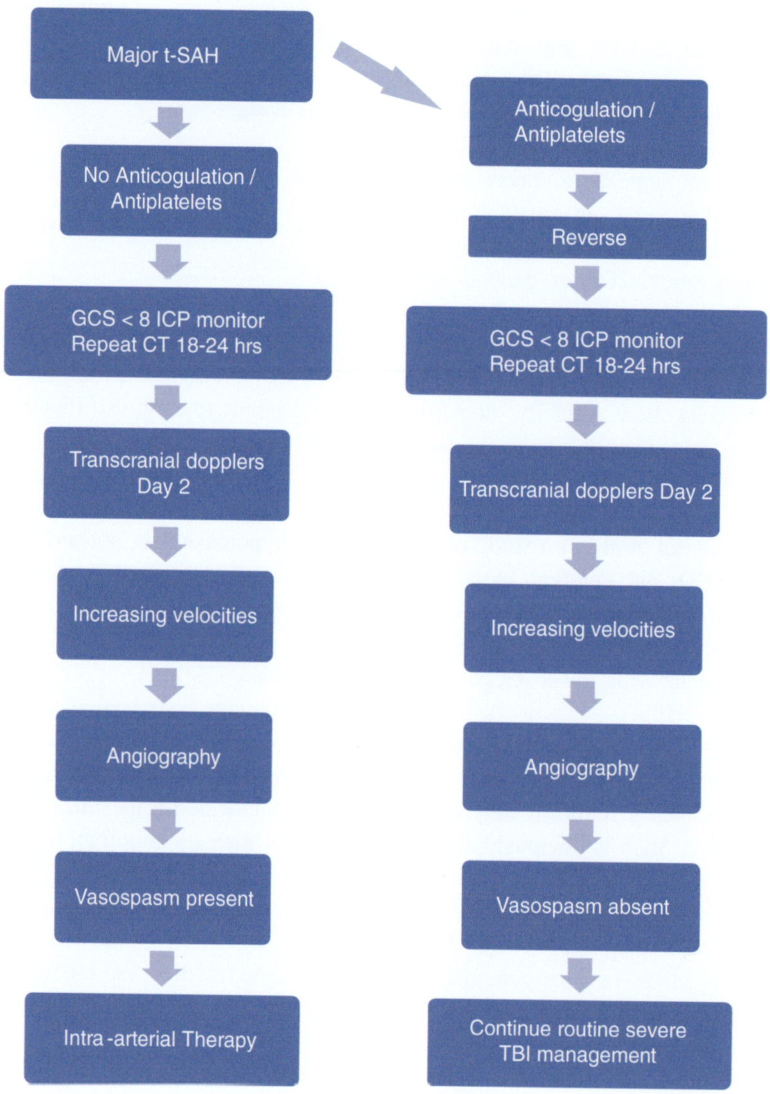

Treatment algorithm—Severe t-SAH

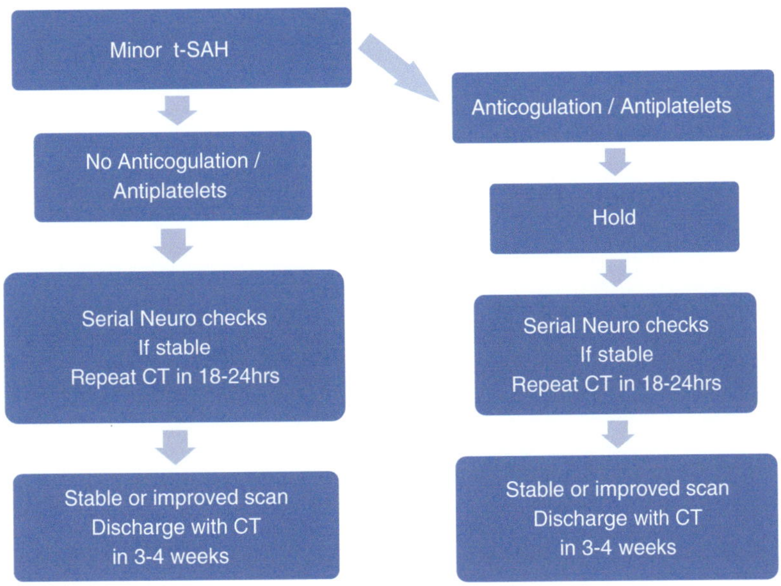

References

1. Freytag E. Autopsy findings in head injuries from blunt forces. Statistical evaluation of 1367 cases. Arch Pathol. 1963;75:402–12.
2. Eisenberg HM, Gary HE, Aidncis EF, et al. Initial CT findings in 753 patients with severe TBI. A report for the NIH Traumatic Coma Data Bank. J Neurosurg. 1990;73:688–98.
3. Mattiol C, Beretta L, Gerevensi S, et al. Traumatic subarachnoid hemorrhages on the computerized tomographic scan obtained at admission, a multicenter assessment of the accuracy of diagnosis and the potential impact on patient outcome. J Neurosurg. 2003;98:37–42.
4. Harders A, Kakarieka A, Braakman R and the German t-SAh Group. J Neurosurg 1996;85:82–89.
5. Hoffman C, Rice D, Sung HY. Persons with chronic conditions: their prevalence and cost. JAMA. 1996;276:1437–9.
6. www.esat.org?tpg/geriatric.PDF-2005.
7. Maung AA, Bhattacharya B, Schuster KM, et al. Trauma patients on new oral anticoagulation agents have lower mortality than those on warfarin. J Trauma. 2016;81:652–75.
8. Kakariek A, Schakel EH. Fritze j. Clinical significance of the finding of subarachnoid blood on CT scan after head injury. Acta Neurochir (Wein). 1994;129:11–5.
9. Kelly DF, Doberstein C, Becker DP. General principles of head injury management. In: Narajan RK, Wilberger JE, Povlishok JT, editors. Neurotrauma. New York, NY: McGraw-Hill; 1996.
10. Greone KA, Jacobwitz R, Marcindo FF. Impact to t-SAH on outcome in nonpenetrating head injury. Part II: relationship to clinical course and outcome variables during acute hospitalization. J Trauma. 1996;41:964–71.
11. Hanlin RE, Demory TA, Kuczen C, et al. Effect of t-SAH on neuropsychologic profiles and vocational outcome following moderate or severe TBI. Brain Inj. 2005;19:257–62.
12. Martin NA, Domberst EM, Zane C, et al. Post-traumatic cerebral arterial spasm, transcranial Doppler ultrasound, cerebral blood flow and angiographic findings. J Neurosurg. 1992;77:575–83.
13. Langham J, Goldfrad C, Teasdale G, et al. Calcium channel blockers for acute traumatic brain injury. Cochrane Database Syst Review 2003;(2):CD000565.
14. Oertel M, Buscardin WJ, Obrist WJ. Post-traumatic vasospasm. The epidemiology, severity, timecourse of an underestimated phenomenon. A prospective study performed in 299 patients. J Neurosurg. 2005;103:812–24.

9 Neuro Critical Care

Mira Ghneim and Deborah M. Stein

Physiological Implications of Aging and Traumatic Brain Injury (TBI)

Geriatric patients represent a unique subset of the trauma patient population that is growing exponentially and has proven to require special considerations in evaluation and management. The current growth in the number and proportion of older adults in the United States is unprecedented in our nation's history. By 2050, it is anticipated that Americans aged 65 or older will number nearly 89 million people, or more than double the number of older adults in the United States in 2010 [1]. Every year one out of three adults greater than 65 years of age sustains a fall [2].

Traumatic brain injury (TBI) among adults aged 65 years is a major public health problem in the United States [3]. The Centers for Disease Control and Prevention (CDC) estimate that at least 1.7 million people sustain a TBI annually [4]. From 2002 to 2006, the CDC estimated that older adults accounted for over 80,000 of the TBI-related hospitalizations per year. This is more than double that of TBI-related hospitalizations for children [5].

A great deal of evidence had defined age as a risk factor for worsened outcomes following TBI and patients 65 years and older are at the highest risk for TBI-associated morbidity and mortality. Their ability to recover from the insult, when compared to their younger counterparts, is limited by reduction in reserve, baseline comorbidities, and functional status and not necessarily the severity of their injury [6–15]. Mortality rates for elderly patients with TBI are nearly double than those seen in the younger population, even for mild injuries. Furthermore, long-term psychological and physical disabilities are frequently observed and are likely secondary to decreased neuronal plasticity. TBI is divided into two phases: primary and secondary brain injury. The primary brain injury is the physical parenchymal damage due to the traumatic event and the resultant shearing and compression of the surrounding brain tissue. The secondary brain injury is a complex process; it can be intra- and extracranial and can exacerbate the sequela of the primary injury. Intracranial injury includes cerebral edema, hematomas, and hydrocephalus and subsequent intracranial hypertension [16, 17]. Extracranial insults are mainly ischemic and include hypotension, hypoxemia, hypercapnia, and fever. While the effects of the primary injury are irreversible, the secondary brain insults are often amenable to prevention or reversal.

M. Ghneim, M.D.
Clinical Assistant Professor, The Department of Surgery, Division of Trauma, Critical Care and Emergency General Surgery, East Carolina University, Brody School of medicine, Greenville, NC, USA
e-mail: ghneimm16@ecu.edu

D.M. Stein
Department of Surgery, University of Maryland school of Medicine, R Adams Cowley shock Trauma Center, University of Maryland Medical Center, Baltimore, MD, USA
e-mail: dstein@umm.edu

A. Rodriguez et al. (eds.), *Geriatric Trauma and Acute Care Surgery*,
https://doi.org/10.1007/978-3-319-57403-5_9

In the geriatric population, these mechanisms may be enhanced due to the comorbidities and physiologic changes that occur with aging. As one ages, there is an overall decrease in number of neurons, a reorganization of the astrocytic gap junctions with a resultant decreased integrity of the blood–brain barrier, increased adherence of the dura mater to the skull, fibrosis and thickening of the meninges, narrowed gyri, and widened sulci with corresponding increase in the size of the subarachnoid space [18]. Atrophy of brain tissue leads to increased susceptibility to vascular damage, increased blood vessel permeability, and diminished ability to autoregulate blood flow. Other normal aging changes include cerebrovascular atherosclerosis and decreased free radical clearance [19]. The former could increase the risk of injury due to secondary insult, and the latter may increase oxidative damage after a TBI [20]. In addition, as part of routine management of chronic conditions, older adults often are on preinjury antiplatelet and anticoagulant therapies that can exacerbate the development of hematomas and hemorrhagic expansion of contusions [19]. As a result, it is necessary to evaluate, treat, and manage the geriatric population as a unique patient group in an attempt to optimize outcomes.

Medical Management of TBI

Over the past 20 years, much has been learned with a remarkable progress in the critical care management of severe TBI. In 1996, the Brain Trauma Foundation (BTF) [21] published the first guidelines on the management of severe TBI that was accepted by the American Association of Neurological Surgeons and endorsed by the World Health Organization Committee in Neurotraumatology and two subsequent revisions published in 2000 [22] and 2007 [23]. While studies have clearly demonstrated that the implementation of protocols for the management of severe TBI, and incorporating recommendations from the guidelines, is associated with substantially better outcomes such as mortality rate, functional outcome scores, length of hospital stay, and costs [24, 25], their direct implications to the geriatric population remain unclear. Per BTF the current recommendations for management of patient with severe TBI are as follows.

Hypotension

Per BTF guidelines SBP <90 mmHg should be avoided (Level II). Histologic evidence of cerebral ischemia has been found in most victims of severe TBI who die, suggesting that cerebral blood flow is reduced in the first hours postinjury [22]. Recent AHA guidelines, based on moderate- to high-quality randomized controlled trials in the general population aged 60 years or older, indicate that accepting higher SBP thresholds in this patient population reduces stroke, heart failure, and coronary heart disease due to improved perfusion [26]. As a result, the SBP >90 recommended by the BTF requires further consideration in the geriatric population, given the potential that it may not be sufficient to maintain adequate cerebral perfusion in the setting of a TBI.

Respiratory Parameters

Hypoxia (PaO_2 <60 mmHg or O_2 saturation <90%) should be avoided (Level III) and prophylactic hyperventilation $PaCO_2$ of 25 or less is not recommended. Hyperventilation reduces ICPs by causing cerebral vasoconstriction. Age-associated reduction in cerebral blood flow has been well established [27, 28]. Therefore it is essential to avoid hyperventilation in the geriatric population to prevent further reduction in cerebral blood flow and potentiation of cerebral ischemia.

ICP Monitoring

Falls represent the most common mechanism of injury in the geriatric population, a low-velocity injury pattern that is not commonly associated with diffuse axonal injury, and intracranial hypertension. Brain atrophy that accompanies the aging process increases the space in the cranial vault allowing more flexibility to accommodate space-occupying lesions and brain swelling. One of the most important and controversial aspects of managing trauma patients with TBI is the utilization of intracranial pressure (ICP) monitors and numerous conflicting studies exist that address this topic. While the BTF guidelines recommend ICP monitoring in severe TBI patients, whether such intervention contributes to outcomes in the elderly patients with TBI has not been fully explored. In 2015 Dang et al. [29] published a retrospective analysis from the National Trauma Database addressing the utilization of ICP monitors in the elderly and examined the associated outcomes. Patients requiring an ICP monitor were younger overall, had higher injury severity, and were more likely to require operative intervention; of those patients with ICP monitoring, overall mortality was significantly higher, and they were less likely to have favorable discharge status. Given the lack of evidence-based recommendations for ICP monitoring in the elderly, the utility of the monitor placement should be determined on a case-by-case basis based on the injury pattern, CT findings, and overall patient injury burden and associated morbidity and mortality.

Management of Increased Intracranial Pressure (ICP)

BTF recommends that ICPs should be monitored in all salvageable patients with severe traumatic brain injury (TBI; Glasgow Coma Scale [GCS] score of 3–8 after resuscitation) and an abnormal computed tomography (CT) scan (see above). An abnormal CT scan of the head is one that reveals hematomas, contusions, swelling, herniation, or compressed basal cisterns or those with a normal brain CT if any two of the following conditions are met: age is >40 years, motor posturing is present, or systolic blood pressure (SBP) after resuscitation is <90 mmHg (Level II) [22].

Normal intracranial pressure in adults is below 15 mm Hg and values that are sustained above 20 mmHg are considered to be pathologic and are associated with poorer outcomes. Under normal conditions, the total volume within the skull remains constant and is determined by the sum of the cerebrospinal fluid, blood, and brain-tissue compartments. The volume of these compartments is tightly regulated, and cerebral blood flow is kept constant by autoregulation. When additional volume is added to the system, such as hematoma or cerebral edema, compensatory mechanisms operate to keep intracranial pressure constant. The relationship between intracranial volume and intracranial pressure is exponential. Initially, pressure increases only slightly with increasing volume, but when the buffering capabilities of the system are exceeded, intracranial pressure rises steeply. This explains the rapid deterioration that is frequently seen in patients with a traumatic intracranial hematoma [30]. As a result BTF recommends ICP treatment to be initiated with the intracranial pressure (ICP) threshold above 20 mmHg (Level II).

Vascular effects of increased intracranial pressure result from impaired cerebral perfusion pressure (CPP) driven by mean arterial blood pressure and intracranial pressure. CPP is the driving force behind cerebral blood flow, but levels required for adequate flow vary among patients. As the CPP decreases, cerebral blood flow may become insufficient for adequate brain-tissue perfusion and oxygenation [31, 32]. Ischemia will induce further cytotoxic edema and result in even higher intracranial pressure. Adverse effects of increased ICP and low CPP on mortality and long-term outcome have been documented in many studies [33–35]. As a result CPP should be maintained above 50 mmHg [9] (Level III) with the caveat that aggressive attempts to maintain CCP >70 should be avoided due to respiratory complications (Level II). The main concern with all such recommendations is that none are specific to the geriatric patient populations who have markedly different cerebral perfusion hemodynamics and variable patterns of intracranial pressure alterations due to normal age-related cerebral atrophy.

Two hyperosmolar agents are currently used clinically to reduce ICP by reversing ongoing brain edema formation: mannitol and HTS. The blood–brain barrier (BBB) is a highly selective permeability barrier; its tight junctions and the paucity of pinocytosis or fenestrations in the capillary endothelium separate the circulating blood from the brain extracellular fluid in the central nervous system. An intact BBB is completely impermeable to sodium and is largely impermeable to mannitol [36].

The BTF guidelines state that mannitol is effective for increased intracranial pressure (ICP) at doses of 0.25–1 g/kg body weight (Level II). The impermeability of the BBB to mannitol allows it to function as an osmotic diuretic. Mannitol draws water into the vascular compartment and then acts as an osmotic diuretic leading to a reduction of circulating blood volume. Intermittent boluses appear to be more effective than continuous infusions. Its adverse effects include hypotension, intravascular volume depletion, rebound cerebral edema, and hyperkalemia. Its effectiveness in the elderly has been questioned in the recent years. Aging is associated with significant changes in BBB, mainly loss of integrity of the tight gap junctions and subsequent increase in permeability. In addition, clinical studies have shown that BBB disruption occurs in humans with severe TBI and may contribute to the occurrence of intracranial hypertension (IH) [37]. This raises the concern that osmotically active molecules, such as mannitol, may leak across the blood–brain barrier and worsen cerebral edema in the severe TBI geriatric population. Additionally, given that it is metabolized and excreted by the kidney, in patients with underlying renal dysfunction and/or congestive heart failure, impaired excretion could lead to worsening of volume overload.

Almost a century ago in 1919, Weed and McKibben [38] first described how hypertonic saline (HTS) reduces brain swelling. HTS initially draws water into the vascular compartment and increases circulating blood volume. HTS has other effects that may serve to reduce ICP. It promotes laminar blood flow by hemodilution. It shrinks erythrocytes, making them more deformable and enhancing their passage through capillaries [39]. Commonly used preparations include 2%, 3%, 5%, 7%, and 23% NaCl. HTS effects result in a biphasic reduction in ICP: first by improving rheological properties, and then by osmotic activity through receptors across the BBB [36]. While there is no randomized controlled clinical trials showing clinically important differences in mortality and neurological outcomes between HTS or mannitol in the management of severe TBI in the young and geriatric trauma population. Nevertheless, HTS appears to avoid hypotension, assist in resuscitation while avoiding volume overload, and have fewer ICP treatment failures. In the geriatric population, its efficacy in reducing ICP and availability in high concentration/low-volume solutions such as 7% NaCl may be paramount in the management of elderly patients with congestive heart failure and severe TBI.

Hypothermia

Therapeutic hypothermia has emerged as a potentially lifesaving treatment for the care of the critically ill. Research in the 1980s using animal models demonstrated the benefits of cooling to 32–34 °C [40, 41], and it has since been proposed that there are a number of potential applications for therapeutic hypothermia [42, 43]. National Health Service (NHS) National Institute for Health and Clinical Excellence (NICE) guidelines were published to support the use of therapeutic hypothermia for hypoxic ischemic encephalopathy [44]. Similarly, NICE guidelines for the use of therapeutic hypothermia in cardiac arrest have also been published. While a number of studies have identified an improvement in outcome with the application of therapeutic hypothermia, the question as to whether therapeutic hypothermia is of benefit in traumatic brain injury (TBI) remains unclear.

The Eurotherm3235 Trial [45] conducted by Andrews et al. addressed whether hypothermia (32–35 °C) for at least 48 h and standard care to control ICP compared to standard care alone reduce death and major disability at 6 months after injury. If ICPs were still inadequately controlled, care was escalated utilizing mannitol, HTS and inotropes, EEG-guided barbiturate coma, and decompressive craniectomy, as deemed appropriate. Patients were rewarmed at 0.25 °C per hour once ICPs were controlled.

Worse outcomes and fewer favorable outcomes were seen in the hypothermia group when compared to the control group, including the need for barbiturate coma and decompressive craniotomy ($p = 0.04$). Given these results, the trial was suspended early since therapeutic hypothermia resulted in a greater risk of death and worse neurological outcomes when compared to standard measure.

Despite failure of therapeutic hypothermia to demonstrate benefit in following TBI, hyperpyrexia increases the brain's metabolic demand and increases the permeability of the BBB potentially worsening the secondary insult. Therefore, one of the goals in management of the patient with severe TBI should be to avoid prolonged periods of hyperpyrexia in the first week postinjury. This should be accomplished with targeted temperature therapy to maintain normothermia with active cooling and medication.

Acetaminophen (APAP) is frequently utilized as an antipyretic agent, and is metabolized by the liver and is known to induce hepatotoxicity. It has been shown that APAP is rapidly and completely absorbed from the gastrointestinal (GI) tract, and neither the rate nor the extent of absorption appears to be age dependent. However, the intrinsic conjugative liver activity, APAP volume of distribution, and pharmacokinetics are known to decrease with age and frailty. As a result APAP metabolism is highly variable in older patients, and dosing should be individualized based on comorbidities and baseline liver function [46, 47].

Nonsteroidal anti-inflammatory drugs (NSAIDs) are also commonly used in the elderly to manage fever and pain. NSAIDs are metabolized in the liver and are protein bound. In the frail elders with hypoalbuminemia NSAIDs exist at higher free drug concentrations leading to toxicity. In addition, many studies have shown that NSAIDs increase the risk of worsened outcomes in older adults. These include GI bleeding as a result of platelet dysfunction, cardiovascular/cerebrovascular, and renal adverse drug events. The risks of NSAIDs need to be balanced by their effectiveness, and diligent monitoring of the patient is essential to prevent adverse events [46, 47].

Seizure Prophylaxis

Without prophylaxis, the incidence of early posttraumatic seizures (PTS) has been estimated to be 4%–25%. In work done by Temkin et al. [48], 4404 patients were randomized to phenytoin (PHE) versus placebo for a year, with 2-year follow-up. Although there was no impact on late PTS, treatment with PHE decreased the clinically recognized early seizure rate significantly from 14.2% down to 3.6%. Based on the available data, the Brain Trauma Foundation Traumatic Brain Injury Guidelines have as a Level II recommendation the use of anticonvulsants to decrease the incidence of early PTS. In 2013 Inaba et al. [49] conducted a prospective observational study comparing the efficacy of levetiracetam (LEV) with that of phenytoin (PHE) for preventing early PTS. Eight hundred and thirteen patients were analyzed. There was no difference in seizure rate (1.5% vs. 1.5%, $p = 0.997$), adverse drug reactions (7.9% vs. 10.3%, $p = 0.227$), or mortality (5.4% vs. 3.7%, $p = 0.236$) between the two groups. With its ease of dosing, lack of need for monitoring, and lesser adverse side effects, LEV may prove to be the drug of choice for early PTS prophylaxis in the elderly population.

Stroke

Stroke is a devastating condition with a high burden of neurologic morbidity and mortality. Currently it is the fourth leading cause of death in the United States. Considerable effort has been invested to develop designated stroke centers with CT scanners in emergency departments, in-house 24/7 stroke teams, and development and implementation of neurological ED pathways that minimize delays in the diagnosis to treatment timeframe. Two main forms of stroke exist, ischemic stroke and hemorrhagic stroke. While ischemic stroke is ten times more common in the Western world, hemorrhagic stroke is associated with much higher morbidity and mortality.

Spontaneous Nontraumatic Intracranial Hemorrhage (ICH)

ICH is associated with worsened outcomes and in 2010 AHA/ASA released the guidelines for management of ICH, which focuses on aggressive medical management. ICH is a medical emergency and rapid neuroimaging is essential for diagnosis and occurs promptly in the emergency department. Subsequent CT angiograms (CTA) are beneficial in the diagnosis and management of underlying vascular abnormalities. Anticoagulation should be promptly reversed with vitamin K, fresh frozen plasma (FFP), and prothrombin complex concentrate (PCC). Recombinant factor (rfVIIa) is not recommended in this setting due to adverse effects of thromboembolic events that outweigh the benefits. Finally DVT prophylaxis should be avoided until 1–4 days after the confirmed cessation of bleeding, and either unfractionated heparin or low-molecular-weight heparin can be used [50].

Patients with ICH should be admitted to the ICU. Blood pressure control focused on maintaining SBP 140–150 mmHg and avoiding lower SBP given the association with worsened outcomes. No seizure prophylaxis is recommended. Continuous EEG monitoring is recommended for patients with worsening mental status or a neurologic exam that is discordant with the injury severity. Clinical seizures should be treated with traditional antiepileptics. In patients with GCS <8, those with clinical evidence of transtentorial herniation or hydrocephalus should undergo ICP monitor placement. The role of surgical intervention is uncertain. Intervention is potentially beneficial in patients with neurologic devastation due to brain stem herniation or hydrocephalus, but the effectiveness of minimally invasive clot evacuation is uncertain and is considered investigational [51].

Ischemic Stroke

Until recently, intravenous tissue-type plasminogen activator (tPA) is the only level 1A treatment for acute ischemic stroke. While 3 h from symptom onset to tPA administration has been the golden standard, multiple recent trials such as ECASS I, ECASS II, ATLANTIS A, and ATLANTIS have challenged the timeline and have tested the use of IV tPA up to 6 h after stroke symptom onset. These trials were able to show that treatment with intravenous rtPA was associated with favorable outcome with a window up to 4.5 h [52–55]. As a result, the current AHA/ASA recommend intravenous (IV) rtPA administration to eligible patients who can be treated in the time period of 3–4.5 h after stroke onset.

Extensive research efforts have been made to develop endovascular devices that would augment recanalization rates. Five studies, Multicenter Randomized Clinical Trial of Endovascular Treatment for Acute Ischemic Stroke in the Netherlands (MR CLEAN), Endovascular Revascularization with Solitaire Device versus Best Medical Therapy in Anterior Circulation Stroke within 8 h (REVASCAT), Endovascular Treatment for Small Core and Proximal Occlusion Ischemic Stroke (ESCAPE), Solitaire TM FR as Primary Treatment for Acute Ischemic Stroke (SWIFT PRIME), and Extending the Time for Thrombolysis in Emergency Neurological Deficits with Intra-Arterial Therapy (EXTEND IA) [56] have demonstrated the importance of mechanical thrombectomy and the efficacy of advanced stent retrievers, as part of endovascular therapy for patients with proximal artery occlusion in the internal carotid and middle cerebral arteries, and improved clinical outcomes.

In 2015, the AHA/ASA published a focused update of the 2013 guidelines for the early management of patients with acute ischemic stroke regarding endovascular treatment within 6 h of symptom onset. The most recent recommendations are as follows: Patients should receive endovascular therapy with a stent retriever if they meet all the following criteria (Level I): Prestroke mRS score 0–1, acute ischemic stroke receiving intravenous r-tPA within 4.5 h of onset, causative occlusion of the ICA or proximal MCA (M1), age ≥18 years, NIHSS score of ≥6, ASPECTS of ≥6; treatment can be initiated (groin puncture) within 6 h of symptom onset [57]. None of these devices or therapies should replace intravenous r-tPA in patients who are candidates for this therapy.

Specific blood pressure management recommendations have been established for patients being considered for fibrinolytic therapy as to avoid the increased risk of intracranial hemorrhage with uncontrolled hypertension in the setting of an acute ischemic stroke. Current AHA/ASA recommendations are as follows: Patients who have elevated blood pressure and are otherwise eligible for treatment with intravenous rtPA should have their blood pressure carefully lowered so that their systolic blood pressure is <185 mmHg and their diastolic blood pressure is <110 mmHg (Class I; Level of Evidence B) before fibrinolytic therapy is initiated [51]. If medications are given to lower blood pressure, the clinician should be sure that the blood pressure is stabilized at the lower level before beginning treatment with intravenous rtPA and maintained below 180/105 mmHg for at least the first 24 h after intravenous rtPA treatment.

Geriatric Patient Consideration in the ICU

Pain Management, Sedation, and Delirium: In the setting of brain injury, it is beneficial to minimize noxious stimuli as to avoid agitation and associated increase in ICP and blood pressure which exacerbate secondary brain injury. Such is achieved with the administration of narcotics. In addition, the need for prolonged ventilation necessitated prolonged sedation. In the elderly, an episode of delirium signals brain vulnerability due to decreased cognitive reserve and is often multifactorial and coexists with dementia [58]. As a result, seemingly benign insults such as a dose of a sedative–hypnotic drug might be enough to precipitate delirium. In the setting of TBI, the baseline brain dysfunction from advanced age and superimposed injury and the sedation required for prolonged intubation potentiates delirium. Therefore it is prudent to minimize sedation, utilize nonnarcotic analgesics, and consider early tracheostomy placement [59].

Early Tracheostomy (ET): The foreseen benefits of performing early tracheostomy for patients with brain injury undergoing prolonged mechanical ventilation include improved patient comfort due to reduced oropharyngeal irritation, improved pulmonary toilet, decreased sedation requirements, and accelerated liberation from mechanical ventilation. Multiple recent studies have suggested that early tracheostomy is associated with reduced ICU and hospital length of stay, reduced ventilator-dependent days, and sedation needs in the setting of both TBI and stroke [60, 61].

Baseline Functional Capacity and Weakness of Critical Illness: Studies have shown that in elderly patients with normal baseline function who are admitted to the ICU, there is a significant reduction in function after surviving a critical illness at discharge and on 1-year follow-up [62]. This functional impairment is more substantial in the setting of functional dependence on admission. It is essential to keep in mind that ICU-acquired weakness contributes to functional impairment and recovery is often slow and incomplete. The negative impact can be reduced with early aggressive physical therapy when deemed appropriate even in the setting of the ICU.

As the geriatric population continues to grow, it is vital to understand that it represents a unique patient population with underlying physiologic changes and comorbidities that present many management challenges in the setting of both TBI and stroke. Furthermore, geriatric-based research is of utmost importance to evaluate the validity of the evidence-based standard-of-care protocols that are implemented in most ICUs and dictate patient care. Finally, a multidisciplinary approach in patient management and the development of in-hospital geriatric services are essential next steps in optimizing patient care and potentially improving outcomes.

References

1. Centers for Disease Control and Prevention. Health related quality of life: nationwide trends. Centers for Disease Control and Prevention Web Site. http://apps.nccd.cdc.gov/HRQOL/TrendV.asp?State=1&Category=3&Measure=2.
2. Centers for Disease Control and Prevention. Falls among older adults: an overview. Home and recreational safety web site. http://www.cdc.gov/HomeandRecreationalSafety/Falls/adultfalls.html.

3. Coronado V, Thomas K, Sattin R, Johnson R. The CDC traumatic brain injury surveillance system characteristics of persons aged 65 years and older hospitalized with a TBI. J Head Trauma Rehabil. 2005;20:215.
4. Faul M, Xu L, Wald M, Coronado V. Traumatic brain injury in the United States: emergency department visits, hospitalization and deaths, 2002–2006. Atlanta: Centers for Disease Control and Prevention: National Center for Injury Prevention and Control; 2010.
5. Coronado V, Johnson R, Faul M, Kegler S. Incidence rates of hospitalization related to traumatic brain injury in the United States, 2002. J Am Med Assoc. 2006;295:201.
6. Susman M, DiRusso SM, Sullivan T, Risucci D, Nealon P, Cuff S, Haider A, Benzil D. Traumatic brain injury in the elderly: increased mortality and worse functional outcome at discharge despite lower injury severity. J Trauma. 2002;53(2):219–23.
7. Tokutomi T, Miyagi T, Ogawa T, Ono J, Kawamata T, Sakamoto T, Shigemori M, Nakamura N. Age-associated increases in poor outcomes after traumatic brain injury: a report from the Japan Neurotrauma Data Bank. J Neurotrauma. 2008;25(12):1407–14.
8. Stocchetti N, Paternò R, Citerio G, Beretta L, Colombo A. Traumatic brain injury in an aging population. J Neurotrauma. 2012;29(6):1119–25.
9. Hukkelhoven CW, Steyerberg EW, Rampen AJ, Farace E, Habbema JD, Marshall LF, Murray GD, Maas AI. Patient age and outcome following severe traumatic brain injury: an analysis of 5,600 patients. J Neurosurg. 2003;99(4):666–73.
10. Mushkudiani NA, Engel DC, Steyerberg EW, Butcher I, Lu J, Marmarou A, Slieker F, McHugh GS, Murray GD, Maas AI. Prognostic value of demographic characteristics in traumatic brain injury: results from the IMPACT study. J Neurotrauma. 2007;24(2):259–69.
11. Thompson HJ, McCormick WC, Kagan SH. Traumatic brain injury in older adults: epidemiology, outcomes, and future implications. J Am Geriatr Soc. 2006;54(10):1590–5.
12. Mosenthal AC, Lavery RF, Addis M, Kaul S, Ross S, Marburger R, Deitch EA, Livingston DH. Isolated traumatic brain injury: age is an independent predictor of mortality and early outcome. J Trauma. 2002;52(5):907–11.
13. Munro PT, Smith RD, Parke TR. Effect of patients' age on management of acute intracranial hematoma: prospective national study. BMJ. 2002;325(7371):1001.
14. Mohindra S, Mukherjee KK, Gupta R, Chhabra R. Continuation of poor surgical outcome after elderly brain injury. Surg Neurol. 2008;69(5):474–7.
15. Bruns J Jr, Hauser WA. The epidemiology of traumatic brain injury: a review. Epilepsia. 2003;44(Suppl 10):2–10.
16. Chesnut RM. Secondary brain insults after head injury: clinical perspectives. New Horiz. 1995;3:366–75.
17. Unterberg AW, Stover JF, Kress B, Kiening KL. Edema and brain trauma. Neuroscience. 2004;129:1021–9.
18. KL MC, Huether SE. Pathophysiology: the biologic basis for disease in adults and children. Mosby: St Lewis ed.; 2006. p. 470–4.
19. Timiras P. The nervous system: structural and biochemical changes. In: Timiras P, editor. Physiological basis of aging and geriatrics. Boca Raton, FL: CRC Press; 2003. p. 99–118.
20. Thompson HJ, Bourbonniere M. Elderly trauma from head to toe. Crit Care Nurs Clin North Am. 2006;18(3):419–31.
21. Bullock R, Chestnut RM, Clifton G, Ghajar J, Marion DW, Narayan RK. Guidelines for the management of severe head injury. J Neurotrauma. 1996;13(11):643–734.
22. Bullock R, Chestnut RM, Clifton G, Ghajar J, Marion DW, Narayan RK. Guidelines for the management of severe traumatic injury. J Neurotrauma. 2000;17:453–553.
23. Bullock R, et al. Guidelines for the management of severe traumatic brain injury. J Neurotrauma. 2007;24(Suppl 1):S1–S106.
24. Fakhry SM, Trask AL, Waller MA, Watts DD. Management of brain-injured patients by an evidence-based medicine protocol improves outcomes and decreases hospital charges. J Trauma. 2004;56(3):492–9.
25. Arabi Y, Haddad S, Tamim H, Al-Dawood A, Al-Qahtani S, Ferayan A, et al. Mortality reduction after implementing a clinical practice guidelines-based management protocol for severe traumatic brain injury. J Crit Care. 2010;25(2):190–5.
26. James PA, Oparil S, Carter PL, Cushman WC, Himmelfarb S, Handler J, Lackland DT, LeFevre ML, MacKenzie TD, Ogedegbe O, Smith SC Jr, Svetkey LP, Taler SJ, Townsend RR, Wright JT Jr, Narva AS, Ortiz E. Evidence-based guideline for the management of high blood pressure in adults report from the panel members appointed to the Eighth Joint National Committee (JNC 8). JAMA. 2014;311(5):507–20.
27. Martin AJ, Friston KJ, Colebatch JG, Frackowiak RS. Decreases in regional cerebral blood flow with normal aging. J Cereb Blood Flow Metab. 1991;11(4):684–9.
28. Sonntag WE, Eckman DM, Ingraham J, Riddle DR. Regulation of cerebrovascular aging. Brain aging: models, methods, and mechanisms. Boca Raton: CRC Press; 2007.
29. Dang Q, Simon J, Catino J, Puente I, Habib F, Zucker L, Bukur M. More fateful than fruitful? Intracranial pressure monitoring in elderly patients with traumatic brain injury is associated with worse outcomes. J Surg Res. 2015;198:482–8.
30. Stocchetti N, Maas AI. Traumatic intracranial hypertension. N Engl J Med. 2014;370:2121–30.
31. Gopinath SP, Robertson CS, Contant CF, et al. Jugular venous desaturation and outcome after head injury. J Neurol Neurosurg Psychiatry. 1994;57:717–23.
32. Nordström CH, Reinstrup P, Xu W, Gardenfors A, Ungerstedt U. Assessment of the lower limit for

cerebral perfusion pressure in severe head injuries by bedside monitoring of regional energy metabolism. Anesthesiology. 2003;98:809–14.
33. Marmarou A, Anderson RL, Ward JD, et al. Impact of ICP instability and hypotension on outcome in patients with severe head trauma. J Neurosurg. 1991;75(Suppl):S59–66.
34. Stocchetti N, Zanaboni C, Colombo A. Refractory intracranial hypertension and "second-tier" therapies in traumatic brain injury. Intensive Care Med. 2008;34:461–7.
35. Vik A, Nag T, Fredriksli OA. Relationship of "dose" of intracranial hypertension to outcome in severe traumatic brain injury. J Neurosurg. 2008;109:678–84.
36. Badaut J, Ashwal S, Obenaus A. Aquaporins in cerebrovascular disease: a target for treatment of brain edema? Cerebrovasc Dis. 2011;31(6):521–31.
37. Jeffcote T, Ho KM. Associations between cerebrospinal fluid concentrations, serum albumin concentrations and intracranial pressure in neurotrauma and intracranial hemorrhage. Anaesth Intensive Care. 2010;38:274–9.
38. Weed LH, McKibben PS. Experimental alteration of brain bulk. Am J Phys. 1919;48:512–30.
39. Hijiya N, Horiuchi K, Asakura T. Morphology of sickle cells produced in solutions of varying osmolarities. J Lab Clin Med. 1991;117(1):60–6.
40. Schuier FJ, Hossmann KA. Experimental brain infarcts in cats. II. Ischemic brain edema. Stroke. 1980;11(6):593–601.
41. Marion DW, White MJ. Treatment of experimental brain injury with moderate hypothermia and 21-aminosteroids. J Neurotrauma. 1996;13:139–47.
42. Rosomoff HL, Kochanek PM, Clark R, DeKosky ST, Ebmeyer U, Grenvik AN, Marion DW, Obrist W, Palmer AM, Safer P, Rosomoff HL, Kochanek PM, Clark R, DeKosky ST, Ebmeyer U, Grenvik AN, Marion DW, Obrist W, Palmer AM, Safer P, White RJ. Resuscitation from severe brain trauma. Crit Care Med. 1996;24:S48–56.
43. Polderman KH. Application of therapeutic hypothermia in the ICU: opportunities and pitfalls of a promising treatment modality. Part 1: indications and evidence. Intensive Care Med. 2004;30:556–75.
44. Therapeutic hypothermia with intracorporeal temperature monitoring for hypoxic perinatal brain injury. http://www.nice.org.uk/nicemedia/live/11315/48809/48809.pdf.
45. Andrews P, Sinclair HL, Rodriguez A, Harris BA, Battison CG, Rhodes JK, Murray GD. Hypothermia for intracranial hypertension after traumatic brain injury. N Engl J Med. 2015;373:2403–12.
46. Hanlon JT, Guay DRP, Ives T. Oral analgesics: efficacy, mechanism of action, pharmacokinetics, adverse effects, drug interactions, and practical recommendations for use in older adults. In: Gibson SJ, Weiner DK, editors. Pain in older persons, progress in pain research and management, vol. 35. Seattle: IASP Press; 2005. p. 205–22.
47. O'Neil CK, Hanlon JT, Marcum ZA. Adverse effects of analgesics commonly used by older adults with osteoarthritis: focus on non-opioid and opioid analgesics. Am J Geriatr Pharmacother. 2012;10(6):331–42.
48. Temkin NR, Dikmen SS, Wilensky AJ, Keihm J, Chabal S, Winn HR. A randomized, double-blind study of phenytoin for the prevention of posttraumatic seizures. N Engl J Med. 1990;323:497–502.
49. Inaba K, Menaker J, Branco BC, Gooch J, vOkoye OT, Herrold J, Scalea TM, DuBose J, Demetriades D. A prospective multicenter comparison of levetiracetam versus phenytoin for early posttraumatic seizure prophylaxis. J Trauma Acute Care Surg. 2013;74(3):766.
50. Morgenstern LB, Hemphill JC 3rd, Anderson C, Becker K, Broderick JP, Connolly ES Jr, Greenberg SM, Huang JN, MacDonald RL, Messé SR, Mitchell PH, Selim M, Tamargo RJ, American Heart Association Stroke Council and Council on Cardiovascular Nursing. Guidelines for the management of spontaneous intracerebral hemorrhage: a guideline for healthcare professionals from the American Heart Association/American Stroke Association. Stroke. 2010;41(9):2108–29.
51. Hemphill JC 3rd, Greenberg SM, Anderson CS, Becker K, Bendok BR, Cushman M, Fung GL, Goldstein JN, Macdonald RL, Mitchell PH, Scott PA, Selim MH, Woo D, American Heart Association Stroke Council; Council on Cardiovascular and Stroke Nursing; Council on Clinical Cardiology. Guidelines for the management of spontaneous intracerebral hemorrhage: a guideline for healthcare professionals from the American Heart Association/American Stroke Association. Stroke. 2015;46(7):2032–60.
52. Hacke W, Kaste M, Fieschi C, von Kummer R, Davalos A, Meier D, Larrue V, Bluhmki E, Davis S, Donnan G, Schneider D, Diez-Tejedor E, Trouillas P. Randomised double-blind placebo-controlled trial of thrombolytic therapy with intravenous alteplase in acute ischemic stroke (ECASS II): second European-Australasian Acute Stroke Study Investigators. Lancet. 1998;352:1245–51. Endorsed by the American Association of Neurological Surgeons, the Congress of Neurological Surgeons, and the Neurocritical Care Society J Stroke 2015;46:1–29.
53. Jauch EC, Saver JL, Adams HP, Bruno A, Connors JJ, Demaerschalk BM, Khatri P, McMullan PW, Qureshi AI, Rosenfield K, Scott PA, Summers DR, Wang DZ, Wintermark M, Yonas H. Guidelines for the early management of patients with acute ischemic stroke: a guideline for healthcare professionals from the American Heart Association/American Stroke Association. The American Academy of Neurology affirms the value of this guideline as an educational tool for neurologists. Endorsed by the American Association of Neurological Surgeons and Congress of Neurological Surgeons. Stroke. 2013;44(3):870–94.
54. Hacke W, Kaste M, Fieschi C, Toni D, Lesaffre E, von Kummer R, Boysen G, Bluhmki E, Höxter G, Mahagne M-H, Hennerici M. Intravenous throm-

bolysis with recombinant tissue plasminogen activator for acute hemispheric stroke: the European Cooperative Acute Stroke Study (ECASS). JAMA. 1995;274:1017–25.
55. Clark WM, Albers GW, Madden KP, Hamilton S. The rtPA (alteplase) 0- to 6-hour acute stroke trial, part A (A0276g): results of a double-blind, placebo-controlled, multicenter study. Thrombolytic Therapy in Acute Ischemic Stroke Study Investigators. Stroke. 2000;31:811–6.
56. Clark WM, Wissman S, Albers GW, Jhamandas JH, Madden KP, Hamilton S. Recombinant tissue-type plasminogen activator (Alteplase) for ischemic stroke 3 to 5 hours after symptom onset: the ATLANTIS Study: a randomized controlled trial: Alteplase thrombolysis for acute noninterventional therapy in ischemic stroke. JAMA. 1999;282:2019–26.
57. Palaniswami M, Yan B. Mechanical thrombectomy is now the gold standard for acute ischemic stroke: implications for routine clinical practice. Intervent Neurol. 2015;4:18–29. Melbourne Brain Centre, Royal Melbourne Hospital, University of Melbourne, Parkville, Vic., Australia
58. Inouye SK, Westendorp RG, Saczynski JS. Delirium in elderly people. Lancet. 2014;383(9920):911–22.
59. Fong TG, Tulebaev SR, Inouye SK. Delirium in elderly adults: diagnosis, prevention and treatment. Nat Rev Neurol. 2009;5(4):210–20.
60. Alali AS, Scales DC, Fowler RA, Mainprize TG, Ray JG, Kiss A, de Mestral C, Nathens AB. Tracheostomy timing in traumatic brain injury: a propensity-matched cohort study. J Trauma Acute Care Surg 2014;76(1):70–6.
61. Bösel J, Schiller P, Hook Y, Andes M, Neumann JO, Poli S, Amiri H, Schönenberger S, Peng Z, Unterberg A, Hacke W, Steiner T. Stroke-related early tracheostomy versus prolonged orotracheal intubation in neurocritical care trial (SETPOINT): a randomized pilot trial. Stroke. 2013;44(1):21–8.
62. Neuman MD, Eckenhoff RG. Functional outcomes after critical illness in the elderly. Crit Care Med. 2015;43(6):1340–1.

Part VI

Spine Injury

Geriatric Cervical Spinal Trauma: History, Presentation, and Treatment

10

Victor Ryan Lewis, Stephen Curran Kane, Ira Martin Garonzik, and James Edmond Conway

Abbreviations

ACDF	Anterior cervical discectomy and fusion
AO	Arbeitsgemeinschaft für Osteosynthesefragen System
AP	Anterior-posterior
AS	Ankylosing spondylitis
ASIA	American Spinal Injury Association's
CCS	Central cord syndrome
CT	Computerized tomography
DDD	Degenerative disc disease
DISH	Diffuse idiopathic skeletal hyperostosis
MVA	Motor vehicle accidents
OPLL	Ossification of the posterior longitudinal ligament
PCDF	Posterior cervical discectomy and fusion
SCI	Spinal cord injury

V.R. Lewis, B.A. (✉) • S.C. Kane, B.S.
Baltimore Neurosurgery and Spine Center, 5051 Greenspring Ave., Suite 101, Baltimore, MD 21219, USA
e-mail: vrlewis1993@gmail.com; kane.stephen.c@gmail.com

I.M. Garonzik, M.D. • J.E. Conway, M.D., Ph.D.
Department of Neurosurgery at Sinai Hospital and Baltimore Neurosurgery and Spine Center, 5051 Greenspring Ave., Suite 101, Baltimore, MD 21219, USA

Baltimore Neurosurgery and Spine Center, 5051 Greenspring Ave., Suite 101, Baltimore, MD 21219, USA

Predispositions to Geriatric Cervical Spinal Trauma

It is estimated that the number of baby boomers reaching the age of retirement, 65 years and older, will amass to 20% of the US population by 2035 [1]. As this population ages, natural degradation, such as osteoporosis and degenerative disc disease (DDD) [2], as well as progressive skeletal disorders, such as diffuse idiopathic skeletal hyperostosis (DISH) [3], ankylosing spondylitis (AS) [4], and ossification of the posterior longitudinal ligament (OPLL) [5] can intensify low-energy trauma to the cervical spine.

Osteoporosis, defined as greater activity in osteoclasts than osteoblasts, is estimated to affect 75 million people throughout Europe, America, and Japan [6]. There are multiple causes of osteoporosis including postmenopausal hypogonadism (type I) [7], hypovitaminosis D due to decreased absorption and activation (type II) [8], decreased activity level [9], calcium insufficiency, renal dysfunction [10], chronic smoking [11], corticosteroid and prescription drug use, and chronic alcoholism [12]. Osteoporosis has been found to affect the vertebral bodies due to increased osteoclastic activity in trabecular bone versus cortical bone [13]. Specifically, a decrease in cross connectivity of trabecular bone weakens the compressive strength of the vertebral bodies making them more susceptible to low-energy fractures [13]. It has been shown that 8.9 million

A. Rodriguez et al. (eds.), *Geriatric Trauma and Acute Care Surgery*,
https://doi.org/10.1007/978-3-319-57403-5_10

osteoporotic fractures occur per year and within the female population 58% of osteoporotic fractures affect the spinal column [14].

Degenerative changes can also affect the discs, facet joints, supporting ligaments, and paraspinal muscles [15]. DDD has historically been the primary sign of aging in the spine. A healthy disc maintains the appropriate balance between the synthesis and degradation of its component matrix elements [16]. As individuals age, endplate calcification causes decreased nutrient flow from surrounding blood supply resulting in decreased hydrostatic pressure and diffuse bulging [17]. Furthermore, changes in axial loading distribution of the spinal column strain the facet joints and anterior aspect of the cervical spine limiting flexion, extension, and torsion maneuvers [18]. This may perpetuate cartilage deterioration within the facet joints in the form of facet hypertrophy, apophyseal malalignment, and spondylolisthesis. The ligaments also experience a progressive thickening and buckling within the spinal canal which can lead to varying degrees of stenosis [19].

DISH is a condition which affects the anterior ligaments, tendons, and endplates of the vertebral body [3]. Many studies have shown that the prevalence of DISH can be as high as 28% for patients over 65 years old [20]. These individuals undergo calcification and ossification of the anterior longitudinal ligament which can lead to spinal stiffness, rigidity, and pain [21, 22]. DISH presents as ossification or calcification of four or more contiguous vertebrae anteriorly with no intervertebral disc height reduction [23]. Additionally, it may present as ankylosing of the spinal vertebrae in the absence of facet joint ankylosis, sacroiliac erosion, sclerosis, or intra-articular osseous fusion [22]. In the geriatric population, DISH increases susceptibility for spinal fractures from low-energy injuries and hyperextension injuries [24]. The rigidity of the spine creates an increased lever arm in patients with fractures which may cause displacement of the spine increasing the susceptibility to further neurological compromise due to instability [22].

OPLL was once thought to be a disease which primarily affects the Asian population, but recent research has found a significant prevalence of OPLL in the non-Asian population [25–27]. OPLL can present in four subtypes based upon the extent to which the condition has developed: (1) focal—localized to the intervertebral disc space, (2) segmental—posterior to each vertebral body but not extending beyond an adjacent intervertebral disc space, (3) continuous—occurs between several levels extending beyond the contained intervertebral disc spaces, and 4) mixed—combination of subtypes (2) and (3) [28]. Kaleb et al. have found the highest prevalence to be the segmental subtype, 39%, followed by mixed, 29%, continuous, 27%, and focal, 5% [25]. The underlying pathophysiology causing OPLL is unknown but current understanding is that the osteoligamentous complex is comprised mainly of laminar bone and fibrous cartilage [26]. It is estimated to be involved in 25% of all patients who present with cervical myelopathy [27].

Neurologically, many disorders can predispose a geriatric individual to low-energy trauma. Parkinson's [29], cognitive impairments, age-related visual impairments, underlying neuromuscular disorders, peripheral neuropathies, and postural instability can predispose a person to floor-level falls [30].

Mechanisms of Injury and Vertebral and Neurological Compromise in Geriatric Cervical Spinal Trauma

Low-energy trauma due to falls from a standing or seated position is the most common method of injury for the geriatric population with the incidence rate ranging from 30 to 73.4% [27, 31–34]. Motor vehicle accidents (MVA) serve as the second most common method of injury [35]. These mechanisms can be further analyzed by assessing the "young elderly" and "old elderly" demographics in which "young elderly" have been found to be more susceptible to cervical trauma as passengers in an MVA while the "old elderly" are more susceptible to falls [36].

One of the more common systems to characterize cervical trauma is the AO (Arbeitsgemeinschaft für Osteosynthesefragen) System [37]. The classification system for C3 through C7 is similar to that of the thoracolumbar spine (see Identification, Treatment, and Prognosis of Geriatric Thoracolumbar Spinal Trauma). These injuries are classified into either compression, distraction, or translational vertebral fracture. However, cervical compression fractures are less common due to the decreased degree of axial loading in the cervical spine [35]. Progressive changes of the osteoligamentous spinal complex such as DISH or AS increase an individual's propensity for distraction or translational fractures [24]. The most common type of cervical fracture found within the geriatric population involves fracture translation of the C2 vertebral body and the odontoid process. This type of fracture is very common due to ground-level falls with hyperextension due to facial-cranial impact with studies reporting a prevalence rate as high as 20% of all cervical fractures [33, 35, 38]. The increased mobility at the C1–2 junction allows for that junction to serve as the lever-arm junction and absorb the greatest amount of force in a ground-level fall [36].

There has been a formal classification and treatment system developed for odontoid fractures. Type I fractures involve the tip of the odontoid and are also the least common type of odontoid fracture [35]. Type II fractures involve a break along the junction line of the odontoid base and the body [35]. Type III fractures involve the odontoid and extend into the vertebral body of C2 [35].

Secondary to osteoligamentous compromise, neurological compression can lead to disorders such as cervical spondylosis with myelopathy [39] or central cord syndrome, cervical radiculopathy, anterior cord syndrome, and Brown-Sequard syndrome. The etiology of the injury dictates the type of neuronal compression and thus corresponds to the individual's symptomology.

Central Cord Syndrome (CCS)

Central cord syndrome is a traumatic spinal cord injury which occurs in the cervical and thoracic spines [40]. It is characterized by increased motor weakness in the upper extremities compared to the lower extremities, bladder dysfunction, and sensory loss below the affected level [41]. The geriatric population has a higher susceptibility to CCS as the major mechanism of injury is hyperextension of the cervical spine [42] and can be intensified by conditions such as OPLL or DISH [43].

Initial Management and Assessment Tools of Geriatric Cervical Spinal Trauma

Following the admission of a trauma patient the primary assessment involves ruling out cervical spine injury. Until this step is taken, all patients must remain in a cervical collar to immobilize the spine, prevent continued injury, and reinforce normal cervical lordosis [44].

The gold standard for cervical spine trauma assessment involves the use of X-rays consisting of three primary views: anterior-posterior (AP), lateral, and open mouth odontoid view. Following this initial assessment, it may be pertinent to obtain additional imaging studies such as computerized tomography (CT) to review in greater detail the bony anatomy [44]. In an effort to be more efficient and increase patient care and overall outcome following cervical spine trauma there has been research implication of a transition from three-view X-rays to CT scan as the primary assessment following trauma. A recent study performed at Lehigh Valley Health Network was able to conclude that CT scans may be used to assess patients without the need for X-rays if they had a negative neurological exam [45].

After a primary assessment, it is essential to obtain a baseline neurological examination. The most accepted system in understanding spinal cord injury is the American Spinal Injury Association's (ASIA) Standards for Neurological and Functional Classification of Spinal Cord Injury [46]. The standards incorporate a sensory and motor exam by systematically testing corresponding nerve root dermatomes and myotomes (summarized in Fig. 10.1). Additionally, the patient may present with autonomic dysreflexia

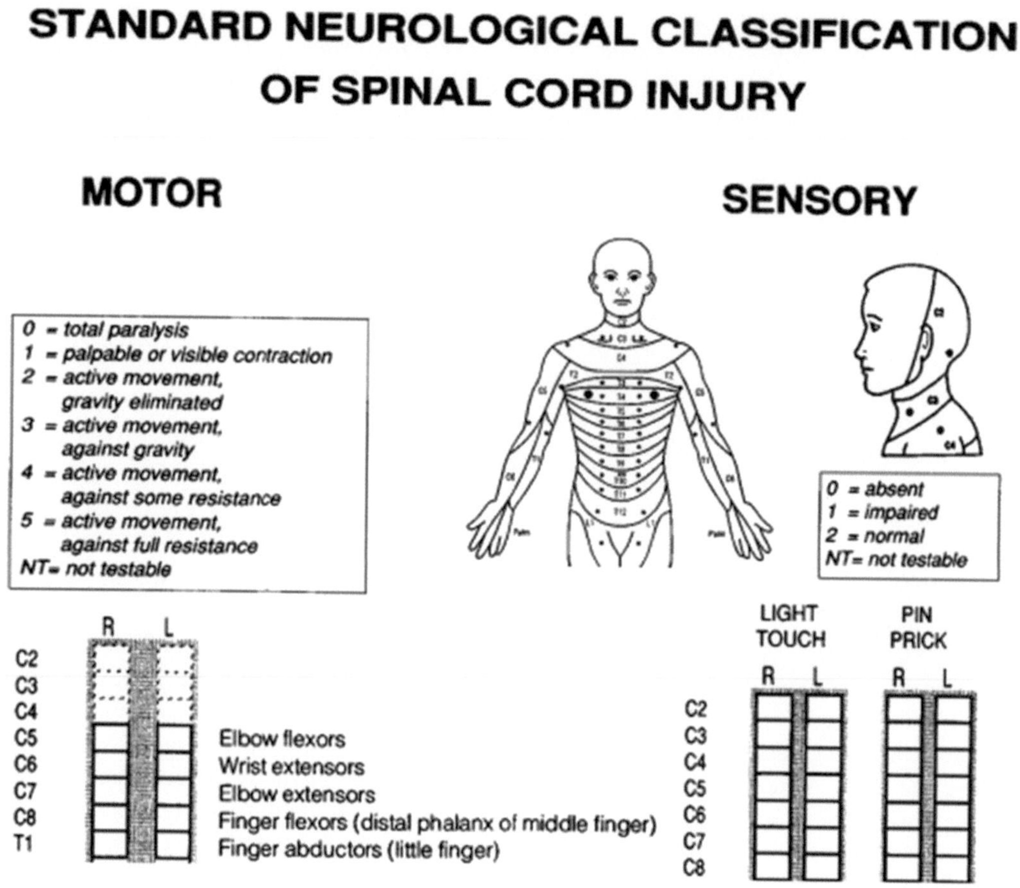

Fig. 10.1 Neurological classification chart (modified from Maynard et al. 1997)

Table 10.1 ASIA impairment rating

Impairment rating	Clinical definition
A	Complete: No sacral sensory or motor preservation
B	Incomplete: Only sensory preservation below level of SCI
C	Incomplete: At least half of the muscles below the level of SCI have a motor grade ≥3
D	Incomplete: Greater than half of the muscles below the level of SCI have a motor grade ≥3
E	Normal: Normal sensory and motor function

from compression of sympathetic innervation projecting caudally [47]. SCI level is defined as the most inferior with a strength grading of ≥3 in conjunction with the superior level being graded 5 (Table 10.1) [46].

Treatment Methods and Prognosis of Geriatric Cervical Spinal Trauma

The most urgent questions facing a treating physician for a patient with geriatric cervical spinal trauma are the following: Does the patient need surgery? Is the surgery urgent? In order to address these questions, systems such as the Subaxial Cervical Spine Injury Classification (SLIC) and severity score have been developed [48], as detailed in Table 10.2. The system allots points and incorporates the osteoligamentous disruption as well as the neurological functional status of the individual. Surgery is only needed if the patient scores greater than 4 on the SLIC. Furthermore, in the geriatric population it is necessary to consider the potential comorbidities of surgery as there are well-documented increased risk for vascular and cardiopulmonary thromboembolic incidents.

Nonsurgical treatment options include immobilization with a cervical collar or halovest, physical and/or occupational therapy, medications (NSAIDS, steroids, muscle relaxers), and corticosteroid injections [49]. Surgical treatments include ACDF, laminectomy with or without lateral mass fixation, odontoid screw fixation, or disc arthroplasty.

Table 10.2 Subaxial cervical spine injury classification (SLIC) and severity score ratings

Morphology	Points
Normal	0
Compression fracture	1–2
Distraction	3
Rotation/translation	4
Discoligamentous complex	
Normal	0
Intermediate	1
Disrupted	2
Neurological status	
Normal	0
Root injury	1
Complete cord injury	2
Partial cord injury	3
Ongoing cord compression	1

In relation to C2 fracture type I and type III fractures have an extremely high union rate and do not usually require aggressive treatment [35]. However, type II fractures are most prevalent and also present with the highest nonunion rate, 12–63%. To help stabilize type II odontoid fractures some patients may undergo internal fixation through an anterior or a posterior approach, such as C2 screw fixation or C1–2 lateral mass screw fixation, as illustrated in Fig. 10.2 [33, 35].

Prognostically, restoration of motor function after a cervical spine injury is positively correlated with age whereas restoration of daily function and ambulation is negatively correlated with age [50, 51]. Furthermore, improvement in bladder function is negatively correlated with traumatic cervical spinal injury [52].

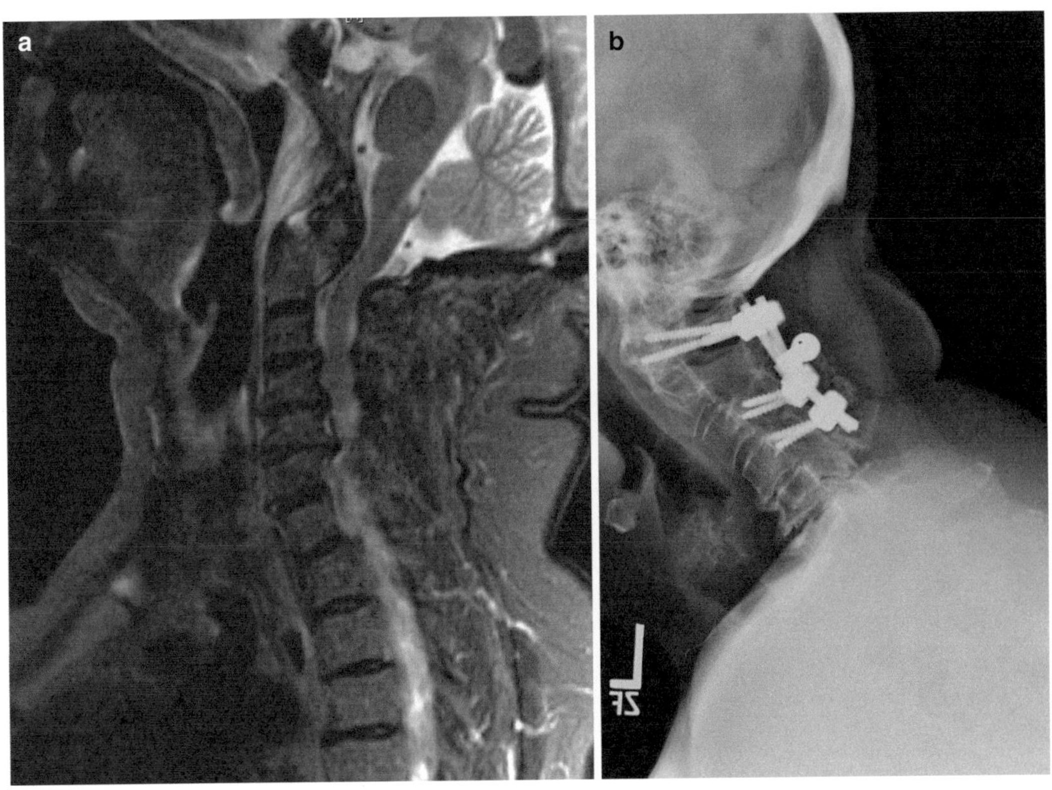

Fig. 10.2 Pre-op MRI (**a**) and post-op X-ray (**b**) illustrating a C2 odontoid fracture and surgical fixation

References

1. Taylor JA, Bussières A. Diagnostic imaging for spinal disorders in the elderly: a narrative review. Chiropr Man Therap. 2012;20:16.
2. Watanabe M, Sakai D, Yamamoto Y, Nagai T, Sato M, Mochida J. Analysis of predisposing factors in elderly people with Type II odontoid fracture. Spine J. 2014;14(6):861.
3. Tanishima S, Takeda C, Hamamoto Y, Kondo Y, Nagashima H. Prompt surgical management for spinal fracture in the elderly aged over 90 years with diffuse idiopathic skeletal hyperostosis to extend their healthy lifespan. Eur J Orthop Surg Traumatol. 2012;22:29–34.
4. Savall F, Mokrane F-Z, Dedouit F, Capuani C, Guilbeau-Frugier C, Rougé D, et al. Spine injury following a low-energy trauma in ankylosing spondylitis: a study of two cases. Forensic Sci Int. 2014;241:123–6.
5. Fujimura Y, Nakamura M, Toyama Y. Influence of minor trauma on surgical results in patients with cervical OPLL. J Spinal Disord. 1998;11:16–20.
6. EFFO, NFO. Who are candidates for prevention and treatment for osteoporosis? Osteoporosis Int. 1997;7:1–6.
7. Lerner U. Bone remodeling in post-menopausal osteoporosis. J Dent Res. 2006;85:584–95.
8. Cherniack EP, Levis S, Troen BR, Hypovitaminosis D. A widespread epidemic. Geriatrics. 2008;63:24–30.
9. Alexander L, Beur SMJD. Lifestyle modifications may help avoid need for pharmacological management of osteoporosis. MD Conf Exp. 2011;11:26–8.
10. Schwarz C, Sulzbacher I, Oberbauer R. Review: diagnosis of renal osteodystrophy. Eur J Clin Investig. 2006;36:13–22.
11. Kelsey JL. Risk factors for osteoporosis and associated fractures. Public Health Rep. 1989;104:14–20.
12. Drake MT, Murad MH, Mauck KF, Lane MA, Undavalli C, Elraiyah T, et al. Risk factors for low bone mass-related fractures in men: a systematic review and meta-analysis. J Clin Endocrinol Metabol. 2012;97:1861–70.
13. Einhorn TA. Bone strength: the bottom line. Calcif Tissue Int. 1992;51:333–9.
14. Johnell O, Kanis JA. An estimate of the worldwide prevalence and disability associated with osteoporotic fractures. Osteoporos Int. 2006;17:1726–33.
15. Todd AG. Cervical spine: degenerative conditions. Curr Rev Musculoskelet Med. 2011;4:168–74.
16. Urban JPG, Mcmullin JF. Swelling pressure of the lumbar intervertebral discs. Spine. 1988;13:179–87.
17. Urban JPG, Holm SH. Intervertebral disc nutrition as related to spinal movements and fusion. Tis Nutr Viabil. 1986:101–19.
18. Kumaresan S, Yoganandan N, Pintar FA, Maiman DJ, Goel VK. Contribution of disc degeneration to osteophyte formation in the cervical spine: a biomechanical investigation. J Orthop Res. 2001;19:977–84.
19. Zhong G, Buser Z, Lao L, Yin R, Wang JC. Kinematic relationship between missed ligamentum flavum bulge and degenerative factors in the cervical spine. Spine J. 2015;15:2216–21.
20. Weinfeld RM, Olson PN, Maki DD, Griffiths HJ. The prevalence of diffuse idiopathic skeletal hyperostosis (DISH) in two large American Midwest metropolitan hospital populations. Skelet Radiol. 1997;26:222–5.
21. Baxi V, Gaiwal S. Diffuse idiopathic skeletal hyperostosis of cervical spine—an unusual cause of difficult flexible fiber optic intubation. Saudi J Anaesth. 2010;4:17.
22. Belanger TA, Rowe DE. Diffuse idiopathic skeletal hyperostosis: musculoskeletal manifestations. J Am Acad Orthop Surg. 2001;9:258–67.
23. Khan AQ, Gupta K, Jameel J, Sherwani M. Diffuse idiopathic skeletal hyperostosis. J Clin Orthop Trauma. 2010;1:47–8.
24. Hir PXL, Sautet A, Gars LL, Zeitoun F, Tubiana JM, Arrivé L, et al. Hyperextension vertebral body fractures in diffuse idiopathic skeletal hyperostosis: a cause of intravertebral fluidlike collections on MR imaging. Am J Roentgenol. 1999;173:1679–83.
25. Kalb S, Martirosyan NL, Perez-Orribo L, Kalani MYS, Theodore N. Analysis of demographics, risk factors, clinical presentation, and surgical treatment modalities for the ossified posterior longitudinal ligament. Neurosurg Focus. 2011;30:E11. https://doi.org/10.3171/2010.12.focus10265.
26. McAfee PC, Regan JJ, Bohlman HH. Cervical cord compression from ossification of the posterior longitudinal ligament in non-orientals. J Bone Joint Surg Br. 1987;69:569–75.
27. Smith ZA, Buchanan CC, Raphael D, Khoo LT. Ossification of the posterior longitudinal ligament: pathogenesis, management, and current surgical approaches. Neurosurg Focus. 2011;30:E10. https://doi.org/10.3171/2011.1.focus10256.
28. Kim T-J, Bae K-W, Uhm W-S, Kim T-H, Joo K-B, Jun J-B. Prevalence of ossification of the posterior longitudinal ligament of the cervical spine. Joint Bone Spine. 2008;75(4):471.
29. Sarkiss CA, Fogg GA, Skovrlj B, Cho SK, Caridi JM. To operate or not? A literature review of surgical outcomes in 95 patients with Parkinson's disease undergoing spine surgery. Clin Neurol Neurosurg. 2015;134:122–5.
30. Fasano A, Plotnik M, Bove F, Berardelli A. The neurobiology of falls. Neurol Sci. 2012;33:1215–23.
31. Bub LD, Blackmore CC, Mann FA, Lomoschitz FM. Cervical spine fractures in patients 65 years and older: a clinical prediction rule for blunt trauma. Radiology. 2005;234:143–9.
32. Fredø H, Bakken I, Lied B, Rønning P, Helseth E. Epidemiology of traumatic cervical spine fractures in the Norwegian population. Global Spine J. 2015. https://doi.org/10.1055/s-0035-1554113.
33. Jabbour P, Fehlings M, Vaccaro AR, Harrop JS. Traumatic spine injuries in the geriatric population. Neurosurg Focus. 2008;25:E16. https://doi.org/10.3171/foc.2008.25.11.e16.
34. Regenbogen V, Rogers L, Atlas S, Kim K. Cervical spinal cord injuries in patients with cervical spondylosis. Am J Roentgenol. 1986;146:277–84.

35. Torretti JA, Sengupta DK. Cervical spine trauma. Indian J Orthop. 2007;41:255–67.
36. Lomoschitz FM, Blackmore CC, Mirza SK, Mann FA. Cervical spine injuries in patients 65 years old and older. Am J Roentgenol. 2002;178:573–7.
37. Moore TA, Vaccaro AR, Anderson PA. Classification of lower cervical spine injuries. Spine. 2006;31:S37–43.
38. London S (2011) ACEP. Geriatric patients fare worse after trauma. https://www.acep.org/content.aspx?id=79746.
39. Jeffreys RV. The surgical treatment of cervical myelopathy due to spondylosis and disc degeneration. J Neurol Neurosurg Psychiatry. 1986;49:353–61.
40. Thompson C, Gonsalves JF, Welsh D. Hyperextension injury of the cervical spine with central cord syndrome. Eur Spine J. 2014;24:195–202.
41. Dahdaleh NS, Lawton CD, El Ahmadieh TY, Nixon AT, El Tecle NE, Oh S, Fessler RG, Smith ZA. Evidence-based management of central cord syndrome. Neurosurg Focus. 2013;35:E6.
42. Aarabi B, Koltz M, Ibrahimi D. Hyperextension cervical spine injuries and traumatic central cord syndrome. Neurosurg Focus. 2008;25(5):E9. https://doi.org/10.3171/FOC.2008.25.11.E9.
43. Taylor AR. The mechanism of injury to the spinal cord in the neck without damage to vertebral column. J Bone Jt Surg Br. 1951;33-B(4):543–7.
44. O'Dowd JK. Basic principles of management for cervical spine trauma. Eur Spine J. 2009;19:18–22.
45. Lehman D, Sandhu RS, Baga L, Hussain F. CT scanning is sufficient to clear the cervical spine of elderly falls less than 5 feet. Poster presented at: Lehigh Valley Hospital; 2011; Allentown, PA.
46. American Spinal Injury Association. Reference manual for the international standards for neurological classification of spinal cord injury. Chicago: American Spinal Injury Association; 2003.
47. Gunduz H, Binak DF. Autonomic dysreflexia: an important cardiovascular complication in spinal cord injury patients. Cardiol J. 2012;19:215–9.
48. Whang PG, Patel AA, Vaccaro AR. The development and evaluation of the subaxial injury classification scoring system for cervical spine trauma. Clin Orthop Relat Res. 2010;469:723–31.
49. Lauweryns P. Role of conservative treatment of cervical spine injuries. Eur Spine J. 2009;19:23–6.
50. Jakob W, Wirz M, van Hedel HJ, et al. Difficulty of elderly SCI subjects to translate motor recovery—"body function"—into daily living activities. J Neurotrauma. 2009;26:2037–44.
51. Kay ED, Deutsch A, Wuermser LA. Predicting walking at discharge from inpatient rehabilitation after a traumatic spinal cord injury. Arch Phys Med Rehabil. 2007;88:745–50.
52. Aito S, D'Andrea M, Werhagen L, et al. Neurological and functional outcome in traumatic central cord syndrome. Spinal Cord. 2007;45:292–7.

11 Identification, Treatment, and Prognosis of Geriatric Thoracolumbar Spinal Trauma

Stephen C. Kane, Victor R. Lewis, James E. Conway, and Ira M. Garonzik

Abbreviations

ASIA	American Spinal Injury Association
BSS	Brown-Séquard syndrome
CES	Cauda equina syndrome
CMS	Conus medullaris syndrome
CT	Computed tomography
DVT	Deep-vein thrombosis
MRI	Magnetic resonance imaging
NSAID	Nonsteroidal anti-inflammatory drug
PE	Pulmonary embolism
SCI	Spinal cord injury
TLF	Thoracolumbar fracture
TLICS	Thoracolumbar injury classification and severity score

S.C. Kane, B.S. (✉) • V.R. Lewis, B.S.
Baltimore Neurosurgery and Spine Center, 5051 Greenspring Ave, Suite 101, Baltimore, MD 21219, USA
e-mail: kane.stephen.c@gmail.com

J.E. Conway, M.D., Ph.D. • I.M. Garonzik, M.D.
Department of Neurosurgery at Sinai Hospital and Baltimore Neurosurgery and Spine Center, 5051 Greenspring Ave, Suite 101, Baltimore, MD 21219, USA

Baltimore Neurosurgery and Spine Center, 5051 Greenspring Ave, Suite 101, Baltimore, MD 21219, USA
e-mail: medassist@baltimoreneurosurgery.com

Geriatric Osteodegenerative, Arthrodegenerative, and Neurodegenerative Predispositions

It is well known that the prevalence of osteoporosis and decreased bone density in the geriatric population is as high as 43.9% [4] and can lead to progressive changes in the vertebral body as well as the neuronal arch, and zygopophenzegal joints, and sagittal or coronal alignment [5]. The causes of geriatric osteoporosis include hypovitaminosis D [6], postmenopausal osteoporosis [7], andropause [8], renal osteodystrophy [9], decreased mechanical stress [10], as well as chronic smoking [11], alcohol [12], or prescription drug use. Specifically, the vertebral body, rich in trabecular bone, has the greatest propensity for degradative changes due to osteoporosis [13]. It has been shown that osteoporosis affects trabecular bone considerably more than cortical bone due to its increased osteoactivity and, specifically, decreases the density of the lateral cross members among trabecular bone [14]. In tandem with low-energy trauma, this could produce an array of fractures including vertebral body and laminar compromise. Furthermore, late-onset hyperossification, such as ankylosing spondylitis, can cause decreased flexibility and increase predisposition to fracture as well [15].

In addition to osteo-degradation, degenerative disk disease has become a hallmark of aging

A. Rodriguez et al. (eds.), *Geriatric Trauma and Acute Care Surgery*,
https://doi.org/10.1007/978-3-319-57403-5_11

individuals and can destabilize the thoracolumbar spine [16]. Ultimately, metabolic changes cause reduced intra-annular hydrostatic pressure [17]. In turn, this creates a "flat-tire" situation in which the disc becomes more likely to rupture, fissure, or tear. Furthermore, this can perpetuate degenerative changes due to the decreased ability of the disc to successfully handle axial loading situations especially in the inferior thoracolumbar spine [18]. In geriatric persons, low-energy impact in any plane can cause disc rupture causing instability with or without neurological compromise.

Neurologically, an array of disorders can predispose a geriatric individual to low-energy trauma. Falls, the most common trauma for elderly persons, can be caused due to degenerative changes such as Parkinson's [19] cognitive impairments, age-related visual impairments, underlying neuromuscular disorders, peripheral neuropathies, and postural instability [20].

Posttraumatic Geriatric Vertebral Fracture

Various mechanisms can cause thoracolumbar fracture (TLF) including compression-type injuries, flexion-distraction injuries, or fracture dislocation injuries. Each individual mechanism can cause an array of TLFs which has been characterized by Denis' three-column system [21]. Denis defines three columns (anterior, middle, and posterior) and characterizes compromise of these accordingly. The anterior column consists of the anterior longitudinal ligament, anterior annulus, and anterior aspect of the vertebral body. The middle column consists of the posterior longitudinal ligament, posterior aspect of the vertebral body, and posterior annulus. The posterior column consists of the ligamentum flavum, the facet joints, and lamina (Fig. 11.1).

Traditionally, elderly patients are more susceptible to low-energy axial loading compression fractures due to degradation of the trabecular bone of the vertebral body [22]. Specifically, violation of the anterior and middle columns (such as endplate fracture, vertebral body collapse, or burst fractures) is typical as up to 80% of axial loading is allocated to the vertebral body and can cause increased kyphosis [23]. Flexion-distraction injuries mainly present after a motor vehicle accident in which the individuals' pelvis is secured but the torso is accelerated forward rapidly causing compression of anterior and middle column in conjunction with fracture of lamina or lesion of the ligamentum flavum. Fracture dislocation injuries are comparable to flexion distraction injuries but include translation with osteoligamentous compromise in the anterior ligaments, disc rupture axially, and facet or pars fracture posteriorly resulting in spondylolisthesis [24]. Typically, TLF occurs in the thoracolumbar junction and lumbar spine rather than the thoracic spine due to the stabilization of the rib cage [25].

X-rays, CT scans, as well as clinical assessment for instability are the gold standard in identifying TLF (Fig. 11.1). It should be noted while attempting to identify a TLF that previous asymptomatic common endplate degradation can appear on radiographic images [26]. This could lead to an inaccurate diagnosis of a posttraumatic fracture rather than a preexisting stable fracture. A T2 flare MRI scan is the most common tool to view vertebral edema deciphering previous degradation versus acute injury.

Treatment for TLF depends on multiple factors including fracture type, fracture severity, degree of neurological compromise, symptom severity, stability, age-related comorbidities, as well as quality of life [27]. In cases with only vertebral body violation and no neurological compromise it may be appropriate to treat merely with medication management (bisphosphonates [28], teriparatide [29, 30], analgesics, or other osteoporosis combative drugs), weight-bearing physical therapy, as well as thoracic-lumbar-sacral orthotics [31]. In cases with increased kyphosis and significant vertebral body compromise it may be appropriate to treat with percutaneous vertebroplasty or kyphoplasty [32]. Treatment using kyphoplasty/vertebroplasty has been controversial in its ability to increase stability and decrease pain [33]. In cases with severe vertebral body collapse, posterior column violation, spondylolisthesis, or severe neurological compromise it is appropriate to consider surgical options including anterior corpectomy with placement of a cage, posterior

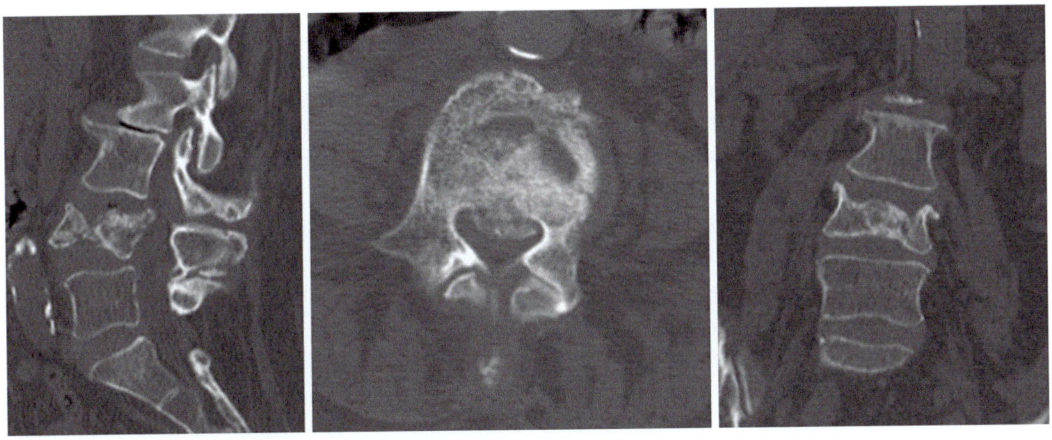

Fig. 11.1 Computed tomography (CT) of a burst fracture after a fall in an 83-year-old female

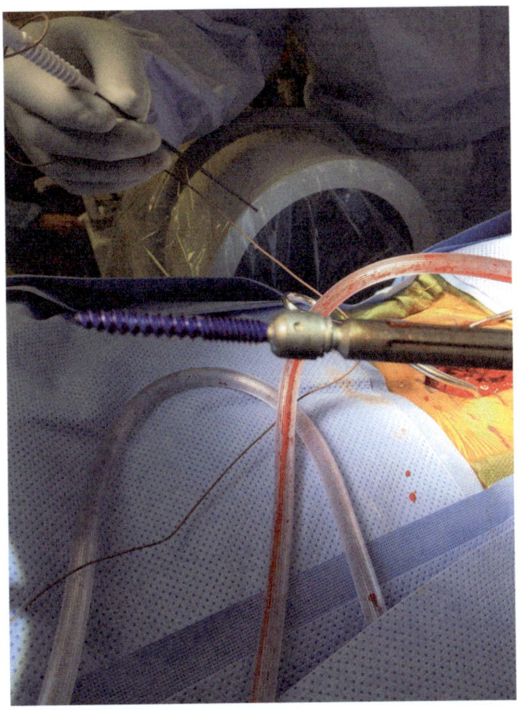

Fig. 11.2 Example of a unicortical pedicle screw with increased cortical threads

stabilization with or without instrumentation, as well as decompression of any ongoing neurological pathology [34]. Due to the poor bone quality of these individuals, it is essential to augment any hardware with autograft and allograft, large-diameter bicortical or unicortical screws (Fig. 11.2), and cement [35].

Posttraumatic Geriatric Neurological Compromise

Thoracolumbar spinal trauma can cause neurological dysfunction secondary to osteoligamentous compromise and/or disc prolapse causing spinal cord injury (SCI) with potential nerve root compression. Most commonly these can present as radiculopathy, anterior cord syndrome, cauda equina syndrome, conus medullaris syndrome, or Brown-Séquard syndrome.

American Spinal Injury Association's (ASIA) Standards for Neurological and Functional Classification of Spinal Cord Injury

After a primary assessment, it is important to obtain a baseline neurological examination. The most accepted system in understanding spinal cord injury is the American Spinal Injury Association's (ASIA) Standards for Neurological and Functional Classification of Spinal Cord Injury [36]. The standards incorporate a sensory and motor exam by systematically testing corresponding nerve root dermatomes and myotomes. The sensory exam consists of bilateral pin prick as well as light-touch sensation and is rated from 0 to 2 (0 = absent, 1 = impaired, 2 = normal). The muscular exam tests bilateral range of motion (ROM) as well as degree of strength against various resistance levels and is graded 0–5 (0 = total paralysis, 1 = palpable or visual contraction, 2 = active movement/full ROM with gravity eliminated, 3 = active movement/full ROM against gravity, 4 = active movement/full ROM against moderate resistance, 5 = active movement/full ROM against full resistance). The myotomes that have not been distinguished are identical to the dermatomes. Formally, the level of SCI is defined muscularly as the most inferior with a grading of ≥3 given that the adjacent superior level is graded a 5 (as muscles are generally innervated by multiple nerve roots). Of note, it should be recognized that inferior nerve roots may have partial preservation of sensation or motor function and should be recorded [36]. It is common among elderly individuals to have contributing symptomatic preexisting degenerative neurocompressive etiology of the thoracolumbar spine which could be most easily clarified through radiographic studies such as MRI as well as diagnostic studies such as EMG/NCV in order to make a correct diagnosis.

Furthermore, the ASIA impairment scale is the gold standard in determining prognosis of SCI. The degree of impairment scale ranges from A to E and is defined as follows: A = Complete: No sacral sensory or motor preservation; B = Incomplete: Only sensory preservation below level of SCI; C = Incomplete: At least half of the muscles below the level of SCI have a motor grade ≥3; D = Incomplete: Greater than half of the muscles below the level of SCI have a motor grade ≥3; E = Normal: Normal sensory and motor function. Prognostically, it has been shown that an individual with an A rating has a 13% chance of returning to incomplete impairment 1 year postinjury [37]. However, an individual with a B rating that maintains pinprick discrimination has a 20–50% chance of regaining ambulation [38].

Anterior Spinal Artery Syndrome (Anterior Cord Syndrome)/Brown-Séquard Syndrome (BSS)

Compression of the anterior spinal artery causing ischemia in the anterior white and gray matter of the spinal cord is termed anterior cord syndrome. Deficits solely present in the spinothalamic tract and corticospinal tracts causing paraplegia (if presenting in the thoracic spine) as well as pain perception dysfunction but spared proprioception and light-touch sensation [39]. Specifically, motor function restoration has a poor prognosis especially if there is minimal recovery within 24 h. There is no current accepted treatment for ischemic damage to the spinal cord.

BSS is well defined as a hemicord syndrome in which the corticospinal tract, ascending fibers in the posterior column, and spinothalamic tract are compressed causing compromise of ipsilateral motor function, ipsilateral proprioception, ipsilateral tactile perception, as well as contralateral pain and temperature perception [40].

Cauda Equina Syndrome (CES)/Conus Medullaris Syndrome (CMS)

Posttraumatic central canal obstruction at the level of the cauda equine (L2-sacrum) due to osteoligamentous material retropulsion posteriorly or significant disc herniation is termed cauada equina syndrome. Symptomatically, the individual would present with motor and sensory disturbance (asymmetric saddle anesthesia and leg weakness), decreased deep tendon reflexes below the injured level, severe low back pain, bowel incontinence, and most commonly urinary retention. Individuals with bladder paralysis or multiple of these symptoms following trauma should undergo emergent MRI to confirm the etiology as well as surgical decompression within 24–48 h of symptom commencement [41]. Interestingly, elderly patients with CES have a significantly poorer sexual function outcome [42].

While very comparable to cauda equina syndrome, conus medullaris syndrome is distinctly different [43]. Symptomatically, the saddle anesthesia presents symmetrically, there is complete absence of lower extremities deep tendon reflexes, and the onset of bladder atonia is accelerated. Due to the location of the compression, the individual may present with upper motor neuron symptomology as well as lower motor neuron dysfunction causing plausible inaccurate diagnosis of cauda equine syndrome or superior spinal cord compression.

Thoracolumbar Radiculopathy

Retropulsion of osteoligamentous material posterolaterally from vertebral body fracture/disc desiccation or vertebral dislocation can cause foraminal stenosis leading to thoracolumbar radiculopathy [44]. Symptomatically, the individual would present with hypoesthesia in the corresponding dermatome, and atrophy of corresponding myotome in the thoracic spine with additional decreased reflexes in the lumbar spine [45]. Palliatively, medication management (opioids, neuropathic agents, NSAIDS) and steroid injections (selective nerve root blocks, epidural steroid injections) could be considered in the absence of structural instability indicating surgical intervention. If the individual fails conservative treatment foraminotomies, laminoforaminotomies, and/or discectomy with or without posterolateral fusion may be needed [46].

Clinical Decision Making in Geriatric Spinal Trauma

In the geriatric population, the main goal of any treatment is to increase mobility as quickly as possible to avoid further degradation and complications. Clinically, the most pressing question upon first evaluation is surgical versus nonsurgical treatment. The most useful system to determine this is the Thoracolumbar Injury Classification and Severity score (TLICS) [47]. The system takes into account the morphology of the injury, neurological compromise, and violation of the posterior column. As a point-based system (Fig. 11.3), it allows for clarity and straightforward decision making. The algorithm dictates a total score of 0–3 as nonoperative, a score of 4 as either operative or nonoperative, and a score of 5 or greater as surgically operable.

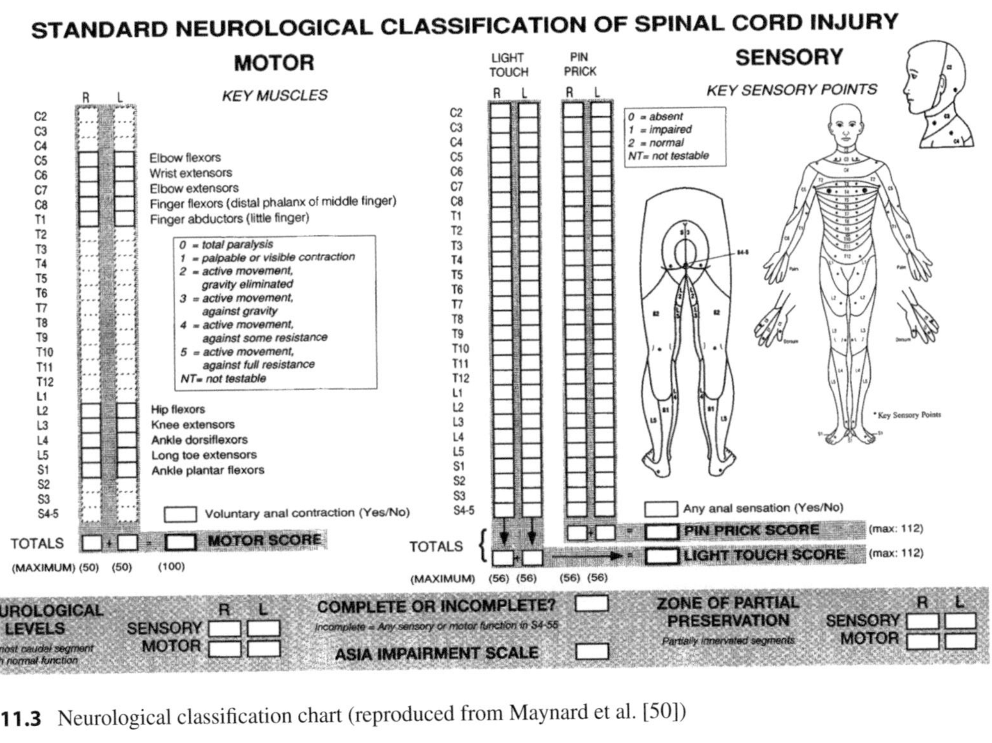

Fig. 11.3 Neurological classification chart (reproduced from Maynard et al. [50])

Parameter	Points
Morphology	
Compression fracture	1
Burst fracture	2
Fracture dislocation	3
Flexion-distraction fracture	4
Neurological compromise	
Normal	0
Nerve root	2
Incomplete spinal cord	3
Complete spinal cord	2
Cauda equina syndrome	3
Posterior column	
Normal	0
Injury suspected	2
Injured	3

Specifically, in elderly patients it is important to take into consideration potential surgical complications. Elderly patients are at a greater risk for a postoperative thromboembolic event (such as a deep-vein thrombosis (DVT) with pulmonary embolism (PE)) and cardiac and respiratory comorbidities [48] as well as further low-energy traumatic events. It has also been shown that patients with Parkinson's are predisposed to requiring a revision spinal surgery [49].

References

1. Ortman JM, Velkoff VA, Hogan H. An aging nation: the older population in the United States, current population reports, P25–1140. Washington, DC: U.S. Census Bureau; 2014.
2. Woods NF, Lacroix AZ, Gray SL, Aragaki A, Cochrane BB, Brunner RL, et al. Frailty: emergence and consequences in women aged 65 and older in the women's health initiative observational study. J Am Geriatr Soc. 2005;53(8):1321–30. Accessed 6 Apr 2016
3. Augat P, Weyand D, Panzer S, Klier T. Osteoporosis prevalence and fracture characteristics in elderly female patients with fractures. Arch Orthop Trauma Surg. 2010;130:1405–10. Accessed 14 Mar 2016
4. Looker AC, Borrud LG, Dawson-Hughes B. Osteoporosis or low bone mass at the femur neck or lumbar spine in older adults: United States, 2005–2008 [Abstract]. NCHS Data Brief. 2012;93:1–8. http://www.cdc.gov/nchs/data/databriefs/db93.pdf. Accessed 14 Mar 2016
5. Flynn MJ, Cody DD. The assessment of vertebral bone macroarchitecture with x-ray computed tomography. Calcif Tissue Int. 1993;53(Suppl 1):S170–5. Accessed 6 Apr 2016
6. Cherniack E, Levis S, Troen B. Hypovitaminosis D: a stealthy epidemic that requires treatment. Geriatrics. 2008;63(4):24–30. 6p. Accessed 14 Mar 2016
7. Lerner U. Bone remodeling in post-menopausal osteoporosis. J Dent Res. 2006;85(7):584–95. Accessed 14 Mar 2016
8. Wespes E, Schulman C. Male andropause: myth, reality, and treatment. Int J Impot Res. 2002;14(1):93. Accessed 14 Mar 2016
9. Schwarz C, Sulzbacher I, Oberbauer R. Diagnosis of renal osteodystrophy. Eur J Clin Invest. 2006;36:13–22. https://doi.org/10.1111/j1365-2362200601666x. Accessed 6 Apr 2016
10. Alexander C, Vico L. Pathophysiology of bone loss in disuse osteoporosis. Bone Joint Spine. 2011;78(6):572–6. Accessed 14 Mar 2016
11. Kelsey JL. Risk factors for osteoporosis and associated fractures. Public Health Rep. 1989;104(Suppl):14–20. Accessed 6 Apr 2016
12. Drake MT, Murad MH, Mauck KF, Lane MA, Undavalli C, Elraiyah T, et al. Risk factors for low bone mass-related fractures in men: a systematic review and meta-analysis. J Clin Endocrinol Metabol. 2012;97(6):1861–70. Accessed 6 Apr 2016
13. Gill SS, Einhorn TA. Bone metabolism and metabolic bone disease. In: Beaty JH, editor. Orthopaedic knowledge update 6. Rosemont: American Academy of Orthopaedic Surgeons; 1998. p. 149–65. Accessed 6 Apr 2016.
14. Einhorn TA. Bone strength: the bottom line. Calcif Tissue Int. 1992;51(5):333–9. Accessed 6 Apr 2016
15. Trent G, Armstrong GW, O'Neil J. Thoracolumbar fractures in ankylosing spondylitis high-risk injuries. Clin Orthop Relat Res. 1988;227:61–6. Accessed 4 Apr 2016
16. Raj PP. Intervertebral disc: anatomy-physiology-pathophysiology-treatment. Pain Pract. 2008;8:18–44. https://doi.org/10.1111/j.1533-2500.2007.00171.x. Accessed 6 Apr 2016
17. Urban JP, Mcmullin JF. Swelling pressure of the lumbar intervertebral discs. Spine. 1988;13(2):179–87. Accessed 6 Apr 2016
18. Adams MA, Mcnally DS, Dolan P. 'Stress' distributions inside intervertebral discs. The effects of age and degeneration. J Bone Joint Surg. 1996;78(6):965–72. Accessed 6 Apr 2016
19. Sarkiss CA, Fogg GA, Skovrlj B, Cho SK, Caridi JM. To operate or not?: A literature review of surgical outcomes in 95 patients with Parkinson's disease undergoing spine surgery. Clin Neurol Neurosurg. 2015;134:122–5. Accessed 4 Apr 2016
20. Fasano A, Plotnik I, Bove F, Berardelli A. The neurobiology of falls. Neurol Sci. 2012;33:1215–23. https://doi.org/10.1007/s10072-012-1126-6. Accessed 6 Apr 2016

21. Denis F. The three column spine and its significance in the classification of acute thoracolumbar spinal injuries. Spine. 1983;8(8):817–31. Accessed 6 Apr 2016
22. Albrand G, Munoz F, Sornay-Rendu E, Duboeuf F, Delmas P. Independent predictors of all osteoporosis-related fractures in healthy postmenopausal women: the OFELY Study. Bone. 2003;32(1):78–85. Accessed 6 Apr 2016
23. Silva MJ, Keaveny TM, Hayes WC. Load sharing between the shell and centrum in the lumbar vertebral body. Spine. 1997;22:140–50. Accessed 6 Apr 2016
24. Bohlman HH. Treatment of fractures and dislocations of the thoracic and lumbar spine. J Bone Joint Surg Am. 1985;67(1):165–9. Accessed 6 Apr 2016
25. Maiman D, Pintar F. Anatomy and clinical biomechanics of the thoracic spine. Clin Neurosurg. 1992;38:296–324. Accessed 6 Apr 2016
26. Reid DC, Hu R, Davis LA, Saboe LA. The nonoperative treatment of burst fractures of the thoracolumbar junction. J Trauma. 1988;28(8):1188–94. Accessed 6 Apr 2016
27. Soultanis KC, Mavrogenis AF, Starantzis KA. When and how to operate on thoracic and lumbar spine fractures? Eur J Orthop Surg Traumatol. 2014;24:443–51. Accessed 21 Mar 2016
28. Cummings SR. Effect of alendronate on risk of fracture in women with low bone density but without vertebral fractures results from the fracture intervention trial. JAMA. 1998;280(24):2077. Accessed 6 Apr 2016
29. Kaback LA, Soung DY, Naik A, Geneau G, Schwarz EM, Rosier RN, O'Keefe RJ, Drissi H. Teriparatide (1-34 human PTH) regulation of osterix during fracture repair. J Cell Biochem. 2008;105:219–26. doi:https://doi.org/10.1002/jcb.21816. Accessed 6 Apr 2016
30. Neer RM, Arnaud CD, Zanchetta JR, et al. Effect of parathyroid hormone (1–34) on fractures and bone mineral density in postmenopausal women with osteoporosis. N Engl J Med. 2001;344(19):1434–41. Accessed 6 Apr 2016
31. Wong C, McGirt M. Vertebral compression fractures: a review of current management and multimodal therapy. J Multidiscip Healthc. 2013;6:205–14. Accessed 21 Mar 2016
32. Firanescu C, Lohle PN, Vries JD, Klazen CA, Juttmann JR, Clark W, Rooij WV. A randomised sham controlled trial of vertebroplasty for painful acute osteoporotic vertebral fractures (VERTOS IV). Trials. 2011;12(1):93. Accessed 6 Apr 2016
33. Kallmes D, Buchbinder R, Jarvik J, Heagerty P, Comstock B, Turner J, Osborne R. Response to "randomized vertebroplasty trials: bad news or sham news?". Am J Neuroradiol. 2009;30(10):1809–10. Accessed 6 Apr 2016
34. Yan D, Wang Z, Lv Y, Baiyila B, Li J. Anterior versus posterior surgical treatment of unstable thoracolumbar burst fracture. Eur J Orthop Surg Traumatol. 2011;22(2):103–9. Accessed 4 Apr 2016
35. Yoshihara H. Surgical options for lumbosacral fusion: biomechanical stability, advantage, disadvantage and affecting factors in selecting options. Eur J Orthop Surg Traumatol. 2013;24(S1):73–82. Accessed 4 Apr 2016
36. American Spinal Injury Association. Reference manual for the International standards for neurological classification of spinal cord injury. Chicago: American Spinal Injury Association; 2003. Accessed 6 Apr 2016
37. Marino RJ, Ditunno JF, Donovan WH, et al. Neurologic recovery after traumatic spinal cord injury: data from the Model Spinal Cord Injury Systems. Arch Phys Med Rehabil. 1999;80:1391–6. Accessed 6 Apr 2016
38. Oleson CV, Burns AS, Ditunno JF, et al. Prognostic value of pinprick preservation in motor complete, sensory incomplete spinal cord injury. Arch Phys Med Rehabil. 2005;86:988–92. Accessed 6 Apr 2016
39. Foo D, Rossier AB. Anterior spinal artery syndrome and its natural history. Paraplegia. 1983;21(1):1–10. Accessed 6 Apr 2016
40. Uhl E, Holtmannspötter M, Tonn J. Improvement of Brown-Sequard syndrome after surgical repair of an idiopathic thoracic spinal cord herniation. J Neurol. 2008;255(1):125–6. Accessed 6 Apr 2016
41. Harrop JS, Hunt GE, Vaccaro AR. Conus medullaris and cauda equina syndrome as a result of traumatic injuries: management principles. Neurosurg Focus. 2004;16(6):1–23. Accessed 25 Mar 2016
42. Ahn UM, Ahn NU, Buchowski JM, Garrett ES, Sieber AN, Kostuik JP. Cauda equina syndrome secondary to lumbar disc herniation. Spine. 2000;25(12):1515–22. Accessed 6 Apr 2016
43. Radcliff KE, Kepler C, Delsotta LA. Current management review of thoracolumbar cord syndromes. Spine J. 2011;11:884–92. Accessed 25 Mar 2016
44. Milette PC. Classification, diagnostic imaging, and imaging characterization of a lumbar herniated disk. Radiol Clin N Am. 2000;38(6):1267–92. Accessed 6 Apr 2016
45. van Rijn JC, Klemetso N, Reitsma JB, Majoie CBLM, Hulsmans FJ, et al. Symptomatic and asymptomatic abnormalities in patients with lumbosacral radicular syndrome: clinical examination compared with MRI. Clin Neurol Neurosurg. 2006;108:553–7. Accessed 6 Apr 2016
46. Hoffman RM, Wheeler KJ, Deyo RA. Surgery for herniated disc: a literature synthesis. J Gen Intern Med. 1993;8:487–95. Accessed 6 Apr 2016
47. Lee JY, Vaccaro AR, Lim MR, Öner F, Hulbert RJ, Hedlund R, Baron EM. Thoracolumbar injury classification and severity score: a new paradigm for the treatment of thoracolumbar spine trauma. J Orthop Sci. 2005;10(6):671–5. Accessed 6 Apr 2016
48. Verlaan JJ, Diekerhof CH, Buskens E, Tweel IV, Verbout AJ, Dhert WJ, Oner FC. Surgical treatment of traumatic fractures of the thoracic and lumbar spine. Spine. 2004;29(7):803–14. Accessed 6 Apr 2016

49. Koller H, Acosta F, Zenner J, Ferraris L, Hitzl W, Meier O, Schmidt R. Spinal surgery in patients with Parkinson's disease: experiences with the challenges posed by sagittal imbalance and the Parkinson's spine. Eur Spine J. 2010;19(10):1785–94. Accessed 4 Apr 2016

50. Jr Maynard FM, Bracken B, Michael & Creasey et al. International standards for neurological and functional classification of spinal cord injury. American Spinal Injury Association. Spinal Cord. 1997;35:266–74. 10.1038/sj.sc.3100432

Part VII

Orthopedic Injury

12 Geriatric Hip Fractures

Ellen P. Fitzpatrick

Introduction

Hip fractures represent a serious source of morbidity and mortality in the elderly population. While hip fractures do occur in the younger population related to high-energy trauma, the majority of hip fractures occur in the elderly related to low-energy falls [1]. Hip fractures have been reported to account for over 350,000 hospital admissions per year [2] and for 72% of total hospital costs for the orthopedic fracture care in the elderly [3–5]. The impact of hip fracture only stands to increase with the aging population. Despite trends toward a decline in the incidence of hip fracture over the past few years, estimates of the number of hip fracture by 2050 are projected to be between 458,000 and 1,037,000 by 2050, with the largest number occurring in females over the age of 65 [6].

Demographics

Risk of hip fractures varies with race, age, and geographic location. Elderly women are at a three times increased risk of hip fracture as compared to elderly men [7]. There is wide variability in the frequency of hip fracture based on race and ethnicity. Rates of hip fractures are highest in Northern European countries [8]. Within the USA, there is significant differences in the frequency of hip fractures based on race. White women are at much higher risk of hip fracture than Asian or African-American. Additional risk factors include advancing age, tobacco and alcohol use, poor general health, a history of falls, history of previous fragility fracture, and low estrogen levels [9].

98% of hip fractures occur in patients over 50 with an average age of 72 [1], with the majority occurring due to low-energy falls [10].

Classifications

The generic term hip fracture encompasses a variety of conditions. Classification of hip fractures is critical for the treating orthopedic surgeon both for purposes of communication and treatment recommendations. Hip fractures are classified based on the location of the fracture as follows:

Femoral Neck Fractures

Femoral neck fracture indicates that a fracture can be classified anatomically as subcapital, transcervical, or basicervical. The critical

E.P. Fitzpatrick, M.D.
Department of Orthopaedic Surgery, UC Davis Medical Center, 4860 Y Street, Suite 3800, Sacramento, CA 95817, USA
e-mail: efitzpatrick@ucdavis.edu

A. Rodriguez et al. (eds.), *Geriatric Trauma and Acute Care Surgery*,
https://doi.org/10.1007/978-3-319-57403-5_12

distinction is between intracapsular and extracapsular, with subcapital and transcervical being the former and basicervical the latter. Intracapsular femoral neck fractures have greater concern regarding healing potential and possibility of avascular necrosis (AVN). The primary blood supply to the femoral head is via the lateral epiphyseal artery, which is the terminal branch of the medial femoral circumflex artery, with second major blood supply provided by the inferior metaphyseal arteries from the lateral femoral circumflex artery and the third major blood supply from the medial epiphyseal branches from the ligamentum teres [11]. Many studies have confirmed that displacement correlates with severity of damage to the blood supply to the femoral neck and risk of AVN. Histologic studies may overestimate the risk of AVN as in situ revascularization can occur [12, 13]. However, due to the risk of fixation failure via AVN or nonunion, intracapsular femoral neck fracture requires consideration of fixation versus replacement, whereas extracapsular hip fractures are typically repaired.

The most widely used historical classifications of femoral neck fractures include the Garden classification and the Pauwels classification system. The Garden classification attempted to group femoral neck fractures based on displacement as it relates to prognosis and incidence of complication. Grade I represents an incomplete or valgus impacted fracture, Grade II a nondisplaced fracture, Grade III a partially displaced fracture, and Grade IV a completely displaced fracture. Displaced fractures (Grade III and Grade IV) are at higher risk of nonunion, AVN, and fixation failure [14]. The Pauwels classification groups femoral neck fractures based on fracture orientation as it relates to shear forces and stability. Pauwels type I is a horizontal fracture (<30 degrees from the horizontal) with low risk of displacement due to lack of shear forces, Pauwels type II is of intermediate inclination (30–50 degrees), and Pauwels type III is a more vertical fracture line (>50 degrees) with more shear forces and higher risk of displacement [15].

Peritrochanteric Femur Fractures

Peritrochanteric femur fracture is a generic term for extra-articular hip fractures which are subdivided based on the location of the fracture. Intertrochanteric hip fractures are fractures involving fractures between the greater and lesser trochanter. Subtrochanteric hip fractures are fractures that extend below the level of the lesser trochanter. These fractures are typically treated with internal fixation, with implant and method determined by fracture pattern. They are extracapsular fracture with robust blood supply and are at minimal risk of disrupting blood supply to the femoral neck [16].

Historically multiple classification systems have been applied to peritrochanteric femur fractures. The key to treatment is distinguishing stable from unstable fractures. Stable fractures tend to be simple patterns with medial apposition. Unstable fractures include reverse obliquity, intertrochanteric fractures with subtrochanteric extension, compromised lateral cortex, and/or posteromedial calcar comminution. The AO/OTA has developed a classification system that classifies intertrochanteric hip fractures on the basis of stability, and helps guide implant choice [16–18].

Evaluation

Clinical Evaluation

As with any injury, a thorough history including mechanism of injury, additional injuries, past medical history including active medical problems and/or any oncologic history, syncopal episodes, history of chest pain, preexisting hip symptoms, and functional status are all critical to evaluation and treatment.

Imaging

Initial evaluation includes standard radiographs, including AP and cross-table lateral of affected hip, as well as AP pelvis for comparison to normal hip. Lateral film can help to assess for posterior femoral neck comminution and displacement.

Cross-table lateral should be performed instead of frog lateral, because the frog lateral is performed by abducting and externally rotating the hip, which can cause further displacement of the fracture. Manual internal rotation view (10–15 degrees) eliminates the anteversion of the femoral neck and allows true AP that can help delineate the fracture pattern, including identifying subtle nondisplaced fractures or impacted fractures. MRI is the imaging modality of choice for detecting occult femoral neck fractures or stress fractures [19]. In a patient with a pacemaker prohibiting MRI, bone scan can be used to detect occult fractures [9].

Preoperative Testing

Routine preoperative testing should include CBC, basic metabolic panel, coagulation studies, urinalysis, EKG, and chest radiographs. Chest radiographs should be performed in all patients with a history of cardiopulmonary disease, as well as in all patients older than 50. There has been a shift to comanagement of hip fracture patients between the orthopedic surgeon and a geriatrician or hospitalist, both in the preoperative and postoperative setting with excellent results. A recent meta-analysis of 18 studies looking at orthogeriatric models showed significant reduction of in-hospital mortality and long-term mortality, and significantly reduced length of stay and time to surgery [20–22].

Hip fracture patients often have significant medical comorbidities requiring further preoperative testing, but delay of surgery has historically been noted to increase morbidity when surgery is delayed more than 48 hours [23], with a recent study showing an odds ratio of 1.13 at 2 days postinjury and 1.33 at 3 days postinjury associated with higher mortality [24]. While these findings may be related to higher risk patients requiring more preoperative evaluation, an effort should still be made to expedite care.

Preoperative testing beyond the routine screening test has been noted to increase the time to surgery and length of hospital stay. A recent retrospective study showed that mean time to surgery for patient undergoing additional tests was nearly twice as long as in nontested patients (73 h vs. 37 h, respectively) and had a 33% longer hospital stay. In only 2 of the 67 patients did test findings alter care [25]. As unnecessary cardiac testing can delay surgery, it should only be performed if it will alter medical care and/or intraoperative monitoring. Additional cardiac testing should be performed in the setting of diminished functional capacity tolerance as represented by metabolic equivalent less than or equal to 4 (e.g., unable to walk a block or do light house work), cardiac risk factors, and abnormalities seen on baseline EKG [9]. Cardiology consults and further cardiac testing should be initiated based on American College of Cardiology (ACC) Foundation and the American Heart Association (AHA) guidelines, which note four discrete cardiac conditions, including severe valvular heart disease, unstable coronary syndromes, decompensated heart failure, and significant arrhythmia. The presence of these conditions indicates that cardiac evaluation may be necessary before a noncardiac surgery [26].

The American Society of Anesthesiologist (ASA) physical status classification determines perioperative risk under anesthesia based on comorbid conditions and functional status and has been shown to directly correlate with inpatient mortality, readmission rates, and complication rates [27].

Treatment

Hip fractures are an operative injury. Nonoperative treatment is reserved for bedridden or nonambulatory patients with limited pain, those with a very limited life expectancy, and those who are unable to tolerate surgery [8, 19, 28, 29]. Nonoperatively treated patients should be mobilized as soon as able with bed to chair to minimize the complications of bedrest such as UTI, thromboembolic disease, urinary tract infections, atelectasis, pulmonary complications, and decubitus ulcers [28]. Even in bedridden patient, surgery should be considered as a pain relief measure and to facilitate transfers if patient is painful and can tolerate surgery.

Surgery is the mainstay of treatment, with goals of allowing early mobilization, return to preinjury function, and pain improvement. Treatment options are dictated by fracture pattern.

Treatment of Femoral Neck Fractures

Despite the prevalence of femoral neck fractures and large body of published literature, there are a limited number of quality randomized controlled trials (RCTs) and reported outcomes are conflicting. Therefore, significant controversy remains regarding optimal treatment algorithms. Treatment options include internal fixation versus arthroplasty.

Stable, nondisplaced, or valgus impacted femoral neck fractures may be considered for internal fixation. In the Garden classification this equates to Garden I or Garden II. These are treated closed, with percutaneous fixation in situ to prevent fracture displacement and allow for early weight bearing [30]. Fixation methods include cannulated screws or sliding hip screw (SHS). Cannulated screws are associated with less surgical time and bleeding than SHS, providing adequate fixation for stable fracture patterns. 6.5, 7.0, or 7.3 cannulated screws are typically utilized in an inverted triangle configuration with three screws. When performed correctly, this configuration provides the greatest stability [31–35]. Sliding hip screws are biomechanically more stable, and should be considered in more unstable fractures such as more vertical fractures with higher shear stress or basicervical fractures [36]. There is still wide variability of implant choice among surgeons. The Fixation Using Alternative Implants for the Treatment of Hip Fractures (FAITH) is an ongoing randomized controlled trial comparing sliding hip screw versus multiple cancellous lag screws followed for a 2-year period in regard to health-related quality of life, function, fracture healing, mortality, and adverse events in patients with stable and unstable femoral neck fractures, seeking to further clarify choice of implant and success rates [37] (Fig. 12.1).

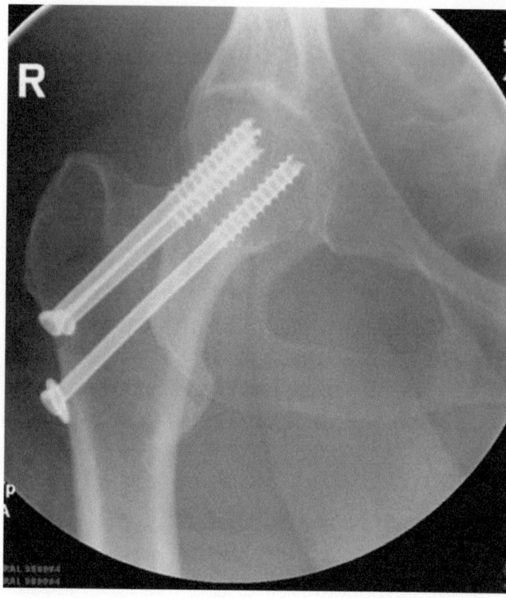

Fig. 12.1 Percutaneous fixation of valgus impacted femoral neck fracture with cannulated screws

One study showed a 90% survival rate with screw fixation in stable femoral neck fractures [38] but internal fixation of displaced femoral neck fractures results in need for reoperation in 30–47% of patients [39–41]; therefore, careful consideration by the surgeon of fracture pattern and risk factors for failure must be considered.

Controversy exists regarding surgical intervention for displaced and unstable femoral neck fractures, i.e., Garden III or Garden IV femoral neck fractures. A Cochrane review in 2003 noted internal fixation results in shorter OR time, less blood loss, lower infection rate, and lower overall complication rate, but much higher risk of reoperation [42]. Another meta-analysis of 20 RCT looking at 3109 patients with displaced femoral neck fractures treated with internal fixation or arthroplasty found that arthroplasty led to fewer surgical complications and reduced incidence of reoperation. However, arthroplasty was at higher risk of deep wound infection, greater blood loss, and longer operating time. Overall there was greater mortality rate in arthroplasty, but it was not statistically significant [43]. Blomfeldt et al. published a RCT comparing mid- to long-term follow-up for internal fixation (IF) versus total hip arthroplasty (THA) in displaced femoral neck fractures in patients older than 70 years old who were relatively independent (no severe cognitive dysfunction, independent living status, ability to walk independently). Main outcomes investigated were hip complications, reoperations, hip function, and health-related quality of life. At 4 years, post-op rate of complications of 4% in THA and 42% in IF were noted, with reoperation of 4% in THA and 47% in IF (34% conversion to THA, 13% screw removal) [41]. While there is a greater role for reduction and internal fixation for displaced femoral neck fractures in younger patients, overall better outcomes are seen with arthroplasty in the geriatric population and recent AAOS guidelines regarding the treatment of geriatric femoral neck fractures report strong evidence to support arthroplasty in displaced femoral neck fractures [44]. Another advantage of arthroplasty is immediate full weight-bearing status, while internal fixation is sometimes associated with restricted weight bearing.

The type of arthroplasty is determined by patient factors such as age, preinjury function, and preexisting hip pain and arthritis. Hemiarthroplasty (HA) has proven as an effective treatment for displaced femoral neck fractures in low-demand patients, allowing early mobilization, pain relief, and good functional recovery [9]. Comparing types of hemiarthroplasty, cemented versus uncemented arthroplasty in a RCT showed similar outcomes in regard to function, dislocation rate, and reoperation at 5-year follow-up [45]. However, Gjertsen reported two times increased rate of reoperation with uncemented hemiarthroplasty primarily due to periprosthetic fracture [46] and Taylor reported higher periprosthetic fracture rate in uncemented HA in the immediate postoperative period and at 2-year follow-up [47]. Use of noncemented or press-fit technique in patients with adequate bone stock has been advocated for shorter operative times and lower blood loss. Although reported rates of periprosthetic fracture risk vary, after review of the literature AAOS clinical guideline recommendations report moderate support for cemented hemiarthroplasty [44] (Fig. 12.2).

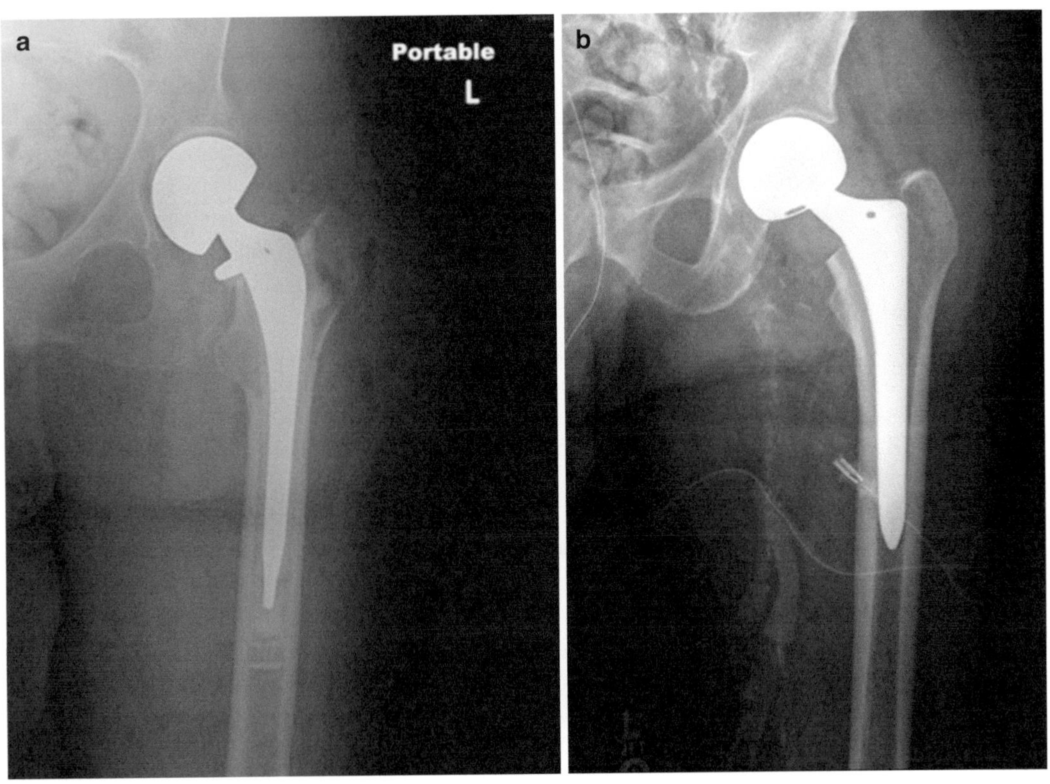

Fig. 12.2 (**a**) Cemented left hip hemiarthroplasty. (**b**) Press-fit hip hemiarthroplasty

Total hip arthroplsty (THA) provides better outcomes in healthier active elderly patients and patients with a history of symptomatic preinjury osteoarthritis [48–51]. Although there is a higher risk of dislocation in acute THA for femoral neck fracture compared with HA, there is still improved results in pain, function, and lower reoperation rate [50, 51]. THA cost is more than that of hemiarthroplasty, but cost is offset by longer implant survival, lower reoperation rate given no acetabular symptom from preexisting arthritis versus ongoing acetabular erosion, and improved functional results [52].

Stress Fractures

Stress fractures are a distinct type of nondisplaced fractures that result from cyclic mechanical loading in the setting of diminished bone quality. As above, MRI is the imaging modality of choice for detection. Tension-sided femoral neck fractures are at high risk of displacement and are recommended for surgical stabilization to avoid associated morbidity of femoral neck fracture displacement. Compression-sided femoral neck fractures are less likely to be displaced, and restricted weight bearing should be considered. Endocrine referral for evaluation of metabolic bone disease should be initiated [53].

Treatment of Peritrochanteric Femur Fractures

The mainstay of peritrochanteric femur fracture treatment is surgery to restore anatomy and allow for healing with controlled compression. This has been achieved via extramedullary or intramedullary devices. Selecting the correct device is based on the stability of the fracture pattern to prevent excessive collapse. In addition to fracture pattern, implant, quality of the bone, and quality the operative reduction all influence the strength of fixation and risk of failure [18].

For intertrochanteric femur fractures, the typical deformity is flexion, shortening, varus, and external rotation. Quality of reduction is critical for stable fixation and using tools such as traction or a fracture table can help correct the above deformities. Varus fixation increases the moment arm on the implant, predisposing to fixation failure. Likewise, varus shortening results in abductor weakness by lengthening the abductor mechanism. Excessive shortening likewise alters hip biomechanics placed at risk of implant cutout. Failure rates have been reported from 9 to 16% [54].

Implant options include traditional extramedullary implants such as sliding hip screws (SHS) and intramedullary implants such as cephalomedullary nails (CMN). Cephalomedullary nails provide the benefit of being a load-sharing implant more closely located to the axis of weight bearing, limiting the amount of femoral neck collapse due to the more medially located nail serving as a buttress effect on the fracture [54–56]. Extramedullary screws rely on the lateral wall to limit compression, so in the setting of lateral wall compromise an intramedullary nail or a side plate is required. Both short and long nails are available. Historically, short nails were associated with higher periprosthetic fracture risk, but improvements have been made to the design of these short CMNs and there is no difference in the complication rate of new short nails compared to long nails in stable fracture patterns [57]. In stable fracture patterns, SHS and CMN have similar outcomes; however CMNs are more expensive [58, 59]. Bridle et al. reported on a series of stable intertrochanteric fractures randomized to SHS versus CMN and found no difference in surgical time, length of stay, mobility, and rate of cutout at 6-month follow-up [60]. In unstable fracture patterns, CMN is required. Failure rates of SHS for unstable fracture patterns are as high as 25% [18]. Reverse obliquity fracture has a high failure rate and fails by medial displacement. While they can have a high failure rate with CMN devices and 95-degree blade plate, not recognizing the instability of this fracture and treating with a SHS result in a 56% failure rate [61] (Fig. 12.3).

Subtrochanteric fractures extend distal to the lesser trochanter and impart instability that is not amenable to fixation with a SHS and requires a trochanteric or femoral reconstruction nail or a

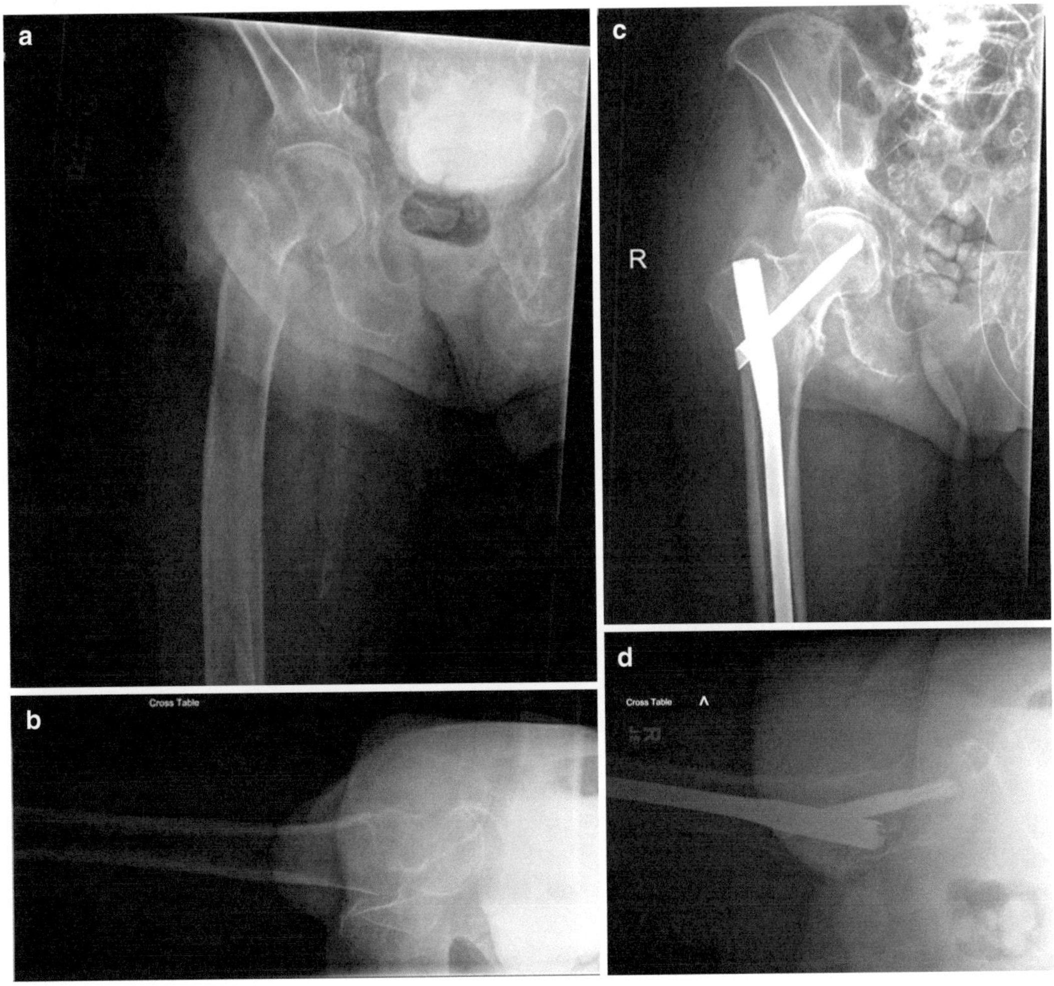

Fig. 12.3 (**a**, **b**) Reverse obliquity peritrochanteric hip fracture. (**c**, **d**) A cephalomedullary nail was selected due to the unstable nature of the fracture pattern

95-degree blade plate. While the identifying factor of the subtrochanteric femur fracture is its distal extension, it can extend up proximally and mimic an intertrochanteric fracture which can lead to incorrect implant selection and subsequent failure [62].

Postoperative Care

Multidisciplinary care with the goal of early mobilization and minimizing complications is becoming the gold standard in geriatric hip fracture patients. Elderly patients are at high risk of postoperative altered mental status and delirium. This is often multifactorial, related to medications, dehydration, baseline dementia, hypoxia, hypoglycemia, and use of restraints. Care should be taken to address underlying causes when possible, provide frequent orientation, maintain day-night cycle, use glasses/hearing aids, and minimize narcotics [63, 64]. Peripheral nerve blocks can help limit narcotic requirements. Seventy percent of hospitalized geriatric patients are at risk or suffer from malnutrition, so identifying this and addressing can help limit malnutrition-related complications, including wound dehiscence, infection, and mortality [65, 66]. Rates of deep vein thrombosis (DVT) have been reported ranging from 30 to 60% in hip fracture [67]. Based on the American College of

Chest Physicians evidence-based clinical practice guidelines, hip fractures should be started on low-molecular-weight heparin within 12 h of surgery and continued for 1 month postoperatively [68]. In the setting of history of syncopal episodes and/or high fall risk, the risk of bleeding event must be considered. Dedicated physical therapy as an inpatient and often discharge to an acute rehab or skilled nursing facility are often required prior to discharge back to independent living situations.

Outcomes

Factors affecting the outcome of femoral neck fractures and peritrochanteric femur factures are dictated by elements intrinsic to the patient including age, sex, past medical history, preinjury functional status, fracture pattern, and then factors related to the treatment including implant selection and rehab protocol.

These fractures have a significant impact on the patient's quality of life. Return to function following hip fracture can be difficult. In one study of hip fractures (femoral neck and peritrochanteric hip fractures) only 57% of patients regained their prefracture functional status and 13% former ambulators were unable to walk [69]. Globally, hip fractures rank in the top ten of causes of disability-adjusted life years lost [71].

Overall, 20% of hip fracture patients die within 1 year of fracture. Compared to age-matched controls, women are at 3.3 times relative risk of death and men are at 4.2 times relative risk [28]. ASA, age, dialysis dependence, obesity, cardiac disease, diabetes, and male sex are all risk factors for mortality following hip fractures. Typically, patients with IT fracture tend to be older and sicker, and have longer hospital stays and worse outcomes at 2 months [70].

Prevention

Given the aging population, prevention is a critical public health concern given the potential socioeconomic burden of hip fractures. Interventions are both nonmedical and medical.

A critical nonmedical intervention is fall prevention. Risk factors for falls include advancing age, weakness, balance problems, visual and cognitive impairment, medication effects, environmental factors, and history of falls. When a fall risk is identified, patient education is key and then taking an interdisciplinary approach to limiting risks including assistive devices, home modifications such as toilet/bed height or shower rails, medication review, gait training, and physical therapy. As most hip fractures are a result of a direct trauma, some have advocated hip protectors which are an orthosis with polypropylene or polyethylene sewn into garments which absorb some of the force in a fall and have been advocated as a simple and cost-effective means of limiting risks [71, 72].

Medical interventions including removing psychotropic medications from patient regimen and unnecessary polypharmacy. Further medical management is focused on combating osteoporosis or secondary causes of osteoporosis. These can include antiresorptive medications such as bisphosphonates, calcium and vitamin D supplementation, estrogen and selective estrogen modulators, calcitonin, and anabolic agents like PTH. Close coordination with primary care physicians and/or endocrinologist can help to combat osteoporosis, and an increased focus on this has been attributed to the downtrending of hip fractures in recent years [73].

While ideally prevention of osteoporosis should be undertaken prior to fracture as a preventive measure, for some patients the first diagnosis of osteoporosis will be at the time of presentation with a fragility fracture. Geriatric hip fracture patients have a high relative risk of second hip fracture, ranging from 2.4 to 5, with 50% occurring within the next 2 years [73–75]. For patients presenting with a fragility fracture, such as a wrist fracture or hip fracture, coordinating programs for osteoporotic workup can decrease likelihood of future fracture and is a cost-effective model [76, 77].

Conclusion

Hip fractures are a complex and life changing event in the geriatric population. Continued efforts and research to improve preventative measures and further randomized controlled trials to improve evidence-based treatment algorithms will be critical in the setting of the aging population.

References

1. Johnell O, Kanis JA. An estimate of the worldwide prevalence and disability associated with osteoporotic fractures. Osteoporos Int. 2006;17:1726–33.
2. American Academy of Orthopaedic Surgeons. Burden of musculoskeletal diseases in the United States: prevalence, societal and economic cost. Rosemont, IL: American Academy of Orthopaedic Surgeons; 2008.
3. Burge R, Dawson-Hughes B, Solomon DH, Wong JB, King A, Tosteson A. Incidence and economic burden of osteoporosis-related fractures in the United States, 2005–2025. J Bone Miner Res. 2007;22(3):465–75.
4. Burge RT, King AB, Balda E, Worley D. Methodology for estimating current and future burden of osteoporosis in state populations: application to Florida in 2000 through 2025. Value Health. 2003;6(5):574–83.
5. Tosteson AN, Burge RT, Marshall DA, Lindsay R. Therapies for treatment of osteoporosis in US women: cost-effectiveness and budget impact considerations. Am J Manag Care. 2008;14(9):605–15.
6. Brown CA, Starr AZ, Nunley JA. Analysis of past secular trends of hip fractures and predicted number in the future 2010–2050. J Orthop Trauma. 2012;26(2):117–22.
7. Wolf JM, Cannada L, Van Heest AE, O'Connor MI, Ladd AL. Male and female differences in musculoskeletal disease. J Am Acad Orthop Surg. 2015;23(6):339–47.
8. Kanis JA, Johnell O, De Laet C, Jonsson B, Oden A, Ogelsby AK. International variations in hip fracture probabilities: implications for risk assessment. J Bone Miner Res. 2002;17:1237–44.
9. Ricci WM, Ostrum RF. Orthopaedic knowledge update: trauma. 5th ed. Rosemont, IL: AAOS; 2016.
10. Jordan KM, Cooper C. Epidemiology of osteoporosis. Best Pract Res Clin Rheumatol. 2002;16(5):795–806.
11. Trueta J, Harrison MHM. The normal vascular anatomy of the femoral head in adult man. J Bone Joint Surg Br. 1953;35:442–61.
12. Konishiike T, Makihata E, Tago H, et al. Acute fracture of the neck of the femur. An assessment of perfusion of the head by dynamic MRI. J Bone Joint Surg Br. 1999;81:596–9.
13. Takeuchi T, Shidou T. Impairment of blood supply to the head of the femur after fracture of the neck. Int Orthop. 1993;17:325–9.
14. Garden RS. Low-angle fixation in fractures of the femoral neck. J Bone Joint Surg Br. 1961;43-B:647–63.
15. Pauwels F. Der schenkelhalsbruch ein mechanisches problem: Grund- lagen des Haeilungsvorganges Prognose und kausale Therapie. Stutt- gart: Ferdinand Enke Verlag; 1935.
16. Kaplan K, Miyamoto R, Levine BR, Egol KA, Zuckerman JD. Hip fractures. An evidence-based review of the literature II: intertrochanteric fractures. J Am Acad Orthop Surg. 2008;16(11):665–73.
17. Egol KA, Marcano AI, Lewis L, Tejwani NC, McLaurin TM, Davidovitch RI. Can the use of an evidence based algorithm for the treatment of intertrochanteric fracture of the hip maintain quality at a reduced cost? Bone Joint J. 2014;960B(9):1192–7.
18. Templeman D, Baumgaertner MR, Leighton RK, Lindsey RW, Moed BR. Reducing complications in the surgical treatment of intertrochanteric fractures. AAOS Instr Course Lect Trauma. 2006;12:187–93.
19. Shmidt AH, Asnis SE, Haidukewych GJ, Koval KJ, Thorngren KG. Femoral neck fractures. AAOS Instr Course Lect Trauma. 2006;11:157–85.
20. Grigoryan KV, Javedan H, Rudolph J. Orthogeriatric care models and outcomes in hip fracture patients: a systematic review and meta-analysis. J Orthop Trauma. 2014;28(3):e49–55.
21. Zuckerman JD, Sakales SR, Fabian DR, Frankel VH. Hip fractures in geriatric patients. Results of an interdisciplinary hospital care program. Clin Orthop Relat Res. 1992;274:213–25.
22. Friedman SM, Mendelson DA, Kates SL, McCann RM. Geriatric co-management of proximal femoral fracture: total quality management and protocol-driven care result in better outcomes for a frail patient population. J Am Ger Soc. 2008;56(7):1349–56.
23. McGuire KJ, Bernstein J, Polsky D, Silber JH. The 2004 Marshall Urist award: delays until surgery after hip fracture increases mortality. Clin Orthop Relat Res. 2004;428:294–301.
24. Ryan DJ, Yoshihara H, Yoneoka D, Egol KA, Zuckerman JD. Delay in hip fracture surgery: an analysis of patient-specific and hospital-specific risk factors. J Orthop Trauma. 2015;29(8):343–8.
25. Bernstein J, Roberts FO, Wiess BB, Ahn J. Preoperative testing for hip fracture patients delay surgery, prolong hospital stays, and rarely dictate care. J Orthop Trauma. 2016;30(2):78–80.
26. Stitgen A, Pludnianyk K, Dulaney-Cripe E, Markert R, Prayson M. Adherence to preoperative cardiac clearance guidelines in hip fracture patients. J Orthop Trauma. 2015;29:500–3.
27. Radcliff TA, Henderson WG, Stoner TJ, Khuri SF, Dohm M, Hutt E. Patient risk factors, operative care, and outcomes among older community-dwelling male veterans with hip fractures. J Bone Joint Surg Am. 2008;90(1):34–42.
28. Anglen JO, Baumgaertner MR, Smith WR, Tornetta P, Ziran BH. Technical tips in fracture care: fractures of the hip. AAOS Instr Course Lect Trauma. 2008;57:17–24.
29. Koval KJ, Zuckerman JD. Hip fractures: 1. Overview and evaluation and treatment of femoral neck fractures. J Am Acad Orthop Surg. 1994;2:141–9.

30. Bjorgul K, Reikeras O. Outcome of undisplaced and moderately displaced femoral neck fractures. Acta Orthop. 2007;78(4):498–504.
31. Maurer SG, Wright KE, Kummer FJ, et al. Two or three screws for fixation of femoral neck fractures? Am J Orthop (Belle Mead NJ). 2003;32:438–42.
32. Zdero R, Keast-Butler O, Schemitsch EH. A biomechanical comparison of two triple-screw methods for femoral neck fracture fixation in a synthetic bone model. J Trauma. 2010;69:1537–44.
33. Selvan VT, Oakley MJ, Rangan A, et al. Optimum configuration of cannulated hip screws for the fixation of intracapsular hip fractures: a biomechanical study. Injury. 2004;35:136–41.
34. Papanastassiou ID, Mavrogenis AF, Kokkalis ZT, et al. Fixation of femoral neck fractures using divergent versus parallel cannulated screws. J Long-Term Eff Med Implants. 2011;21:63–9.
35. Walker E, Mukherjee DP, Ogden AL, et al. A biomechanical study of simulated femoral neck fracture fixation by cannulated screws: effects of placement angle and number of screws. Am J Orthop (Belle Mead NJ). 2007;36:680–4.
36. Aminian A, Gao F, Fedoriw WW, Zhang LQ, Kalainov DM, Merk BR. Vertically oriented femoral neck fractures: mechanical analysis of four fixation techniques. J Orthop Trauma. 2007;21(8):544–8.
37. FAITH Investigators. Fixation using alternative implants for the treatment of hip fractures (FAITH): design and rationale for a multi-centre randomized trial comparing sliding hip screws and cancellous screws on revision surgery rates and quality of life in the treatment of femoral neck fractures. BMC Musculoskelet Disord. 2014;15:219.
38. Gjertsen JE, Fevang JM, Matre K, Vinje T, Engesaeter LB. Clinical outcome after undisplaced femoral neck fractures. Acta Orthop. 2011;82(3):268–74.
39. Skinner P, Riley D, Ellery J, et al. Displaced subcapital fractures of the femur: a prospective randomized comparison of internal fixation, hemiarthroplasty and total hip replacement. Injury. 1989;20:291–3.
40. Heetveld MJ, Rogmark C, Frihagen F, et al. Internal fixation versus arthroplasty for displaced femoral neck fractures: what is the evidence? J Orthop Trauma. 2009;23:395–402.
41. Blomfeldt R, Tornkvist H, Ponzer S, Soderqvist A, Tidermark J. Comparison of internal fixation with total hip replacement for displaced femoral neck fractures: randomized, controlled trial performed at four years. J Bone Joint Surg Am. 2005;87A(8):1680–8.
42. Masson M, Parker MJ, Fleischer S. Internal fixation versus arthroplasty for intracapsular proximal femoral fractures in adults. Cochrane Database Syst Rev. 2003;2:CD0017808.
43. Wang J, Jiang B, Marshal RJ, Zhang P. Arthroplasty or internal fixation for displaced femoral neck fracture: which is the optimal alternative for elderly patients? A meta-analysis. Int Orthop. 2009;33:1179–87.
44. Roberts KC, Brox WT, Jevsevar DS, Sevarino K. AAOS clinical practice guidelines summary: management of hip fractures in the elderly. JAAOS. 2015;23(2):138–40.
45. Langslet E, Fihagen F, Opland V, Madsen JE, Nordsletten L, Figved W. Cemented versus uncemented hemiarthroplasty for displaced femoral neck fractures: 5-year follow-up of randomized controlled trial. Clin Orthop Relat Res. 2014;472:1291–9.
46. Gjertsen JE, Lie SA, Vinje T, Engesaeter LB, Hallan G, Matre K, Furnes O. More re-operations after uncemented than cemented hemiarthroplasty used in the treatment of displaced fractures of the femoral neck: an observational study of 11,116 hemi- arthroplasties from a national register. J Bone Joint Surg Br. 2012;94:1113–9.
47. Taylor F, Wright M, Zhu M. Hemiarthroplasty of the hip with and without cement: a randomized clinical trial. J Bone Joint Surg Am. 2012;94:577–83.
48. Leighton RK, Schmidt AH, Collier P, Trask K. Advances in the treatment of intracapsular hip fractures in the elderly. Injury. 2007;38(Suppl 3):524–34.
49. Unger AC, Dirksen B, Renken FG, Wilde E, Willkomm M, Schulz AP. Treatment of femoral neck fracture with a minimal invasive surgical approach for hemiarthroplasty-clinical and radiological results in 180 geriatric patients. Open Orthop J. 2014;8:225–31.
50. Burgers PT, Van Geene AR, Van den Bekerom MP, et al. Total hip arthroplasty versus hemiarthoplasty for displaced femoral neck fracture in healthy elderly: a meta-analysis and systematic review of randomized trials. Int Orthop. 2012;36(8):1549–60.
51. Zi-Sheng A, You-Shui G, Zhi-Zhen J, Ting Y, Chang-Qing Z. Hemiarthroplasty vs primary total hip arthroplasty for displaced fractures of the femoral neck in the elderly: a meta-analysis. J Arthroplast. 2012;27(4):583–90.
52. Carroll C, Stevenson M, Scope A, et al. Hemiarthroplasty and total hip arthroplasty for treating primary intracapsular fracture of the hip: a systematic review and cost-effectiveness analysis. Health Technol Assess. 2011;15:1–74.
53. Egol KA, Koval KJ, Kummer F, Frankel VH. Stress fractures of the femoral neck. Clin Orthop Relat Res. 1998;348:72–8.
54. Adams CI, Robinson CM, Court-Brown CM, McQueen MM. Prospective randomized controlled trial of an intramedullary nail versus dynamic screw and plate for intertrochanteric fractures of the femur. J Orthop Trauma. 2001;15(6):394–400.
55. Curtis MJ, Jinnah RH, Wilson V, Cunningham BW. Proximal femoral fractures: a biomechanical study to compare intramedullary and extramedullary fixation. Injury. 1994;25(2):99–104.
56. Reindle R, Harve EJ, Berry GK, Rahme EL. Intramedullary versus extramedullary fixation for unstable intertrochanteric femur fractures. J Bone Joint Surg Am. 2015;97:1905–12.

57. Boone C, Carlberg KN, Koueiter DM, et al. Short versus long intramedullary nails for treatment of intertrochanteric femur fracture (OTA 31-A1 and A2). J Orthop Trauma. 2014;28(5):e96–e100.
58. Radford PJ, Needoff M, Webb JK. A prospective randomised comparison of the dynamic hip screw and the gamma locking nail. J Bone Joint Surg Br. 1993;75:789–93.
59. Saudan M, Lübbeke A, Sadowski C, Riand N, Stern R, Hoffmeyer P. Pertrochanteric fractures: is there an ad- vantage to an intramedullary nail? A randomized, prospective study of 206 patients comparing the dynamic hip screw and proximal femoral nail. J Orthop Trauma. 2002;16:386–93.
60. Bridle SH, Patel AD, Bircher M, Calvert PT. Fixation of intertrochanteric fractures of the femur: a randomized prospective comparison of the gamma nail and the dynamic hip screw. J Bone Joint Surg Br. 1991;73:330–4.
61. Haidukewych GJ, Israel TA, Berry DJ. Reverse obliquity fractures of the intertrochanteric region of the femur. J Bone Joint Surg Am. 2001;83:643–50.
62. Lundy DA. Subtrochanteric Femoral Fractures. J Am Acad Orthop Surg. 2007;15:663–71.
63. Inouye SK, Zhang Y, Jones RN, Kiely DK, Yang F, Marcantonio ER. Risk factors for delirium at discharge: development and validation of a predictive model. Arch Intern Med. 2007;167:1406–13.
64. Schlitzkus LL, Melin AA, Johanning JM, Schenarts PJ. Perioperative Management of elderly patients. Surg Clin North Am. 2015;95(2):391–415.
65. Wallace JI, Schwartz RS, LaCroix AZ, Uhlmann RF, Perlman RA. Involuntary weight loss in older outpatients: incidence and clinical significance. J Am Geriatr Soc. 1995;43(4):329–37.
66. Koval KJ, Maurer SG, Su ET, Aharanoff GB, Zuckerman JD. The effect of nutritional status on outcome after hip fracture. J Orthop Trauma. 1999;13(3):164–9.
67. Ennis RS. Postoperative deep vein thrombosis prophylaxis: a retrospective analysis in 1000 consecutive hip fracture patients treated in a community hospital setting. J South Orthop Assoc. 2003;12(1):10–7.
68. Falck-Ytter Y, Francis CW, Johanson NA, Curley C, Dahl OE, Schulman S, Ortel TL, Pauker SG, Colwell CW Jr, American College of Chest Physicians. Prevention o VTE in orthopedic surgery patients: antithrombotic therapy and prevention of thrombosis, 9th ed: American College of Chest Physicians Evidence-Based Clinical Practice Guidelines. Chest. 2012;141(2 Suppl):e278S–325S.
69. Mariconda M, Costa GG, Cerbasi S, Recano P, Orabona G, Bambacorta M, Misasi M. Factors predicting mobility and the change in activities of daily living after hip fracture: a 1 year prospective Cohort Study. J Orthop Trauma. 2016;30(2):71–7.
70. Clyburn TA, Heydemann JA. Fall prevention in the elderly: analysis and comprehensive review of methods used in hospital and in home. J Am Acad Orthop Surg. 2011;19:402–9.
71. Lin JT, Lane JM. Prevention of hip fractures: medical and nonmedical management. AAOS Instr Course Lect Trauma. 2006;13:195–203.
72. Center JR, Bliuc D, Nguyen TV, et al. Risk of subsequent fracture after low-trauma fracture in men and women. JAMA. 2007;297:387–94.
73. Klotzbuecher CM, Ross PD, Landsman PB, et al. Patients with prior fractures have an increased risk of future fractures: a summary of the literature and statistical synthesis. J Bone Miner Res. 2000;15:721–39.
74. Schroder HM, Petersen KK, Erlandsen M. Occurrence and incidence of the second hip fracture. Clin Orthop. 1993;289:166–9.
75. Majumdar SR, Johnson JA, Lier DA, et al. Persistence, reproducibility, and cost-effectiveness of an intervention to improve the quality of osteoporosis care after a fracture of the wrist: results of a controlled trial. Osteoporos Int. 2007;18:261–70.
76. Maetzel A, Sander B, Elliot-Gibson V, et al. Targeting fragility fractures in an orthopaedic treatment unit: cost effectiveness of a dedicated coordinator. J Bone Miner Res. 2004;19:S319.
77. Cooper C, Campion G, Melton LJ. Hip fractures in the elderly: a world-wide projection. Osteoporos Int. 1992;2:285–9.
78. Fox KM, Magaziner J, Hebel JR, Kensora JE, Kashner TM. Intertrochanteric versus femoral neck hip fracture: differential characteristics, treatment, and sequelae. J Gerontol. 1999;54(12):M635–40.

13 Geriatric Acetabulum Fractures

Daniel T. Altman and Edward R. Westrick

Introduction

Acetabular fractures in the elderly are estimated to account for 10–20% of all osteoporotic pelvis fractures and represent the fastest growing segment of pelvic trauma [1].

The incidence of acetabular fractures in the Medicare population alone has increased by 29% since 1998 [2]. As the population ages, this number will likely continue to grow. Although age older than 60 years was defined as a contraindication to surgery in Judet and Letournel's 1964 text [3], this was redacted in their second edition in 1981 [4]. Devastating functional results have been demonstrated with nonoperative management involving bedrest or traction [5, 6]. Today, the majority of patients benefit from operative management due to the inherent instability of their fractures and the need for mobilization. That being said, treatment is decided on a case-by-case basis depending on patients' overall functional status, with the ultimate goal of early mobilization. Although mortality rates following acetabular fractures have improved over the past 25 years, recent studies show 1-year mortality of approximately 16% [7] and 5-year mortality of 29.5% [8], thereby demonstrating the devastating nature of these injuries and the need for timely and accurate diagnosis and treatment. There is not much literature available to determine the proper treatment of acetabulum fractures in the geriatric population; however, options continue to expand.

Mechanism

In contrast to younger patients, geriatric acetabulum fractures frequently result from low-energy mechanisms. In their 2010 study, Ferguson et al. [9] reported that 49.8% of their geriatric study population sustained their injury in a fall. Only 37.4% of fractures resulted from a motor vehicle accident, in contrast to 66% in their younger population. Because of this difference in mechanisms, only 29.8% of the geriatric population had an associated injury, compared to 49.1% of the younger study population.

Fall from standing height causes a direct impact on the greater trochanter, which displaces the femoral head medially into pelvis, causing impaction of the anterior column and quadrilateral plate. The femoral head then medializes to the anterior column and impacts the posteromedial portion of the roof [10, 11]. As a result, anterior column, associated both column, and anterior column/posterior

D.T. Altman, M.D. (✉) • E.R. Westrick, M.D.
Department of Orthopaedic Surgery, Drexel University College of Medicine, Allegheny General Hospital, Allegheny Health Network, 1307 Federal Street, 2nd floor, Pittsburgh, PA 15212, USA
e-mail: daltman@wpahs.org; Altmangregory@hotmail.com; ewestric@wpahs.org; edward.westrick@ahn.org

A. Rodriguez et al. (eds.), *Geriatric Trauma and Acute Care Surgery*,
https://doi.org/10.1007/978-3-319-57403-5_13

hemitransverse with medial protrusion of the femoral head are the most common fracture patterns [9]. Posterior wall fractures are uncommon and are associated with posterior hip dislocations. Posterior column fractures are similarly uncommon due to the comparatively good bone quality of the column [9].

Due to osteoporosis and poor bone quality, geriatric acetabulum fractures tend to be highly comminuted and demonstrate metaphyseal impaction [12]. Marginal impaction of either the anteromedial or the posteromedial joint surfaces is common, occurring in about 40–56% of fractures [9, 13]. The "gull sign" was described by Anglen et al. [14] and represents impaction of a portion of the subchondral bone of the anteromedial roof into the osteopenic supporting bone. This results from medial displacement of the femoral head, causing central or superior dome impaction. In their paper, Anglen et al. had a 100% rate of fixation failure in patients demonstrating this radiographic finding. Although further studies have improved this percentage [14], it remains a harbinger of poor outcome [13]. Comminution of the posterior wall with more than three fragments is also an indicator of early fixation failure [9, 15]. Zha et al. [15] had early loss of reduction in 33% of patients. Although reduction was able to be achieved initially, multiple fracture fragments made maintenance of reduction difficult. Posterior dislocation of the hip, femoral head impaction, and quadrilateral plate fracture are also negative indicators of successful fracture fixation [1].

Diagnosis

AP and Judet radiographs of the pelvis should be obtained in all geriatric patients presenting with hip or groin pain [16]. However, poor bone quality can decrease the diagnostic capability of radiographs, and CT scan should be used if clinical suspicion exists [17]. Schicho et al. [18] diagnosed 15 acetabular fractures with CT scan that had previously been missed on plain radiographs. If clinical suspicion remains after negative CT scan, MRI should be obtained. Henes et al. [19] demonstrated 100% sensitivity and specificity in MRI diagnosis of acetabular fractures, whereas CT demonstrated 100% specificity and 96.4% sensitivity for left-sided fractures and 68.8% for right-sided fractures.

Although associated injuries are not as common in geriatric patients, a full primary and secondary survey should be obtained. Fractures resulting from a low-energy mechanism such as a fall should be regarded as fragility fractures and an appropriate workup consisting of vitamin D levels, detection of secondary causes of osteoporosis, and an inpatient DEXA scan for baseline bone mineral density should be performed [20].

Initial Management

Once initial primary and secondary surveys have been completed in accordance with ATLS principles, management should focus on stabilization of the patient, prevention of injury propagation, and prompt medical risk stratification and optimization. Initial priority is given to the overall hemodynamic stability and resuscitation of the elderly patient. Oftentimes, although appearing to be hemodynamically stable, elderly patients can be subclinically under-resuscitated, with depleted intravascular volume.

Close evaluation of the radiographs will guide decision making for the best way to initially stabilize the injury. Continued cartilage impaction or joint instability calls for skeletal traction to avoid further displacement, cartilage abrasion, and vascular compromise to the femoral head, and to aid in patient comfort.

Early and aggressive involvement of a medical team is also a key factor to a successful outcome. A thorough medical, surgical, and social history will allow for risk stratification and better treatment and decision making. A comprehensive medical evaluation including standard labs (chemistry, complete blood count, coagulation profile), EKG, and a preoperative chest radiograph in conjunction with appropriate involvement of cardiac, pulmonary, renal consultation will aid in the medical optimization for the patient.

Treatment

The goals of treatment of geriatric acetabular fractures are as follows:

1. Early mobilization and pain control to prevent complications of bedrest
2. Optimization of hip joint function
3. Minimizing of complications from surgical or nonsurgical treatment [21]

A full history and physical examination should be completed with a focus on the patient's associated injuries, medical history, prior ambulatory and functional status, living situation, and history of arthritic hip pain prior to medical decision making [2].

Pagenkopf et al. [22] created an algorithm for acetabulum surgery in the older adult, which they defined as age over 50.

Copied from Carroll, Eben A., et al. "Treatment of acetabular fractures in an older population." *Journal of Orthopaedic Trauma* 24.10 (2010): 637–644.

There still exists considerable inconsistency in the treatment of displaced geriatric acetabular fractures. Significant site variation was demonstrated in a study of 15 US level I trauma centers participating in the Major Extremity Trauma Research Consortium (METRC) [23]. Sixty percent (162/269) of patients 60 years or older were surgically treated, with age younger than 80, high-energy mechanism, femoral head impaction, and incongruity of the hip joint significantly associated with receiving operative treatment.

Nonoperative Treatment

Nonoperative treatment may be indicated in both column fractures exhibiting secondary congruence. Because all fracture fragments are separated from the intact ilium, they settle around the femoral head, with the head acting as a template to

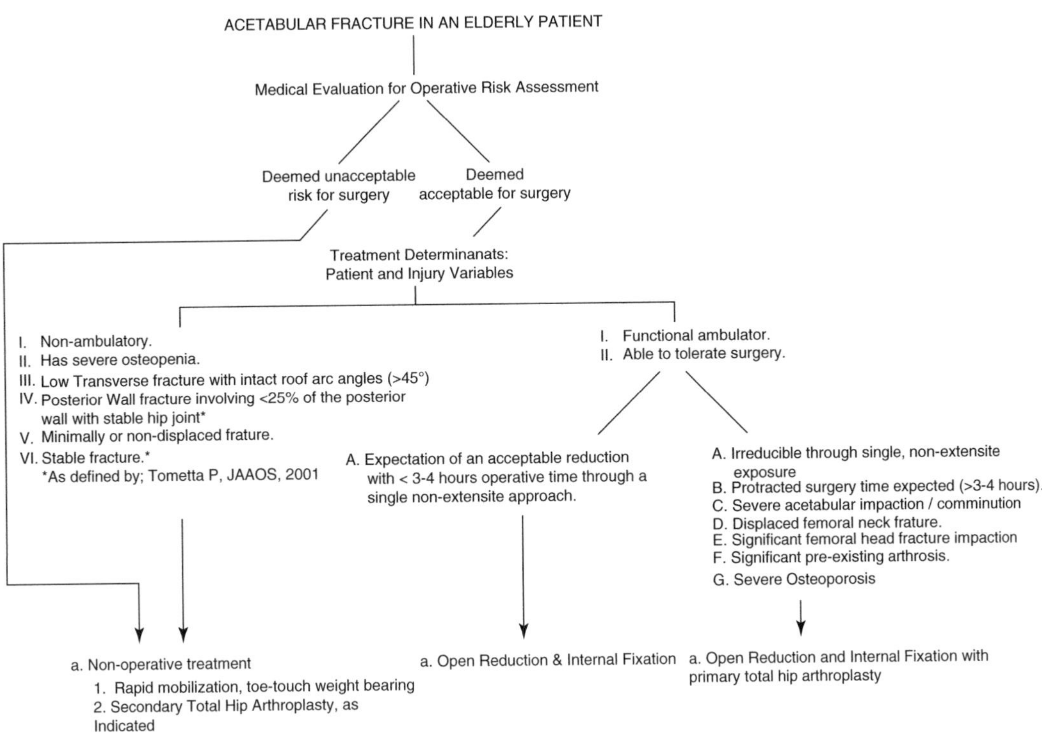

produce an acceptable hip joint [24]. Nonoperative management may also be trialed in fractures that simultaneously meet all of the following criteria: less than 2 mm of displacement, an intact roof arc angle of 45°, intact subchondral ring, involvement of less than 20% of the posterior wall, stability of the hip joint, and preservation of the hip joint [6, 25, 26]. In addition, nonoperative management is preferred and generally necessary for patients who are medically unfit for surgery or functionally incapacitated. Butterwick's protocol for nonoperative patients [26] involved a short period of bedrest for pain control followed by toe-touch weight bearing for 6 weeks with subsequent progression to full weight bearing. Deep-vein thrombosis prophylaxis was recommended until the patient is fully weight bearing.

Minimally Invasive (Percutaneous) Fixation

Due to the extensive exposure and subsequent large blood loss with open procedures, methods have been developed to perform a more minimally invasive approach to acetabulum fractures. Percutaneous fixation was first described by Starr et al. in 1998 [27] as an adjunct to open fixation. Indications have expanded since then and percutaneous fixation can now be used either as a stand-alone procedure or in conjunction with other procedures such as open reduction or total hip arthroplasty. Percutaneous fixation can be used for any column fractures, but posterior wall fractures are contraindicated [28]. Reduction may need to be obtained using either percutaneously placed clamps or a limited open approach. In general, percutaneous acetabular fixation is best for minimally displaced, potentially unstable fractures involving a single-column (posterior or anterior), anterior column posterior hemitransverse fractures, or transverse-type fractures. This technique may also be used to preserve bone stock and serve as a temporizing surgery prior to total hip arthroplasty in patients unable to undergo arthroplasty acutely [29]. Disadvantages of minimally invasive fixation include limited access to the fracture site with subsequent decreased ability to adequately reduce the fracture and apply stable implants. Screw purchase in osteoporotic bone is unpredictable and the procedure is technically challenging, with narrow safe zones for screw placement and potential for hemorrhage or neurologic injury with improper placement [30].

At our institution, we use the method for percutaneous fixation described by Starr et al. [27]. To place a posterior column screw, the hip and knee are positioned in flexion with the hip in slight external rotation to decrease tension on the sciatic nerve [31]. The central or medial portion of the ischial tuberosity is used as a starting point for the cannulated screw guidewire; this wire is then drilled cephalad up the posterior column. Iliac and obturator radiographs are used to ensure intraosseous placement. Once the wire has been appropriately positioned, the outer cortex of the ischial tuberosity is drilled and the correct length partially threaded 6.5 or 7.3 mm screw is inserted, ensuring that all threads cross the fracture site.

Anterior column screws can be placed in an antegrade (cephalad to caudad) or retrograde (caudad to cephalad) manner [32]. For retrograde placement, a mini-Pfannenstiel incision is made proximal to the pubic symphysis and the cannulated screw guidewire is inserted through the ipsilateral pubic tubercle, aimed posterior and inferior to the anterior inferior iliac spine. The wire is then passed cephalad up the superior pubic ramus. Inlet iliac oblique radiographs are obtained to ensure that the guidewire does not penetrate the inner cortex of the ramus, and outlet obturator oblique radiographs are used to prevent penetration of the hip joint. Following appropriate wire placement, the outer cortex is again drilled and the correct size 6.5 or 7.3 mm partially threaded cannulated screw is advanced, again ensuring that all threads cross the fracture site.

For antegrade screws, the starting point is at the junction of a line drawn along the lateral border of the femur through the greater trochanter and a line from the pubic symphysis through the anterior inferior iliac spine [28]. The guidewire is then passed down the superior pubic ramus to the pubic symphysis. Again, frequent inlet iliac oblique and outlet obturator oblique radiographs are obtained before the outer cortex is drilled and the correct size partially threaded screw inserted.

A study by Gary et al. [33] showed a 25% conversion rate to total hip arthroplasty (THA) at a mean time of 1.4 years, with no statistically significant difference between percutaneous and open procedures. These results were corroborated in 2012 [34], where again functional outcomes and rates of conversion to total hip arthroplasty in patients treated with percutaneous fixation were not significantly different from patients treated with formal open reduction internal fixation. This was likely because elderly patients generally tolerate slight malalignment of the hip joint better due to lower functional demands and better pain tolerance as well as reluctance to undergo further surgery.

Open Reduction Internal Fixation

Open reduction and internal fixation (ORIF) through an open approach remains the treatment of choice for markedly displaced fractures and gross incongruency of the hip joint [35]. In fractures demonstrating marginal impaction, an open reduction is necessary to improve reduction and preserve hip joint function [36]. Malreduction has been shown to contribute to poor results and early conversion to total hip arthroplasty in several studies [15, 37, 38]. However, open reduction internal fixation is challenging in elderly patients as it necessitates a larger exposure with potential for greater blood loss and neurovascular damage. In addition, previous hernia repair, abdominal surgery, or prostate or bladder surgery can cause scarring in the areas of planned incisions. Because of this, limited incision approaches have been trialed [12, 39–41].

Almost any fracture pattern involving the anterior column may be approached via either an ilioinguinal or Stoppa approach. Fractures involving the posterior wall or isolated posterior column require a Kocher-Langenbeck approach [42]. In fractures involving the anterior column with displacement of the quadrilateral plate, the Stoppa approach provides direct access and visualization of these fragments. Comparison of the full ilioinguinal and Stoppa approaches demonstrated statistically significant rates of acceptable reduction in the Stoppa group as well as shorter operative time. No difference was detected in the frequency of postoperative complications, which consisted mainly of surgical site infections and nerve palsy [43]. LaFlamme et al. [12] reported their results with a combined Stoppa and lateral window of the ilioinguinal approach in patients over age 60 with an acute displaced fracture of the anterior column. Significant loss of reduction was seen in two patients; however, the majority had a good functional outcome. Limited use of the ilioinguinal approach involving only the lateral two windows has also been used successfully. Jeffcoat et al. [40] reported on their results in patients over age 55 treated using this approach. In their analysis of fractures of the anterior column cephalad to the midportion of the pubic ramus, the limited incision group had shorter operative time and decreased blood loss but no difference in functional outcome or quality of reduction when compared to fractures treated with the full ilioinguinal approach.

Once the approach of choice has been performed, reduction begins with disimpaction of the medialized femoral head using traction via a proximal femoral Schanz pin. Reduction and fixation of high anterior column fractures can then be completed through the lateral ilioinguinal window. Internal rotation of the anterior column is usually needed to correct the deformity. The impacted roof segments should be disimpacted via a bone tamp placed through a cortical window [26]. Regarding fixation, implant failure with plates and screws is more common in the elderly patient, as deterioration of cortical and trabecular bone with aging and osteoporosis causes reduction in construct strength [44]. Lag screws alone are inadequate in osteoporotic bone. Neutralization plates are required for column fixation and buttress plates are necessary for wall fractures. Although locking implants are typically used in osteoporotic bone, their use is limited in pelvic fractures due to the need for variable angle screw placement and contouring of plates.

Peter [45] described his experience with buttress plating of the quadrilateral surface to prevent medial displacement in older patients. He used an overcontoured 7–10 hole 3.5 mm reconstruction plate with an angle of approximately 80° positioned perpendicularly across the pelvic brim. He did not have any early or late implant failures in his series. Archdeacon et al. [46] treated 38 patients aged 70 and older with protrusion-type fractures with an infrapectineal buttress plate and a pelvic brim plate. Twenty patients had an anatomic reduction, 14 had an imperfect reduction, and 4 had a poor reduction on plain radiographs. None sustained early loss of fixation. At 12 months postoperatively, five patients had received a total hip arthroplasty.

O'Toole et al. [47] examined the rate of conversion of ORIF to THA. Twenty-eight percent of patients treated initially with ORIF required conversion at an average of 2.2 years following their index procedure. There were no statistically significant radiographic differences between patients who required conversion and those who did not.

Total Hip Arthroplasty

When fractures are associated with poor bone quality, articular comminution, femoral head impaction, and injury to the weight bearing dome, achieving satisfactory reduction and stable fixation may not be possible [48]. Acute THA is generally beneficial in patients with severe nonreconstructible comminution related to poor bone density, femoral head lesions, impaction fractures consisting of greater than 40% of the dome, femoral head and/or neck fractures, and preexisting severe degenerative arthritis [49]. Acute THA allows for immediate full weight bearing and reduces the occurrence of delayed surgery for posttraumatic onset of osteoarthritis [50]. However, it is a technically demanding procedure with potential for large blood loss, infection, dislocation, and neurologic damage. Another challenge is achieving acetabular component stability. The uncontained acetabular fragments preclude effective cement pressurization or press-fit cementless fixation of the acetabular component. In addition, there is limited contact surface between the acetabular component and the host hip bone [51]. This has led to early radiographic loosening in up to 21% of cases [52]. As a result, several ancillary techniques have been trialed, including antiprotrusion cages, cable fixation, plate fixation, and cup-cage constructs [50–52].

ORIF and THA

The "combined hip procedure" involves operative stabilization of an acetabular fracture followed by acute placement of a total hip arthroplasty. When fracture comminution is associated with osteopenia, achieving adequate bone stock for a subsequent total hip arthroplasty may be difficult. Fracture fixation increases the available surface area for fixation of the acetabular cup [1]. It is a technically difficult procedure that is often performed with both a trauma surgeon and an arthroplasty surgeon. There is potential for high transfusion rates, lengthy anesthesia times, and technical difficulties even in experienced hands [50]. Rickman et al. [53] reported their results with 24 patients treated with the combined hip procedure. In 20 patients, the anterior column was stabilized initially through a modified Stoppa approach before the posterior column was stabilized through a Kocher-Langenbeck approach and a THA performed. The remaining four patients were treated exclusively through a Kocher-Langenbeck approach. They allowed full weight bearing postoperatively. Radiographically, no component migration was seen in any patient at 1-year follow-up. There was one case of superficial wound infection, one symptomatic deep venous thrombosis, and one inpatient death from myocardial infarction. Boraiah et al. [48] had similar results in their study using ORIF and THA through the Kocher-Langenbeck approach. Osteotomy of the femoral neck and excision of the femoral head were performed before ORIF of the displaced column fractures. Femoral head autograft was used to augment the posterior wall prior to acetabular component implantation. Patients were touchdown weight bearing for 8 weeks and allowed to weight bear as tolerated 12 weeks after the surgery. One patient who developed superficial wound infection was successfully treated with antibiotics. One patient required revision of the THA 3 weeks after the index surgery due to recurrent hip dislocation. At the time of final follow-up, there was no radiographic evidence of loosening of the acetabular component. One uncemented femoral stem showed osteolysis but no subsidence.

Cup-Cage Construct

In cases involving an associated both column acetabular fracture or acetabular protrusion, the small contact area can preclude almost any form of fixation. Because cup-cage constructs have been successfully used for cases of pelvic discontinuity, they have also been trialed as an alternative to ORIF [54–56]. Solomon et al. [51] used an oversized acetabular component with screws inserted only into the ilium and a cup-cage construct with femoral head autograft. Postoperatively all patients were allowed to weight bear as tolerated. Using radiostereometric analysis at 1 year postsurgery, they noted that 33% of acetabular components developed proximal migration or sagittal rotations above the suggested limits of migration for primary THA. As a result, they added screw fixation of the acetabular component to the ischial tuberosity and the superior pubic ramus to increase the surface contact area.

Delayed THA

Converting an initial procedure to an arthroplasty is a difficult procedure, as is performing an arthroplasty for posttraumatic arthrosis from failed nonoperative treatment. These situations should not be undertaken lightly, as there are many obstacles. Scarring, heterotopic bone, retained hardware, acetabular deformity, acetabular nonunion, potential deep infection, and osteonecrosis of the femoral head [57] are all frequently reported complications. Additionally, arthroplasty remains challenging due to difficulty with fixation of the acetabular components [1]. However, arthroplasty may be necessary in patients with failed fixation or intractable pain from arthrosis.

Schnaser et al. [58] reviewed 17 patients with acetabulum fractures who went on to require a total hip replacement. Thirteen fractures were initially treated by ORIF, three were treated nonoperatively, and one was treated with an acute THA. Eleven of the 17 failures occurred within 5 years of fixation. One patient in the nonoperative group underwent THA 18 months after injury. Following revision surgery, they noted that the procedure was more challenging with a higher rate of complications and more blood loss when compared with a primary THA. Two patients dislocated in the immediate postoperative period, with one requiring revision acutely. When compared with controls, patients who had THA after an acetabular fracture had significantly higher musculoskeletal function assessment scores and significantly lower Harris hip scores, indicative of worse functional level.

Morison et al. [59] also reported worse results in patients requiring a delayed THA. The 10-year survivorship of the prosthesis was lower in patients with a previous acetabular fracture than in the matched cohort. There were no differences in the 10-year implant survival rate for those patients whose acetabular fracture was initially treated nonoperatively and those treated with initial ORIF. Patients with previous acetabular fractures also had a higher likelihood of developing infection, dislocation, or heterotopic ossification following total hip arthroplasty.

Conclusion

As the population continues to age, acetabulum fractures in the geriatric population will likely continue to increase in frequency. Due to the devastating nature of this injury, not only is appropriate treatment necessary, but also prevention of further fragility fractures. Geriatric acetabular fractures demonstrate different fracture patterns and fracture characteristics compared to acetabular fractures in younger patients and should be treated differently. Although nonoperative management remains a possibility, there are many options for surgical treatment of these fractures that should be weighed on a case-by-case basis.

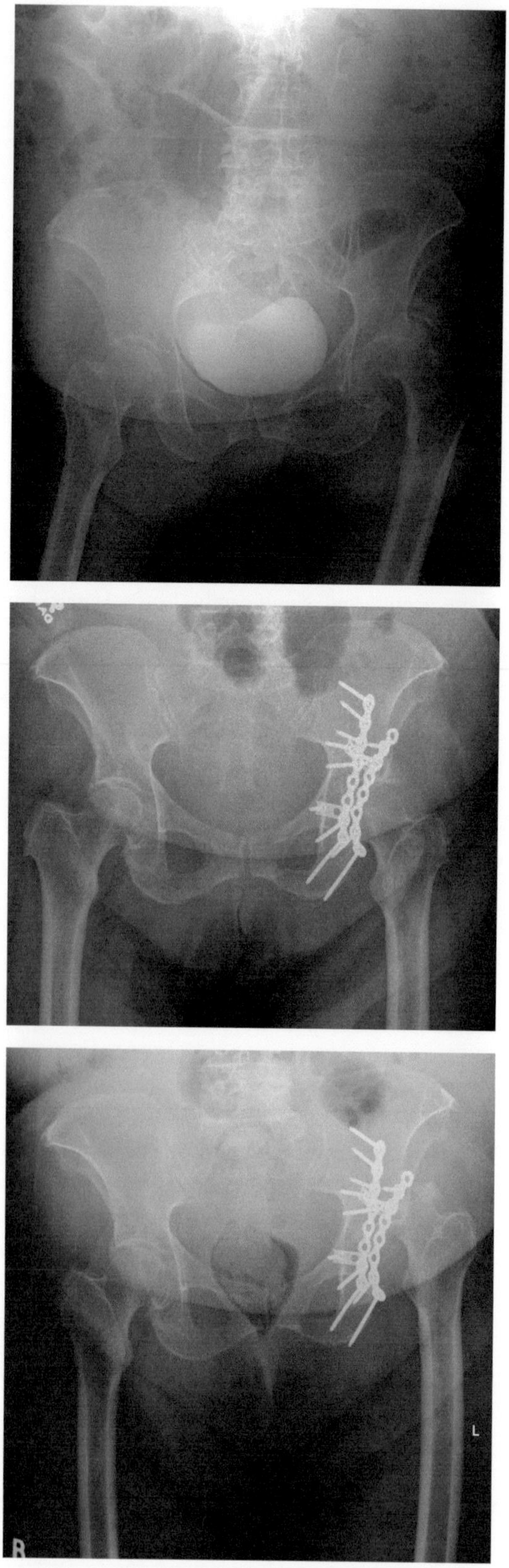

Radiographs of a 67-year-old lady demonstrating comminution of the posterior wall with posterior dislocation of the femoral head. Although her initial 2-week radiographs demonstrate maintained reduction, she sustained a dislocation with catastrophic implant failure at 6 weeks postoperatively.

References

1. Buller LT, Lawrie CM, Vilella FE. A growing problem: acetabular fractures in the elderly and the combined hip procedure. Orthop Clin N Am. 2015;46(2):215–25.
2. Hayes PJ, et al. Operative treatment of acetabular fractures in the Medicare population. Orthopedics. 2013;36(8):e1065–70.
3. Judet R, Judet J, Letournel E. Fractures of the acetabulum: classification and surgical approaches for open reduction. Preliminary report. J Bone Joint Surg Am. 1964;46:1615–46.
4. Letournel E, Judet R. Fractures of the acetabulum. Berlin: Springer; 1981.
5. Spencer RF. Acetabular fractures in older patients. J Bone Joint Surg Br. 1989;71(5):774–6.
6. Matta JM, et al. Fractures of the acetabulum: a retrospective analysis. Clin Orthop Relat Res. 1986;205:230–40.
7. Gary JL, et al. Effect of surgical treatment on mortality after acetabular fracture in the elderly: a multicenter study of 454 patients. J Orthop Trauma. 2015;29(4):202–8.
8. Scarcella N, Schnaser E, Vallier HA. Results and complications in elderly patients with acetabular fractures. Curr Orthop Pract. 2016;27(4):388–92.
9. Ferguson TA, et al. Fractures of the acetabulum in patients aged 60 years and older. J Bone Joint Surg Br. 2010;92(2):250–7.
10. Zelle BA, Cole PA. Open reduction and internal fixation of complex geriatric acetabular fracture. Operat Tech Orthop. 2011;21:286–92.
11. Cornell CN. Management of acetabular fractures in the elderly patient. HSS J. 2005;1(1):25–30.
12. Laflamme GY, Hebert-Davies J, Rouleau D, et al. Internal fixation of osteopenic acetabular fractures involving the quadrilateral plate. Injury. 2011;42(10):1130–4.
13. Carroll EA, et al. Treatment of acetabular fractures in an older population. J Orthop Trauma. 2010;24(10):637–44.
14. Anglen JO, et al. The "Gull Sign": a harbinger of failure for internal fixation of geriatric acetabular fractures. J Orthop Trauma. 2003;17(9):625–34.
15. Zha G-C, Sun J-Y, Dong S-J. Predictors of clinical outcomes after surgical treatment of displaced

acetabular fractures in the elderly. J Orthop Res. 2013;31(4):588–95.
16. Alton TB, Firoozabadi R. Management of pelvic ring fractures in the geriatric patient. Curr Geriatr Rep. 2014;3(2):101–8.
17. Masciocchi C, et al. Imaging of insufficiency fractures. In: Geriatric imaging. Berlin, Heidelberg: Springer Berlin Heidelberg; 2013. p. 83–91.
18. Schicho A, et al. Conventional AP-radiographs are not reliable in detecting acetabular and proximal femur fractures in the elderly. J Osteopor Phys Act. 2015;3(142):2.
19. Henes FO, et al. Comparison of diagnostic accuracy of magnetic resonance imaging and multidetector computed tomography in the detection of pelvic fractures. Eur J Radiol. 2012;81(9):2337–42.
20. Farmer RP, et al. Osteoporosis and the orthopaedic surgeon: basic concepts for successful co-management of patients' bone health. Int Orthop. 2014;38(8):1731–8.
21. Henry PDG, Kreder HJ, Jenkinson RJ. The osteoporotic acetabular fracture. Orthop Clin N Am. 2013;44(2):201–15.
22. Pagenkopf E, et al. Acetabular fractures in the elderly: treatment recommendations. HSS J. 2006;2(2):161–71.
23. Manson T, et al. Variation in treatment of displaced geriatric acetabular fractures among 15 level I Trauma Centers. J Orthop Trauma. 2016;30(9):457–62.
24. Tornetta P. Displaced acetabular fractures: indications for operative and nonoperative management. J Am Acad Orthop Surg. 2001;9(1):18–28.
25. Sen RK, Veerappa LA. Long-term outcome of conservatively managed displaced acetabular fractures. J Trauma Acute Care Surg. 2009;67(1):155–9.
26. Butterwick D, et al. Acetabular fractures in the elderly: evaluation and management. J Bone Joint Surg Am. 2015;97(9):758–68.
27. Starr AJ, Reinert CM, Jones AL. Percutaneous fixation of the columns of the acetabulum: a new technique. J Orthop Trauma. 1998;12(1):51–8.
28. Bozzio AE, et al. Percutaneous fixation of anterior and posterior column acetabular fractures. Orthopedics. 2014;37(10):675–8.
29. von Keudell A, Tobert D, Rodriguez EK. Percutaneous fixation in pelvic and acetabular fractures: understanding evolving indications and contraindications. Oper Tech Orthop. 2015;25(4):248–55.
30. Puchwein P, et al. Percutaneous fixation of acetabular fractures: computer-assisted determination of safe zones, angles and lengths for screw insertion. Arch Orthop Trauma Surg. 2012;132(6):805–11.
31. Azzam K, et al. Percutaneous retrograde posterior column acetabular fixation: is the sciatic nerve safe? A cadaveric study. J Orthop Trauma. 2014;28(1):37–40.
32. Peng Y, et al. Comparison of anterograde versus retrograde percutaneous screw fixation of anterior column acetabular fractures. Int J Comput Assist Radiol Surg. 2016;11(4):635–9.
33. Gary JL, et al. Survivorship of the native hip joint after percutaneous repair of acetabular fractures in the elderly. Injury. 2011;42(10):1144–51.
34. Gary JL, et al. Functional outcomes in elderly patients with acetabular fractures treated with minimally invasive reduction and percutaneous fixation. J Orthop Trauma. 2012;26(5):278–83.
35. Matta JM. Fractures of the acetabulum: accuracy of reduction and clinical results in patients managed operatively within three weeks after the injury. J Bone Joint Surg Am. 1996;78(11):1632–45.
36. Borrelli J Jr, et al. Assessment of articular fragment displacement in acetabular fractures: a comparison of computerized tomography and plain radiographs. J Orthop Trauma. 2002;16(7):449–56.
37. Bastian JD, et al. Mid-term results in relation to age and analysis of predictive factors after fixation of acetabular fractures using the modified Stoppa approach. Injury. 2013;44(12):1793–8.
38. Meena UK, et al. Predictors of postoperative outcome for acetabular fractures. Orthop Traumatol Surg Res. 2013;99(8):929–35.
39. Ruchholtz S, et al. The two-incision, minimally invasive approach in the treatment of acetabular fractures. J Orthop Trauma. 2013;27(5):248–55.
40. Jeffcoat DM, et al. Operative treatment of acetabular fractures in an older population through a limited ilioinguinal approach. J Orthop Trauma. 2012;26(5):284–9.
41. Abo-Elsoud M, et al. Short-segment fixation through a limited ilioinguinal approach for treating anterior acetabular fractures: a historical-control study. Int Orthop. 2014;38(7):1469–75.
42. Routt MLC, Winquist RA. Simultaneous anterior and posterior surgical exposures in the operative treatment of acetabular fractures—The technique. Oper Tech Orthop. 1993;3(1):71–9.
43. Shazar N, et al. Comparison of acetabular fracture reduction quality by the ilioinguinal or the anterior intrapelvic (modified rives–Stoppa) surgical approaches. J Orthop Trauma. 2014;28(6):313–9.
44. von Rüden C, Augat P. Failure of fracture fixation in osteoporotic bone. Injury. 2016;47:S3–S10.
45. Peter RE. Open reduction and internal fixation of osteoporotic acetabular fractures through the ilioinguinal approach: use of buttress plates to control medial displacement of the quadrilateral surface. Injury. 2015;46:S2–7.
46. Archdeacon MT, et al. Treatment of protrusio fractures of the acetabulum in patients 70 years and older. J Orthop Trauma. 2013;27(5):256–61.
47. O'Toole RV, et al. How often does open reduction and internal fixation of geriatric acetabular fractures lead to hip arthroplasty? J Orthop Trauma. 2014;28(3):148–53.
48. Boraiah S, et al. Open reduction internal fixation and primary total hip arthroplasty of selected acetabular fractures. J Orthop Trauma. 2009;23(4):243–8.
49. Mears DC, Velyvis JH. Acute total hip arthroplasty for selected displaced acetabular fractures. J Bone Joint Surg Am. 2002;84(1):1–9.
50. Bellis D, Giovanni U, Legnani C, Calori GM. Acute total hip replacement for acetabular fractures:

a systematic review of the literature. Injury. 2014;45(2):356–61.
51. Solomon LB, et al. Does cup-cage reconstruction with oversized cups provide initial stability in THA for osteoporotic acetabular fractures? Clin Orthop Relat Res. 2015;473(12):3811–9.
52. Sarkar MR, et al. Acute total hip replacement for displaced acetabular fractures in older patients. Eur J Trauma. 2004;30(5):296–304.
53. Mark Rickman MD, et al. Managing acetabular fractures in the elderly with fixation and primary arthroplasty: aiming for early weightbearing. Clin Orthop Relat Res. 2014;472(11):3375.
54. Ballester Alfaro JJ, Sueiro Fernández J. Trabecular metal buttress augment and the trabecular metal cup-cage construct in revision hip arthroplasty for severe acetabular bone loss and pelvic discontinuity. Hip Int. 2010;20:S119–27.
55. Amenabar T, et al. Promising mid-term results with a cup-cage construct for large acetabular defects and pelvic discontinuity. Clin Orthop Relat Res. 2016;474(2):408–14.
56. Gross AE. Severe bone loss and pelvic discontinuity: the cup cage solution. Bone Joint J. 2014;96(Suppl 8):62.
57. Sierra RJ, et al. Acetabular fractures. Bone Joint J. 2013;95(11 Suppl A):11–6.
58. Schnaser E, Scarcella NR, Vallier HA. Acetabular fractures converted to total hip arthroplasties in the elderly: how does function compare to primary total hip arthroplasty? J Orthop Trauma. 2014;28(12):694–9.
59. Morison Z, et al. Total hip arthroplasty after acetabular fracture is associated with lower survivorship and more complications. Clin Orthop Relat Res. 2016;474(2):392–8.

14 Geriatric Long Bone Fractures

Jessica G. Kingsberg and Daniel T. Altman

Introduction

Long bone fractures in the elderly are uncommon. According to a retrospective database review performed by Keller et al. [1], fractures of the ribs, distal radius, pelvic ring, facial bones, proximal humerus, clavicle, ankle, and sacrum were the most common fractures in patients over age 65. Although uncommon, fractures of the tibial and femoral diaphysis can have devastating functional effects on elderly patients and have increased rates of morbidity and mortality compared to equivalent fractures in younger patients [2]. Schatzker et al. [3] in their 1974 review of 68 patients with distal femur fractures recommended cast treatment for all elderly patients with easily reducible fractures and described using internal fixation in patients with osteoporosis as "doomed" due to the risks of implant failure, malunion, and nonunion. Since that time, treatment of elderly patients with diaphyseal fractures of the tibia and femur has changed dramatically. That being said, true fixation may be difficult without supplemental fixation. Treatment depends on the patient's overall functional status with the goal of early mobilization and pain control.

J.G. Kingsberg, M.D.
Silver State Orthopedics, 3196 South Maryland Pkwy, Suite 112, Las Vegas, NV 89109, USA
e-mail: jkingsberg@gmail.com

D.T. Altman, M.D. (✉)
Allegheny Health Network, Drexel University College of Medicine, Philadelphia, PA 19129, USA
e-mail: daltman@wpahs.org;
Altmangregory@hotmail.com

Evaluation and Management

Falls constitute 75% of all geriatric traumas, with the frequency of blunt trauma much higher than that of penetrating trauma [4]. Because fractures in nonambulatory and bedridden patients may result from minimal trauma, radiographs should be carefully scrutinized if these patients are reporting limb pain [5]. Radiographs of osteoporotic bone may be difficult to interpret, but generally patients with a fracture of the long bones have less subtle radiographs. Nondisplaced fractures may still be missed due to reduced sensitivity in patients with osteopenia. If radiographs are negative, CT scan may be obtained to further evaluate bony anatomy. Because low-energy injuries frequently result from torsional injury to the diaphysis, CT may also be used to evaluate the extent of the fracture and determine the presence or absence of intra-articular extension. MRI may be used for subtle nondisplaced fractures of the diaphysis, although these are rare. Salminen et al. [6] noted that 32 out of 50 patients admitted to their facility with a low-energy femur fracture

A. Rodriguez et al. (eds.), *Geriatric Trauma and Acute Care Surgery*,
https://doi.org/10.1007/978-3-319-57403-5_14

had a fracture of the left femur. The fracture was in the middle third of the femur in 33 patients and was a spiral configuration in 29, transverse in 10, oblique-transverse in 7, and oblique in 4 patients. These low-energy fractures are usually closed and have less internal soft-tissue stripping, although soft-tissue damage may still be present. Comminution is almost always noted in high- and low-energy fractures in the elderly population secondary to their thinner and weaker outer cortices, less hematopoietic activity, and greater overall brittleness of the bone [7, 8].

Following diagnosis, the overwhelming majority of geriatric patients with a long bone fracture are admitted to an inpatient unit. Due to proximal muscle weakness and balance issues, many elderly patients are unable to care for themselves when faced with weight-bearing restrictions. It is common for many geriatric patients to be admitted to an internal medicine service, but this has been shown to be costly and cause excessive and unnecessary testing [9]. Even in patients with low-energy mechanisms of injury, surgery is often delayed secondary to perceived need for unnecessary cardiology consultation or echocardiogram [10]. This delay in surgery can have catastrophic results. To begin with, removing the elderly patient from their regular environment and placing them in the hospital disrupts their sleep-wake cycle, which causes confusion and delirium. These symptoms are often then treated with medications such as sedatives, which can increase confusion and make falls more likely [11]. This effect can also be magnified with narcotic treatment, which may cause not only confusion and delirium, but also gastrointestinal side effects. Lack of mobilization may also have a debilitating effect on geriatric patients. Because of their increased ventilation perfusion mismatch at rest, they are at particular risk of atelectasis if they also have rib fractures. This leads to hypoxia and possibly mechanical ventilation, which brings with it risks of tracheomalacia and ventilator-associated pneumonia [12]. Elderly patients are also more likely to develop skin breakdown and pressure ulcers from bedrest [13].

Early stabilization of long bone fractures has been supported since the 1980s with Johnson et al. [14] reporting a fivefold reduction in the rate of adult respiratory distress syndrome in patients treated with early fixation compared to late. In 1985, Seibel et al. [15] demonstrated that femur fracture fixation within 24 h was associated with a decreased mortality rate. In a classic article published in 1989, Bone et al. [16] demonstrated that reamed intramedullary nailing within 24 h was not only safe, but led to a shorter hospitalization compared to delayed treatment. These principles apply to elderly patients as well as younger patients. When early definitive treatment is not possible in the elderly, external fixation may be safely used for geriatric patients and has proven to be cost effective and simple, causing minimal trauma to skin and soft tissues [17]. It can also be revised to facilitate the healing process. Unfortunately, external fixation also has several drawbacks in elderly patients. Screw fixation is decreased in osteoporosis, which causes decreased primary stability at the bone-implant interface, increased initial loosening, and overall decreased functional strength of the construct [18]. These issues plague traction pins as well, with poor purchase even in the shaft of the femur.

Femoral Shaft Fractures

In the elderly, femoral shaft fractures may result from either high-energy or low-energy mechanisms. Low-energy femur fractures generally result from a fall from standing height; these affect the midshaft femur less often than the proximal and distal femur. High-energy fractures usually result from a motor vehicle accident, similar to younger patients [2]. Patel et al. [19] identified a 1-year mortality rate of 21% in geriatric patients who sustained a high-energy femoral shaft fracture, with patients demonstrating increased postoperative complications, longer hospital length of stay, greater percentage of discharges to rehabilitation facilities, and more accompanying long bone fractures. The association between surgical delay and mortality in geriatric patients was found to be stronger in geriatric patients than in younger patients. [20] Cantu et al. explored this relationship and found that for elderly patients with an isolated femur fracture, surgical delay beyond 48 h was associated with nearly five times greater mortality risk compared with surgery within 12 h.

Immediate Management

Although traction may be utilized initially during resuscitation or for a short period of time in the critically ill patient, it carries with it the risks of immobilization described earlier. Because patients are unable to move in bed, they are at even greater risk of developing decubitus ulcers, pneumonia, or other complications of bedrest. In addition, traction is unwieldy for patients who must undergo multiple procedures prior to their eventual surgery. External fixation may be used as an alternative, particularly in a patient who is polytraumatized or underresuscitated. Many external fixators are compatible with magnetic resonance imaging, which is especially useful in polytraumatized patients who need to undergo MRIs or other advanced imaging procedures [21]. However, both external fixation and traction are difficult to use to maintain length and reduction in elderly patients due to their weakened bone quality and its effect on the bone-pin interface. In addition, there are risks of pin tract infection, both superficial and deep. There are no recent studies on the use of external fixation for definitive treatment of femoral shaft fractures in elderly patients; it is recommended to perform an additional method of fixation up to 2 weeks later [22].

Plate Fixation

Compression plating is difficult to perform in most geriatric fracture patterns due to fracture comminution. Attempting compression plating in the face of comminution and poor bone quality generally results in shortening of the diaphysis and lack of appropriate cortical contact [23]. In large areas of comminution, bridge plating is recommended instead [24]. Indications for plating include a large open associated wound, complex femoral shaft and neck fractures, and theoretical risk to cardiopulmonary systems with reaming [22, 25]. Bridge plating may also be performed in a percutaneous manner to avoid disrupting the blood supply to the fracture fragments of the femoral shaft. Weight bearing is generally restricted for several weeks, although range of motion at the hip and knee is allowed in the early postoperative period.

Khursheed et al. [26] reported their results with minimally invasive plate osteosynthesis (MIPO) techniques with locking screws for extra-articular distal femoral shaft fractures in 25 patients over aged 60. None of their patients developed delayed union or nonunion and MIPO was felt to be a good option for elderly patients despite comminution and osteoporosis.

Complications may arise using MIPO due to atrophic tissues and poor soft-tissue envelope. Implant loosening in osteoporotic bone may occur, as can alteration of metaphyseal soft tissues. Frankhauser et al. [27] reported irritation of the iliotibial band by the implant as the main cause for implant removal in 23.4% of cases.

Intramedullary Nailing

Fractures resulting from low-energy trauma in patients older than 50 years of age account for as much as 85% of all distal femur fractures [28]. For that reason, retrograde intramedullary nailing and supracondylar nail fixation have both been used for treatment of these distal fractures. Intramedullary nailing demonstrates superior axial stability to plate constructs [29], making it especially useful for elderly patients who have difficulty following weight-bearing restrictions. Minimal soft-tissue stripping is also an advantage of these procedures [30]. Retrograde nails are also useful in the treatment of femoral fractures proximal to a total knee prosthesis as they avoid soft-tissue stripping and potential contamination of the implant [31] (Fig. 14.1).

With retrograde nailing, reduction of the fracture site is generally obtained through external manipulation of the leg or percutaneous clamping, although it is sometimes necessary to perform an open reduction at the fracture site through a lateral approach. The femur is then reamed sequentially and the nail is seated 3–5 mm deep to the distal articular cartilage extending to the level of the lesser trochanter. Proximal and distal interlocking screws are placed. Following surgery, the patient is generally allowed to weight bear as tolerated and hip and knee motion is encouraged. In fractures of the midshaft or proximal shaft of the femur, antegrade nailing obtains better control of the fracture site. The starting point is the piriformis fossa or just medial to the tip of the greater trochanter.

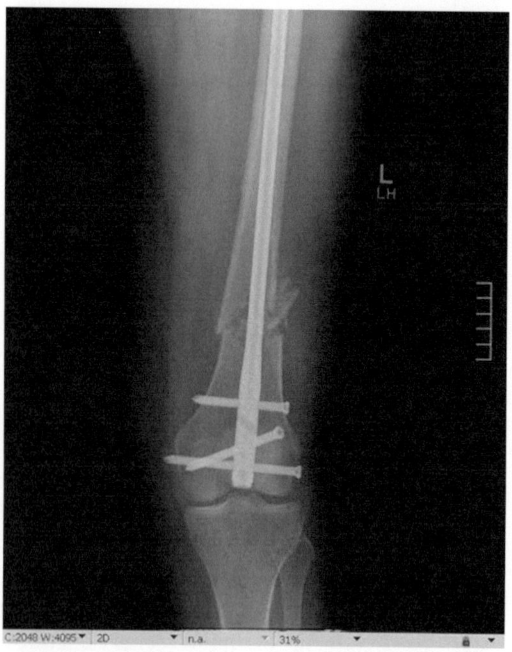

Fig. 14.1 Radiograph of a 65-year-old female with a high-energy distal femoral shaft fracture treated with retrograde intramedullary nail fixation

Neubauer et al. [32] reported a 97.8% union rate of femoral fractures treated with retrograde nail fixation. The most common complication was loosening of distal locking bolts in three patients, followed by a periprosthetic fracture after 15 months, septic nonunion, subcutaneous bleeding, and recurvatum of >5° in one patient each.

Bliemel et al. [33] performed an analysis of polyaxial angle-stable locking plate versus a retrograde intramedullary nail in a human cadaveric bone model. They noted that the load to failure for both implants in geriatric femur cadavers was much higher than that experienced with normal ambulation.

Tibial Shaft Fractures

Diaphyseal fractures of the tibia are uncommon in the elderly population but represent a devastating injury. Clement et al. [34] determined that the 120-day and 1-year unadjusted mortality rate of a tibial shaft fracture was 17% and 27%, respectively. Their research also showed that fractures of the diaphysis of the tibia occurred predominantly in women (73%) and were sustained in a fall (61%). Elderly women were also found to have more severe injuries, with an increased rate of open fractures and greater risk of nonunions. Ritchie et al. [35] evaluated 23 patients aged over 60 with open tibial shaft fractures and found a final amputation rate of 47%, demonstrating the severity of these injuries. Although they concluded that age was not a contraindication to attempted limb salvage in open injuries of the tibia, they had a 100% amputation rate in grade IIIC injuries of the tibia, proving the catastrophic effect of this injury.

Immediate Management

Low-energy tibia fractures in the elderly typically present as long spiral oblique fractures. As is the case with younger patients, high-energy fractures are generally transverse and represent a more unstable fracture pattern [36]. In contrast to femoral shaft fractures, tibial shaft fractures may be treated nonoperatively under certain circumstances. Although indications for closed treatment of tibial shaft fractures are somewhat arbitrary, most authors agree that nonoperative treatment is only appropriate for fractures at least 5 cm away from the plateau and plafond. In addition, fractures must be stable after reduction, and demonstrate at least 50% cortical overlap, less than 1 cm shortening, and less than 5 degrees varus/valgus angulation or anterior/posterior angulation. Internal rotation should not exceed 10 degrees and external rotation should not exceed 20 degrees [37]. Although fractures may be treated nonoperatively with casting followed by treatment in a patellar tendon-bearing brace, elderly patients generally have frail skin, which makes prolonged casting difficult. Close follow-up with frequent skin checks must be arranged and the cast must remain well padded over bony prominences [13].

External fixation may also be trialed in patients with tibial shaft fractures, but this carries with it similar risks to that of patients with femoral shaft fractures and should be used mainly as a temporizing measure and not for definitive fixation.

Plate Fixation

After a tibial shaft fracture, the periosteal blood supply becomes the major nutrient vessel. Because of this, plate fixation of the tibia is rarely performed, as this would involve disrupting the vascularity. Although percutaneous plating techniques have been trialed, plating of the tibia is best indicated for extreme proximal and distal segments of the tibia [38]. Although subcutaneous and minimally invasive plating techniques have been developed, these still run the risk of skin compromise and even skin breakdown. Lau et al. [39] demonstrated a 15% rate of deep infection following MIPO fixation of distal tibia fractures in elderly patients and 52% of patients eventually underwent implant removal. They felt that although the overall clinical outcome was very good, late wound infection and impingement were still common complications.

Intramedullary Nailing

Intramedullary nailing is the preferred treatment for fractures of the tibial shaft. The advantages to intramedullary nailing include preservation of the periosteal blood supply, decreased soft-tissue stripping, and immediate weight bearing. Disadvantages include anterior knee pain and difficulty utilizing the technique with extreme proximal or distal fractures [40].

There have been no studies specifically studying the effects of intramedullary nailing on tibial shaft fractures in geriatric patients.

Conclusion

Fractures of the femoral and tibial diaphysis are uncommon injuries in the elderly population but treatment principles generally follow the same patterns as those of diaphyseal fractures in younger patients. Emphasis is placed on mobility and preservation of blood supply, with the goal of early weight bearing. The majority of diaphyseal fractures may be treated with load-sharing intramedullary implants, which preserve the periosteal blood supply while limiting soft-tissue stripping.

References

1. Keller JM, et al. Geriatric trauma: demographics, injuries, and mortality. J Orthop Trauma. 2012;26(9):e161–5.
2. Enninghorst N, et al. Population-based epidemiology of femur shaft fractures. J Trauma Acute Care Surg. 2013;74(6):1516–20.
3. Schatzker J, Horne G, Waddell J. The Toronto experience with the supracondylar fracture of the femur, 1966–1972. Injury. 1974;6(2):113–28.
4. Sterling DA, O'Connor JA, Bonadies J. Geriatric falls: injury severity is high and disproportionate to mechanism. J Trauma Acute Care Surg. 2001;50(1):116–9.
5. Sadro CT, et al. Geriatric trauma: a radiologist's guide to imaging trauma patients aged 65 years and older. Radiographics. 2015;35(4):1263–85.
6. Salminen S, et al. Specific features associated with femoral shaft fractures caused by low-energy trauma. J Trauma Acute Care Surg. 1997;43(1):117–22.
7. Cummings SR, et al. Risk factors for hip fracture in white women. N Engl J Med. 1995;332(12):767–74.
8. Tinubu J, Scalea TM. Management of fractures in a geriatric surgical patient. Surg Clin N Am. 2015;95(1):115–28.

9. Bernstein J, et al. Preoperative testing for hip fracture patients delays surgery, prolongs hospital stays, and rarely dictates care. J Orthop Trauma. 2016;30(2):78–80.
10. Marcantonio A, et al. The clinical and economic impact of preoperative transthoracic echocardiography in elderly patients with hip fractures. Bull Hosp Joint Dis. 2015;73(4):239–42.
11. Naylor MD, et al. Comparison of evidence-based interventions on outcomes of hospitalized, cognitively impaired older adults. J Comp Eff Res. 2014;3(3):245–57.
12. Umei N, et al. Impact of mobilisation therapy on the haemodynamic and respiratory status of elderly intubated patients in an intensive care unit: a retrospective analysis. Intensive Crit Care Nurs. 2016;35:16–21.
13. Al-Nuaimi Y, Sherratt MJ, Griffiths CEM. Skin health in older age. Maturitas. 2014;79(3):256–64.
14. Johnson KD, Cadambi A, Burton Seibert G. Incidence of adult respiratory distress syndrome in patients with multiple musculoskeletal injuries: effect of early operative stabilization of fractures. J Trauma Acute Care Surg. 1985;25(5):375–84.
15. Seibel R, Border JR, et al. Blunt multiple trauma (ISS 36), femur traction, and the pulmonary failure-septic state. Ann Surg. 1985;202(3):283.
16. Bone LB, et al. Early versus delayed stabilization of femoral fractures. A prospective randomized study. J Bone Joint Surg Am. 1989;71(3):336–40.
17. Andruszkow H, et al. External fixation in the elderly. Injury. 2015;46:S7–S12.
18. Seebeck J, et al. Effect of cortical thickness and cancellous bone density on the holding strength of internal fixator screws. J Orthop Res. 2004;22(6):1237–42.
19. Patel KV, et al. High-energy femur fractures increase morbidity but not mortality in elderly patients. Clin Orthop Relat Res. 2014;472(3):1030–5.
20. Cantu RV, Graves SC, Spratt KF. In-hospital mortality from femoral shaft fracture depends on the initial delay to fracture fixation and injury severity score-a retrospective cohort study from the NTDB 2002–2006. J Trauma Acute Care Surg. 2014;76(6):1433.
21. Tuttle MS, et al. Safety and efficacy of damage control external fixation versus early definitive stabilization for femoral shaft fractures in the multiple-injured patient. J Trauma Acute Care Surg. 2009;67(3):602–5.
22. Nowotarski PJ, et al. Conversion of external fixation to intramedullary nailing for fractures of the shaft of the femur in multiply injured patients. J Bone Joint Surg Am. 2000;82(6):781–8.
23. Seligson D, et al. Plating of femoral shaft fractures. A review of 15 cases. injury. 2001;14:17.
24. Nayak RM, et al. Minimally invasive plate osteosynthesis using a locking compression plate for distal femoral fractures. J Orthop Surg. 2011;19(2):185.
25. Watson JT, Moed BR. Ipsilateral femoral neck and shaft fractures: complications and their treatment. Clin Orthop Relat Res. 2002;399:78–86.
26. Khursheed O, et al. Results of treatment of distal extra: articular femur fractures with locking plates using minimally invasive approach—experience with 25 consecutive geriatric patients. Musculoskelet Surg. 2015;99(2):139–47.
27. Fankhauser F, et al. Minimal-invasive treatment of distal femoral fractures with the LISS (Less Invasive Stabilization System): a prospective study of 30 fractures with a follow up of 20 months. Acta Orthop Scand. 2004;75(1):56–60.
28. Dunlop DG, Brenkel IJ. The supracondylar intramedullary nail in elderly patients with distal femoral fractures. Injury. 1999;30:475–84.
29. Wähnert D, et al. Long-term stability of angle-stable versus conventional locked intramedullary nails in distal tibia fractures. BMC Musculoskelet Disord. 2013;14(1):1.
30. Yoon RS, et al. Outcomes following combined intramedullary nail and plate fixation for complex tibia fractures: a multi-centre study. Injury. 2015;46(6):1097–101.
31. Meneghini RM, et al. Modern retrograde intramedullary nails versus periarticular locked plates for supracondylar femur fractures after total knee arthroplasty. J Arthroplast. 2014;29(7):1478–81.
32. Neubauer T, et al. Retrograde femoral nailing in elderly patients: outcome and functional results. Orthopedics. 2012;35(6):e855–61.
33. Bliemel C, et al. Distal femoral fractures in the elderly: biomechanical analysis of a polyaxial angle-stable locking plate versus a retrograde intramedullary nail in a human cadaveric bone model. Arch Orthop Trauma Surg. 2015;135(1):49–58.
34. Clement ND, et al. The outcome of tibial diaphyseal fractures in the elderly. Bone Joint J. 2013;95(9):1255–62.
35. Ritchie AJ, et al. Type III tibial fractures in the elderly: results of 23 fractures in 20 patients. Injury. 1991;22(4):267–70.
36. McBirnie J. The epidemiology of tibial fractures. Bone Joint J. 1995;77(3):417–21.
37. Schmidt AH, Finkemeier CG, Tornetta P. Treatment of closed tibial fractures. J Bone Joint Surg Am. 2003;85(2):352–68.
38. Coles CP, Gross M. Closed tibial shaft fractures: management and treatment complications. A review of the prospective literature. Can J Surg. 2000;43(4):256.
39. Lau TW, et al. Wound complication of minimally invasive plate osteosynthesis in distal tibia fractures. Int Orthop. 2008;32(5):697–703.
40. Finkemeier CG, et al. A prospective, randomized study of intramedullary nails inserted with and without reaming for the treatment of open and closed fractures of the tibial shaft. J Orthop Trauma. 2000;14(3):187–93.

Part VIII

Cardiothoracic Injury

15 Cardiac Trauma

Benjamin Moran, Lars Ola Sjoholm, and Amy J. Goldberg

Introduction

Cardiac trauma to the geriatric population is rare. A 10-year registry review of the Pennsylvania Trauma Outcomes from 2006 to 2015 showed only 458 patients over 65 with cardiac injury [1]. The geriatric patient is exposed to the same amount of force as their younger counterparts, but has less physiologic reserve to combat the effects of traumatic stress. There are few studies and guidelines about specific management of geriatric cardiac trauma due to its uncommon nature. When comparing the younger myocardium to an aged and injured counterpart, injuries to the elder heart can be difficult to manage with very high rates of mortality.

B. Moran, M.D.
Department of Surgery, Lewis Katz School of Medicine at Temple University, Philadelphia, PA, USA

L.O. Sjoholm, M.D.
Department of Surgery, Trauma Program, Lewis Katz School of Medicine at Temple University, Philadelphia, PA, USA

A.J. Goldberg, M.D., F.A.C.S. (✉)
Department of Surgery, Lewis Katz School of Medicine at Temple University, Philadelphia, PA, USA
e-mail: Amy.Goldberg@tuhs.temple.edu

Physiologic and Pathologic Effects of Aging

To effectively treat geriatric cardiac injury, the physician must understand the pathologic and physiologic effects of aging on the heart. Physiologic aging is unique in that it affects every individual. The effect is variable in the population, with patients being "young" 75-year-olds, and "old" 50-year-olds. This differs from the pathologic effects of aging, those being modifiable and preventable disease processes like coronary artery disease [2]. The total amount of cardiac myocytes decreases with age, leading to the overall decline of cardiac function by 50% between the ages of 20 and 80 years [2, 3]. The elasticity of the aorta and great vessels declines over time causing decreased compliance, stiff vessels, and increased afterload which results in left ventricular hypertrophy [2]. Increased vascular afterload, arterial-ventricular load mismatching, and decreased ventricular inotropic reserve cause reduced exercise tolerance [4]. Cardiac autonomic regulation is impaired as baroreceptors and intrinsic catecholamines have a decreased effect on myocardial tissue [2, 4]. The depressed response to catecholamines may be compounded by preexisting beta-blocker use, leading to fixed heart rates, which prevents cardiac output from rising to achieve adequate tissue perfusion when most necessary [5]. The aging myocardium serves to mask the classical effects of hypovolemia in these patients making triage and treatment a challenge.

A. Rodriguez et al. (eds.), *Geriatric Trauma and Acute Care Surgery*,
https://doi.org/10.1007/978-3-319-57403-5_15

Physiologic effects of aging	
Declining cardiac function [3]	Decreased and fixed cardiac output
Myocyte depletion [2]	Decreased contractility
	Decreased cardiac output
	Less inotropic reserve
Decreased aortic and great vessel elasticity [2]	Decreased arterial compliance
	Increased afterload
	Left ventricular hypertrophy
Impaired response to catecholamines [2, 4]	Decreased response in stress
	Lower HR and BP

The pathologic effects on coronary artery disease, heart disease, and valvular disease must be considered in treating geriatric patients. As the population ages over 40, men have a 49% and women have a 32% lifetime risk of developing coronary heart disease [6, 7]. Women typically lag in cardiac events behind men by about 10 years; however the rates rise as menopause occurs. The manifestation of coronary artery disease in women increases 3:2 compared to men aged 65–94 [7, 8]. The prevalence of valvular disease increases with age, as 11.7% of patients over the age of 75 have moderate to severe valve disease [9]. The effects of coronary and valvular heart disease can impair myocardial function and perfusion which may lead to deleterious effects during stress and trauma. Plaque and calcification in coronary artery disease may act as lead points for arterial dissection in blunt cardiac trauma [10].

Mechanism and Incidence

In Pennsylvania from 2006 to 2015 patients over 65 represented 20% of all cardiac injuries sustained in trauma. The overall mortality in this age group was 35%. In patients over 65 blunt mechanism was the cause of cardiac injury 90% of the time, where penetrating injury was the primary mechanism in 10%. This differed from injury mechanisms in all age groups where blunt mechanism accounted for 60% of all injuries and penetrating injury accounted for 40%. Myocardial infarction (MI) occurred in association with cardiac trauma in 2.9% of patients over 65. Cardiac injuries with a concurrent MI in this age group were very lethal with a mortality approaching 50% [1].

Penetrating cardiac injuries most commonly result from stab wounds and gun shots. The injury pattern follows the anatomy of the myocardium. Roughly one-third of the heart lies to the right of midline and two-thirds lie to the left. In the anterior-posterior dimension the right ventricle encompasses the majority of the anterior surface of the heart while the left atrium comprises the posterior aspect [11]. This anatomy creates a descending order of injury incidence, with the right ventricle (40–43%), left ventricle (34–40%), right atrium (18–24%), and left atrium (3–5%) [11, 12]. These are deadly injuries, with an overall mortality of 47%.

Blunt cardiac injury (BCI) occurs with compression of the thoracic cavity leading to direct energy transfer to the myocardium. Rapid acceleration and deceleration incidents create myocardial injury as the heart swings and pivots against the sternum and spinal canal. These forces are most often seen in motor vehicle collisions as the sternum strikes the steering wheel. The energy transfer is intensified in the geriatric patient as intercostal muscle mass decreases and bone density of the ribs decreases the protective effect of the thoracic cavity [13]. Myocardial contusion occurs often in blunt chest trauma, with rates reported between 16 and 76% [14]. Blunt injury may manifest in a variety of ways. Arrhythmias are common, with sinus tachycardia seen most often followed by ventricular, atrial premature contractions and atrial fibrillation [15]. Valve and myocardial rupture can result from thoracic impact. Myocardial rupture is a devastating injury with near-100% mortality. It is most commonly found during autopsies in cases from non-penetrating chest injury. Rates of cardiac chamber rupture in decreasing frequency include right atrium (40%), right ventricle (31%), left atrium (25%), and lastly left ventricle (12.5%) [16]. Right ventricular rupture occurs most often followed by the left ventricle, right atrium, and left atrium. Valvular rupture is often a result of papillary muscle rupture leading to immediate insufficiency which may precipitate myocardial tress and hypotension. The aortic valve is injured most commonly, followed by mitral, tricuspid, and pulmonic with rupture occurring more frequently in patients with preexisting valve disease [17]. Coronary artery occlusion and dissection can result from direct impact of the chest. Preexisting plaques rupture causing intimal flaps which results in dissection and occlusion [10].

Invasive procedures can cause iatrogenic injury to the myocardium. Central lines, cardiac catherization, endovascular repair, transcatheter-based valve repairs, and pericardiocentesis may all injure the heart. Central lines may puncture the innominate-caval confluence, causing cardiac tamponade and necessitating the need for surgery [18]. Myocardial hematomas may result from cardiac catherization procedures [10]. Chest compressions during cardiopulmonary resuscitation can lead to cardiac injury.

Electrocution may lead to cardiac damage, through occupational exposures or accidents at home. Electrical energy causes disruption of the ventricular conduction system and heat damage to the myocardium. Ventricular fibrillation and cardiac standstill may occur with increasing amounts of energy transfer and duration of current applied to these patients. Additionally, there has been reports of direct myonecrosis and coronary vasospasm precipitated from electrocution [19, 20].

Evaluation

Initial evaluation follows advanced trauma support guidelines, beginning with airway, breathing, and circulation. The heart rate and blood pressure exhibited in the geriatric trauma patient may be misleading. Preexisting pathological and physiological effects of aging and concomitant medication use, specifically beta-blockade, may lead to a fixed cardiac output. A normotensive patient can be physiologically hypotensive.

In penetrating trauma caused by firearms it is important to understand the missile trajectory. This is achieved by rolling the patient early on, identifying all wounds and obtaining plain X-rays. For stab wounds, if the injury is located in the "cardiac box" there needs to be a high index of suspicion for cardiac injury. These landmarks are defined as the area between the borders of both nipples, sternal notch, and xiphoid. The cardiac view of the focused assessment with sonography for trauma (FAST) exam is crucial in identifying the presence of pericardial fluid in both blunt and penetrating injuries. If fluid is present, the patient may need to be further evaluated with pericardial window. Computerized tomography may be of use in the blunt geriatric trauma patient in order to evaluate pericardial fluid composition by measuring Hounsfield units.

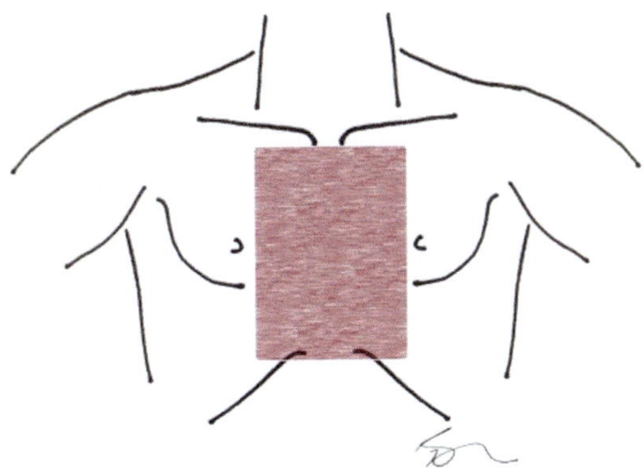

Cardiac Box: Defined area between borders – superior/inferior: sternal notch/xiphoid. Lateral edges – nipples

BCI must be considered when a patient has sustained significant force to the thoracic cavity. There are no specific correlations between fracture pattern and BCI. In isolated sternal fractures there is no clear correlation with cardiac injury, and therefore all patients do not need screening [21, 22]. Thus the physician must be vigilant and have a high index of suspicion for BCI when there is appropriate mechanism. Suggested screening guidelines for BCI consist of obtaining an electrocardiogram and a troponin I value. If both the electrocardiogram and troponin I levels are normal, BCI may safely be ruled out. If there are new ECG changes or troponin elevation the patient should be admitted for monitoring [21]. An echocardiogram is not beneficial as a screening tool; however it is useful in identifying injuries in patients who have hypotension, murmurs, and/or arrhythmias. An echocardiogram is the diagnostic test of choice in patients with BCI; however computerized tomography or magnetic resonance imaging may be used to differentiate acute myocardial infarction from BCI [21, 23].

Treatment

Penetrating Cardiac Injury

Penetrating cardiac injury is an uncommon entity in the elderly. Penetrating injuries necessitate operative intervention with cardiac exposure best accomplished by either a left anterior-lateral thoracotomy or a median sternotomy. Median sternotomy is often reserved for precordial stab wounds; this will allow access to the heart but will not allow for adequate access to the lungs or aortic cross clamping. A left anterolateral thoracotomy provides rapid cardiac exposure, which may be accomplished as a resuscitative thoracotomy in the trauma bay or operating room. An incision is made in the fifth intercostal space from the sternum to the midaxillary line. Exposure provides immediate pericardial decompression and allows for aortic cross clamping. If there is myocardial injury there are a variety of ways to perform cardiac repair. Finger occlusion and stapling with a skin stapler can be used to obtain temporary control. Definitive repair is achieved with suturing with a nonabsorbable suture material done with or without pledgets. If the injury is close to the coronary artery, care must be taken to avoid iatrogenic injury [24].

Blunt Cardiac Injury

Patients who present to the hospital with blunt cardiac injury generally have injuries that are less severe, as most patients who have suffered ventricular rupture are pronounced at the scene of injury. The most common injuries following blunt cardiac injury are myocardial stunning, intramural hematoma, myocardial wall rupture, valve injury, and coronary injury. Patients that have sustained myocardial wall rupture have near-100% mortality rate. Pericardial tamponade may present in patients with atrial or ventricular wall rupture. These patients require immediate decompression and cardiac repair. There is a role for emergency department thoracotomy in this patient group.

In blunt cardiac injury patients should have a baseline ECG obtained at the time of admission and continuous cardiac monitoring for dysrhythmias. Sinus tachycardia, ventricular and atrial premature contractions followed by atrial fibrillation are the most common dysrhythmias seen in BCI [10]. If there is unexplained hypotension or arrhythmias a transthoracic echocardiogram is useful to determine overall cardiac function [21]. BCI is usually self-limiting and treated with supportive care. In extreme cases inotropic or mechanical support may be necessary.

Intramural hematoma (IH) is another injury pattern, often an incidental finding seen on echocardiogram. This may also be present on CT or MRI. IH is less often seen after a trauma incident, but seen more commonly after percutaneous coronary interventions or cardiac surgery. These injuries are associated with premature ventricular contractions and transient bundle branch blocks. The right ventricle followed by the left ventricle are the most common sites. IH usually has a benign course, is self-limiting, and resolves within 4–12 weeks [10].

Valvular injury may result following blunt chest trauma. Diagnosis is achieved by echocardiogram [10]. The aortic valve is injured most frequently, followed by mitral, tricuspid, and pulmonic with rupture occurring more frequently in patients with preexisting valve disease [17]. Blunt force causes papillary muscle rupture, chordae, or injury to the leaflets leading to acute valvular regurgitation [10]. These patients need early supportive care with emergent or delayed valve surgery determined by clinical stability and cardiac function. Papillary muscle rupture causes dynamic fluid shifts in the heart which can precipitate ventricular failure. An early cardiothoracic consultation is recommended, as 57% of patients sustaining mitral valve rupture required valve replacement [14]. Tricuspid valve rupture and regurgitation are often well tolerated, and may present in a delayed fashion. First-, second- and third-degree heart blocks are associated with tricuspid valve rupture [10].

Coronary artery injury occurs when direct impact over the left anterior descending or the left main coronary artery causes an acute dissection. Dissected segments rarely occur in healthy arteries; however they occur in disease segments. Plaque rupture initiates intimal tearing which then precipitates atrial dissection. This can lead to complete occlusion and infarction. Infarction usually involves the apex, septum, or both as the septal and distal LAD branches occlude and thrombose, leading to ST elevations on ECG. Prompt coronary revascularization is necessary in these circumstanc es [10].

Arrhythmias associated with cardiac injury	
Penetrating cardiac injury	Sinus tachycardia, supraventricular tachycardia, ST segment changes, ventricular tachycardia, ventricular fibrillation [24]
Blunt cardiac injury	Sinus tachycardia, ventricular, atrial premature contractions, atrial fibrillation [10]
Intramural hematoma	PVC, bundle branch block [10]
Valvular injury	First-degree, second-degree, complete heart block [10]
Coronary artery injury	ST segment elevation [10]
Electrocution	Sinus tachycardia, bundle branch blocks, ST segment and T wave changes, prolonged QT, supraventricular tachycardia, atrial fibrillation, ventricular tachycardia/fibrillation [24]

Summary

Cardiac injury in the geriatric population has not been thoroughly studied but appears to be rare. It is associated with high morbidity and mortality. The most important aspect when caring for these patients is understanding the physiologic reserve of the geriatric patient and providing close continuous monitoring and supportive care.

References

1. Pennsylvania Trauma Outcome Study 2006. In: Disclaimer: these data were provided by the Pennsylvania Trauma Systems Foundation, Mechanicsburg, PA; 2015. The foundation specifically disclaims responsibility for any analyses, interpretations, or conclusions.
2. Cheitlin MD. Cardiovascular physiology-changes with aging. Am J Geriatr Cardiol. 2003;12(1):9–13.
3. Lewis MC, Abouelenin K, Paniagua M. Geriatric trauma: special considerations in the anesthetic management of the injured elderly patient. Anesthesiol Clin. 2007;25(1):75–90, ix.
4. Ferrara N, Komici K, Corbi G, Pagano G, Furgi G, Rengo C, et al. β-adrenergic receptor responsiveness in aging heart and clinical implications. Front Physiol. 2014;4:396.
5. Neideen T, Lam M, Brasel KJ. Preinjury beta blockers are associated with increased mortality in geriatric trauma patients. J Trauma. 2008;65(5):1016–20.
6. Lerner DJ, Kannel WB. Patterns of coronary heart disease morbidity and mortality in the sexes: a 26-year follow-up of the Framingham population. Am Heart J. 1986;111(2):383–90.
7. Gordon T, Kannel WB, Hjortland MC, McNamara PM. Menopause and coronary heart disease. The Framingham Study. Ann Intern Med. 1978;89(2):157–61.
8. Lloyd-Jones D, Adams RJ, Brown TM, Carnethon M, Dai S, De Simone G, et al. Executive summary: heart disease and stroke statistics--2010 update: a report from the American Heart Association. Circulation. 2010;121(7):948–54.
9. Nkomo VT, Gardin JM, Skelton TN, Gottdiener JS, Scott CG, Enriquez-Sarano M. Burden of valvular heart diseases: a population-based study. Lancet Lond Engl. 2006;368(9540):1005–11.
10. Yousef R, Carr JA. Blunt cardiac trauma: a review of the current knowledge and management. Ann Thorac Surg. 2014;98(3):1134–40.
11. Kang N, Hsee L, Rizoli S, Alison P. Penetrating cardiac injury: overcoming the limits set by Nature. Injury. 2009;40(9):919–27.
12. Wall MJ, Mattox KL, Chen CD, Baldwin JC. Acute management of complex cardiac injuries. J Trauma. 1997;42(5):905–12.
13. Keough V, Letizia M. Blunt cardiac injury in the elderly trauma patient. Int J Trauma Nurs. 1998;4(2):38–43.
14. Pasquier M, Sierro C, Yersin B, Delay D, Carron P-N. Traumatic mitral valve injury after blunt chest trauma: a case report and review of the literature. J Trauma. 2010;68(1):243–6.
15. Marcolini EG, Keegan J. Blunt Cardiac Injury. Emerg Med Clin North Am. 2015;33(3):519–27.
16. Brathwaite CE, Rodriguez A, Turney SZ, Dunham CM, Cowley R. Blunt traumatic cardiac rupture. A 5-year experience. Ann Surg. 1990;212(6):701–4.

17. Liedtke AJ, DeMuth WE. Nonpenetrating cardiac injuries: a collective review. Am Heart J. 1973;86(5):687–97.
18. Baumgartner FJ, Rayhanabad J, Bongard FS, Milliken JC, Donayre C, Klein SR. Central venous injuries of the subclavian-jugular and innominate-caval confluences. Tex Heart Inst J. 1999;26(3):177–81.
19. Fineschi V, Di Donato S, Mondillo S, Turillazzi E. Electric shock: cardiac effects relative to non fatal injuries and post-mortem findings in fatal cases. Int J Cardiol. 2006;111(1):6–11.
20. Shetty BSK, Kanchan T, Acharya J, Naik R. Cardiac pathology in fatal electrocution. Burns. 2014;40(7):e45–6.
21. Clancy K, Velopulos C, Bilaniuk JW, Collier B, Crowley W, Kurek S, et al. Screening for blunt cardiac injury: an Eastern Association for the Surgery of Trauma practice management guideline. J Trauma Acute Care Surg. 2012;73(5 Suppl 4):S301–6.
22. Athanassiadi K, Gerazounis M, Moustardas M, Metaxas E. Sternal fractures: retrospective analysis of 100 cases. World J Surg. 2002;26(10):1243–6.
23. Vignon P, Boncoeur MP, François B, Rambaud G, Maubon A, Gastinne H. Comparison of multiplane transesophageal echocardiography and contrast-enhanced helical CT in the diagnosis of blunt traumatic cardiovascular injuries. Anesthesiology. 2001;94(4):615–22. discussion 5A
24. Mattox KL, Moore E. Trauma. 7e ed. Newyork: McGraw-Hill Education/Medical; 2012. p. 1248.

16 Geriatric Thoracic Vascular Injury

David Elliott and Aurelio Rodriguez

A 75-year-old male is the restrained driver of a motor vehicle broadsided by a pickup truck. There is only mild intrusion to the driver's side door. The patient appears stable and minimally injured on initial evaluation, although two posterior rib fractures are apparent on a suboptimal chest radiograph.

Is this patient more or less likely than patient half his age to harbor a thoracic vascular injury? Should he undergo further studies at this point to exclude such an injury, and, if so, which one(s)?

If the patient has sustained a blunt aortic injury (BAI) from this trauma, what are his chances of survival? Is he likely to have other injuries as well? Would he be best served by repair by thoracotomy, thoracic endovascular aortic repair (TEVAR), or observation with medical control but without surgery?

D. Elliott, M.D. (✉)
Médecins Sans Frontières/Doctors Without Borders, Richmond, VA, USA
e-mail: delliott@icloud.com

A. Rodriguez, M.D., F.A.C.S.
Drexel University College of Medicine, University of Maryland School of Medicine, Baltimore, MD, USA
e-mail: arod@zoominternet.net

Epidemiology

Regardless of age, thoracic vascular injury (TVI)—in particular, BAI—remains a major cause of mortality in trauma victims, despite recent advances in diagnostic and therapeutic strategies. Although, compared to the nongeriatric cohort, geriatric patients have a lower likelihood of incurring vascular injuries overall, the vascular injuries sustained are much more likely to be TVI, especially blunt TVI. TVI carries a mortality of 43% in trauma victims under the age of 65 years, and 66% in those over 65 years: higher than vascular injuries in any other body region for both age groups (Fig. 16.1) [1].

In an autopsy study of all blunt traumatic deaths in Los Angeles County in 2005, 34% had sustained BAI, and 80% of those died at the scene of the injury [2]. All had associated injuries, including blunt cardiac (44%) and intra-abdominal (74%) as well as rib fractures (86%).

A similar autopsy study out of Athens, Greece, reporting on all blunt and penetrating deaths due to injury to the thoracic aorta or its branches (13% of all trauma-related deaths) found that 83% incurring BAI expired at the scene, while 100% of gunshot victims and 80% of knife-wound victims with TVI died at the scene. BAI constituted 92% of all blunt TVI (isthmus and descending segments), whereas aortic injuries occurred in 81% of TVI victims with gunshot wounds, primarily within the ascending segment,

A. Rodriguez et al. (eds.), *Geriatric Trauma and Acute Care Surgery*,
https://doi.org/10.1007/978-3-319-57403-5_16

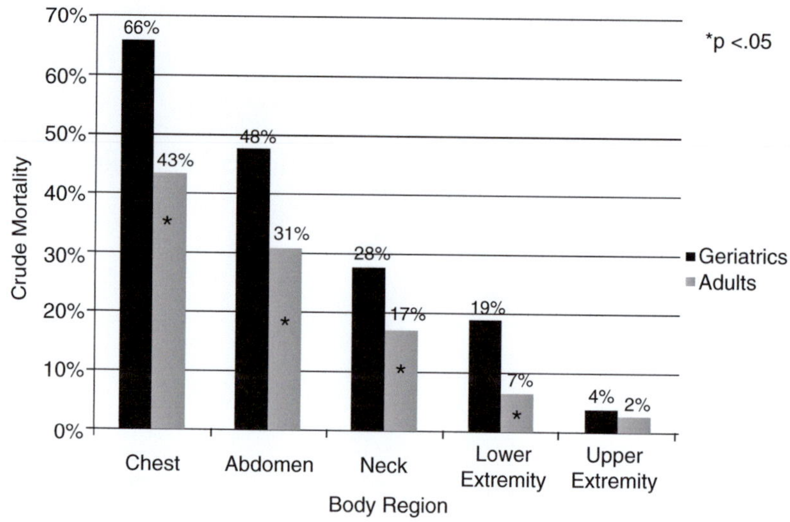

Fig. 16.1 Mortality among geriatric and nongeriatric adult patients, stratified by location of vascular injury (reproduced from Konstantinidis et al., J Trauma 2011)

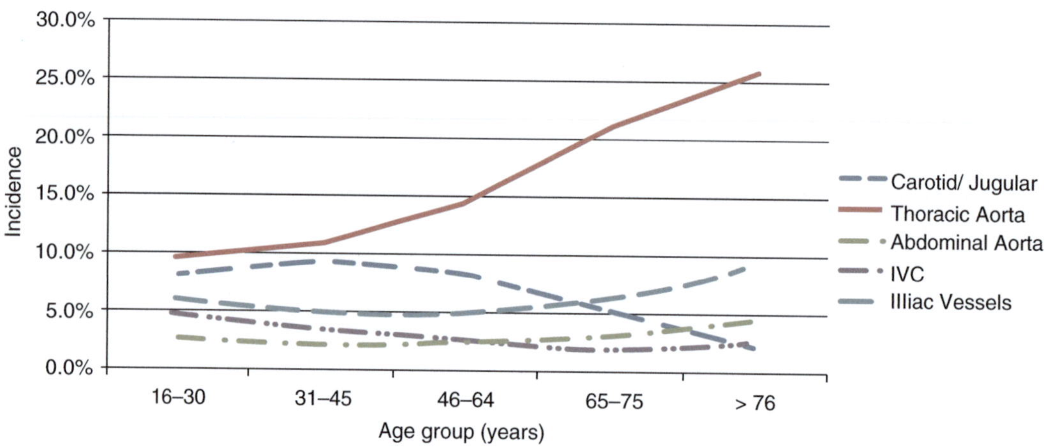

Fig. 16.2 Incidence of major truncal vascular injuries, stratified by location and age. *IVC* inferior vena cava (reproduced from Konstantinidis et al., J Trauma 2011)

and in only 26% of TVI deaths due to knife wounds (the majority occurring in aortic arch branches) [3].

Looking specifically at the geriatric age group in an analysis of the National Trauma Databank, Konstantinidis and colleagues showed that BAI constituted 33% of all geriatric vascular injuries, that the incidence of BAI steadily increased with age (Fig. 16.2), and that the geriatric cohort demonstrated a fourfold higher risk for mortality after vascular injury than their younger counterparts [1]. The authors concluded, "Given this high incidence and the increased mortality that is associated with traumatic aortic rupture in geriatric patients compared with their younger counterparts, a high clinical suspicion for this injury must always be present when assessing this particular age group of patients" [1].

Similar results were found by McGwin and colleagues, utilizing an analysis of the National Automotive Sampling System [4]. 85% of BAI victims died at the scene, consistent with other studies, and not differing between the geriatric and younger age groups. Most notable, however, were the findings that in-hospital mortality increased for BAI victims greater than 60 years of age; that a third of the geriatric BAI patients were in motor vehicles which sustained collisions which were not frontal;

and that geriatric patients sustained BAI at significantly lower velocity of impact ("delta-V") than the nongeriatric cohort. These latter findings suggest that the clinician must maintain a high index of suspicion for BAI in the geriatric patient despite involvement in a low-velocity collision.

The findings in both these studies, that geriatric trauma victims have a higher incidence of TVI (especially BAI) as well as a higher chance of in-hospital mortality should they reach the hospital alive, are supported by two other studies, one showing a ninefold increased risk of in-hospital death in geriatric trauma patients due to all causes (but especially higher incidences of chest, intracranial, and spinal injuries) [5] and the other showing a 40-fold increased risk of mortality for operative repair of BAI in "old patients" (greater than 55 years of age, and before the advent of TEVAR) [6].

Diagnosis

In the 10 years between 1997 and 2007, a mark shift occurred in the modalities chosen for diagnosis of TVI, especially BAI. The use of aortography for diagnosis plummeted, from 87 to 8%, as did the need for transesophageal echocardiography (12 to 1%); both were replaced by CT scan, which now predominates as the means for BAI diagnosis (35% in 1997; 93% in 2007; Fig. 16.3) [7]. In addition to its accuracy in diagnosis, CT also offers the advantages of rapidity of diagnosis, and ability to elicit additional intrathoracic injuries. Aortography still is essential, however, both for diagnosis when CT scanning is equivocal or suboptimal and for placement of the stent graft when TEVAR is utilized for treatment.

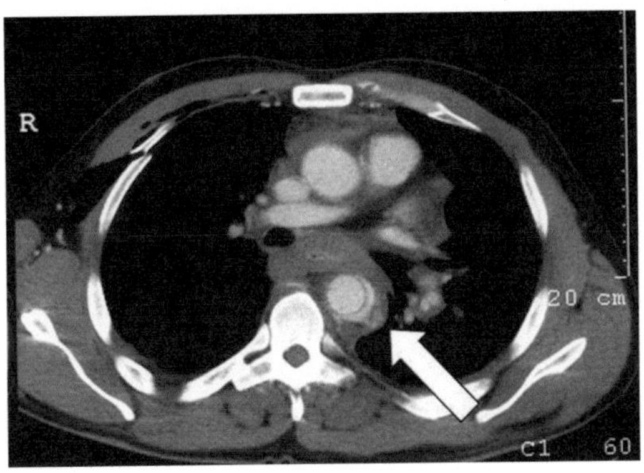

Fig. 16.3 Preoperative CT scan showing BAI with *arrow* pointing to rupture at isthmus (reproduced from Nano et al., J Cardiothorac Surg 2011) [25]

Treatment

As with means for diagnosis, in the last two decades the means for treatment of TVI has also undergone a marked shift: from open surgery (thoracotomy) to endovascular (TEVAR), which involves remote (generally femoral artery) deployment of an expandable stent graft to cover, exclude, and repair the aortic defect, under arteriographic guidance (Fig. 16.4) [7–9, 11–17]. This shift to the endovascular approach has been accompanied by a marked decrease in mortality and paraplegia, by liberalized indications for intervention (including age, comorbidities, additional injuries, physiologic status), and by an increase in graft-related complications.

Three published reports of prospective observational multicenter studies sponsored and conducted by the American Association for the Surgery of Trauma (AAST) [7–9] give a clear and contrasting picture of the results of open repair and TEVAR for BAI. One compared a late twentieth-century standard of care to more modern results, and found that use of open repair fell from 100% of cases to 35%, as TEVAR increased in utilization from 0 to 65%, with a resultant fall in procedural mortality from 22 to 13%, and fall in perioperative paraplegia from 8.7 to 1.6%, but accompanied by a TEVAR graft-related complication rate of 20% [7].

The second report detailed analysis of the most recent AAST multicenter data. As compared to open repair, TEVAR of BAI significantly resulted in lower mortality (7.2% vs. 23.5%), paraplegia (0.8% vs. 2.9%), acute renal failure (8.3% vs. 10.4%), and use of blood products (9.5 vs. 12 units). Given the predominance of geriatric patients assigned to TEVAR, the adjusted odds ratio for mortality for open repair (vs. TEVAR) was 8.4, and that for use of blood products, 5.0 [9].

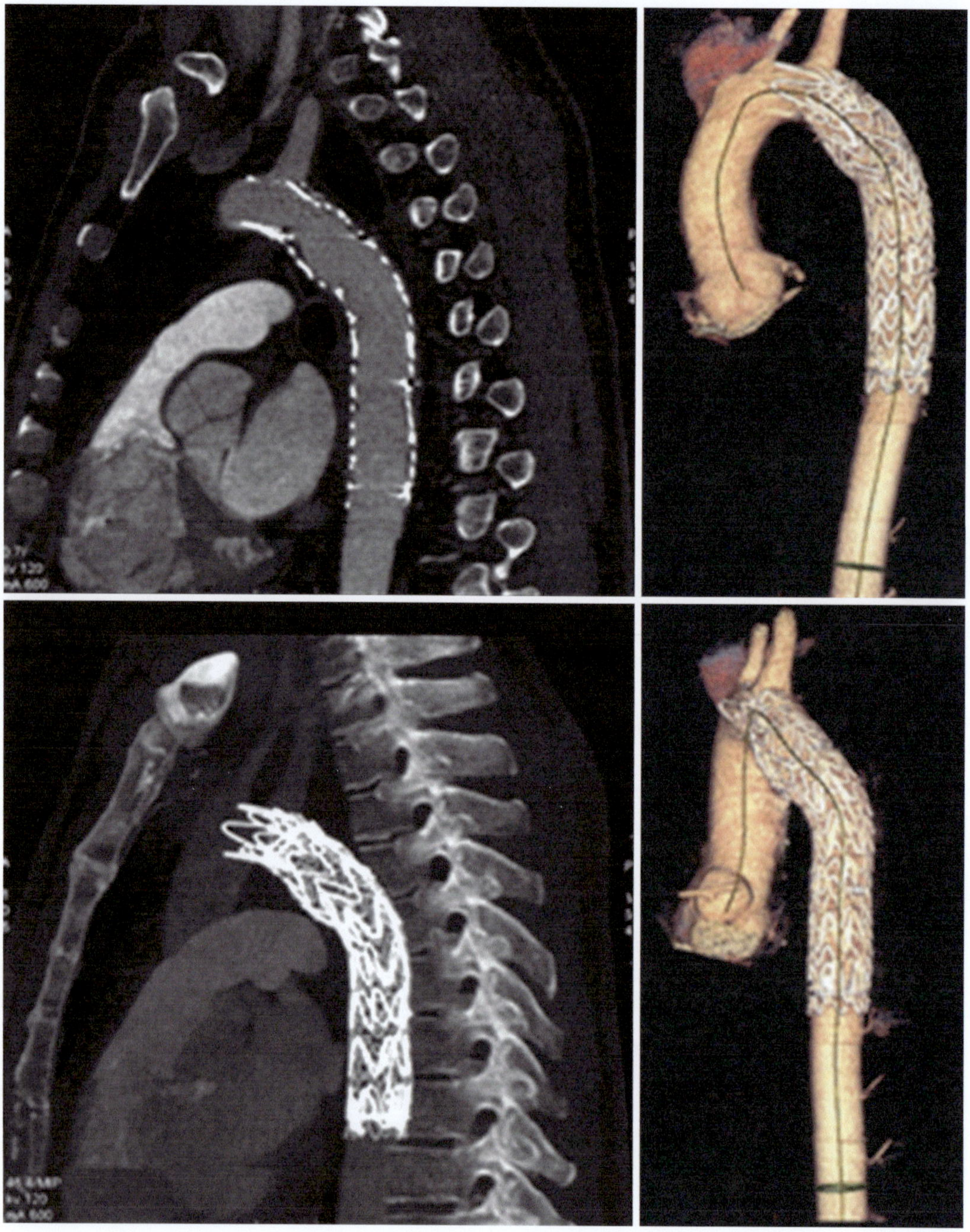

Fig. 16.4 Postoperative CT scan of TEVAR graft properly positioned in thoracic aorta; left subclavian artery is patent (reproduced from Nano et al., J Cardiothorac Surg 2011) [25]

The third report of these AAST data concerned the advisability of early (<24 h) versus delayed (>24 h) repair of BAI. Adjusting for other variables, the authors found that those patients who received delayed BAI repair had a lower mortality, irrespective of associated injuries, but incurred a longer ICU stay and more complications. Of particular note, in multivariate regression analysis, age >55 years did not prove to be a factor in outcome, regardless of associated injuries or timing of intervention [8]. Given the high percentage of BAI repaired by TEVAR in this study, this provides a stark contrast to age-related outcomes previously reported after open surgery [6].

A number of other recent retrospective studies also corroborate the superiority of TEVAR over open repair of BAI. One meta-analysis of 17 published studies, which included BAI patients who underwent 220 TEVAR and 369 open surgical procedures, matched for age but not for injury severity (the TEVAR patients had significantly higher ISS scores), demonstrated significantly lower 30-day mortality (8% vs. 20%) and paraplegia (0% vs. 7%) rates for the TEVAR group [10]. Another group of authors analyzed 7 years of data from the National Inpatient Sample, a nationwide administrative database of inpatient admissions that reflects national trends, and found that TEVAR has significantly extended the inclusion criteria for operative treatment of BAI (including geriatric patients and those with severe comorbidities, associated injuries, and shock), and in the process lowered the overall mortality for the injury [11]. A separate analysis of the National Trauma Databank over two time periods (2002–2006 and 2008) showed a marked increase over time in the percentage of traumatic vascular repairs performed by endovascular means (1 to 11% overall, 1 to 17% blunt; Fig. 16.5), and regression analysis confirmed that early endoscopic repairs of BAI and blunt carotid and subclavian injuries resulted in a 35% reduction in mortality, even in geriatric patients and those with higher ISS and lower GCS scores (Fig. 16.6) [12].

Many other recent studies have added evidence to the preference of TEVAR for treatment of BAI. In a meta-analysis of 33 published articles with 699 BAI patients (half repaired by TEVAR, half by open surgery), Tang and colleagues reported that TEVAR carried half the mortality of open surgery (7.6% vs. 15.2%), no paraplegia, and much lower risk of stroke (0.8% vs. 5.3%) [13]. Of particular interest, they noted that TEVAR proved especially suitable for geriatric patients, whose aortas generally enlarge with age (>23 mm), making the available endografts designed for aneurysmal disease more technically and clinically satisfactory. Watson and colleagues, in a single-center retrospective study spanning 14 years, found similar improved outcomes with TEVAR compared to open repair, reporting significantly lower rates of mortality (7% vs. 42%), renal failure requiring hemodialysis (0% vs. 9%), and paraplegia (0% vs. 6%); no breakout for geriatric patients was performed [14]. In another meta-analysis, this one including 139 studies of 7768 BAI patients covering 20 years of evolving treatment, Murad and

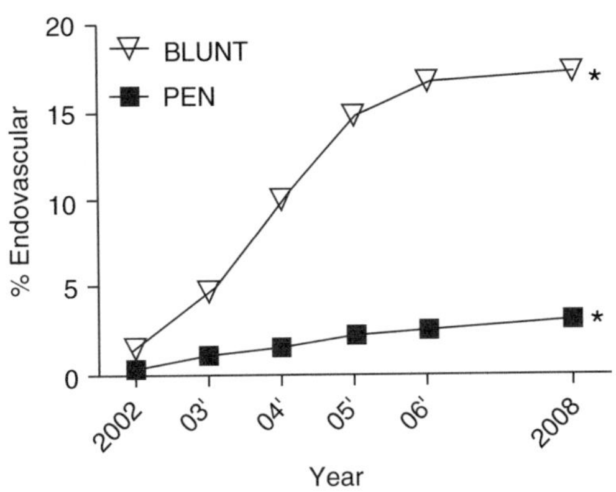

Fig. 16.5 Six-year trend: frequency of utilizing endovascular repair for vascular injuries, stratified by blunt versus penetrating mechanism. Significance: * = $p < 0.05$ (reproduced from Avery et al., J Trauma 2012)

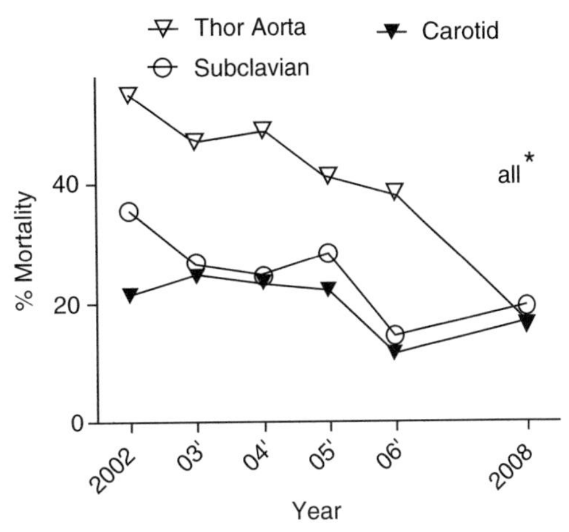

Fig. 16.6 Six-year trend of mortality rate for specified types of arterial injuries. Significance: * = $p < 0.05$ (reproduced from Avery et al., J Trauma 2012)

colleagues confirmed the superiority of TEVAR over open repair and nonoperative management with respect to mortality (9% vs. 19% vs. 46%, respectively), paraplegia (3% vs. 9% vs. 3%), and renal failure (3% vs. 8% vs. 5%) [15]. This study showed no difference in the three treatment groups with regard to stroke rate. Open repair carried a higher graft infection rate than TEVAR (11% vs. 3%), but TEVAR resulted in graft failure (leak, collapse, or rupture) in 10% of cases, which necessitated additional operations.

Based on the results of this last study, the Society of Vascular Surgery (SVS) published a position paper recommending TEVAR as the preferred treatment of BAI; in justifying this recommendation, "the committee placed a significantly higher value on preventing catastrophic complications of thoracic aortic repair (death, stroke, and spinal cord ischemia) and a lower value on potential adverse events such as endoleak, need for reintervention, and device failures. The committee also placed less value on possible late-term outcomes that remain unknown at this time." [16] In this article, the SVS also put forward its consensus for guidelines for the use of TEVAR for BAI (Table 16.1).

One of the SVS recommendations for TEVAR of BAI includes "selective [as opposed to mandatory] revascularization of the left subclavian artery." [16] This issue is addressed because 30% of stent graft placement by TEVAR results in total or partial coverage of the left subclavian artery (LSA) [15], which can lead to arterial occlusion and arm ischemia requiring urgent left carotid-to-subclavian bypass grafting. One prospective, nonrandomized, multicenter trial examining this issue found that the LSA was covered in 29 of 50 TEVAR graft placements for BAI

Table 16.1 Society for Vascular Surgery-recommended guidelines for use of TEVAR for BAI (reproduced from Lee et al., J Vasc Surg 2011)

Guideline	Consensus	Grade of recommendation 1—strong 2—weak	Quality of evidence A—high B—moderate C—low or very low
Choice of treatment	We suggest that endovascular repair be performed preferentially over open surgical repair or nonoperauve management	**2**	C
Timing of repair	We suggest urgent (<24 hours) repair, and at the latest prior to hospital discharge	**2**	C
Management of minimal aortic injury	We suggest expectant management with serial imaging for type I injuries	**2**	C
Type of repair in the young patient	We suggest endovascular repair regardless of age if anatomically suitable	**2**	C
Management of left subclavian artery	We suggest selective revascularization of the left subclavian artery	**2**	C
Systemic heparinization	We suggest routine heparinization but at a lower dose than in elective TEVAR	**2**	C
Spinal drainage	We do not suggest routine spinal drainage	**2**	C
Choice of anesthesia	We suggest general anesthesia	**2**	C
Femoral access technique	We suggest open femoral exposure	**2**	C

(58%); 3 of the 29 (10%) required carotid-to-subclavian bypass grafting for arm ischemia and claudication [17]. A meta-analysis of this issue, sponsored by the SVS and involving 51 studies with 3365 patients, found that LSA coverage during TEVAR graft placement increased the risk 47-fold for arm ischemia and 11-fold for vertebrobasilar ischemia: of the patients with BAI who underwent TEVAR graft placement with LSA coverage, a total of 5 of 57 (9%) developed arm ischemia and 1 of 47 (2%) vertebrobasilar ischemia [18].

Tang and colleagues [13] assert that there is one subset of BAI patients in whom TEVAR with LSA coverage mandates prophylactic carotid-to-subclavian bypass grafting: those patients who have had prior coronary artery bypass grafting using the left internal mammary artery, as this vessel originates from the LSA.

Similar to the SVS, the Eastern Association for the Surgery of Trauma (EAST) has also adopted and published a set of guidelines for BAI, utilizing meta-analysis of 51 peer-reviewed articles published between 1998 and 2013; EAST strongly recommends the use of CT for BAI diagnosis and the use of TEVAR for BAI repair, and it suggests its preference for delayed repair of BAI, especially in the presence of other life-threatening injuries, as long as the blood pressure is controlled with anti-impulse (antihypertensive) medication [19].

One currently debated topic in the treatment of BAI concerns the use of nonoperative therapy for minimal aortic injury. Starnes and colleagues from Seattle based treatment strategy on a novel CT grading scheme. Discovering that, in their series, "no patient with a normal external contour of the aorta died of their BAI," they successfully employed nonoperative therapy for all intimal tears and nonprogressive intimal flaps, and based urgency of operative therapy on the presence of hypotension or periaortic hematomata (>2 cm) in BAI patients with an abnormal aortic external contour (pseudoaneurysm or free extravasation) [20]. The fundamentals of this treatment strategy were corroborated by Rabin and colleagues [21], Smeds and colleagues [22], and DuBose and colleagues [23].

Recently, the FDA has approved two second-generation commercially available thoracic aortic endograft systems for the treatment of BAI. Industry improvements with these newer devices that should lower the rate of previously published TEVAR-related complications include (a) expanding stent graft choices down to an aortic diameter of 16 mm; (b) increasing the aortic arch angulation and proximal wall conformability; and (c) improving percutaneous peripheral access with smaller delivery profiles and preclose technique devices. These three factors should expand TEVAR use to a broader range of patients (especially younger ones with smaller diameter aortas and tight radius of curvature of the aortic arch) and concomitantly reduce the risk of endoleak, LSA coverage, and iliofemoral access-site injury [23, 24].

Conclusions

Although relatively uncommon, thoracic vascular injuries are highly lethal after both blunt and penetrating trauma, regardless of age. In particular, blunt aortic injury still carries an 85% mortality at the scene, in both the geriatric and younger age groups. For the blunt trauma victim of geriatric age, (a) the incidence of BAI increases linearly with advancing years, (b) BAI can occur at much lower levels of blunt impact, and (c) BAI has traditionally incurred a greater chance of mortality once a live patient reaches the hospital.

Recent years have seen significant progress in the diagnosis, treatment, and chance of survival for geriatric patients sustaining BAI. CT scan has become the diagnostic modality of choice, obviating the need for time-consuming, resource-intensive, invasive aortography to rule in or out this injury. TEVAR has become the preferred means for treatment of BAI and other blunt TVI, resulting in improved survival rates, most dramatically in geriatric patients, eliminating the risks of open surgery. Primarily due to TEVAR, advanced age is no longer a significant factor in deciding whether to perform repair for BAI, even when combined with numerous comorbidities or other severe injuries.

Nonetheless, published studies of TEVAR relate a high rate of procedure-related complications, such as endoleak, arm ischemia due to LSA coverage, and insertion-site injury, necessitating additional procedures in up to 20% of patients. The fact that significantly more geriatric patients now survive this extremely lethal injury makes such complications seem less important; however, efforts to minimize such TEVAR side effects are crucial. Recent product innovations by industry are addressing these issues, and published reports of improvements are forthcoming. Long-term follow-up studies of BAI patients treated with TEVAR are lacking; such will undoubtedly prove critical in both refining the technique and validating whether endovascular stent graft placement can endure as a safe and effective form of treatment.

Recent studies have confirmed a place for nonoperative therapy for BAI. Agreement seems to exist that those injuries showing only intimal tear or intimal flap on CT rarely cause mortality, and can be medically managed (with anti-impulse medication). Disagreement exists on how best to handle small BAI pseudoaneurysms, but delaying therapy until severe associated injuries are addressed seems appropriate.

Finally, it should be noted that there exist very few published, peer-reviewed studies concerning TVI in the geriatric population, especially articles containing data for injuries other than BAI. Researchers and clinicians are encouraged to focus more efforts on studying such lethal injuries in the aged, particularly as those of the "baby boomer" generation reach their seventh decade of life.

References

1. Konstantinidis A, Inaba K, Dubose J, Barmparas G, Lam L, Plurad D, et al. Vascular trauma in geriatric patients: a national trauma databank review. J Trauma. 2011;71:909–16.
2. Teixeira P, Inaba K, Barmparas G, Georgiou C, Toms C, Noguchi T, et al. Blunt thoracic aortic injuries: an autopsy study. J Trauma. 2011;70:197–202.
3. Dosios T, Salemis N, Angouras D, Nonas E. Blunt and penetrating trauma of the thoracic aorta and aortic arch branches: an autopsy study. J Trauma. 2000;49:696–703.
4. McGwin G, Reiff D, Moran S, Rue L. Incidence and characteristics of motor vehicle collision – related blunt thoracic aortic injury according to age. J Trauma. 2002;52:859–66.
5. Bauzá G, LaMorte W, Burke P, Hirsch E. High mortality in elderly drivers is associated with distinct injury patterns: analysis of 187,869 injured drivers. J Trauma. 2008;64:304–10.
6. Camp P, Rogers F, Shackford S, Leavitt B, Cobean R, Clark D. Blunt traumatic thoracic aortic lacerations in the elderly: an analysis of outcome. J Trauma. 1994;37:418–23.
7. Demetriades D, Velmahos G, Scalea T, Jurkovich G, Karmy-Jones R, Teixeira P, et al. Diagnosis and treatment of blunt thoracic aortic injuries: changing perspectives. J Trauma. 2008;64:1415–9.
8. Demetriades D, Velmahos G, Scalea T, Jurkovich G, Karmy-Jones R, Teixeira P, et al. Blunt traumatic thoracic aortic injuries: early or delayed repair—results of an American Association for the Surgery of Trauma Prospective Study. J Trauma. 2009;66:967–73.
9. Demetriades D, Velmahos G, Scalea T, Jurkovich G, Karmy-Jones R, Teixeira P, et al. Operative repair or endovascular stent graft in blunt traumatic thoracic aortic injuries: results of an American Association for the Surgery of Trauma Multicenter Study. J Trauma. 2008;64:561–71.
10. Xenos E, Abedi N, Davenport D, Minion D, Hamdallah O, Sorial E, et al. Meta-analysis of endovascular vs open repair for traumatic descending thoracic aortic rupture. J Vasc Surg. 2008;48:1343–51.
11. Hong M, Feezor R, Lee A, Nelson P. The advent of thoracic endovascular aortic repair is associated with broadened treatment eligibility and decreased overall mortality in traumatic thoracic aortic injury. J Vasc Surg. 2011;53:36–43.
12. Avery L, Stahlfeld K, Corcos A, Scifres A, Ziembicki J, Varcelotti J, et al. Evolving role of endovascular techniques for traumatic vascular injury: a changing landscape? J Trauma. 2012;72:41–7.
13. Tang G, Tehrani H, Usman A, Katariya K, Otero C, Perez E, et al. Reduced mortality, paraplegia, and stroke with stent graft repair of blunt aortic transections: a modern meta-analysis. J Vasc Surg. 2008;47:671–5.
14. Watson J, Slaiby J, MD TM, Marcaccio E, Chong T. A 14-year experience with blunt thoracic aortic injury. J Vasc Surg. 2013;58:380–5.
15. Murad M, Rizvi A, Malgor R, Carey J, Alkatib A, Erwin P, et al. Comparative effectiveness of the treatments for thoracic aortic transaction. J Vasc Surg. 2011;53:193–9.
16. Lee A, Matsumura J, Mitchell S, Farber M, Greenberg R, Azizzadeh A, et al. Endovascular repair of traumatic thoracic aortic injury: clinical practice guide-

lines of the Society for Vascular Surgery. J Vasc Surg. 2011;53:187–92.

17. Khoynezhad A, Azizzadeh A, Donayre C, Matsumoto A, Velazquez O, White R, et al. Results of a multicenter, prospective trial of thoracic endovascular aortic repair for blunt thoracic aortic injury (RESCUE trial). J Vasc Surg. 2013;57:899–905.
18. Rizvi A, Murad H, Fairman R, Erwin P, Montori V. The effect of left subclavian artery coverage on morbidity and mortality in patients undergoing endovascular thoracic aortic interventions: a systematic review and meta-analysis. J Vasc Surg. 2009;50:1159–69.
19. Fox N, Schwartz D, Salazar J, Haut E, Dahm P, Black J, et al. Evaluation and management of blunt traumatic aortic injury: a practice management guideline from the Eastern Association for the Surgery of Trauma. J Trauma Acute Care Surg. 2015;78:136–46.
20. Starnes B, Lundgren R, Gunn M, Quade S, Hatsukami T, Tran N. A new classification scheme for treating blunt aortic injury. J Vasc Surg. 2012;55:47–54.
21. Rabin J, DuBose J, Sliker C, Connor J, Scalea T, Griffith B. Parameters for successful nonoperative management of traumatic aortic injury. J Thorac Cardiovasc Surg. 2014;147:143–50.
22. Smeds M, Wright M, Eidt J, Moursi M, Escobar G, Spencer H, et al. Delayed management of grade III blunt aortic injury: series from a level-I trauma center. J Trauma Acute Care Surg. 2016;80(6):947–51. Epub ahead of print
23. DuBose J, Leake S, Brenner M, Pasley J, O'Callaghan T, Luo-Owen X, et al. Contemporary management and outcomes of blunt thoracic aortic injury: a multicenter retrospective study. J Trauma Acute Care Surg. 2015;78:360–9.
24. Adams J, Kern J. Blunt thoracic aortic injury: current issues and endovascular treatment paradigms. Endovasc Today. 2014;13:38–42.
25. Nano N, Mazzaccaro D, Malacrida G, Occhiuto M, Stegher S, Tealdi D. Delayed endovascular treatment of descending aorta stent graft collapse in a patient treated for post- traumatic aortic rupture: a case report. J Cardiothorac Surg. 2011;6:76–81.

17 Thoracic Trauma in the Elderly

T. Robert Qaqish, JoAnn Coleman, and Mark Katlic

Introduction

As our population continues to age, the management of the "geriatric trauma patient" will become more commonplace in emergency departments across the country. In a report of the National Automotive Sampling System/Crashworthiness Data System (1998–2007) the relationship between occupant's age and incidence of thoracic injuries was measured [1]. The authors found that occupants 75+ had a higher percentage of moderate to severe (abbreviated injury score, AIS 2+) thoracic injuries than the three other age groups studied (25–44, 45–64, 65–74) in a tow-away crash. Moreover, the threshold for thoracic injury in older adults was lower when compared to their younger counterparts. Seventy-five percent of occupants greater than 75 years of age sustained a AIS 2+ thoracic injuries at a crash delta-v (Delta-V (Δv) is a measure of the severity of a traffic collision, defined as the change in velocity between precollision and postcollision trajectories of a vehicle [2]) of 37 km/h (23 mph) or less whereas the same AIS of thoracic injury in 75% of patients aged 25–44 was sustained at a crash delta-v of 46 km/h (28.6 mph). Furthermore, the ratio of thoracic injuries to other causes of death was highest in patients greater than 75 (Fig. 17.1). Although the above study represents one, albeit a common mechanism of trauma, motor vehicle collision (MVC), it underscores and provides perspective regarding our geriatric trauma patients that suffer from thoracic injuries.

The Thorax as We Age

Unlike other intra-thoracic or intra-abdominal organs, the lungs are in direct contact with the atmosphere. Over a person's lifetime, this poses a number of environmental insults, most notably, first- and second-hand tobacco smoke. Oxidative stress within the airways is a key component that drives airway inflammation with the downstream effects, such as accumulation of ROS, culminating in the eventual decline in lung function [3].

As we age, the lung undergoes both structural and physiologic changes over time. The lung becomes more stiff which translates into a less compliant lung. Moreover, the elastic recoil of the lung parenchyma is dampened. This is secondary to disruption of collagen and elastin fibers

T. Robert Qaqish, M.Sc., M.D.
J. Coleman, D.N.P., A.C.N.P., A.O.C.N.
M. Katlic, M.D., M.M.M., F.A.C.S. (✉)
Department of Surgery, Sinai Hospital of Baltimore, 2401 West Belvedere Avenue, Hoffberger Building/Suite 42, Baltimore, MD 21215, USA
e-mail: tqaqish@lifebridgehealth.org; jocolema@lifebridgehealth.org; mkatlic@lifebridgehealth.org

A. Rodriguez et al. (eds.), *Geriatric Trauma and Acute Care Surgery*,
https://doi.org/10.1007/978-3-319-57403-5_17

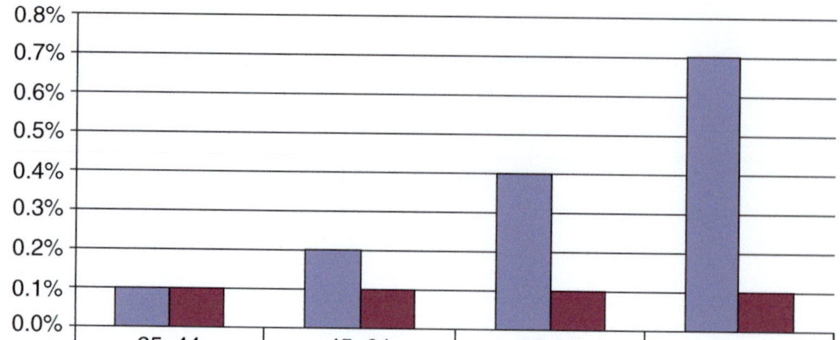

	25–44	45–64	65–74	75+
Thorax	0.1%	0.2%	0.4%	0.7%
Other	0.1%	0.1%	0.1%	0.1%

Fig. 17.1 The ratio of mortality from chest injuries to other injuries increases proportional to age in patients involved in a tow-away crash MVC (reprinted with permission [1])

that ultimately leads to dilatation of alveolar ducts and subsequent reduction of surface area and gas exchange. As a result, there is a greater tendency for the small airways to collapse [4]. In healthy elderly individuals, this may be of no consequence; however in an elderly patient who suffers from acute chest trauma, pulmonary reserve is further restricted and less tolerant to injury. As a result, the manifestations of so-called senile emphysema flourish.

Compliance of the chest wall is a measure of the thoracic cavity's ability to expand and contract. The compliance of an elderly patient's chest wall is decreased secondary to ossification of costal cartilages and calcification of the articular surfaces of ribs [5]. The mobility of the chest wall is further impaired from vertebral body collapse from osteoporosis [5]. As a consequence, the thoracic rib cage is more brittle and less pliable during blunt trauma. This not only predisposes the chest wall to fracture (rib, sternum) but may also predispose to more severe chest wall injuries (flail chest, thoracic spine fracture) and resultant morbidity and mortality.

The structural changes described above alter the chest wall dynamics and in consequence impair the respiratory cycle. Forced expiratory volume in 1 second (FEV1) and forced vital capacity (FVC) are reduced with age. Residual volume (RV) and functional residual capacity (FRC) increase with age as the elastic recoil of the terminal airways is compromised. The elderly adult breathes at higher tidal volumes forcing a greater energy expenditure on the muscles of respiration [6]. Alveoli collapse at lower lung volumes in the elderly leading to greater ventilation/perfusion mismatch. Pulmonary capillary blood volume and capillary density are also decreased [5].

Immune-related changes are also present in the elderly lung. Reduced mucociliary clearance further exposes the lung to environmental insults. Chemotaxis and bactericidal activity of neutrophils is reduced in the elderly [7]. Such phenomena may predispose the lung to infection and render it more susceptible to environmental insult.

Thus, the elderly patient's respiratory system is inherently vulnerable to injury. When an elderly patient suffers trauma to the thoracic cavity, the injuries are often more severe than their younger counterparts. Furthermore, the sequelae that follow these injuries often result in a more turbulent clinical course.

Rib Fractures

After life-threatening conditions that require emergent therapy during the primary survey are managed, the secondary survey can help identify potential injuries to the chest wall prior to more sophisticated diagnostic modalities such as computed tomography (CT) are employed.

It is important to palpate all aspects of the chest wall, including the upper abdomen, during the secondary survey of the Advanced Trauma

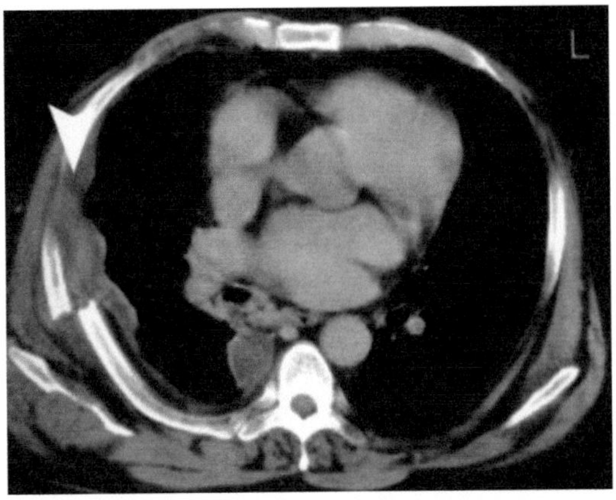

Fig. 17.2 *Arrowhead* indicating extrapleural hematoma associated with right-sided rib fractures (reprinted with permission [8])

Life Support (ATLS) algorithm. The multitrauma patient often possesses distracting injuries, and the provider may not immediately observe the clinical manifestations of rib fractures such as splinting or paradoxical chest wall motion. Ecchymosis, abrasions, and seat belt injuries should alert the clinician that there may be underlying bony injury to the thoracic cage. However, the absence of physical manifestations on the patient's chest or back does not serve as reassurance that rib fractures do not exist. Furthermore, a negative upright chest X-ray as an adjunct to the primary survey should also not reassure the provider that rib fractures are absent as up to 50% of chest X-rays may fail to identify rib fractures (Fig. 17.2) [8]. In addition, the elderly have blunted responses to hypoxia and hypercarbia which may result in a delayed presentation as clinical signs of respiratory compromise may not be immediately apparent.

Rib fractures represent the most common thoracic injury as a result of blunt chest trauma in the elderly. In a retrospective cohort study from Taiwan where 1621 thoracic trauma patients were reviewed over a 9-year period (mean age 51.2), 78.5% had rib fractures [9]. Approximately 75% of the rib fracture patients had three or fewer rib fractures with left-sided rib fractures being more common and the fifth and sixth ribs fractured most often. In this study, patients between 65 and 74 were identified as a risk factor associated with rib fractures (OR 2.41, 1.6–3.6, <0.001). Moreover, the number of rib fractures was positively associated with hemothorax, pneumothorax, and hemopneumothorax. Mortality was not significantly associated with increasing rib fractures; however, it has been demonstrated elsewhere [10].

Similar data has been reproduced in the United States. In a retrospective 10-year study in Ohio, 3095 elderly patients were admitted for blunt trauma, of which 12% of patients suffered from blunt chest trauma [10]. Sixty-five percent of patients suffered from rib fractures, with 50% of the patients presenting with falls as their primary mechanism of injury. There was a linear relationship associated with a higher number of rib fractures and overall mortality. In the elderly, the mortality was twice that compared to adults (18% vs. 9%, $p = 0.03$), Fig. 17.3. This was supportive of other reports where mortality was higher in elderly patients with increasing rib fractures and risk of pneumonia increased 27% for each rib fracture in patients greater than 65 years of age [11].

Although falls are the predominant mechanism of trauma in our elderly patients, blunt chest trauma from MVCs represents a large portion of traumatic admissions [12]. Moreover, seat belts, steering wheels, armrest, and side panels are often responsible for rib and sternum fractures during MVCs.

Multiple rib fractures in the elderly also predispose patients to adverse events during their evaluation and treatment for blunt chest trauma. In a small retrospective review of 99 trauma patients with isolated blunt trauma to the chest, 16.2% developed an adverse event that included pneumonia (most common), transfer to the intensive care unit for hypoxia, unanticipated endotracheal intubation, ARDS, or death from pulmonary sequelae. Risk factors for developing any of the above-mentioned sequelae included age greater than 85, initial SBP less than 90, hemothorax, pneumothorax, greater or equal to three rib fractures, or pulmonary contusion [13].

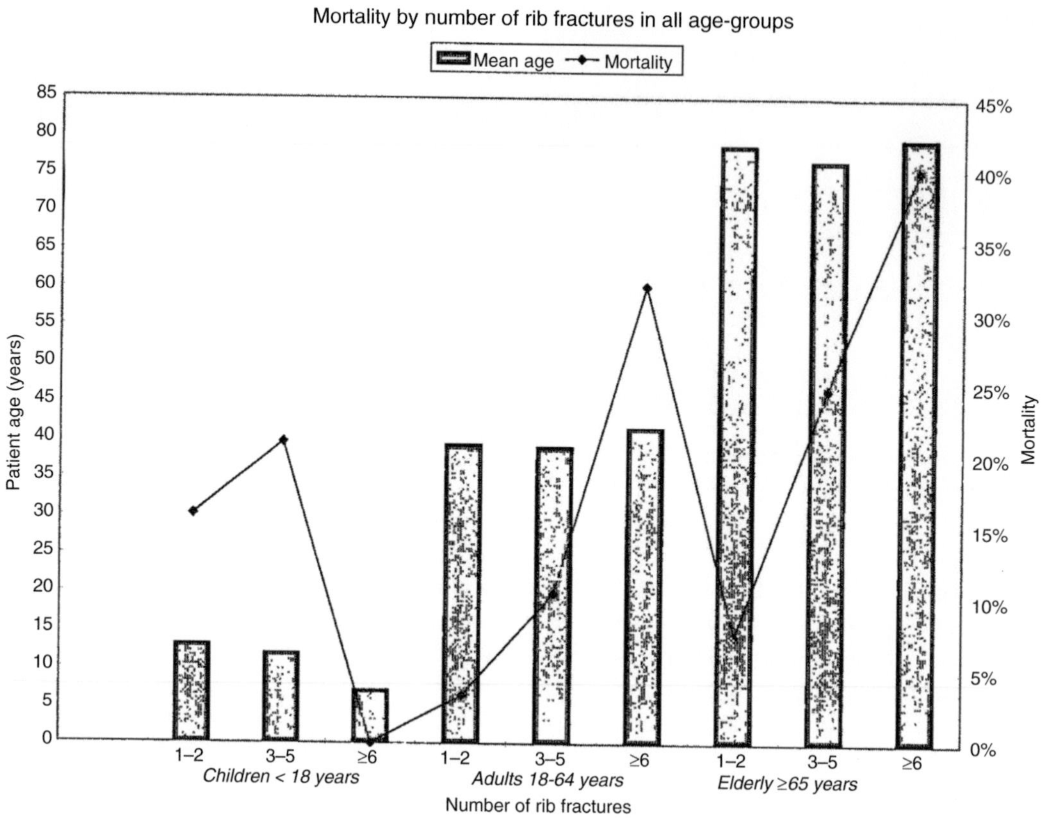

Fig. 17.3 Mortality associated with rib fractures is greatest in elderly trauma patients (reprinted with permission [10])

Rib Fracture Management

Analgesia and aggressive pulmonary toilet are the tenets of rib fracture management and apply across all patient populations. Management of rib fracture-associated pain helps prevent splinting and subsequent atelectasis and helps prevent the elderly population's already heightened risk of suffering from pulmonary sequelae. Continuous hemodynamic monitoring, supplemental oxygen, and pulse oximetry are also paramount in caring for the elderly patient with bony thoracic injury.

Multiple options exist for the management of rib fracture-associated pain. Oral and intravenous narcotics are the mainstays of therapy where the intravenous route has many forms including nursing administered versus patient-controlled routes (i.e., patient-controlled analgesia, PCA). Extrathoracic modes of therapy are also employed such as epidural analgesia in which an anesthetic agent is injected into the epidural space to assist with pain control. Nonsteroidal anti-inflammatory drugs (NSAIDs) are commonly administered in younger patients with rib fractures; however their use in elderly individuals needs to be heavily balanced in light of baseline renal dysfunction and history and risks of peptic ulcer disease.

Intravenous narcotics are effective in managing fracture-associated pain and are often used first line in managing patients with rib fractures. Respiratory depression as well as central nervous and hemodynamic consequences are not uncommon with the use of intravenous narcotics. Moreover, the elderly patient's underlying cognitive impairment (i.e., dementia, Alzheimer's) must be taken into consideration when prescribing narcotic therapy in the inpatient setting.

Level I recommendations from the Eastern Association for the Surgery of Trauma (EAST) advocate early implementation of epidural anesthesia (EA) as the preferred method of analgesia for severe blunt trauma resulting in rib fractures [14]. Contraindications to EA include coagulopathy, unstable spinal trauma, an uncooperative patient, infection overlying the puncture site, and increased intracranial pressure. In the multitrauma elderly patient, consideration should also be given when serial abdominal examinations are performed while conservatively managing an intra-abdominal process. Epidural anesthesia in this setting may disguise clinical abdominal findings.

The rationale for the use of EA stems from studies demonstrating increased pO_2, improved spirometry parameters including FRC, lung compliance, and vital capacity [15]. EA is able to maintain adequate analgesia while not influencing the patient's level of sedation. This allows the patient to participate more frequently in pulmonary physical therapy [16].

Alternate forms of pain management options exist and include intercostal nerve block, intrapleural anesthesia, and thoracic paravertebral blockade.

Intercostal nerve blocks depend on the infiltrating agent to bath the posterior compartment of the intercostal space. This is typically achieved via percutaneous injection or catheter placement and requires multiple anatomic injections above and below the affected rib segments. This achieves unilateral analgesia, and improves peak expiratory flow rates and volumes without significant effects on hemodynamics; however it requires palpation overlying the fractured ribs and repeated injections [17, 18].

Intrapleural anesthesia involves placement of a local anesthetic into the pleural space via an indwelling catheter [19]. The diffusion, and essentially the effectiveness of the anesthetic, is gravity dependent. Thus patient positioning, presence of hemothorax or pneumothorax, and tube thoracostomy may impair its effectiveness.

Thoracic paravertebral blockade involves percutaneous injections in close proximity to the thoracic vertebrae for unilateral thoracic analgesia. The injections produce unilateral somatic and sympathetic blockade without the inherit risks of spinal cord injury or need to palpate along the fractured rib segments [20–23].

Although the preferred delivery of analgesia is epidural anesthesia, clinical factors as well as resource limitations often dictate the intervention the patient receives. The analgesic options are numerous and should often combine multiple modalities of pain control with the overarching goal of encouraging as much patient participation in pulmonary physiotherapy as well as facilitate patient mobility.

Flail Chest

Flail chest is the result of double fractures to three or more contiguous ribs or combined sternal and rib fractures. A nonintegrated chest wall is one that occurs when there are multiple single-rib fractures [24]. The clinical manifestations on physical exam result in an inward displacement of the affected segment during inspiration and outward movement during expiration termed "paradoxical" chest wall movement. As a result of this gross deformity of the chest wall, the dynamics of the chest wall and diaphragm are altered compromising the respiratory parameters of lung function. The patient's inspiratory capacity is limited and the vital capacity may decrease by more than 50%. The deformity restricts the lung, decreases its compliance, and ultimately results in impaired gas exchange (Fig. 17.4). In the elderly patient, where the respiratory reserve is already reduced, an insult such as an unstable chest wall is often devastating to the patient's respiratory system and is often associated with a high morbidity and mortality.

In a review of the National Trauma Bank Data between 2007 and 2009, 354,945 blunt trauma patients with injury severity scores (ISS) of 9 or greater were extracted [25]. One percent (3467/354,945) had a documented flail chest injury. The mean age was 52.5 years and mean ISS was 30.4. The most common mechanism of injury was MVC (79%) and falls being the second most common (16%). Data regarding the remainder of the clinical cohort and outcomes is outlined in Fig. 17.5. Severe head injury (defined as an Abbreviated Injury Score of three or greater and Glasgow Coma Scale (GCS) less

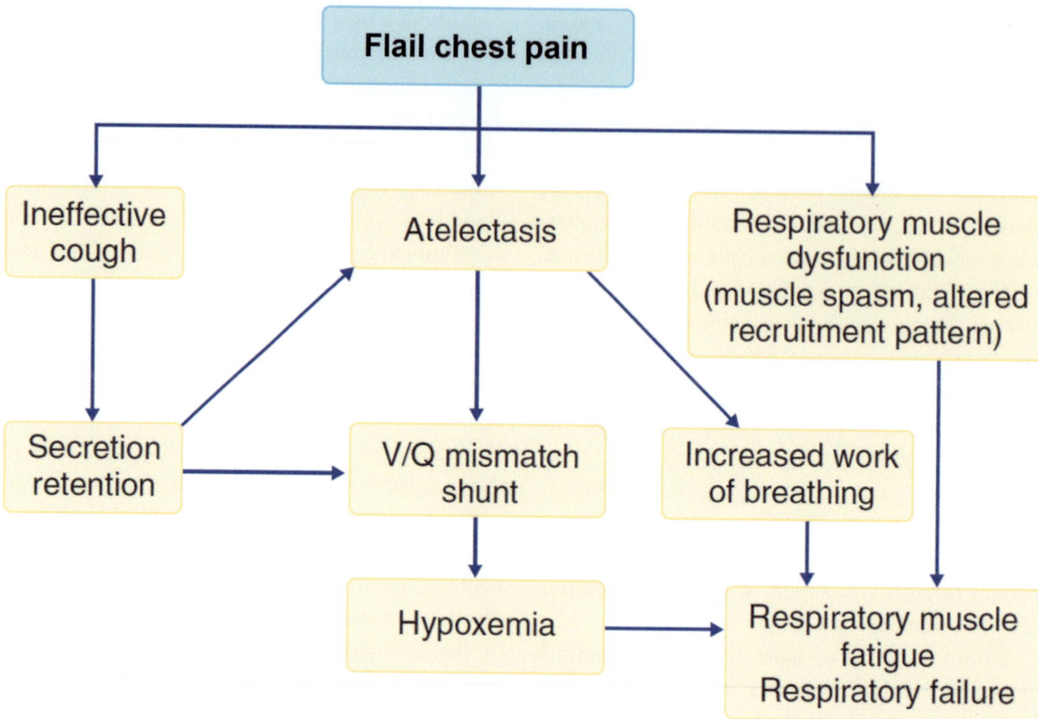

Fig. 17.4 Factors involved in the pathophysiology of respiratory failure in patients with flail chest (reprinted with permission [24])

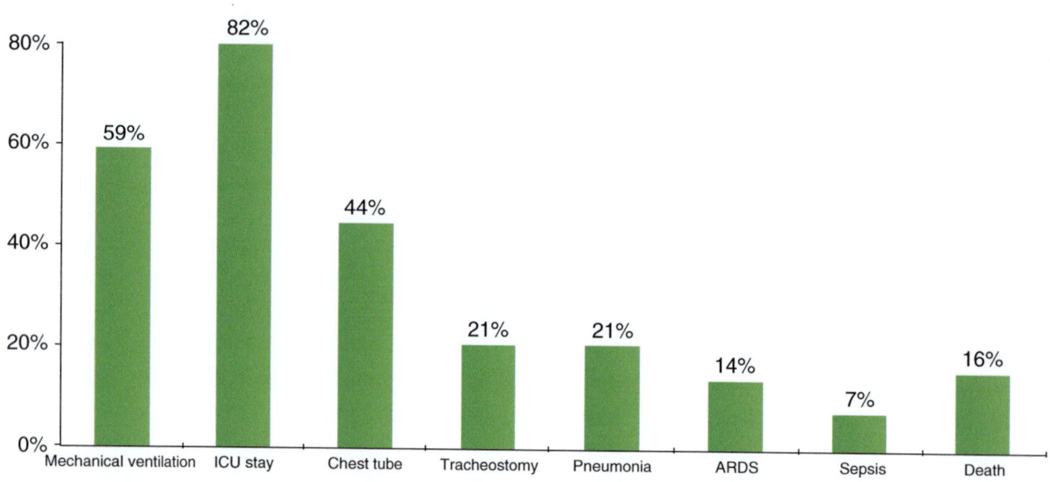

Fig. 17.5 Outcomes, morbidity, and mortality for 3467 patients identified with flail chest injury (reprinted with permission [25])

than or equal to four) occurred in 15% of patients with FC and 54% had documented lung contusions. Patients with severe head injuries required longer ventilatory support/ICU stay and ultimately had worse outcomes. Elderly patients were unfortunately not subcategorized in this study for analysis.

In a retrospective review of 58 trauma patients admitted with flail chest, patients above the age of 55 (n = 26) had a 58% mortality whereas mortality reported for patients less than or equal to 55 ($n = 32$) was 16% [26]. Contrastingly, in a retrospective review by Athanassiadi et al., in which 250 patients presenting with flail chest were studied (mean age 58.3 ± 16.5 years) age did not affect mortality; however it did affect the length of hospitalization. Although flail chest is a relatively uncommon thoracic injury, it is a marker of more severe chest trauma and often mandates a longer and more morbid hospitalization, especially in the elderly.

The current literature on the surgical management of flail chest is relatively scant. The studies that do exist are mostly small and retrospective and include a wide range of patient demographics, including age. Nonetheless, the data from a number of these studies were reviewed in a meta-analysis by Slobogean and colleagues [27]. From the 11 studies reviewed, a total of 753 patients comprised the study pool and the literature data spanned between 1965 and 2008. Nine studies were retrospective and two were prospective and randomized. The pooled studies demonstrated multiple benefits to operative fixation of flail chest that included decreased odds for mortality, tracheostomy, pneumonia, sepsis, and chest deformity. Although small and mostly retrospective in nature, the pooled data suggested that operative repair reduced the number of mean ventilator days, ICU, and hospital days. Furthermore, another meta-analysis reported similar findings in that operative fixation improves the outcomes related to resource expenditure, mortality, and morbidity [28]. Currently, patients with flail chest are mostly managed conservatively just as other patients with rib fractures, with analgesia and pulmonary toilet representing the most crucial aspects of treatment.

In a more recent randomized control trial by Marasco et al., 22 patients with traumatic flail requiring mechanical ventilation were randomized to receive operative fixation, and 23 received nonoperative management (mean age 57.8 ± 17.1 vs. 59.3 ± 10.4 with patients greater than 80 excluded secondary to osteoporotic rib segments precluding rib fixation) [29]. This study supported the findings of older literature in that those who received rib fixation had reduced ventilation requirements (duration of noninvasive ventilation postextubation, 3 h [0–25] versus 50 [17–102] $p = 0.01$) and ICU stay (324 h [238–380 h] versus 448 h [323–647] $p = 0.03$). There were no significant differences in spirometry results at 3 months post hospitalization between the two groups in their study; however their study population was older (mean age 58) than the two previously reported randomized trials (mean ages 45 [30] and 38 [31]).

There are a number of clinical trials that are currently evaluating the efficacy of the operative management of flail chest and rib fractures, two of which are North American studies (ClinicalTrials.gov identifiers: NCT01367951, NCT02635165, NCT02132416, NCT02595593). The results from these studies may bolster the encouraging, albeit small, above-mentioned literature supporting operative repair of flail chest.

Sternal Fractures

With the introduction of seat belt legislation, sternal fractures (SF) have been on the rise [32]. In a review from the data from the National Trauma Data Bank, 32,742 records of patients with sternal fractures were analyzed [33]. In this study by Yeh et al., 84% of the patients were involved in a MVC and falls accounted for 8%. The mortality associated with isolated SF was 3.5%; however poorer outcomes were associated with comorbidities as well as associated injuries. Increasing age was also one factor.

The diagnostic accuracy of chest X-ray (CXR) relative to chest computed tomography in the evaluation of sternal fractures is low. In a review of 14,553 patients from the NEXUS Chest (Jan 2009 to Dec 2012) and NEXUS Chest CT (Aug 2011 to May 2013) which were two multicenter observational cohorts of blunt trauma patients, 292 were diagnosed with sternal fractures (2.0%). Two hundred seventy-five of the 292 patients had both CXRs and chest CTs. From this group that had both imaging modalities, 257 (93.4%) had sternal fractures only seen on CT. Thus, with trauma algorithms that are CT driven, we are surely to see a rise in the incidence of sternal fractures in our patients who suffer from blunt chest trauma.

In the evaluation of an elderly trauma patient, the clinician should be alerted to the associated injuries that may be associated with sternal fractures. In the review by Yeh et al., from 32,742 patients with sternal fractures, approximately 70% and 30% had associated rib fractures and pulmonary contusions, respectively—both of which were found to be predictors of mortality (OR 2.06 and OR 1.41, $p < 0.001$).

Surgical interventions for sternal fractures are uncommon. In a small review by Velissaris et al., of 73 patients with traumatic sternal fractures, 3 underwent surgical correction with positive outcomes [34]. Indications for repair include severe unrelenting, intractable pain, respiratory insufficiency or ventilator dependence, sternal deformity/instability, and nonunion or hunched posture with limited range of motion.

The data on sternal fracture repair is not exhaustive. In a review of 12 publications by Harston and Roberts, 76 cases of sternal fractures were reviewed [35]. The techniques for repair varied amongst the population of surgeons as did the indications. Not all studies made specific reference to complications; however in the seven studies that did ($n = 64$), 12 patients suffered from complications. The most common was surgical removal of hardware secondary to pain. Furthermore, the authors found that only 35.5% of the patients had long-term follow-up. Accordingly, further prospective studies should be conducted before guidelines and algorithms are created to assist the clinician in surgically treating patients with sternal fractures.

Associated Injuries and Pulmonary Sequelae

Elderly patients commonly have more than one injury to the thorax as a result of thoracic trauma. In a retrospective cohort study by Bulger et al., trauma patients with rib fractures greater than 65 ($n = 277$) were compared to similarly injured patients less than 65 ($n = 187$) [11]. The incidence of hemothorax and pulmonary contusion in elderly patients (greater than 65) was 25% and 27%, respectively, and was not statistically significant from the incidence of hemothorax and pulmonary contusion that occurred in patients <65. Interestingly, pneumothorax in association with rib fractures occurred less frequently in patients greater than 65 (34 vs. 44%). Moreover, two retrospective studies that investigated isolated rib fractures in elderly trauma patients found that pulmonary contusions and hemothorax can be found in up to 20% and 13%, respectively, in patients with isolated rib fractures [36, 37].

The accepted initial management of traumatic hemothorax is tube thoracostomy. The inability of the first chest tube to adequately drain the hemothorax should not prompt additional placement of a secondary tube. Video-assisted thoracoscopic surgery (VATS) is recommended in these instances where a hemothorax is retained [38]. Ideally, this should be performed early (3–7 days of hospitalization) to decrease the risks of empyema; however there are reports where this is successfully performed later during the patient's hospitalization [39].

Post-traumatic hemothorax can be successfully treated with VATS drainage even in elderly patients. In a retrospective review in which 60 patients (mean age 63.2) underwent VATS for post-traumatic hemothorax, the outcomes of the elderly population within this review (15 patients) were examined [39]. Ninety-three percent of the elderly population underwent successful VATS drainage of their hemothorax with no inpatient mortalities. The elderly patients were greater than 80, mostly suffered from blunt thoracic trauma (87%), and had a median delay between trauma and VATS of 16 days (range 1–45 days). The outcomes reported included median hospital stay after VATS (20 days), number of patients requiring ICU-level care (9/15), mean ICU stay (11.8 days), and postoperative mechanical ventilation (5/15). The authors concluded that the morbidity and extended prolonged hospitalizations may be improved if patients are referred earlier for surgical management rather than later.

The management of patients with pulmonary contusions requires a careful evaluation of the patient's fluid and resuscitation status. Although level 1 recommendations do not exist for the management of pulmonary contusions, the EAST guidelines support the administration of fluids to maintain tissue perfusion, i.e., avoid and correct shock and avoid unnecessary overadministration [40]. Unfortunately, management guidelines for pulmonary contusions in the elderly do not exist; however a careful examination of the patient's volume status, including consideration of echocardiographic findings, results from serial chest radiographs, as well as laboratory surrogates for the patient's volume and resuscitation status will help the clinician tailor the elderly trauma patient's treatment accordingly.

The most frequent pulmonary sequelae as it relates to blunt chest trauma is pneumonia. Pneumonia was observed in 31% of elderly patients treated over a 10-year period admitted with rib fractures [11]. Moreover, pneumonia contributes to the overall mortality to an elderly patient's clinical course and not surprisingly represents a significant morbidity.

Concluding Remarks

The elderly trauma patient is often more severely injured and as a consequence may have a more prolonged and volatile clinical course. This is no different as it pertains to thoracic injuries in this age group. Our elderly patients are more vulnerable to injury and are limited in their tolerance to traumatic insult. The clinician responsible for the care and evaluation of the elderly thoracic trauma patient should have a high index of suspicion while judiciously assessing the patient for bony injury in all components of the chest wall. Greater attention to associated intrathoracic injuries may also prepare the clinician for common pulmonary sequelae that accompany blunt thoracic trauma.

As the geriatric trauma literature grows and professional societies continue to place emphasis on the care of the elderly, trauma-related outcomes in our elderly population should continue to improve.

References

1. Hanna R, Hershman L. Evaluation of thoracic injuries among older motor vehicle occupants. 2009. Technical Report. NHTSA US DOT HS 811 101.
2. Shelby SG. Delta-v as a measure of traffic conflict severity. 2011. http://onlinepubs.trb.org/onlinepubs/conferences/2011/RSS/1/Shelby,S.pdf. Accessed 1 June 2016.
3. Rahman I, Morrison D, Donaldson K, MacNee W. Systemic oxidative stress in asthma, COPD, and smokers. Am J Respir Crit Care Med. 1996;154:1055–60.
4. Verbeken EK, Cauberghs M, Mertens I, Clement J, Lauweryns JM, Van de Woestijne KP. The senile lung: comparison with normal and emphysematous lungs. Chest. 1992;101:793–9.
5. Davies GA, Bolton CE. Age related changes in the respiratory system. In: Brocklehurst's textbook of geriatric medicine and gerontology. Philadelphia: Elsevier; 2010. p. 97–100.
6. Anthonisen NR, Danson J, Robertson PC, Ross WR. Airway closure as a function of age. Respir Physiol. 1970;8:58–65.
7. Gomez CR, Boehmer ED, Kovacs EJ. The aging innate immune system. Curr Opin Immunol. 2005;17:457–62.
8. Ziegler DW, Agarwal NN. The morbidity and mortality of rib fractures. J Trauma. 1994;37:975–9.
9. Lin FC, Li RY, Tung YW, Jeng KC, Tsai SC. Morbidity, mortality, associated injuries, and management of traumatic rib fractures. J Chin Med Assoc. 2016;79(6):329–34.
10. Sharma OP, Oswanski MF, Jolly S, Lauer SK, Dressel R, Stombaugh HA. Perils of rib fractures. Am Surg. 2008;74:310–4.
11. Bulger EM, Arneson MA, Mock CN, Jurokovich GJ. Rib fractures in the elderly. J Trauma. 2000;48(6):1040–7.
12. Bansal V, Conroy C, Chang D, Tominaga GT, Coimbra R. Rib and sternum fractures in the elderly and extreme elderly following motor vehicle crashes. Accid Anal Prev. 2011;43:661–5.
13. Lotfipour S, Kaku SK, Vaca FE, Patel C, Anderson CL, Ahmed SS, Menchine MD. Factors associated with complications in older adults with isolated blunt chest trauma. West J Emerg Med. 2009;10:79–84.
14. Simon BJ, Cushman J, Barraco R, Lane V, Luchette FA, Miglietta M. Pain management guidelines for blunt thoracic trauma. J Trauma. 2005;59:1256–67.
15. Karmakar MJ, Ho AM. Acute pain management of patients with multiple rib fractures. J Trauma. 2003;54:615–25.
16. Dittmann M, Ferstl A, Wolff G. Epidural analgesia for the treatment of multiple rib fractures. Eur J Intensive Care Med. 1975;1:71–5.
17. Pedersen VM, Schulze S, Hoier-Madsen K, Halkier E. Air flow meter assessment of the effect of intercostal nerve blockade on respiratory function in rib fractures. Acta Chir Scand. 1983;149:119–20.

18. Karmakar MJ, Critchley AH, Ho AM, Gin T, Lee TW, Yim AP. Continuous thoracic paravertebral infusion of bupivacaine in patients with multiple rib fractures. Chest. 2003;123:424–31.
19. Kvalheim L, Reiestad F. Interpleural catheter in the management of postoperative pain. Anesthesiology. 1984;61:A231.
20. Karmakar MK. Thoracic paravertebral block. Anesthesiology. 2001;95:771–80.
21. Haenel JB, Moore FA, Moore EE, Sauaia A, Read RA, Burch JM. Extrapleural bupivacaine for amelioration of multiple rib fractures. J Trauma. 1995;38(1):22–7.
22. O'Kelly E. Continuous pain relief for multiple fractures ribs. Br J Anaesth. 1981;53:989–91.
23. Richardson J, Sabanathan S, Mearns AJ, Shah RD, Goulden C. A prospective randomized comparison of interpleural and paravertebral analgesia in thoracic surgery. Br J Anaesth. 1995;75:405–8.
24. Mccool D. Diseases of the diaphragm, chest wall, pleura and mediastinum. In: Goldman L, Schafer AI, editors. Goldman-Cecil Medicine. Philadelphia: Elsevier Health Sciences; 2016. p. 627–37.
25. Dehghan N, de Mestral C, McKee MD, Schemitsch EH, Nathens A. Flail chest injuries: a review of outcomes and treatment practices from the National Trauma Data Bank. J Trauma Acute Care Surg. 2014;76(2):462–8.
26. Albaugh G, Kann B, Puc MM, Vemurlapalli P, Marra S, Ross S. Age-adjusted outcomes in traumatic flail chest injuries in the elderly. Am Surg. 2000;66:978–81.
27. Slobogean GP, MacPherson CA, Sun T, Pelletier ME, Hameed SM. Surgical fixation versus non-operative management of flail chest: a meta-analysis. J Am Coll Surg. 2013;216:302–11.
28. Leinicke JA, Elmore L, Freeman BD, Colditz GA. Operative management of rib fractures in the setting of flail chest: a systematic review and meta-analysis. Ann Surg. 2013;258(6):914–21.
29. Marasco SF, Davies AR, Cooper J, Varma D, Bennett V, Nevill R, et al. Prospective randomized controlled trial of operative rib fixation in traumatic flail chest. J Am Coll Surg. 2013;216:924–32.
30. Tanaka H, Yukioka T, Yamaguti Y, Shimizu S, Goto H, Matsuda H, et al. Surgical stabilization of internal pneumatic stabilization? A prospective randomized study of management of severe flail chest patients. J Trauma. 2002;52(4):727–32.
31. Granetzny A, Abd El-Aal M, Emam E, Shalaby A, Boseila A. Surgical versus conservative treatment of flail chest. Evaluation of the pulmonary status. Interact Cardiovasc Thorac Surg. 2005;4(6):583–7.
32. Budd JS. Effect of seat belt legislation on the incidence of sternal fractures seen in the accident department. Br Med J (Clin Red Ed). 1985;291(6498):785.
33. Yeh DD, Hwabejire JO, DeMoya MA, Alam HB, King DR. Sternal fracture – an analysis of the National Trauma Data Bank. J Surg Res. 2014;186(1):39–43.
34. Velissaris T, Tang AT, Patel A, Khallifa K, Weeden DF. Traumatic sternal fracture: outcome following admission to a Thoracic Surgical Unit. Injury. 2003;34:924–7.
35. Harston A, Roberts C. Fixation of sternal fractures: a systemic review. J Trauma. 2011;71(6):1875–9.
36. Barnea Y, Kashtan H, Skornick Y, Werbin N. Isolated rib fractures in elderly patients: mortality and morbidity. Can J Surg. 2002;45(1):43–6.
37. Elmistekawy EM, Hammad AA. Isolated rib fractures in geriatric patients. Ann Thor Med. 2007;2(4):166–8.
38. Mowery NT, Gunter OL, Collier BR, Diaz JJ, Haut E, et al. Practice management guidelines for management of hemothorax and occult pneumothorax. J Trauma. 2011;70(2):510–8.
39. Schweigert M, Beron M, Dubecz A, Stadlhuber AR, Stei H. Video-assisted thoracoscopic surgery for posttraumatic hemothorax in the very elderly. Thorac Cardiovasc Surg. 2012;60(7):474–9.
40. Simon B, Ebert J, Bokhari F, Capella J, Emhoff T. Management of pulmonary contusion and flail chest: an Eastern Association for the Surgery of Trauma practice management guideline. J Trauma Acute Care Surg. 2012;73(5):S351–61.

18 Esophageal Injury

Mathew A. Van Deusen, Mark Crye, and Jonathan Levy

Anatomic Considerations

The esophagus is a tubular muscular structure, approximately 25–30 cm in length. There are three discrete anatomic divisions of the esophagus. The cervical esophagus begins at the pharyngeoesophageal junction and ends at the thoracic inlet. The thoracic portion of the esophagus begins at the thoracic inlet and ends at the diaphragmatic hiatus. The intra-abdominal portion of the esophagus begins at the diaphragmatic hiatus and ends at the gastroesophageal junction. There are three prominent areas of anatomic narrowing that naturally occur. The first is at the level of the cricopharyngeus muscle, which occurs in the cervical esophagus at the level of the cricoid cartilage. The second area is found in the intrathoracic portion of the esophagus, as it courses behind the aorta and left mainstem bronchus. The final location of anatomic narrowing can be found at the level of the diaphragmatic hiatus, where the intra-abdominal portion of the esophagus begins.

M.A. Van Deusen, M.D. • M. Crye, M.D.
Department of Cardiovascular and Thoracic Surgery, Allegheny Health Network, 320 East North Avenue, Pittsburgh, PA 1521, USA
e-mail: mathew.vandeusen@ahn.org

J. Levy, M.D.
Department of General Surgery, Allegheny Health Network, 320 East North Avenue, Pittsburgh, PA 1521, USA

Initial Evaluation

The initial evaluation of any trauma patient begins with the appropriate and rapid assessment of airway, breathing, and circulation. Immediate operative exploration may be necessary in patients with blunt or penetrating injury involving the neck or chest. In the hemodynamically stable patient, without indications for immediate operative exploration, computed axial tomography (CT) scanning is the best modality for the initial evaluation of esophageal trauma. Radiographic evaluation alone is inadequate, as it has been found to be only 15% sensitive [1]. Helical CT scan has been shown to be 100% sensitive and 85% specific in the identification of major aerodigestive injury, primarily due to the improved ability to visualize subtle pneumomediastinum as an indicator of potential esophageal or tracheobronchial injury [2]. Pneumomediastinum alone is not a sensitive indicator of esophageal trauma, as almost 90% of trauma patients found to have pneumomediastinum on CT scan do not have any esophageal injury [1]. Because pneumomediastinum is so nonspecific for esophageal trauma, further evaluation of the aerodigestive tracts with bronchoscopy and endoscopy may be necessary [3]. Not all patients require direct visualization, however. Given the relatively low incidence of esophageal injury, the rate of negative endoscopy would be prohibitively high if all patients

A. Rodriguez et al. (eds.), *Geriatric Trauma and Acute Care Surgery*,
https://doi.org/10.1007/978-3-319-57403-5_18

with pneumomediastinum underwent endoscopic evaluation. Additional CT findings specific to esophageal injury may include esophageal thickening, periesophageal fluid, mediastinal inflammation, and pleural effusion [2]. Additionally, helical CT scan is of tremendous value in the evaluation of other potential injuries and sources of chest pain, which can be a useful diagnostic tool in the elderly patient with multiple comorbidities and risk factors [2].

Additional Radiographic and Endoscopic Evaluation

When esophageal injury is suspected based on clinical findings and CT scan, the gold standard for further testing is a contrast esophagogram with fluoroscopy. This can be supplemented by direct endoscopic evaluation if inconclusive, or if not obtainable. Water-soluble contrast should be used initially to rule out large perforations, as barium may cause significant mediastinal fibrosis if it is allowed to escape into the mediastinum. If negative, this may be followed by barium swallow study, which is more sensitive and specific than water-soluble contrast and has been shown to identify more injuries than water-soluble contrast alone [4]. While contrast esophagogram is sensitive for esophageal injury, there is still a significant false-negative rate. It may always not be possible to obtain, as it requires a neurologically intact patient with an adequate swallowing mechanism. Aspiration of water-soluble contrast can cause significant pneumonitis or pulmonary edema [4]. This is an especially important consideration in the elderly population, as these patients may already have baseline dysphagia. CT esophagogram with oral contrast is becoming an acceptable alternative to fluoroscopic imaging.

Endoscopic evaluation may be particularly useful in the diagnosis of esophageal injury following penetrating trauma. Direct visualization of the mucosa of the esophagus may be necessary in patients who cannot tolerate further imaging studies and in patients who have inconclusive radiographic studies.

In patients where there is a clinical suspicion of esophageal injury, associated with positive findings on CT scan, proceeding to endoscopic evaluation or to operative exploration may be the appropriate initial intervention. Clinical signs and symptoms of esophageal injury may include crepitus, chest pain, dysphagia, blood in orogastric or nasogastric secretions, hoarseness, and classic signs of injury such as tachypnea and tachycardia [1, 5, 6]. Unfortunately, in some cases there may be no overt signs of injury. Of these clinical findings and symptoms, dyspnea and hoarseness were seen to be up to 90% specific in the evaluation of aerodigestive injury [1].

Management

General

The mechanism, extent, and location of the injury are important factors in determining the necessary management. All patients should also be placed on broad-spectrum antibiotics to cover both gram-negative and gram-positive flora escaping from the GI tract. In the case of blunt esophageal injury, if the patient is stable and there is only a suggestion of esophageal trauma (small amount of pneumomediastinum, contained perforation), then the patient can often be managed nonoperatively with close observation and expectant management [1, 4]. Patients with penetrating esophageal injury or unstable patients with significant blunt trauma associated with possible esophageal injury are typically managed surgically. Similarly, in patients with significant contamination following iatrogenic injury, surgical intervention is warranted.

Injury of the Cervical Esophagus

Injuries to the cervical esophagus are much more common than injuries to the thoracic esophagus as a result of the forces acting on the esophagus in rapid deceleration injuries associated with blunt trauma and the relatively exposed area of the neck in penetrating trauma. With any cervical esophageal injury, the treatment of choice is open drainage via an oblique left neck incision at the anterior sternocleidomastoid border [2, 4]. While small studies have examined the possibility of expectant management, the morbidity associated with a cervical neck incision and primary drainage and repair is extremely low and generally considered very safe [4]. Dissection is carried down to identify the carotid sheath, which is reflected laterally. Care must be taken to avoid injury to the recurrent laryngeal nerve, which is located within the tracheoesophageal groove. Blunt finger dissection is utilized to form a plane between the trachea and esophagus, taking care to avoid injury to the membranous trachea. A nasogastric tube can be helpful to identify the esophagus, as tissues and planes can be distorted with significant inflammation and contamination in the setting of perforation. Retroesophageal dissection is performed bluntly between the esophagus and vertebral body. A Penrose drain can be utilized to facilitate traction on the esophagus at this point, and an attempt at locating the perforation should be undertaken. If the location of injury is identified, the muscular layer must be opened longitudinally, proximally, and distally, to fully visualize the extent of the mucosal disruption. The mucosa and submucosal layers are then reapproximated utilizing interrupted absorbable suture. The muscular layer is then closed in a running fashion with nonabsorbable suture. Once the perforation is closed, the repair is buttressed with a muscle flap from either the sternocleidomastoid or a strap muscle. Whether the location of injury can be found or not, it is critical to ensure that blunt dissection is carried down into the thoracic inlet to assist with mediastinal drainage. A Jackson-Pratt drain can then be guided down into the mediastinum and brought out through a separate neck stab incision. In severe trauma where the cervical esophagus cannot be repaired, the injured area can be brought to/near the skin and act as a temporary side esophagostomy [4]. The distal lumen of the esophagus can even be sutured closed to prevent further contamination as the patient recovers enough to have the perforation heal or be closed in a delayed fashion.

Thoracic Esophageal Injury

For thoracic esophageal injuries, operative drainage and primary repair are the standards of care. Intrathoracic perforation can progress to mediastinal sepsis if not treated early, which can lead to fatal consequence. The most important step is to ensure wide drainage of the mediastinal contamination. This can be performed via an open thoracotomy or minimally invasive thoracoscopic approach, based on the stability of the patient and the expertise of the surgeon. Surgical repair is often undertaken via open thoracotomy. The position of the patient (right lateral decubitis versus left lateral decubitis) is dependent on the location of the injury. For injuries to the proximal intrathoracic esophagus, the incision should be made on the right side, as the arch of the aorta and great vessels prevent exposure of the proximal esophagus [2, 4]. Injuries of the distal intrathoracic esophagus should generally be approached via a left thoracotomy. In all patients with intrathoracic perforations, endoscopy is critical to identify the exact location of the lesion and the extent of mucosal injury. As in surgical repair of cervical esophageal perforations, the area of injury should ideally be closed primarily without tension in two layers of nonabsorbable suture. Viable tissue should be routinely used to buttress the surgical repair. Options for coverage include intercostal muscle flaps, pleural and pericardial flaps, diaphragm flaps, flaps involving the fundus of the stomach, and omental flaps. For any case in which the thoracic esophagus cannot be closed primarily, either due to excess tension or gross contamination, the esophagus may be managed with repair around a T-tube. This strategy can provide controlled drainage of esophageal contents until a formal repair can be obtained or adequate healing can occur. Adequate drainage of the pleural space is necessary. In the event of severe tissue loss where repair is not possible, diversion can be performed with a cervical esophagostomy, esophageal debridement, and resection as needed. Creation of a gastrostomy tube and enteral access with a jejunostomy tube may be necessary [2, 4]. Traumatic injuries of the intra-abdominal portion of the esophagus can be managed similarly, through an abdominal approach, typically performed for management of associated intra-abdominal injuries.

Iatrogenic Injury

Esophageal injury is most likely to occur as a result of medical intervention. Iatrogenic injury related to endoscopic intervention is the most common cause of esophageal perforation, encompassing up to 60% of all cases. Additional causes that have been reported include injury from placement of nasogastric or orogastric tubes, and injury associated with surgery of the cervical or thoracic spine, airway procedures, and cardiac procedures. As previously mentioned, the most common locations of perforation within the esophagus are the areas of anatomic narrowing. A high index of suspicion is required to identify the injury regardless of the location. This may be challenging in the geriatric population. Chronic illnesses, polypharmacy, altered sensorium, and anatomic changes are all factors that can make identifying and treating esophageal injuries more problematic.

Evaluation of patients with concern for iatrogenic esophageal perforation should include a detailed history of the procedures. Signs and symptoms at presentation can be nonspecific. These may include chest or abdominal pain, fever, leukocytosis, dyspnea, and crepitus. The severity of the symptoms may also be variable and is often related to the duration of time from perforation to presentation. Thorough physical examination and laboratory analysis should be performed. A detailed review of medication usage is critical, including the use of anticoagulation and antiplatelet therapies. Physical exam and vital signs may be blunted in the geriatric population due to chronic illnesses, relative immune suppression, and effects of medications such as beta-blockers. Radiographic and endoscopic evaluation, as in patients with blunt or penetrating esophageal injury, is often needed. Management of iatrogenic esophageal perforation may include observation, endoscopic therapies, or operative intervention, similar to that of traumatic esophageal injury.

Endoscopic Intervention

With improved endoscopic visualization and techniques, there has been growing support for endoscopic management of esophageal injuries. Esophageal stent placement in stable patients with traumatic esophageal injury may be a consideration [2]. While this has been examined more commonly in patients with spontaneous and iatrogenic esophageal perforations, the idea that trauma patients can quickly be managed with a stent has great appeal. However, there has been no direct study examining primary repair versus stent placement. Secondary complications of esophageal stenting may include perforation, bleeding, and stricture. More importantly, the majority of patients with traumatic esophageal injury have other associated vascular and tissue injuries which mandate operative management [4].

Postoperative Management

Postoperatively, all patients should be monitored closely for signs of ongoing sepsis. Patients should be continued on appropriate broad-spectrum antibiotics and maintained NPO. Postoperative imaging including an upper gastrointestinal study is routinely performed to assess for persistent extravasation prior to resuming oral nutrition [2, 4]. In the elderly population, care should again be taken to ensure that no baseline dysphagia exists, as this can lead to aspiration and potential pulmonary compromise. In addition, many elderly patients have either a baseline dementia which may be exacerbated following traumatic injury or prolonged recovery from illness or a new delirium while in the hospital. Either of these may interfere with the patient's ability to swallow in a coordinated fashion. In those patients, repeat endoscopy can be performed to examine the repair.

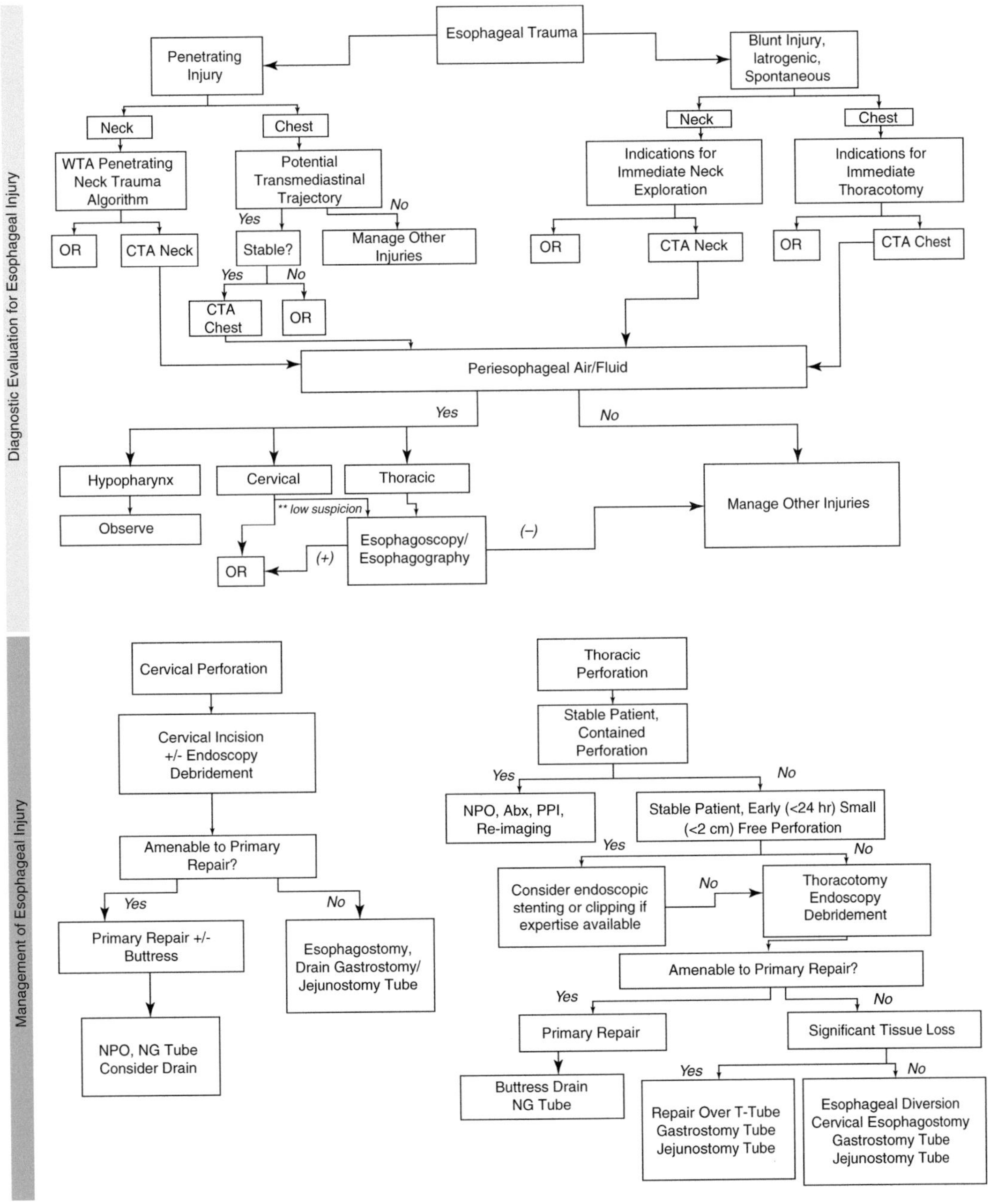

Fig. 1. From Western Trauma Association Critical Decisions in Trauma: Diagnosis and management of esophageal injuries. Biffl W, et al. Journal of Trauma and Acute Care Surgery. June 2015. 79(6):1089–95.

References

1. Dissanaike S, Shalhub S, Jurkovich GJ. The evaluation of pneumomediastinum in blunt trauma patients. J Trauma. 2008;65(6):1340–5. http://www.ncbi.nlm.nih.gov/pubmed/19077624
2. Brinster CJ, et al. Evolving options in the management of esophageal perforation. Ann Thorac Surg. 2004;77(4):1475–83. http://www.annalsthoracicsurgery.org/article/S0003-4975(03)01708-9/pdf
3. Keogh IJ, Rowley H, Russell J. Critical airway compromise caused by neck haematoma. Clin Otolaryngol Allied Sci. 2002;27(4):244–5.
4. Biffl WL, et al. Western Trauma Association Critical Decisions in Trauma: diagnosis and management of esophageal injuries. J Trauma Acute Care Surg. 2015;79(6):1089–95. http://journals.lww.com/jtrauma/Citation/2015/12000/Western_Trauma_Association_Critical_Decisions_in.31.aspx
5. Rathlev NK, et al. Evaluation and management of neck trauma. Emerg Med Clin North Am. 2007;25(3):679–94. http://www.emergpa.net/wp/wp-content/uploads/2012/02/Emerg-Med-Clin-N-Am-2007-Neck-Injuries.pdf
6. Fadoo F, et al. Helical CT eosphagography for evaluation of suspected esophageal perforation or rupture. AJR Am J Roentgenol. 2004;182(5):1177–9. http://www.ajronline.org/doi/pdf/10.2214/ajr.182.5.1821177

Part IX

Abdominal Injury

19 Liver Trauma

Adrian W. Ong and Rao R. Ivatury

Initial Approach to Liver Injuries

In patients with suspected intra-abdominal injuries after blunt trauma, immediate operation is indicated in the setting of refractory shock with hemoperitoneum demonstrated on ultrasound or diagnostic peritoneal lavage. Otherwise computerized tomographic (CT) scanning should almost always be done if possible. If a liver injury is identified on CT, the decision to pursue nonoperative management (NOM) hinges on the severity of the physiologic derangement, and the presence or absence of peritonitis. CT characteristics of the liver injury such as grade of liver injury, presence of a vascular "blush" or contrast extravasation, the degree of hemoperitoneum, and presence of associated injuries should also be considered in the decision to pursue NOM. Angioembolization is an important modality which can be utilized as the primary therapeutic intervention when NOM is pursued, or as an adjunct to operative management where hemostasis is less than satisfactory. The decision to proceed with angiography in the latter scenario is usually made on the basis of operative findings and clinical course although a recent study has also demonstrated some value in postoperative CT scanning to guide the need for angiography [1].

In most (70–90%) of the patients presenting with blunt liver injuries, NOM can be attempted with a high success rate [2, 3]. Despite the fact that higher grade (American Association for the Surgery of Trauma [AAST] Organ injury Scale grades 3–5) liver injuries are more likely to require operative intervention, the failure rate is low (about 6–8%) for NOM when properly selected [4, 5].

For patients with penetrating abdominal injuries, urgent operation is largely necessary in gunshot wounds, and less so for stab wounds. In the stable patient with a documented trajectory through the liver on CT and a very low suspicion of hollow viscus injury by examination and CT findings, NOM is an acceptable strategy [6]. In one series, NOM was attempted in only 15% of patients with penetrating liver injuries, with a low (3%) failure rate [7]. Another study found that of 36 penetrating liver injuries selected for NOM, the success rate was 86% [8].

A.W. Ong, M.D. (✉)
Department of Surgery, University of Pennsylvania, Philadelphia, PA, USA

Department of Surgery, Reading Health System, Sixth Avenue and Spruce Street, Reading, PA 19611, USA
e-mail: Adrian.ong@readinghealth.org

R.R. Ivatury, M.D.
Virginia Commonwealth University, Richmond, VA, USA
e-mail: raoIvatury@gmail.com

A. Rodriguez et al. (eds.), *Geriatric Trauma and Acute Care Surgery*,
https://doi.org/10.1007/978-3-319-57403-5_19

The Geriatric Patient: Initial Approach

In elderly patients with blunt liver injuries, there is no available evidence demonstrating that NOM is detrimental or that the NOM strategy should be somehow modified. In a multicenter study of severe (AAST OIS grades 4 and 5) blunt liver injuries undergoing NOM, where NOM was defined by "a clear note in the medical record committing the patient to NOM or by the fact that an operation was booked later than 3 hours after the diagnosis," there was no difference in mean age as to who underwent immediate operation as opposed to a trial of NOM. Out of 262 patients, 23 (8.8%) failed NOM. Patients 55 years and older formed 10.3% ($n = 27$) of the entire cohort and only 1 of 27 (4.3%) failed NOM [4]. Recent guidelines by prominent societies [9, 10] have not considered age an important factor in the decision to pursue NOM of blunt liver injuries (Fig. 19.1).

In the largest recent study of isolated severe (AIS of 4 or greater) blunt liver injuries from the National Trauma Data Bank, attempted NOM (defined as no surgery in the first 6 hours) occurred in 73% of 3267 patients with a failure rate of 6.5% [11]. Failed NOM was independently associated with 30-day in-hospital mortality after controlling for confounders (crude survival rate 78.8% vs. 92.9%, hazard rate, 1.7; 95% confidence interval [C.I.] 1.1–2.6). Age (odds ratio 1.02, [95% C.I. 1.01–1.03]) was a predictor of NOM failure, others being male sex, systolic blood pressure <90 mmHg, Injury Severity Score, Glasgow Coma Scale score, and need for hepatic angioembolization. Putting this into practical terms, for every 10 years of age, the odds of failure of NOM changed by 1.02^{10} or 1.22. If the NOM failure rate was 6.5% at age 30, the corresponding rates would be 11% at age 60 and 13.3% at age 70 with the other variables in the study being equal. These hypothetical figures give some reassurance to clinicians that although age is associated with failure of NOM, NOM is still an acceptable strategy in the elderly with severe blunt liver injuries.

There is no available evidence to suggest that age is a contraindication to NOM of selected patients with penetrating injuries. In recent published guidelines [6, 10] there is no mention of age as a contraindication for this strategy. The decision to manage patients nonoperatively for penetrating injuries should be made by an experienced surgeon with the ability to provide vigilant follow-up.

The Geriatric Patient: Operative Management of Liver Injury

There is no available evidence to suggest that different operative techniques should be used in elderly patients as opposed to younger patients to control bleeding from the injured liver. However, in general, the elderly have a poorer outcome when operative management is necessary compared to younger patients. Lustenberger et al. [12] compared 34 patients ≥55 years of age to 124 younger patients with head-Abbreviated Injury Score (AIS) of ≤2 who received initial damage control laparotomy for predominantly blunt (>90%) injuries: in-hospital mortality rate was significantly higher for elderly patients (29% vs. 4.8%) with the main causes of death being hemorrhagic shock and multi-organ system failure.

Studies comparing younger to older patients in terms of techniques of liver hemostasis in trauma are also lacking. Liver resection, an uncommon technique in trauma, has been evaluated in one study: Tsugawa et al. [13] compared 29 patients >70 years of age and 71 younger patients undergoing anatomic liver resection. The older patients were more severely injured and had a lower mean GCS. The majority of the resections involved right hepatectomy (52% in the older patients vs. 63% in younger patients). Survival was significantly lower in the older group (66% vs. 80%). There were no intraoperative deaths or deaths related to exsanguination in either group. The authors concluded that anatomic resection might still be a viable option in the elderly with blunt liver trauma. This study,

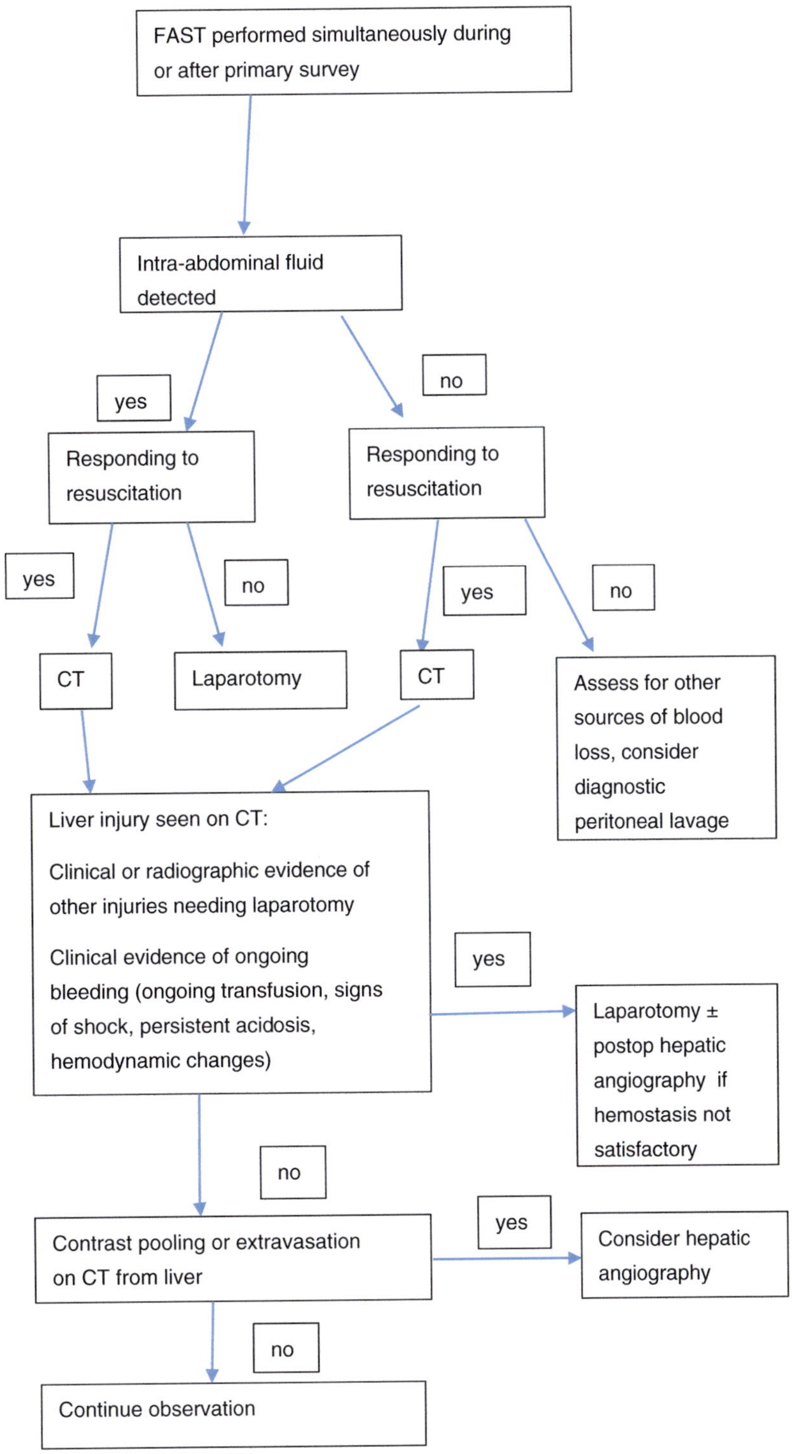

Fig. 19.1 Blunt liver injury: initial management

however, was notable for its frequent utilization of anatomic liver resection (100/487 or 21%) for blunt liver trauma and poorer outcomes in the elderly.

In contrast, there is more data on elective liver resections. In general, studies show a higher but still acceptable postoperative mortality rate for the elderly compared to younger patients [14–17]. However, in major liver resections (≥3 liver segments), the elderly may have poorer outcomes. Reddy et al. [18] found that for major resections, postoperative mortality rates were 8.4% for patients ≥65 years old and 1.5% in patient 50 years and younger. Age was an independent predictor of postoperative mortality (odds ratio of 1.43 for every 10 years' increase in age). Other predictors included male sex, simultaneous procedure, diagnosis of malignancy, and American Society of Anesthesiologists (ASA) grade. On the other hand, Menon et al. [19] similarly evaluated patients 70 years and older compared to younger patients who underwent major resections with similar 30-day mortality rates (7.9% vs. 5.4%), ICU length of stay, and postoperative complication rates. In this study, ASA grade III and intraoperative transfusion of more than 3 units of blood were predictive of overall survival, not age. Studies of elective liver resection need to be interpreted with caution because of selection bias: details of selection of elderly patients for these major liver procedures are not always available.

Complications of Hepatic Trauma

There are several well-described complications of liver trauma: delayed hemorrhage [4, 5], bile leak manifesting as bile ascites or biloma [4, 20], hepatic necrosis [21], hepatic failure [5, 19], abscess [5, 22–24], and hemobilia [25, 26]. These complications are more likely to be associated with higher grade liver injuries, whether operatively or nonoperatively managed. Studies comparing hepatic-related complication rates and outcomes of management of these complications between the elderly and younger patients are lacking.

Summary

The approach to the geriatric patient with liver injury should follow the same principles as that for younger patients. It is important to recognize that although age is associated with failure of NOM in blunt liver injuries NOM is still an acceptable strategy in elderly patients with low NOM failure rates. When operative intervention is necessary, the elderly have poorer outcomes in general. There is very scant evidence available comparing elderly and younger patients in terms of operative techniques, except perhaps liver resection. There is very scant evidence comparing elderly to younger patients in terms of liver-related complications after liver trauma.

References

1. Kutcher ME, Weis JJ, Siada SS, et al. The role of computed tomographic scan in ongoing triage of operative hepatic trauma: a western trauma association multicenter retrospective study. J Trauma Acute Care Surg. 2015;79:951–6.
2. Velmahos GC, Toutouzas K, Randin R, et al. High success with nonoperative management of blunt hepatic trauma. Arch Surg. 2003;138:475–81.
3. Malhotra AK, Fabian TC, Croce MA, et al. Blunt hepatic injury: a paradigm shift from operative to nonoperative management in the 1990s. Ann Surg. 2000;231(6):804–13.
4. Van der Wilden GM, Velmahos GC, Emhoff T, et al. Successful nonoperative management of the most severe blunt liver injuries. A multicenter study of the research consortium of New England centers for trauma. Arch Surg. 2012;147:423–8.
5. Kozar RA, Moore FA, Cothren CC, et al. Risk factors for hepatic morbidity following nonoperative management. Multicenter Study Arch Surg. 2006;141:451–9.
6. Como JJ, Bokhari F, Chiu WC, et al. Practice management guidelines for selective nonoperative management of penetrating abdominal trauma. J Trauma. 2010;68:721–33.
7. Schnüriger B, Talving P, Barbarino R, et al. Current practice and the role of the CT in the management of penetrating liver injuries at a level I trauma center. J Emerg Trauma Shock. 2011;4:53–7.
8. Demetriades D, Hadjizacharia P, Constantinou C, et al. Selective nonoperative management of penetrating abdominal solid organ injuries. Ann Surg. 2006;244:620–8.
9. Stassen NA, Bhullar I, Cheng JD, et al. Nonoperative management of blunt hepatic injury: an eastern Association for the Surgery of trauma practice

management guideline. J Trauma Acute Care Surg. 2012;73:S288–93.
10. Coccolini F, Montori G, Catena F, et al. Liver trauma: WSES position paper. World J Emerg Surg. 2015;10:39.
11. Polanco PM, Brown JB, Puyana JC, et al. The swinging pendulum: a national perspective of nonoperative management in severe blunt liver injury. J Trauma Acute Care Surg. 2013;75:590–5.
12. Lustenberger T, Talving P, Schnuriger B, et al. Impact of advanced age on outcomes following damage control interventions for trauma. World J Surg. 2012;36:208–15.
13. Tsugawa K, Koyanagi N, Hashizume M, et al. Anatomic resection for severe blunt liver trauma in 100 patients: significant differences between young and elderly. World J Surg. 2002;26:544–9.
14. Huang J, Li B-K, Chen G-H, et al. Long-term outcomes and prognostic factors of elderly patients with hepatocellular carcinoma undergoing hepatectomy. J Gastrointest Surg. 2009;13:1627–35.
15. Kondo K, Chijiiwa K, Funagayama M, et al. Hepatic resection is justified for elderly patients with hepatocellular carcinoma. World J Surg. 2008;32:2223–9.
16. Oishi K, Itamoto T, Kobayashi T, et al. Hepatectomy for hepatocellular carcinoma in elderly patients aged 75 years or more. J Gastrointest Surg. 2009;13:695–701.
17. Phan K, An VVG, Ha H, et al. Hepatic resection for malignant liver tumors in the elderly: a systematic review and meta-analysis. ANZ J Surg. 2015;85:815–22.
18. Reddy SK, Barbas AS, Turley RS, et al. Major liver resection in elderly patients: a multi-institutional analysis. J Am Coll Surg. 2011;212:787–95.
19. Menon KV, Al-Mukhtar A, Aldouri A, et al. Outcomes after major hepatectomy in elderly patients. J Am Coll Surg. 2006;203:677–83.
20. Bala M, Gazalla SA, Faroja M, et al. Complications of high grade liver injuries: management and outcome with focus on bile leaks. Scand J Trauma Resusc Emerg Med. 2012;20:20.
21. Dabbs DN, Stein DM, Scalea TM. Major hepatic necrosis: a common complication after angioembolization for treatment for high grade liver injuries. J Trauma. 2009;66:621–9.
22. Croce MA, Fabian TC, Menke PG, et al. Nonoperative management of blunt hepatic trauma is the treatment of choice for hemodynamically stable patients. Results of a prospective trial. Ann Surg. 1995;221:744–55.
23. Fabian TC, Croce MA, Stanford GG, et al. Factors affecting morbidity following hepatic trauma. A prospective analysis of 482 injuries. Ann Surg. 1991;213:540–8.
24. Bender JS, Geller ER, Wilson RF. Intra-abdominal sepsis following liver trauma. J Trauma. 1989;29:1140–5.
25. Krige JE, Bornman PC, Terblanche J. Therapeutic perihepatic packing in complex liver trauma. Br J Surg. 1992;79:43–6.
26. Carmona RH, Peck DZ, Lim RC. The role of packing and planned reoperation in severe hepatic trauma. J Trauma. 1984;24:779–84.

20 Optimal Management of Blunt Splenic Injury in the Geriatric Patient

James M. Haan

The spleen is the most commonly injured organ from blunt abdominal trauma. Historically, due to high nonoperative mortality rates, splenectomy was the treatment of choice in the early 1900s [1]. In 1919 Bullock recognized overwhelming post-splenectomy sepsis (OPSS) as an uncommon, but lethal, condition, with studies indicating a 1–2% incidence of OPSS with a mortality rate of 50–80% [2–5]. This infectious concern led to the advent of surgical splenic conservation in the 1950s and 1960s [6]. In 1968, nonoperative management of children with splenic injury was first described [7]. In the 1980s, this nonoperative management of splenic injury in children became the standard of care, even in those requiring transfusion [8]. This success paved the way for the use of nonoperative management of injured spleens in hemodynamically stable adults [9–33]. Advanced age as defined by either age greater than 55 or 65 years was initially felt to mandate surgery as risk of failure in nonoperative and operative patients with limited reserves would lead to unacceptably high mortality. Many studies debate the risk of nonoperative failure with the routine use of splenic operative techniques in the elderly trauma population versus the risk of laparotomy in this group [25–33]. This chapter reviews the diagnosis and management options of elderly patients with splenic injury.

J.M. Haan, M.D.
Trauma Services, Trauma Services Via Christi Hospitals, Via Christi Hospitals St. Francis Campus, 929 N St. Francis Street, Wichita, KS, USA
e-mail: james_haan@via-christi.org

Evaluation

The elderly trauma patient undergoes initial history and physical examination. The determination of hemodynamic stability is critical in management of the spleen; hemodynamically unstable patients, especially elderly patients, should undergo primary surgical therapy. In many instances the finding of left upper quadrant pain, shock, and ± positive FAST will lead to exploration for presumed splenic injury. Historically shock had been defined as systolic blood pressure less than 90 mmHg. In recent years, the concept of occult shock was noted especially in the elderly. Eastridge et al. attempted to define shock based on the review of the National Trauma Data Bank. Their review defines a new set point in the injured elderly for shock of 110 mmHg with biochemical markers of shock occurring in the elderly at 117 mmHg [34]. Based on this, the clinician must take care to carefully consider primary operative therapy in elderly patients presenting with SBP not only less than 90 but also even 110 mmHg, especially if vitals do not immediately normalize resuscitation. Additionally, even in those considered stable

A. Rodriguez et al. (eds.), *Geriatric Trauma and Acute Care Surgery*,
https://doi.org/10.1007/978-3-319-57403-5_20

based on vital signs, evaluation for occult shock using lactate or arterial blood gas with base deficit should be performed. In those patients with biochemical shock markers greater than six, there should be a serious consideration of primary surgical therapy, especially in those with higher grade splenic injury and/or limited physiologic reserves.

Diagnosis

In those deemed hemodynamically stable, the diagnosis of splenic injury is made with contrast CT. Contrast reaction and renal injury are of concern but effects are relatively rare, even in elderly trauma patients [35–37]. Adequate but judicious volume loading pre- and postprocedure should be performed to minimize renal toxicity risks. The routine use of non-contrast abdominal CT in trauma is to be condemned as it will miss significant organ injury [38]. Additionally, even in those scans in which injury is demonstrated, it cannot detect many markers for nonoperative failure such as contrast extravasation, injury grade, and pseudoaneurysm [38–42]. Abdominal CT with a detailed evaluation of the extent of injury is critical in making a treatment plan.

Treatment Selection

After determining continued hemodynamic stability, patient frailty, and descriptive abdominal CT characteristic of the splenic injury, treatment is then determined. Accepting that age is not a contraindication to nonoperative management, it is admitted in most studies that the nonoperative failure rate will be higher than in younger patients with rates varying from a low of 6% up to 33% based on screening criteria [25–33]. Prior studies describe the importance of volume of hemoperitoneum, associated intra-abdominal injuries, neurologic injury, splenic injury grade, and abdominal CT evidence of vascular injury (pseudoaneurysm, extravasation contained or into peritoneum) [9–33, 38–42]. All these predictive factors have been evaluated for failure in overall trauma patients with splenic injury but only in limited studies are they specifically evaluated in the elderly subgroup [25–35]. Untreated PSA were thought to have a 50% failure rate without intervention with 15–75% seen on delayed imaging [38–41]. There are ongoing multicenter trials to see if this rate of delayed pseudoaneurysm with high nonoperative failure rate remains true in the latest generation multidetector CT scanners. In considering nonoperative management, it is important to consider that free intraperitoneal extravasation has a 90% success rate with angiographic embolization but 50% will become unstable prior to treatment [43]. Arteriovenous fistula has a 40% failure rate even with successful angiography [43, 44]. As such, primary operative therapy is recommended in these groups.

Angiography

In those with CT evidence of vascular injury and higher grade injury, angioembolization should be used to increase salvage rates. There remains some debate regarding angioembolization and splenic salvage. There is a large volume of literature supporting angioembolization for pseudoaneurysm, extravasation, and increasing injury grade defined grades 3–5 [40–54]. Main coil or proximal splenic artery embolization is preferred to decrease symptoms of infarction as well as repeat embolization is needed [43, 51]. Prior studies describe missed or delayed pseudoaneurysm on follow-up imaging in patients undergoing selective distal technique. This can require additional invasive therapies while those patients undergoing main splenic artery embolization are already treated even if a new pseudoaneurysm is seen. Proximal splenic artery embolization decreases gland perfusion pressure thereby allowing injuried vessels to clot increasing splenic salvage [46]. In selective, superselective, or distal embolization, only the specific pseudoaneurysm is treated. The incidence of delayed pseudoaneurysm is debated but in the 15–75% range based on current literature [45, 55, 56]. This, coupled with the inherent gland infarction from selective/distal embolization and equivalent efficacy, makes the proximal embolization approach preferred, especially in the elderly [43]. As noted in prior studies combination of selective and main coil embolization has a high complication rate and must be avoided [44]. When Ong et al. reviewed elderly patients with splenic injury they found an overall nonoperative failure rate of 15% with a greater than 50% failure rate for AAST OIS splenic injury grades 3–5 in the elderly without interventions [27]. Mortality in this and prior studies was linked to increasing age and failure of nonoperative management [25–33]. With this in mind angiographic screening for high-grade injury seems to improve outcomes in the majority of studies. Although prophylactic embolization is debated, in recent studies age was used to perform prophylactic embolization with improved salvage and has been used at our institution with good results for high-grade injuries [43, 51, 52].

Operation

As in all trauma adequate exposure and mobilization are critical in trauma laparotomy. Midline incision xiphoid to pubis is used in all acute operations. In documented isolated splenic injury, a left subcostal can be used, but as abdominal CT can miss pancreatic and hollow visceral injury, this incision should be reserved for delayed failures of nonoperative management with no other organ concerns. Clot is evacuated and four quadrants are packed to allow resuscitation with compressive hemostasis. If packs do not control hemorrhage, rapid control of hilum is performed. In most of these cases the massively injured spleen is already mobilized by the force of the accident allowing rapid access to hilum. The spleen is stabilized by multiple ligaments in the left upper quadrant. The phrenicolienal and lienorenal are avascular and may be rapid taken bluntly or sharply. Care must be taken not to go too far medially as the inferior polar vessel and collaterals from the dorsal pancreatic artery can be seen close to this area. Large vessels may be present in the lienocolic ligament. Care must be taken to also identify and ligate the short gastric vessels between the greater curve of the stomach and the superior pole of the spleen. Postoperative bleeding after splenectomy is uncommon but when it occurs it usually is from improper ligation of a short gastric or misses an avulsed vessel in the initial exploration. Although many vessel ligation systems are popular in elective splenectomy, this author has had to reexplore patients in which the supposedly coapted short gastric had reopened and bled. Additionally in patients who have failed a proximal splenic artery embolization, splenectomy should be performed as the mobilization process; ligating the short gastrics and pancreatic collaterals will devascularize the spleen leading to postoperative infarction.

The now mobilized spleen is displaced into the midline and packs are placed behind to maintain this position and provide retroperitoneal hemostasis. Now the surgeon can occlude the hilum posteriorly using fingers near the pancreatic tail to minimize blood loss while evaluating the extent of injury.

The surgeon now determines the extent of injury and patient stability. In minimal injury such as low-grade capsular tears, hemostatic agents and cautery can be used. Higher grade splenic injury may require ligation of individual distal vessels or even polar vessel to control bleeding. After allowing gland demarcation of ischemic tissue, partial resection is performed leaving a rim of devitalized tissue. Mattress sutures over pledgets are placed for additional hemostasis in rim residual devitalized tissue. Residual capsule or omentum may be placed on the cut end as well using the mattress ends to secure. Unless there is minimal injury or isolation to a limited area of gland, splenectomy with individual splenic artery and vein ligation is preferred for two reasons. First with the limited reserves in the elder, the potential need for a second surgery due to bleeding must be avoided at all costs. Incidence of overwhelming post-splenectomy sepsis is low, and the elderly patient have far fewer years left to potionally experience it. Therefore the risk of rebleed in attempts to salvage a severly injuried spleen outweigh the benefit of complicated splenic salvage surgeries. In the elderly this likely is very low while the morbidity and mortality of rebleed following laparotomy are high. With this in mind, other conservation techniques such as wrapping the pulverized spleen in mesh should not be used in this patient population. After removal a laparotomy pad is spread over the raw retroperitoneum and rolled up lateral to medial with control of all bleeding points as exposed from beneath the pad, or "taking a walk on the splenic bed." The pancreas is then carefully examined for signs of contusion/laceration. Drains should be placed only if there are concerns of pancreatic injury and potential for leak.

Post-injury Management

In the past, prolonged bedrest to allow the vessels to clot and stabilize was recommended. There were additional concerns regarding delayed bleed or rupture. Early mobilization and limited hospital observation are advocated based on the following. In those with splenic injury, there is usually an associated thoracic injury or rib fractures. This mandates good pain control, pulmonary toilet, and early mobilization to prevent pneumonia. This is especially critical in the elderly as this is the number one cause of mortality following trauma. Additionally, the majority of studies, of nonoperative failures, occur within 72 h [9–33, 39–60]. One recent study using the National Trauma Data bank noted that 95% of failures in the elderly occurred at 48 h [27]. We recommend early aggressive monitoring with serial abdominal exams and blood counts performed every 8 h to detect occult signs of bleeding. When two stable exams and hematocrits occur, routine lab and physician exam are decreased to daily unless change from patient baseline. Based on this and our prior studies, patients with grades 1 and 2 without interventions are discharged at 48 h while those with higher grade injuries, treated operatively, or with angioembolization, are discharged at 72 h. An area of debate remains in the utility of delayed imaging prior to discharge. There is good evidence that grades 1 and 2 injuries without vascular injuries can be discharged at 24–48 h without repeat imaging [27, 58]. A more difficult question is the utility in higher grade splenic injury. As stated earlier, 15–75% of pseudoaneurysms were seen on delayed imaging in prior studies. Current large studies are ongoing regarding the rate of delayed pseudoaneurysm and its significance. Until these results return, specifically in the elderly, repeat imaging on day 3 prior to discharge may be indicated in those not undergoing angioembolization in grades 3–5 or with evidence of vascular injury [43, 51, 58–60]. The advantage to the aggressive use of angiography and main coil embolization is that no follow-up imaging or therapy is needed. Angiography still appears more sensitive than CT. We believe that many of the classic delayed pseudoaneurysms were present and in spasm on initial CT. These are identified as pseudoaneurysm or as vessel truncation on admission and would be treated initially. Even if delayed pseudoaneurysms were seen on CT in main coil group, the patient is already treated and requires no further interventions [43, 51].

Postoperative complications include most frequently atelectasis, effusion, and pneumonia as above [61, 62]. Subphrenic abscess occurs in 3–13% usually in patients with concomitant bowel and pancreatic injuries [61, 62]. Close monitoring in the elderly especially with associated injuries is critical as leukocytosis is common following splenectomy limiting lab utility. Screening procalcitonin may assist in determining infection from post-splenectomy state. Additionally with diminished immune function, the elderly may not be febrile and physical complaints may be limited even with infection. As stated reoperation for bleeding is low between 2.5 and 1% [62–65].

In those patients undergoing embolization, a significant portion will experience post-embolization syndrome. Attributed to the body's reaction to infarcted splenic tissue, the patient experiences left upper quadrant pain, low-grade fever at usually 38°C, and mild leukocytosis 10,500–12,000. These symptoms should improve with time and NSAIDs may benefit. If signs and symptoms are greater than above, standard infection must be assessed with chest X-ray, cultures, procalcitonin, and white cell differential. If pain is significant or no other source, abdominal CT is performed to assess for abscess. Of note, in the embolization group, small collections of air can be seen without infection. If large pockets of splenic air are seen, however, splenic infection can be presumed and the patient should undergo splenectomy [66].

Immunization for patients undergoing splenectomy is widely accepted with data recommending waiting at least 2 weeks from injury to maximize antibody response [67]. Most data indicate that the severely injured and embolized spleen both recover immunologic function [67–72]. However the majority of studies use indirect markers of immune function. Streptococcal vaccination is already recommended in this age group. As many have lost their immune response to Haemophilus with time, we routinely vaccinate for both in follow-up. The utility of booster vaccines is unclear, but as these are recommended in this age group, we routinely perform them.

OPSS

As stated, splenic conservation stems from the recognition of overwhelming post-splenectomy sepsis (OPSS). This is a rare but often fatal complication of the asplenic state. The risk is highest in children undergoing splenectomy with cancer, a described lifetime incidence of 2%. It is accepted to be lower in the adult population under 1%.

Protocol

The recommended abbreviated protocol is early operation for SBP <90 with serious consideration of operative therapy for SBP <110 or lactate/base deficit ≥6. Contrast ACT to delineate the extent of injury. Patients with low-grade injury (one to two) undergo observation with serial examination and hematocrit for 24–48 h. Patients undergo admission angiography for grades 3–5 or evidence of vascular injury (PSA, extravasation, vessel truncation). Operative therapy is preferred if active extravasation into peritoneal cavity or arteriovenous fistula. Embolization is performed for all signs of vascular injury and prophylactic embolization in grades 3–5 is recommended in this elderly group. Discharge at 72 h unless other injuries preclude with follow-up at 2 weeks for patients undergoing splenectomy or embolization.

Conclusion

As both age and increasing splenic injury grade of three or greater are predictors of non-operative failure, a more aggressive use of angioembolization and operative therapy is needed. The elderly may arrive with systolic blood pressure of 110 mmHg or less or biochemical markers of occult, but significant shock, warranting early consideration of operative therapy. In those with higher grade injury or signs of vascular injury, angiographic proximal splenic artery embolization remains a valuable adjunct to splenic salvage.

References

1. Land-Sudden J. Observation on the surgery of the spleen. Br J Surg. 1912;1:157.
2. Morris DH, Bullock FD. The importance of the spleen in resistance to infection. Ann Surg. 1919;70:153.
3. Gopal V, Bisno AL. Fulminant pneumococcal infections in "normal" asplenic host. Arch Intern Med. 1977;137:1526.
4. Leonard AS, Giebink GS, Baesl TJ, Krivit W. The overwhelming post-splenectomy infection problem. World J Surg. 1980;4:1423.
5. Krivit W. Overwhelming post-splenectomy infection. Am J Hematol. 1977;2:193.
6. Campos CH. Segmental resections of the spleen. O Hospital (Rio de Janeiro). 1961;62:187.
7. Upadhyaya P, Simpson JS. Splenic trauma in children. Surg Gynecol Obstet. 1968;126:677.
8. Pearl RH, Wesson DE, Spence LJ, Filler RM, et al. Splenic injury: a 5-year update with improved results and changing criteria for conservative management. J Pediatr Surg. 1989;24(5):428–31.
9. Luna GK, Dellinger EP. Nonoperative observation therapy for splenic injuries: a safe therapeutic option? Am J Surg. 1987;153(5):462–8.
10. Brasel KJ, DeLisle CM, Olson CJ, Borgstrom DC. Splenic injury: trends in evaluation and management. J Trauma. 1998;44(2):283–6.

11. Pachter HL, Guth AA, Hofstetter SR, Spencer FC. Changing patterns in the management of splenic trauma: the impact of nonoperative management. Ann Surg. 1998;227(5):708–19.
12. Koury HI, Peschiera JL, Welling RE. Non-operative management of blunt splenic trauma: a 10-year experience. Injury. 1991;22(5):349–52.
13. Pachter HL, Spencer FC, Hofstetter SR, Liang HG, et al. Experience with selective operative and nonoperative treatment of splenic injuries in 193 patients. Ann Surg. 1990;211(5):583–91.
14. Longo WE, Baker CC, McMillen MA, Modlin IM, et al. Nonoperative management of adult blunt splenic trauma: criteria for successful outcome. Ann Surg. 1989;210(5):626–9.
15. Cogbill TH, Moore EE, Jurkovich GJ, Morris JA, et al. Nonoperative management of blunt splenic trauma: a multicenter experience. J Trauma. 1989;29(10):1312–7.
16. Renzulli P, Gross T, Schnuriger B, et al. Management of blunt injuries to the spleen. Br J Surg. 2010;97(11):1696–703.
17. Steele M, Lim RC Jr. Advances in management of splenic injuries. Am J Surg. 1975;130(2):159–65.
18. Lucas CE. Splenic trauma. Choice of management. Ann Surg. 1991;213(2):98–112.
19. Cathey KL, Brady WJ, Butler K, Blow O, et al. Blunt splenic trauma: characteristics of patients requiring urgent laparotomy. Am Surg. 1998;64(5):450–4.
20. Nix JA, Costanza M, Daley BJ, Powell MA, et al. Outcome of the current management of splenic injuries. J Trauma. 2001;50(5):835–42.
21. Velmahos GC, Chan LS, Kamel E, et al. Nonoperative management of splenic injuries: have we gone too far? Arch Surg. 2000;135(6):674–81.
22. Peitzman A, Heil B, Rivera L, Federle M, et al. Blunt splenic injury in adults: multi-institutional study of the Eastern Association for the Surgery of trauma. J Trauma. 2000;49(2):177–89.
23. Velmahos GC, Zacharias N, Emhoff TA, et al. Management of the most severely injured spleen: a multicenter study of the research consortium of New England Centers for Trauma (ReCONECT). Arch Surg. 2010;145(5):456–60.
24. Zarzaur BL, Kozar R, Myers JG, Claridge JA, Scalea TM, Neideen TA, Maung AA, et al. The splenic injury outcomes trial: an American Association for the Surgery of Trauma Multi-Institutional Study. J Trauma. 2015;79(3):335–42.
25. Bhullar IS, Frykberg ER, Siragusa D, Chesire D, et al. Age does not affect outcomes of nonoperative management of blunt splenic trauma. J Am Coll Surg. 2012;214(6):958–64.
26. Bee TK, Croce MA, Miller PR, Pritchard FE, et al. Failure of splenic nonoperative management: is the glass half empty or half full? J Trauma. 2001;50(2):230–6.
27. Ong AW, Eilertson KE, Reilly EF, Geng TA, et al. Nonoperative management of splenic injuries: significance of age. J Surg Res. 2016;201(1):134–40.
28. Cocanour CS, Moore FA, Ware DN, Marvin RG, Duke JH. Age should not be a consideration for nonoperative management of blunt splenic injury. J Trauma. 2000;48(4):606–10.
29. Barone JE, Burns G, Svehlak SA, Tucker JB, et al. Management of blunt splenic trauma in patients older than 55 years. J Trauma. 1999;46(1):87–90.
30. Albrecht RM, Schermer CR, Morris A. Nonoperative management of blunt splenic injuries: factors influencing success in age >55 years. Am Surg. 2002;68(3):227–30.
31. Godley CD, Warren RL, Sheridan RL, McCabe CJ. Nonoperative management of blunt splenic injury in adults: age over 55 years as a powerful indicator for failure. J Am Coll Surg. 1996;183(2):133–9.
32. Myers JG, Dent DL, Stewart RM, Gray GA, et al. Blunt splenic injuries: dedicated trauma surgeons can achieve a high rate of nonoperative success in patients of all ages. J Trauma Injury. 2000;48(5):801–5.
33. Jeremitsky E, Smith RS, Ong AW. Starting the clock: defining nonoperative management of blunt splenic injury by time. Am J Surg. 2013;205(3):298–301.
34. Eastridge BJ, Salinas J, McManus JG, et al. Hypotension begins at 110 mm Hg: redefining "hypotension" with data. J Trauma. 2007;631:291.
35. Vassiliu P, Sava J, Toutouzas KG, Velmahos GC. Is contrast as bad as we think? Renal function after angiographic embolization of injured patients. J Am Coll Surg. 2002;194(2):142–6.
36. Colling KP, Irwin ED, Byrnes MC, et al. Computed tomography scans with intravenous contrast: low incidence of contrast-induced nephropathy in blunt trauma patients. J Trauma. 2014;77(2):226–30.
37. Hsieh TM, Tsai TH, Liu YW, Hsieh CH. Risk factors for contrast-induced nephropathy and their association with mortality in patients with blunt splenic injuries. Int J Surg. 2016;35:69–75.
38. Murken DR, Weiss JJ, Hill GC, et al. Radiographic assessment of blunt splenic injury without contrast: is contrast truly needed? Surgery. 2012;152(4):676–82.
39. Schurr MJ, Fabian TC, Gavant M, Croce MA, et al. Management of blunt splenic trauma: computed tomographic contrast blush predicts failure of nonoperative management. J Trauma. 1995;39(3):507–12.
40. Wong YC, Wang LJ, See LC, Fang JF, et al. Contrast material extravasation on contrast-enhanced helical computed tomographic scan of blunt abdominal trauma: its significance on the choice, time, and outcome of treatment. J Trauma. 2003;54(1):164–70.
41. Sclafoni SJA, Shaftan G, Scalea TM, et al. Nonoperative salvage of computed tomography-diagnosed splenic injuries: utilization of angiography for triage and embolization for hemostasis. J Trauma. 1995;39(5):818–27.
42. Shanmuganathan K, Mirvis S, Boyd-Kranis R, Scalea TM. Nonsurgical management of blunt splenic injury: use of CT criteria to select patients for angiography and potential endovascular therapy. Radiology. 2000;217(1):75–82.
43. Sabe AA, Claridge JA, Rosenblum DI, et al. The effects of splenic artery embolization on nonoperative

management of blunt splenic injury: a 16 year experience. J Trauma. 2009;67:565–72.
44. Haan JM, Bochicchio GV, Kramer N, Scalea TM. Nonoperative management of blunt splenic injury: a 5-year experience. J Trauma. 2005; 58(3):492–8.
45. Davis KA, Fabian TC, Croce MA, Gavant ML, et al. Improved success in nonoperative management of blunt splenic injuries: embolization of splenic artery pseudoaneurysms. J Trauma. 1998;44(6):1008–13.
46. Brault-Noble G, Charbit J, Chardon P, Barral L, Guillon F, Taourel P, Millet I. Age should be considered in the decision making of prophylactic splenic angioembolization in nonoperative management of blunt splenic trauma: a study of 208 consecutive patients. J Trauma. 2012;73(5):1213–20.
47. Requarth J, Miller P. The splenic artery stump pressure is affected by arterial anatomy after proximal embolotherapy in blunt splenic injury. J Trauma. 2012;73(5):1221–4.
48. Hagiwara A, Yukioka T, Ohta S, et al. Nonsurgical management of patients with blunt splenic injury: efficacy of transcatheter arterial embolization. Am J Radiol. 1996;167:159–66.
49. Wei B, Hemmila MR, Arabi S, et al. Angioembolization reduces operative intervention for blunt splenic injury. J Trauma. 2008;64:1472–7.
50. Haan J, Marmery H, Shanmuganathan K, Scalea TM. Experience with main coil embolization and significance of new or persistent pseudoaneursym; reembolize, operate, or observe. J Trauma. 2007;63(3):615–9.
51. Haan J, Scott J, Boyd-Kranis RL, Ho S, Kramer M, Scalea TM. Admission angiography for blunt splenic injury: advantages and pitfalls. J Trauma. 2001;51(6):1161–5.
52. Clancy TV, Ramshaw DG, Maxwell JG, Covington DL, et al. Management outcomes in splenic injury: a statewide trauma center review. Ann Surg. 1997;226(1):17–24.
53. Banerjee A, Duane TM, Wilson SP, Haney S, et al. Trauma center variation in splenic artery embolization and spleen salvage: a multicenter analysis. J Trauma Acute Care Surg. 2013;75(1):69–74.
54. Haan J, Ilahi ON, Kramer M, Scalea TM. Protocol-driven nonoperative management in patients with blunt splenic trauma and minimal associated injury decreases length of stay. J Trauma. 2003;55(2):317–21.
55. Muroya T, Ogura H, Shimuzu K, et al. Delayed formation of splenic pseudaneurysm following nonoperative management in blunt splenic injury: Multi-Institutional Study in Osaka, Japan. J Trauma Acute Care Surg. 2013;73(5):1213–20.
56. Weinburg JA, Lockhart ME, Parmar AD, et al. Computed tomography identification of latent pseudoaneursym after blunt splenic injury: pathology or technology? J Trauma. 2010;68(5):1112–6.
57. Haan JM, Biffl W, Knudson MM, Davis DA, et al. Splenic embolization revisited: a multicenter review. J Trauma. 2004;56(3):542–7.
58. Thaemert BC, Cogbill TH, Lambert PJ. Nonoperative management of splenic injury: are follow-up computed tomographic scans of any value? J Trauma. 1997;43(5):748–51.
59. Uecker J, Pickett C, Dunn E. The role of follow-up radiographic studies in nonoperative management of spleen trauma. Am Surg. 2001;67(1):22–5.
60. Ellison EC, Fabri PJ. Complications of splenectomy. Surg Clin North Am. 1983;63:1313.
61. Livingston CD, Sirinek KR, Levine BA, et al. Traumatic splenic injury. Arch Surg. 1982;117:670.
62. Shackford SR, Molin M. Management of splenic injuries. Surg Clin North Am. 1990;70:595.
63. Beal SL, Spisso JM. The risk of splenorrhaphy. Arch Surg. 1988;123:1158.
64. Ghosh S, Symes JM, Walsh TH. Splenic repair for trauma. Br J Surg. 1988;75:1139.
65. Haan J, Bochicchio G, Kramer M, Scalea TM. Air following splenic embolization: infection or incidental finding? Am Surg. 2003;69(12):1036–40.
66. Shatz DV, Romero-Steiner S, Elie CM, Holder PF, Carlone GM. Antibody responses in postsplenectomy trauma patients receiving the 23-valent pneumococcal polysaccharide vaccine at 14 versus 28 days postoperatively. J Trauma. 2002;53(6):1037–42.
67. Bessoud B, Duchosal M, Siegrist S, et al. Proximal splenic artery embolization for blunt splenic injury: clinical, immunologic, and ultrasound-doppler follow-up. J Trauma. 2007;62(6):1481–6.
68. Olthof DC, Lammers AJ, van Leeuwen EM, Hoekstra JB, et al. Antibody response to a T-cell-independent antigen is preserved after splenic artery embolization for trauma. Clin Vaccine Immunol. 2014;21(11):1500–4.
69. Malhotra AK, Carter RF, Lebman DA, Carter DS, et al. Preservation of splenic immunocompetence after splenic artery angioembolization for blunt splenic injury. J Trauma Injury. 2010;69(5):1126–30.
70. Oller-Sales B, Troya-Diaz J, Martinez-Arconada MJ, Rodriguez N, et al. Post traumatic splenic function depending on severity of injury and management. Transl Res. 2011;158(2):118–28.
71. Connell NT, Brunner AM, Kerr CA, Schiffman FJ. Splenosis and sepsis: the born-again spleen provides poor protection. Virulence. 2011;2(1):4–11.
72. Walusimbi MS, Dominguez KM, Sands JM, Markert RJ, McCarthy MC. Circulating cellular and humoral elements of immune function following arterial embolization or splenectomy in trauma patients. Injury. 2012;43(2):180–3.

Check for updates

21 Hollow Viscus Injury in Geriatric Trauma: Damage Control, Surgical Management, and Critical Care

Arturo R. Maldonado† and Juan L. Peschiera

Introduction

Hollow viscus injury (HVI) in elderly trauma patients is a source of high morbidity and mortality. Age-related declines in organ function, end-stage comorbidities, and long-standing metabolic syndrome sequelae lower survival in these patients [1–5]. The higher mortality in frail elderly patients leads to a poor outcome correlation with Injury Severity Scores (ISS) when compared to younger patients [5, 6]. From 2013 to 2014, trauma was the seventh most common cause of mortality for patients over the age of 65, and 13.5% of those deaths were related to motor vehicle crashes (MVCs) [1–3, 7]. This subset of patients with higher mortality can be expanded to include patients aged 45–56 which showed increased mortality and increased rates of decubitus ulcers, renal failure, sepsis, wound infections, abscesses, and multi-organ failure [8–10]. In addition, morbidity is also higher in elderly trauma patients with 88% of the patients not able to return to pre-injury level of mobility, activity, and independence [11, 12]. When mortality of patients with HVI was compared to non-HVI patients, patients with HVI had a higher mortality and severely injured elderly patients had the highest mortality [13, 14]. The high mortality associated with HVI in all age groups accentuates the importance of having a high index of suspicion and prompt expert management of all patients that suffer from HVI, especially the elderly.

The Eastern Association for the Surgery of Trauma (EAST) HVI study analyzed registry data from 95 trauma centers. Out of 2632 patients, the incidence of stomach injury was 4.3% and small bowel perforation from blunt trauma was 0.3% [13]. Though the incidence for HVI from blunt trauma is low, the impact of gastric, small bowel, and large bowel perforation on morbidity and mortality is significant. With the escalation of morbidity and mortality in the elderly, even with best management, HVI in geriatric patients is devastating.

Despite differences in obesity rates and comorbidities among patients from different nations, HVI remains a worldwide problem [15]. HVI does not escape disparities in healthcare, with patients of low socioeconomic status having 7.1% more anastomotic leaks, 11.4% more fascial dehiscence, and 13.8% more abscesses than higher status [16]. Though computer tomography (CT) scanning technology has improved significantly, early diagnosis and management of HVI remain clinically challenging [17].

†Author was deceased at the time of publication

A.R. Maldonado, M.D., Ph.D., F.A.C.S.
J.L. Peschiera, M.D. (✉)
Bethesda North Trauma Center, Bethesda North Hospital, 10500 Montgomery Road, Cincinnati, OH 45245, USA
e-mail: art@arturo.ws; jpeschiera@gmail.com

A. Rodriguez et al. (eds.), *Geriatric Trauma and Acute Care Surgery*,
https://doi.org/10.1007/978-3-319-57403-5_21

Mechanisms of Injury

Geriatric patients are more likely to be severely injured from motor vehicle crashes (MVCs) compared to younger patients [18]. In addition, blunt abdominal injury and concomitant operative fractures increase the risk of sepsis and multi-organ failure [19]. Though seatbelts increase survival from MVC, seatbelts have increased the incidence of HVI [20]. Three-point restraints have 4.38-fold more risk of HVI compared to no belt and two-point lap belt restraints have 10-fold increased risk [21]. Seatbelts are associated with high-energy transfer to the abdomen which can result in a flexion distraction injury-related fracture called a Chance fracture. A Chance fracture is a transverse fracture of the posterior elements of a vertebral body between T12 and L4. First described by G.Q. Chance in 1948, the vertebra most commonly fractured through this mechanism is L2 [22]. A subgroup analysis of patients with chance fractures showed that 62.5% of patients had concomitant HVI [21]. Though gastric injury from improper seatbelt use is rare, there is a case report of a 65-year-old woman who suffered from gastric mucosal lacerations, pneumatosis of the stomach, and massive bleeding [23]. The presence of a transected rectus abdominis or abdominal wall hernia after improper seatbelt placement and MVC has been associated with major bowel devascularization and morbidity [24, 25]. Seatbelt syndrome-related HVI is a worldwide problem with increasing incidence in developing countries [26, 27].

Most of these seatbelt-related HVIs occur because lap belts are inappropriately worn above the pelvic anterior superior iliac spines (ASIS), on the anterior abdominal wall, and not across the hips below the abdomen. Similarly, the shoulder harness can lead to additional injuries if not worn or placed below the arm instead of across the chest and shoulder. Aggressive campaigns exist to improve compliance and correct use of child seats and seat belts in pediatric patients [27–30]. These efforts have decreased morbidity and mortality in pediatric patients [31]. To decrease preventable MVC-related HVI in adult and geriatric patients, major educational campaigns focused on the correct use and placement of lap and harness belts need to be created and implemented for adults and the elderly.

HVI occurs more commonly after penetrating trauma than blunt trauma. Of penetrating injuries, 68–80% of small-bowel injuries occur from gunshot wounds (GSW) and 20–32% from stabbings or impalements [32]. Like small bowel, 75% of large-bowel injuries occur from penetrating trauma [33]. Ivatury et al. reported that 80% of rectal injuries were caused by GSW, 6% by transanal injury, and stab wounds <3% [34]. Though penetrating trauma occurs less often in geriatric patients, the elderly wounded have twice the length of stay in the ICU compared to non-elderly patients and worse morbidity and mortality [35].

Multi-Organ Dysfunction and HVI in the Elderly

Trauma management and outcomes in geriatric patients, and especially those who suffer from HVI, are complicated by impaired physiologic reserve. There is a large impact on gastrointestinal perfusion because of impaired cardiopulmonary function, central, and peripheral vascular disease. A significant number of patients arrive on medications that further decrease cardiac output such as beta-blockers and calcium-channel blockers. In trauma patients with heart disease and cardiac stents, preexisting hemorrhage risk exists from antiplatelet agents, such as acetylsalicylic acid (ASA) and clopidogrel. Some patients present on anticoagulants such as warfarin, dabigatran, rivaroxaban, apixaban, and edoxaban [36–40]. These agents increase or have the potential to increase blood loss, morbidity, and mortality in trauma patients [41–43]. To complicate the management of drug-enhanced exsanguination, some of these agents do not have efficient reversal agents, and may require dialysis for removal. Most reversal protocols involve reversal using FFP or prothrombin complex concentrates (PCC) which have shown improvement in outcomes with potential for thromboembolism complications under retrospective evaluation [44].

Prospective randomized trials evaluating outcomes after treatment with FFP and PCC in trauma patients need to be performed [45–52]. Idarucizumab, a monoclonal antibody to dabigatran, has been recently approved by the FDA as an antidote and its impact on trauma outcomes is yet to be elucidated. Several experimental drugs are under investigation for the reversal of factor Xa inhibitors such as andexanet alfa (PRT064445) and aripazine (PER977), but are not available for general clinical use in the United States [40, 53]. Volume loss from hemorrhage combined with low ejection fraction and a combination of beta-blockers and or calcium-channel blockers contributes to the patient's inability to compensate for worsening shock [54].

Treatment of shock, not hemoglobin, is the initial trigger of transfusion in the immediate period after trauma and a massive transfusion protocol is activated if clinically indicated [55]. Though some controversy exists regarding trauma outcomes, almost 40% of US trauma surgeons routinely use tranexamic acid (TXA) in patients that present with hemorrhagic shock because the majority of studies report decreased mortality, transfusion requirements, coagulopathy, or multi-organ failure in adult and pediatric patients after tranexamic acid treatment [56–65].

Initial Management and Diagnosis

On presentation to the trauma center, the American College of Surgeons Advanced Trauma Life Support (ATLS) protocol is initiated and the patient's airway, breathing, and circulation are assessed while the trauma team simultaneously places the patient on a cardiac monitor, pulse oximetry, and capnography; obtains blood for testing; and inserts two large-bore intravenous catheters (IVs) [66]. Assuming that airway and breathing are normal, hypotension would be treated with 1 L of saline, and if severe emergency uncross-matched O blood released for transfusion. Studies have shown that the physical exam does not reliably assist in the diagnosis of HVI [67, 68]. Though the presence of a seatbelt sign is highly suggestive of HVI, absence of the sign does not rule out HVI [69]. Obvious signs such as evisceration after penetrating trauma or peritonitis are not common. Blood on digital rectal exam, proximity perianal wounds, or projectile trajectories would increase the index of suspicion and warrant further workup for HVI [70].

Laboratory Studies

A CBC with differential would give a baseline assessment of preexisting leukocytosis or anemia from an uncompensated sample if the patient presented immediately after HVI and hemorrhage. This assay could reveal if the patient has preexisting thrombocytopenia. Though nonspecific for duodenal or pancreatic injury, an amylase may be helpful. A basic metabolic panel would be assessed for metabolic acidosis, possible existence of acute and or chronic kidney disease, and any electrolyte abnormality such as hypokalemia from diuretic therapy or hyponatremia from thiazide therapy, hypovolemia, proton pump inhibitors, or heart failure [71–73].

Imaging Studies and ATLS Adjuncts

First published by Spanish surgeons, the ultrasound (U/S) has been in clinical use for the purposes of trauma care since 1953 [74–77]. In the last two decades, it has been widely adopted as the adjunct of choice in the unstable trauma patient for the rapid identification of peritoneal hemorrhage and pericardial tamponade. The Focused Assessment with Sonography for Trauma (FAST) examines the peritoneal cavity for free fluid in the right flank in the hepatorenal recess of Morison's pouch, the left flank in the subphrenic perisplenic space, and suprapubic area posterior to the bladder in men or in the pouch of Douglas in women. The fourth FAST position is the subxiphoid view with the probe pointed towards the left shoulder to assess for a pericardial effusion between the liver and the heart [78–80]. With additional training, the probe can also be used to assess for pleural effusions, pneumothorax, and preload assessment by visualizing the vena cava. With the additional pleural assessment, the FAST acronym has been modified to Extended Focused Assessment with Sonography for Trauma (EFAST). Using computed tomography (CT) of the chest as the gold standard, the ultrasound showed a 28% higher sensitivity for pneumothorax detection than chest X-ray (CXR) [81, 82]. Advantages of FAST over DPL are that FAST is noninvasive and can be easily repeated, and additional organs can be assessed. The disadvantages are the operator dependence of quality, learning curve, and lower sensitivity and specificity compared to diagnostic peritoneal lavage (DPL), but close to equivalent with improvements in ultrasound technology and training [83–87]. In 1997, a prospective study by McKenney and colleagues showed that abdominal U/S could replace the invasive DPL abdominal assessment in the unstable, blunt trauma patient [88]. However, if the FAST exam is repeatedly equivocal or an ultrasound device is not available, a DPL may be needed in the unstable blunt trauma patient.

At some American and European metropolitan trauma centers, DPL is still in use [89, 90]. To prevent bladder and stomach injuries, catheters are inserted to drain the bladder and stomach prior to the surgical procedure. The DPL can be done minimally invasively with an over-wire catheter kit. However, if a kit is not available, the DPL can be done with a scalpel, retractors, an 18-gauge angiocatheter, a 1 L saline bag, IV tubing with bidirectional flow, and a peritoneal dialysis catheter. Open and percutaneous methods of DPL are equivalent in accuracy and safety when performed by a trauma surgeon, though technical difficulty or adhesions may require an open technique [91, 92]. After prepping and draping with aseptic technique, lidocaine with epinephrine is injected in the planned incision site to prevent a false-positive reading from incisional bleeding. The surgeon cuts down to the linea alba, above or below the umbilicus depending on body habitus, presence of pelvic fracture, or gravid uterus. An 18-gauge angiocatheter is inserted in a 45° angle towards caudally or cephalad. Aspiration of 10 mL of blood from the peritoneal cavity is diagnostic for peritoneal hemorrhage. If there is any bile-stained fluid or food particles, then injury to hollow viscus is identified. If there is no evidence of injury on aspiration, a soft peritoneal dialysis catheter is inserted into the peritoneal cavity and a liter of saline in adults or 10–15 mL/kg in children is infused by gravity [93]. Once it is completed, the bag is held below the patient and allowed to fill by gravity. At least 30% of the peritoneal effluent is sent to the lab and assayed for RBCs, WBC, amylase, and alkaline phosphatase. If >100,000 RBC/mm^3, then it is considered positive for peritoneal hemorrhage. With a RBC cutoff of 100,000 RBC/mm^3, the negative laparotomy rate was 0.2–4.1% and the false-negative rate was 0–1.2% [94, 95]. If WBC > 500/mm^3, amylase >20 IU/L, or alkaline phosphatase >3 IU/L, then the DPL is considered positive for HVI [96]. The fascia is closed if the open technique was used. Advantages of DPL are that it has slightly better sensitivity, specificity, and predictive values compared to U/S. The disadvantages are that it is invasive and can cause intestinal, aortic, or bladder injury depending on technique and the needle angle of attack, though complication rates are <2% [95, 97].

If the patient is hemodynamically unstable, then the patient is taken to the operating room for peritoneal hemorrhage control. If the patient is an immediate responder to intravenous resuscitation and the blood pressure is stable, then a CT of the abdomen and pelvis (CTA/P) is obtained with intravenous (IV) contrast. Free fluid is present in 68.8% of HVI cases, and in 29–38% of hollow viscus perforation. Absence of free fluid does not rule out HVI. Injury of the mesentery may present as fat stranding. Pneumatosis indicates bowel necrosis and free air indicates perforated hollow viscus. Sensitivity, specificity, and predictive values for HVI vary from institution to institution, but CT can detect up to 80% of HVI cases. Livingston and colleagues performed a four-trauma-center, prospective study that analyzed 2299 patients and reported that no admission for observation was necessary if the CTA/P was normal because of a negative predictive value of 99.63% [98].

Perioperative Management

After ATLS primary and secondary surveys, initial intravenous resuscitation, and diagnosis of hollow viscus perforation, type and screen, empiric broad-spectrum antibiotics are initiated, a central venous introducer sheath is inserted, and the patient is taken to the operating room. A thermal-regulated rapid infusion pump is placed on standby and the blood bank is notified in case of activation of the massive transfusion protocol (MTP). If the MTP is activated and the injury occurred <3 h from presentation, 1 g of tranexamic acid is administered over 10 min. Some surgeons will employ an autotransfusion blood salvage device despite bacterial contamination of blood from HVI. Multiple studies and a 2015 Cochrane database systematic review report that filtered, bacterial contaminated, autologous blood does not alter clinical outcomes and lowers transfusion requirements in trauma patients. These findings suggest that the infectious and transfusion reaction risks from heterologous blood components are a greater risk to the trauma patient and increase healthcare costs [99–103].

As the surgical team scrubs, sequential compression devices (SCDs) are placed and catheters are inserted to decompress bladder and stomach. Multiple studies have shown that prompt surgical management leads to better outcomes. Though a greater than 24-h delay has not been clearly shown to increase mortality in patients, there is consensus that worse infectious complications occur with operative delay including anastomotic leaks, abscesses, and sepsis [104–106].

Because anesthesia resuscitation methods vary greatly even within the same institution, communication between then trauma surgeon and the anesthesia team is critical. In addition to verifying preoperative antibiotics, the authors discuss the resuscitation plan, usually a balanced crystalloid and blood product resuscitation, to prevent massive crystalloid infusions. Predominantly crystalloid resuscitations lead to intra-abdominal edema, abdominal hypertension, and possibly abdominal compartment syndrome. Also, the patient is serially assessed for the trauma "triad of death": hypothermia (temperature < 36 °C), metabolic acidosis (pH < 7.2), and coagulopathy if not already present.

Damage Control Resuscitation and Surgery

At the initial stages of the trauma triad of death, the definitive operative repairs must be abandoned for a damage control operation and temporary abdominal closure (TAC) utilized. Failure to recognize or heed the trauma triad of death at INR >1.5 will lead to 47.8% mortality and, if the INR reaches three or greater, certain death [107–114]. The authors have had success closing open abdomens covered with a commercially available negative-pressure TAC device (ABThera, Kinetic Concepts Inc., San Antonio, TX) which prevents loss of abdominal domain as long as the device is deployed correctly and washouts are performed every 1–2 days. As washout interval increases in duration, the risk of adhesions causing loss of abdominal domain and preventing primary fascial closure increases. A 2014 prospective, multicenter study showed that second-look operations >24 h from initial operation decreased the rate of primary fascial closures and >48 h showed a trend towards more intra-abdominal complications [115].

The patient is prepped neck to knees and a midline incision laparotomy is created if the FAST was suggestive of peritoneal hemorrhage or hollow viscus injury. All four quadrants are packed and time is given to anesthesia to catch up with resuscitation now that bleeding is relatively controlled. After the patient is euvolemic, the cleanest packs are removed first. All hemorrhage is stopped and perforations are controlled to prevent further soilage. If the patient is exhibiting the lethal triad of death, or has received a massive transfusion protocol, then hollow viscus anastomoses will be avoided at this operation because anastomotic failures will occur in up to 40% of patients resulting in leaks and fistulas [116]. Perforations are either stapled off, closed with umbilical tape, or vessel loops [117]. A temporary abdominal closure device is utilized and the patient is transferred to the ICU for continued resuscitation and warming. After 24–48 h of resuscitation and stabilization, the patient is taken back to the OR. If there is still significant edema and the abdomen cannot be closed, then stomas are created. If minimal edema and the fascia can be closed without tension, then an ileocolic anastomosis is created for perforations to the right of the middle colic pedicle. For perforations to the left of the middle colic and above the peritoneal reflection, most surgeons would perform either stapled or two-layered hand-sewn repairs. Rectal injuries are treated with a Hartmann's procedure with diverting colostomy and pelvic closed suction drains are placed. Additional indications for diversion are massive fecal soilage or ongoing massive transfusion as discussed above.

If the patient can be closed at the second operation and GI tract edema has mostly resolved, repairs and resections are performed. If the patient cannot be closed on the second washout operation, then an aggressive fluid mobilization strategy is pursued in between washouts to decrease bowel and mesenteric edema and allow for fascial closure of the abdomen. Because mobilization of excess total body water is a slow process, preventing large-volume crystalloid resuscitations with a balanced use of non-crystalloid solutions and blood products has been shown to improve rates of primary fascial closure [118].

Pitfalls of temporary abdominal closure include improper application of the temporary abdominal closure (TAC) appliance whether commercially available or created at the time of surgery. If the device does not sufficiently cover the small intestines, then significant retraction of the abdominal wall and adhesions would create complex and permanent abdominal wound because of loss of abdominal domain. If timing between washouts increases past 48–72 h, then bowel adhesions may prevent peritoneal closure. Lack of fluid mobilization in between washouts will prolong closure beyond 7 days and the probability of successful peritoneal closure will be significantly decreased. In addition, overutilizing crystalloids and insufficient transfusion of blood products in the initial resuscitation period increase the time to peritoneal fascial closure from 2.4 to 7.2 days and increase the number of washout laparotomies from 2.7 to 4.3 [118, 119]. Because of the complexities of open abdomen management, classifications and evidence-based management guidelines have been created to maximize the rate of primary fascial closures, decrease morbidity, and improve survival of patients who require an open abdomen after damage control surgery [120–123].

Hollow Viscus Injury Scales and Surgical Repairs

> *"In all cases of abdominal contusions the prognosis should be guarded, and the patients ought to be kept under careful observation. Upon the least suspicion of rupture immediate laparotomy is the only course to be followed."* Emanuel J. Senn M.D., 1904 [124].

The first laparotomy for blunt HVI was performed by M. Bouilly M.D. in 1883 on a 29-year-old man kicked by a horse [125]. Dr. Bouilly performed a 5-in. small-bowel resection, created a single-layered primary anastomosis with No. 0 silk in a Lembert fashion, and closed the abdomen with silver wire. The patient had bowel recovery on postoperative day (POD) 3 and survived until POD 11. On POD 10, to determine how to repair the enterocutaneous fistula that appeared, Dr. Bouilly digitally explored the patient's fistula at the bedside which created a free perforation, peritoneal sepsis, septic shock, and death within 24 h [124, 125]. In 1889, John Croft M.D. performed the first successful repair for HVI in a 14-year-old boy kicked by a horse. He performed a 1-in. small-bowel resection of the ileum for a small perforation, repaired it primarily in a two-layered fashion, and washed out the abdomen with a dilute carbolic acid solution for a total operative time of 1 h and 45 min. His patient recovered successfully [124–126]. Per Sir Zachary Cope's 1914 report on early diagnosis and treatment of ruptured intestine and surgical repair of HVI, including complex duodenal injuries, became the standard of care after Dr. Croft succeeded in 1889 [127].

The American Association for the Surgery of Trauma (AAST) Organ Injury Scales (OIS) for abdominal GI tract is shown in Tables 21.1, 21.2, 21.3, 21.4, and 21.5 [128]. Principles of surgery must be followed to decrease risks of surgical complications. Performing tension-free anastomoses and not sewing ischemic viscus together have improved surgical success and clinical outcomes. Traditional perfusion assessments of hollow viscus after injury are subjective assessments of color, degree of pulsatile flow in the mesentery, and bleeding cut edges. Because these measures are indirect, subjective, and qualitative measurements of organ perfusion, anastomotic failures occur throughout the gastrointestinal tract, most commonly in the rectum and esophagus. The use of intraoperative fluorescence angiography is currently being investigative as a direct measurement of perfusion and preliminary data shows reduced anastomotic failures [129–131].

Table 21.1 Stomach injury scale

Grade[a]	Injury	ICD-9	AIS-90
1	Contusion or hematoma Partial thickness laceration	863.0/1	2
II	Laceration	863.0/1	3
	<2 cm in GE junction or pylorus		
	<5 cm in proximal 1/3 stomach		
	<10 cm in distal 2/3 stomach		
III	Laceration	863.0/1	3
	>2 cm in GE junction or pylorus		
	>5 cm in proximal 1/3 stomach		
	>10 cm in distal 2/3 stomach		
IV	Tissue loss or devasoularization <2/3 stomach	863.0/1	4
V	Tissue loss or devasoularization >2/3 stomach	863.0/1	4

[a]Advance one grade for multiple injuries up to grade III. GE (gastroesophageal). Adapted from Moore et al., American Association for the Surgery of Trauma Organ Injury Scaling, 2010

Table 21.2 Duodenum injury scale

Grade[a]	Injury	ICD-9	AIS-90
I	Hematoma involving single portion of duodenum Partial thickness laceration without perforation	863.21	2 3
II	Hem atoma Involving more than one portion Laceration <50% of circumference	863.21	2 4
III	Laceration	863.21	4
	50–75% of circumference of D2		4
	50%–100% of circLtnterence of D1, D3, D4		
IV	Disruption >75% of circumference of D2 Involving ampulla or distal common bile duct	863.21	5
V	Massive disruption of duodenopancreatic complex Devascularization of duodenum	863.21	5 5

[a]Advance one grade for multiple injuries up to grade III. D1 (1st portion of duodenum), D2 (2nd portion of duodenum), D3 (3ed portion of duodenum), D4 (4th portion of duodenum). Adapted from Moore et al., American Association for the Surgery of Trauma Organ Injury Scaling, 2010

Table 21.3 Small bowel injury scale

Grade[a]	Injury	ICD-9	AIS-90
I	Contusion or hematoma without devascularization Partial thickness laceration without perforation	863.20	2 2
II	Laceration <50% of circumference	863.30	3
III	Laceration > 50% of circumference without transection	863.30	3
IV	Transection of the small bowel	863.20	4
V	Transection of the small bowel with segmental tissue loss Devascularized segment	863.30	4 4

[a]Advance one grade for multiple injures up to grade II. Adapted from Moore et al. American Association for the Surgery of Trauma Organ Injury Scaling, 2010

Table 21.4 Colon injury scale

Grade[a]	Injury	ICD-9[b]	AIS-90
I	Contusion or hematoma without devascularization Partial thickness laceration without perforation	863.40-863.44	2 2
II	Laceration <50% of circumference	863.50-863.54	3
III	Laceration >50% of circumference without transection	863.50-863.54	3
Iv	Tran section of the bowel	863.50-863.54	4
V	Transection of the bowel with segmental tissue loss Devascularized segment	863.50-863.54	4 4

[a]Advance one grade for multiple injures up to grade III
[b]863.41, 863.5 - ascending; 863.42, 863.52—transverse; 863.45, 863.53—descending; 863.44, 863.54—sigmoid. Adapted from Moore et al. American Association for the Surgery of Trauma Organ Injury Scaling, 2010

Table 21.5 Rectum injury scale

Grade[a]	Injury	ICD-9	AIS-90
I	Contusion or hematoma without devascularization Partial thickness laceration	863.45	2 2
II	Laceration <50% of circumference	863.45	3
III	Laceration > 50% of circumference	863.55	4
IV	Full-thickness laceration with extension into the perineum	863.55	5
V	Devascularized segment	863.55	5

[a]Advance one grade for multiple injures up to grade III. Adapted from Moore et al., American Association for the Surgery of Trauma Organ Injury Scaling, 2010

The low-grade, uncomplicated, stomach, small-bowel, and colon injuries can be primarily repaired or resected with a primary stapled anastomosis using Lembert sutures as a second layer of reinforcement. Rectal injuries can be primarily repaired and diverted as discussed previously with avoidance of the more difficult three-stage Hartmann's procedure and diverting colostomy. If there is significant bowel edema, most surgeons would avoid a stapled anastomosis and perform either a hand-sewn two-layered anastomosis or diverting stoma as required.

Based on the degree of injury and devascularization, gastric repair injuries are either primarily repaired or reconstructed after resection of devitalized tissue. Injuries involving the pylorus can be repaired using a pyloroplasty technique to prevent gastric outlet obstruction. Depending on the nature of the gastric injuries, Billroth I or Roux-en-Y gastrojejunostomy is usually chosen for reconstruction. Billroth II reconstructions are usually avoided because of the significant morbidity associated with postoperative retrograde bile reflux and impaired quality of life. Primary repairs are performed using stapled or hand-sewn techniques.

Because of complication rates associated with duodenal repairs, duodenal hematoma grades I and II (Table 21.2) are initially treated conservatively for 2 weeks with nasogastric tube (NGT) decompression, total parenteral nutrition (TPN), and weekly gastrografin studies. Repair of low-grade duodenal injuries of the first, third, and fourth parts of the duodenum (D1, D3, and D4) has a <2% postoperative fistula rate and the rate increases with grade of injury [132]. A tension-free repair is critical for success and the duodenum must be mobilized. Longitudinal injuries are closed transversely to prevent duodenal stricture. Omentum is accepted as the best tissue to be used to buttress the duodenal repair as is done with a Graham patch for perforated peptic ulcers [133]. If the omentum is not sufficient to buttress a duodenal repair, alternative options are jejunal serosa, gallbladder wall, or falciform ligament [134, 135].

About 20% of duodenal injuries are moderate to high grade, grades III–V (Table 21.2), and require complex repairs. The second part of the duodenum (D2) contains the major duodenal papilla which connects to the biliopancreatic ampulla where the sphincter of Oddi prevents retrograde reflux. The biliopancreatic ampulla is the common channel of the common bile duct (CBD) and pancreatic duct confluence. Because of the proximity of the biliary and pancreatic outflow tracts, injuries to this area are difficult to repair. In

1914, Sir Zachary Cope reported the need for gastrojejunostomy when repairing complex duodenal injuries [127]. To minimize morbidity and mortality, these complex repairs must be performed as a staged procedure when the patient exhibits hypothermia, acidosis, and coagulopathy [107–114]. Patients with associated mesenteric vascular or pancreatic injury are at higher risk for duodenal leak. If the duodenal injury is of high grade, grades IV and V (Table 21.2), an omental or a serosal patch repair is not feasible, and there is major mesenteric devascularization, or concomitant pancreatic injury, the majority of surgeons would perform a pyloric exclusion procedure [136–142]. In a pyloric exclusion, the pylorus is closed either externally with a linear non-cutting stapler or sutured closed with 0 absorbable suture through a gastrotomy. A loop gastrojejunostomy was originally described, but a Roux-en-Y gastrojejunostomy is commonly created to restore gastrointestinal continuity with a lower risk of bile reflux. The excluded duodenum is decompressed via a distal retrograde jejunoduodenostomy tube and a gastrojejunostomy feeding tube through the anastomosis or feeding jejunostomy may be placed. Studies have reported lower fistula rates of 0.5% vs. 19.3% with and without pyloric exclusion, for severe combined duodenal and pancreatic injuries [132]. Mortality for moderate to severe duodenal injuries has decreased to 1.6–10.5% with use of pyloric exclusion, proximal drainage, and distal retrograde intraluminal drainage [117, 142]. Vagotomy for prevention of marginal ulcers is not performed because of the efficacy of proton pump inhibitors (PPIs) [143, 144]. Less popular than pyloric exclusion and more labor intensive is the duodenal diverticulization in which the duodenal is defunctionalized and the hepatopancreaticobiliary system is externally drained. Diverticulization involves vagotomy, antrectomy, gastrojejunostomy, biliary T-tube drainage, duodenal primary repair, and lateral duodenostomy drainage [145, 146]. Though diverticulization was reported in the literature prior to pyloric exclusion, there are insufficient studies to suggest superiority over pyloric exclusion for the most complex pancreaticoduodenal injuries. Obliteration of the duodenum and pancreatic head which is reported in <3% of patients has been successfully treated with staged repair, control of hemorrhage, and contamination with wide drainage, followed by Whipple pancreaticojejunostomy (PJ) reconstruction [147]. Reported as early as 1965, the modern-day trauma Whipple procedure is associated with significant morbidity of 84% and mortality of 28% even with damage control surgery because of the cumulative severity of associated visceral and vascular injuries [148–151]. Pancreaticogastrostomy (PG) has been compared to PJ in multiple randomized controlled trials (RCTs) and meta-analyses and found to be relatively equivalent in postoperative fistula rates, 12.3% vs. 11.1%, morbidity and mortality [152–155]. A study of five trauma patients that underwent PG alone or after failed PJ reconstruction showed reasonable outcomes despite massive transfusion and long operative times. PG is a viable alternative to PJ for complex reconstruction, especially in elderly patients [147, 156, 157]. Some studies suggest that there is worse postoperative exocrine dysfunction and pancreatic duct strictures with PG, so PJ may be the better procedure in younger patients despite non-inferiority in RCTs and multiple meta-analyses [158, 159].

If there is <50% loss of jejunal, ileal, or colon lumen, grades I and II (Tables 21.3 and 21.4), the authors prefer to perform a primary repair in two layers, 3–0 absorbable running suture for the inner layer and 4–0 silk Lembert sutures for the outer layer in a transverse fashion to prevent stricture. A resection and enteroenterostomy, ileocolostomy, or colocolostomy anastomosis is performed if there is >50% loss of bowel lumen, grades III–V (Tables 21.3 and 21.4).

In healthy patients under elective conditions, rectal anastomoses have a 3–26% leak rate [160]. Massive transfusions and concomitant comorbidities increase the leak rate to 42% or greater [161]. Some advocate a loop-diverting colostomy with a skin-level bridge device that is matured immediately with the proximal lumen sutured so that it is 100% diverting [162]. This approach allows for an easier procedure to return the patient to gastrointestinal continuity, assuming that the patient was stable and the surgeon performed a primary rectal anastomosis. Some acute-care surgeons prefer to perform a Hartmann's procedure with colostomy diversion in the setting of massive transfusions or massive fecal contamination. Wide drainage with closed-suction drains or sump drains is considered based on degree of fecal contamination.

To prevent surgical site infections (SSI) after massive fecal contamination, most surgeons will close the fascia, but leave the skin partially open. Drains may be used in the subcutaneous tissue to obliterate dead space lateral to the incision. Removal of projectiles is usually not done except if they traverse a hollow viscus prior to ending in subcutaneous tissues. Necrotizing fasciitis can occur from contaminated bullets and projectiles left in the soft tissues after penetrating intestines [163].

Postoperative Management

Hypoperfusion after trauma and surgery contributes to secondary injury of compromised hollow viscus. Even if the patient is successfully resuscitated and repaired, there is a risk of anastomotic failure from perioperative hypoxia and/or hypotension [164]. Elderly patients that are frail have preexisting malnutrition, hypoalbuminemia, and low oncotic pressure which lead to increased third spacing, anasarca, and intestinal anastomotic leak [164–166]. Unfortunately, indiscriminate use of diuretic therapy and hypovolemia to improve pulmonary function and minimize ventilator time in the immediate postoperative period can have disastrous consequences. Diuresis in a third-spacing trauma patient who has poor cardiac output, impaired perfusion from atherosclerosis, and low oncotic pressure will likely create an ischemic hollow viscus repair [167, 168]. Dehydration is compensated by splanchnic vasoconstriction which impairs arterial inflow to the gastrointestinal tract even further. Brief, repetitive, and persistent ischemic insults to any hollow viscus repair will increase the probability of breakdown and catastrophic leak.

A balanced resuscitation strategy to prevent excessive fluid overload, maintain effective oncotic pressures, and provide for sufficient oxygen transport capacity is critical for preventing hollow viscus repair complications. Patients with chronic hypertension are prone to end-organ hypoperfusion. A MAP of 65 mmHg may be insufficient for hollow viscus perfusion, especially in elderly patients with a baseline MAP >100 mmHg [169, 170]. In patients with uncontrolled hypertension, hemodynamics should be maintained at a mean arterial pressure (MAP) of 75–85 mmHg instead of a MAP >65 mmHg because of the increased risk of acute kidney injury, hollow viscus hypoperfusion, morbidity, and mortality [169, 170]. Because of the unreliability of vital signs to predict perfusion outcomes in geriatric patients, all geriatric patients should have lactic acid levels drawn until trending towards normal to avoid occult hypoperfusion [171, 172].

After traumatic hemorrhage is controlled, a hemoglobin concentration of 7 g/dL, which may provide adequate oxygen-carrying capacity for a young healthy patient, could potentiate the ischemic insult in the elderly patient with cardiopulmonary and peripheral vascular disease. Therefore, elderly patients with severe cardiopulmonary disease may require a greater hemoglobin concentration. If in doubt, use a goal-directed approach with indirect measures of perfusion such as mixed venous oxygen saturation of >65% and resolution of lactic acidosis to obtain adequate oxygen delivery and perfusion [173–176].

Because the stress of trauma, shock, and work of breathing increase the risk of paroxysmal atrial fibrillation (Afib) with rapid ventricular response (RVR) in patients with preexisting arrhythmogenicity, magnesium and phosphate levels are ordered and treated. In patients at high risk for postoperative Afib with RVR, short-term prophylactic amiodarone therapy should be initiated immediately postoperatively. Afib with RVR would further exacerbate the gastrointestinal hypoperfusion because of diminished cardiac output. Judicious use of beta-blockers or calcium-channel blockers and combination therapy with class III antiarrhythmics such as amiodarone can prevent additional hypotension and subsequent secondary injury to the hollow viscus at risk [177].

Proximal GI injuries, especially in the stomach and duodenum, benefit from NGT decompression to prevent vomiting, aspiration complications, and gastroduodenal distension. In addition, gastric distension could precipitate massive bleeding from the short gastrics if one of the sutures is compromised. Efforts at prevention of multi-organ dysfunction, ileus, and Ogilvie's syndrome are made by replacing electrolytes, preventing massive fluid shifts, keeping the patient euvolemic, and minimizing drugs with antimotility activity such as narcotics and anticholinergics. Enteral feeds are initiated as soon as gastric residuals have decreased and bowel recovery is in progress. A potential pitfall of early enteral feedings is simultaneous vasopressor use. The reduced splanchnic inflow combined with the increase in oxygen, nutrient metabolism, and waste removal can exceed perfusion capacity and put the patient at risk for anastomosis ischemia, necrosis, and leak.

Stress ulcer prophylaxis with PPIs is critical, especially when a pyloric exclusion is performed in which the stomach may be overproducing acid. Because of posttraumatic hypercoagulability, immobility, total body excess water which is typical in multi-trauma patients, and intra-abdominal hypertension, HVI patients are at high risk for thromboembolic events. Based on the degree of coagulopathy seen at the time of operation, heparin or Lovenox is given for DVT prophylaxis. Fluids and medications are optimized for optimal anastomosis perfusion and healing.

Postoperative Complications

If the leak after hollow viscus repair is minimal and imaging shows a contained abscess, percutaneous drainage may be sufficient treatment in addition to antibiotics and nutrition. However, high-output fistulas from massive hollow viscus leaks identified in the early postoperative period generally benefit from early operative intervention. Delays in surgical diversion led to higher mortality because of infectious complications such as sepsis, shock, and multi-organ failure [104–106].

Low-output fistulas with <50 mL output per day are usually managed nonoperatively because of the increased risks for morbidity and mortality from reoperation. Management strategies include making the patient NPO, TPN, antibiotics if indicated, a gradual transition to enteral feeds, and placing drainage appliance to protect the skin. If slow feeds do not convert the fistula to high output, the feeds are increased to goal while the TPN is weaned off. This reduces the risks of central line infections, bacteremia, sepsis, and multi-organ failure inherent in long-term TPN therapy. Severely injured trauma patients with tube or needle feeding jejunostomy have a 4% complication rate with more leaks from the tube than the needle [178]. HVI-related low-output fistulas close in 55% of patients and if persistent are amenable to endoscopic treatment with covered endoscopic stents, absorbable biologic plugs, and fibrin glue [104, 179].

Severe HVI complicated by comorbidities, occult postoperative hypoperfusion, or postoperative vasopressor use can lead to postoperative strictures [180]. Management will depend on the location of the stricture, whether the patient has enough physiologic reserve to undergo revision surgery, or if the stricture can be managed short-term with an endoscopic stent. Especially in the distal large-bowel obstruction, endoscopic stents have made it possible for patients to be bowel prepped, undergo elective surgery, and avoid a colostomy. Because of the high rate and variety of complications associated with stomas, including obstruction, herniation, peristomal abscesses, bowel necrosis, and altered patient quality of life, surgical strategies including endoscopic stents are used to avoid stoma creation when possible [181, 182]. In addition, patients over 70 years old have a lower probability that their stoma will be reversed [183].

Surgical site infection (SSI) is one of the most common complications after operative blunt trauma, occurring in up to 9.3% of patients repaired primarily and up to 50% in patients requiring intestinal diversion [184, 185]. SSIs after contaminated HVI repairs or stoma closures are prevented generally by closing the fascia, but leaving the skin partially open. Some surgeons close the lateral edges and leave the center open, while others place loose sutures to bring the skin closer together [186]. The flora of these infections is usually polymicrobial and broad-spectrum antibiotics are empirically initiated [187]. If the SSI is associated with a deep organ space infection (DOSI) postoperatively because of anastomotic leak, the patient could develop necrotizing fasciitis, especially in immunocompromised individuals. Prompt intervention with diversion, cultures, biopsy, washout, debridement, antibiotics, and nutrition optimization is critical [188]. Large defects with significant fluid losses often benefit from negative-pressure therapy prior to definitive closure [189].

Short bowel syndrome (SBS) occurs when an individual with normal bowel function loses >50% of small intestine, <200 cm of small and large bowel, or less in someone with baseline compromised bowel function such as Crohn's disease. Of all adult patients with SBS, 8% of cases occurred because of traumatic injury [190]. Trauma-related SBS occurs from major devascularization injuries that obliterate major branches of the superior mesenteric artery (SMA) in 38% of trauma patients. The remainder of trauma SBS are caused by bowel necrosis from posttraumatic shock or extensive resections of injured small bowel [191].

In SBS patients, diarrhea from malabsorption of fluid, electrolytes, and nutrients causes large fluid loses, electrolyte abnormalities, enteral bicarbonate loss, and acid-base derangements [192]. The patients are infused with total parenteral nutrition (TPN) chronically which can cause liver and renal failure in addition to central venous access complications, such as line sepsis [193–195]. These patients also require vitamin, mineral, and trace element supplementation intravenously because of significant enteral losses.

Enteral feeding protocols are initiated to maximize intestinal adaptation which can take months to years, depending on baseline bowel function and length remaining [196, 197]. To potentiate intestinal adaptation and increase mucosal surface area, patients can now be treated with a recently FDA-approved drug called teduglutide. Teduglutide is a glucagon-like peptide-2 (GLP2) analog, a gut peptide hormone endogenously synthesized from proglucagon that stimulates intestinal proliferation and nutrient metabolism, reduces bone reabsorption, and is protective to the enteric nervous system [198, 199]. Because the proteolytic binding site of GLP2 is mutated in teduglutide, the half-life is increased from 7 min to 2 h which potentiates its downstream signal transduction efficacy [200].

Prevention of short bowel syndrome includes deploying temporary intravascular shunts (TIVS) to reestablish SMA perfusion in unstable patients undergoing damage control surgery, avoiding resection of partially viable bowel, placing a TAC appliance, and performing the complex SMA reconstruction at the second-look operation [201]. Microvascular reconstruction is successful in preserving small-bowel length in some patients [202]. If all else fails, small-bowel transplantation may be necessary in eligible elderly patients, currently patients with an age in the lower 60s [203, 204].

Conclusions and Future Directions

Worldwide, hollow viscus injury is a rare but deadly traumatic event in elderly patients, a patient population prone to higher morbidity and mortality [1–4, 6]. To decrease mortality and healthcare costs of seatbelt syndrome-related HVI in patients of advanced age, greater efforts worldwide are needed in creating and instituting prevention programs aiming to educating adults and seniors in the correct use and placement of lap and harness belts in motor vehicles [25].

Because of the low incidence of HVI in blunt trauma and the difficulty in making a clinical diagnosis, the traumatologist must keep a high index of suspicion [13, 125–127]. The use of multimodal diagnostic approaches including FAST and high-fidelity CT scans is essential for early diagnosis [17, 74, 80, 81, 98, 205]. CT protocols focused on evaluation of sarcopenia severity are being investigated with preliminary results suggesting that these protocols can predict mortality at 6 months [206]. Prognosis may inform the surgeon's decision not to operate if the sarcopenic severity and clinical circumstances suggest that an operation would be a futile effort. These sarcopenia protocols are experimental and need to be validated with prospective clinical trials.

Early intervention is critical for most HVI to decrease infectious complications that lead to high morbidity and mortality [207]. Damage control resuscitation, staged surgical repairs, frequent organ perfusion assessments, judicious perioperative management, and medical optimization of comorbidities have been shown to improve hollow viscous repair outcomes and patient survival [107–114]. As the laparoscopic technology and surgeon's skills become more advanced, there may be a greater role in the future for laparoscopic surgery in the management of traumatic hollow viscus injury, especially in the hemodynamically stable elderly patient population. Real-time intraoperative fluorescence angiography may become the standard of care if it can reproducibly decrease hollow viscus repair complications in future prospective RCTs [129–131].

References

1. Oreskovich MR, Howard JD, Copass MK, Carrico CJ. Geriatric trauma: injury patterns and outcome. J Trauma. 1984;24(7):565–72.
2. Schwab CW, Kauder DR. Trauma in the geriatric patient. Arch Surg. 1992;127(6):701–6.
3. Tornetta P III, Mostafavi H, Riina J, Turen C, Reimer B, Levine R, et al. Morbidity and mortality in elderly trauma patients. J Trauma. 1999;46(4):702–6.
4. Ferrera PC, Bartfield JM, D'Andrea CC. Outcomes of admitted geriatric trauma victims. Am J Emerg Med. 2000;18(5):575–80.
5. Hashmi A, Ibrahim-Zada I, Rhee P, Aziz H, Fain MJ, Friese RS, et al. Predictors of mortality in geriatric trauma patients: a systematic review and meta-analysis. J Trauma Acute Care Surg. 2014;76(3):894–901.
6. Sterling DA, O'Connor JA, Bonadies J. Geriatric falls: injury severity is high and disproportionate to mechanism. J Trauma. 2001;50(1):116–9.
7. Maldonado AR. 2013–2014 Causes of death in patients over 65 years of age, WISQARS database query. Atlanta: National Center for Injury Prevention and Control, Centers for Disease Control and Prevention; 2016.
8. Holcomb JB, McMullin NR, Kozar RA, Lygas MH, Moore FA. Morbidity from rib fractures increases after age 45. J Am Coll Surg. 2003;196(4):549–55.
9. Kuhne CA, Ruchholtz S, Kaiser GM, Nast-Kolb D. Mortality in severely injured elderly trauma patients—when does age become a risk factor? World J Surg. 2005;29(11):1476–82.
10. Adams SD, Cotton BA, McGuire MF, Dipasupil E, Podbielski JM, Zaharia A, et al. Unique pattern of complications in elderly trauma patients at a level I trauma center. J Trauma Acute Care Surg. 2012;72(1):112–8.
11. Kelley-Quon L, Min L, Morley E, Hiatt JR, Cryer H, Tillou A. Functional status after injury: a longitudinal study of geriatric trauma. Am Surg. 2010;76(10):1055–8.
12. Intiso D, Di Rienzo F, Grimaldi G, Lombardi T, Fiore P, Maruzzi G, et al. Survival and functional outcome in patients 90 years of age or older after hip fracture. Age Ageing. 2009;38(5):619–22.
13. Watts DD, Fakhry SM. Incidence of hollow viscus injury in blunt trauma: an analysis from 275,557 trauma admissions from the East multi-institutional trial. J Trauma. 2003;54(2):289–94.
14. Hong J, Wang SY, Qian L, Chen ZY. Diagnosis and treatment of duodenal injury: a clinical analysis. Hepato-Gastroenterology. 2015;62(139):641–6.
15. Jha NK, Yadav SK, Sharma R, Sinha DK, Kumar S, Kerketta MD, et al. Characteristics of hollow viscus injury following blunt abdominal trauma; a Single Centre Experience from Eastern India 2014. Bull Emerg Trauma. 2014;2(4 Oct):156–60.
16. Hazlitt M, Hill JB, Gunter OL, Guillamondegui OD. Disparities in trauma: the impact of socioeconomic factors on outcomes following traumatic hollow viscus injury. J Surg Res. 2014;191(1):6–11.
17. Bhagvan S, Turai M, Holden A, Ng A, Civil I. Predicting hollow viscus injury in blunt abdominal trauma with computed tomography. World J Surg. 2013;37(1):123–6.
18. Carter PM, Flannagan CA, Reed MP, Cunningham RM, Rupp JD. Comparing the effects of age, BMI and gender on severe injury (AIS 3+) in motor-vehicle crashes. Accid Anal Prev. 2014;72:146–60.
19. Nahm NJ, Como JJ, Vallier HA. The impact of major operative fractures in blunt abdominal injury. J Trauma Acute Care Surg. 2013;74(5):1307–14.
20. Appleby JP, Nagy AG. Abdominal injuries associated with the use of seatbelts. Am J Surg. 1989;157(5):457–8.
21. Anderson PA, Rivara FP, Maier RV, Drake C. The epidemiology of seatbelt-associated injuries. J Trauma. 1991;31(1):60–7.
22. Chance GQ. Note on a type of flexion fracture of the spine. Br J Radiol. 1948;21(249):452.
23. Mori H, Tsushimi T, Kobara H, Nishiyama N, Fujihara S, Matsunaga T, et al. Seatbelt syndrome with gastric mucosal breaks and intra-gastric wall air leakage. Intern Med. 2015;54(20):2599–601.
24. Patel K, Doolin R, Suggett N. Blunt transection of rectus abdominis following seatbelt related trauma with associated small and large bowel injury. Int J Surg Case Rep. 2013;4(11):958–60.

25. Thompson NS, Date R, Charlwood AP, Adair IV, Clements WD. Seat-belt syndrome revisited. Int J Clin Pract. 2001;55(8):573–5.
26. Torba M, Hijazi S, Gjata A, Buci S, Madani R, Subashi K. Seat belt syndrome, a new pattern of injury in developing countries. Case report and review of literature*. G Chir. 2014;35(7–8):177–80.
27. Nugmanova ZS, Ussatayeva G, McNutt LA. Seatbelt and child-restraint use in Kazakhstan: attitudes and behaviours of medical university students. Inj Prev. 2015;21(e1):e109–12.
28. Macpherson AK, Brussoni M, Fuselli P, Middaugh-Bonney T, Piedt S, Pike I. An evaluation of evidence-based paediatric injury prevention policies across Canada. BMC Public Health. 2015;15:707.
29. Will KE, Decina LE, Maple EL, Perkins AM. Examining the relative effectiveness of different message framing strategies for child passenger safety: recommendations for increased comprehension and compliance. Accid Anal Prev. 2015;79:170–81.
30. Chen X, Yang J, Peek-Asa C, McGehee DV, Li L. Parents' knowledge, attitude, and use of child restraints, Shantou, China. Am J Prev Med. 2014;46(1):85–8.
31. Truong WH, Hill BW, Cole PA. Automobile safety in children: a review of North American evidence and recommendations. J Am Acad Orthop Surg. 2013;21(6):323–31.
32. Salim A, Teixeira PG, Inaba K, Brown C, Browder T, Demetriades D. Analysis of 178 penetrating stomach and small bowel injuries. World J Surg. 2008;32(3):471–5.
33. Nallathambi MN, Ivatury RR, Shah PM, Gaudino J, Stahl WM. Aggressive definitive management of penetrating colon injuries: 136 cases with 3.7 percent mortality. J Trauma. 1984;24(6):500–5.
34. Ivatury RR, Licata J, Gunduz Y, Rao P, Stahl WM. Management options in penetrating rectal injuries. Am Surg. 1991;57(1):50–5.
35. Nagy KK, Smith RF, Roberts RR, Joseph KT, An GC, Bokhari F, et al. Prognosis of penetrating trauma in elderly patients: a comparison with younger patients. J Trauma. 2000;49(2):190–3; discussion 3–4.
36. Schulman S, Kearon C, Kakkar AK, Mismetti P, Schellong S, Eriksson H, et al. Dabigatran versus warfarin in the treatment of acute venous thromboembolism. N Engl J Med. 2009;361(24):2342–52.
37. Bauersachs R, Berkowitz SD, Brenner B, Buller HR, Decousus H, Gallus AS, et al. Oral rivaroxaban for symptomatic venous thromboembolism. N Engl J Med. 2010;363(26):2499–510.
38. Buller HR, Prins MH, Lensin AW, Decousus H, Jacobson BF, Minar E, et al. Oral rivaroxaban for the treatment of symptomatic pulmonary embolism. N Engl J Med. 2012;366(14):1287–97.
39. Agnelli G, Buller HR, Cohen A, Curto M, Gallus AS, Johnson M, et al. Oral apixaban for the treatment of acute venous thromboembolism. N Engl J Med. 2013;369(9):799–808.
40. Siegal DM, Curnutte JT, Connolly SJ, Lu G, Conley PB, Wiens BL, et al. Andexanet alfa for the reversal of factor Xa inhibitor activity. N Engl J Med. 2015;373(25):2413–24.
41. Reynolds FD, Dietz PA, Higgins D, Whitaker TS. Time to deterioration of the elderly, anticoagulated, minor head injury patient who presents without evidence of neurologic abnormality. J Trauma. 2003;54(3):492–6.
42. Rossaint R, Bouillon B, Cerny V, Coats TJ, Duranteau J, Fernandez-Mondejar E, et al. The European guideline on management of major bleeding and coagulopathy following trauma: fourth edition. Crit Care. 2016;20(1):100.
43. von Heymann C, Rosenthal C, Kaufner L, Sander M. Management of direct oral anticoagulants-associated bleeding in the trauma patient. Curr Opin Anaesthesiol. 2016;29(2):220–8.
44. Grottke O, Aisenberg J, Bernstein R, Goldstein P, Huisman MV, Jamieson DG, et al. Efficacy of prothrombin complex concentrates for the emergency reversal of dabigatran-induced anticoagulation. Crit Care. 2016;20(1):115.
45. van Aart L, Eijkhout HW, Kamphuis JS, Dam M, Schattenkerk ME, Schouten TJ, et al. Individualized dosing regimen for prothrombin complex concentrate more effective than standard treatment in the reversal of oral anticoagulant therapy: an open, prospective randomized controlled trial. Thromb Res. 2006;118(3):313–20.
46. Cartmill M, Dolan G, Byrne JL, Byrne PO. Prothrombin complex concentrate for oral anticoagulant reversal in neurosurgical emergencies. Br J Neurosurg. 2000;14(5):458–61.
47. Taberner DA, Thomson JM, Poller L. Comparison of prothrombin complex concentrate and vitamin K1 in oral anticoagulant reversal. Br Med J. 1976;2(6027):83–5.
48. Joseph B, Amini A, Friese RS, Houdek M, Hays D, Kulvatunyou N, et al. Factor IX complex for the correction of traumatic coagulopathy. J Trauma Acute Care Surg. 2012;72(4):828–34.
49. Innerhofer P, Westermann I, Tauber H, Breitkopf R, Fries D, Kastenberger T, et al. The exclusive use of coagulation factor concentrates enables reversal of coagulopathy and decreases transfusion rates in patients with major blunt trauma. Injury. 2013;44(2):209–16.
50. Yanamadala V, Walcott BP, Fecci PE, Rozman P, Kumar JI, Nahed BV, et al. Reversal of warfarin associated coagulopathy with 4-factor prothrombin complex concentrate in traumatic brain injury and intracranial hemorrhage. J Clin Neurosci. 2014;21(11):1881–4.
51. Mangram A, Oguntodu OF, Dzandu JK, Hollingworth AK, Hall S, Cung C, et al. Is there a difference in efficacy, safety, and cost-effectiveness between 3-factor and 4-factor prothrombin complex concentrates among trauma patients on oral anticoagulants? J Crit Care. 2016;33:252–6.

52. Martin DT, Barton CA, Dodgion C, Schreiber M. Emergent reversal of vitamin K antagonists: addressing all the factors. Am J Surg. 2016;211(5):919–25.
53. Yorkgitis BK. Non-vitamin K antagonist oral anticoagulant reversal: hope is on the horizon. Am J Surg. 2016;212:160–4.
54. Rosenthal RA, Kavic SM. Assessment and management of the geriatric patient. Crit Care Med. 2004;32(4 Suppl):S92–105.
55. Sisak K, Manolis M, Hardy BM, Enninghorst N, Bendinelli C, Balogh ZJ. Acute transfusion practice during trauma resuscitation: who, when, where and why? Injury. 2013;44(5):581–6.
56. Shakur H, Roberts I, Bautista R, Caballero J, Coats T, Dewan Y, et al. Effects of tranexamic acid on death, vascular occlusive events, and blood transfusion in trauma patients with significant haemorrhage (CRASH-2): a randomised, placebo-controlled trial. Lancet. 2010;376(9734):23–32.
57. Cap AP, Baer DG, Orman JA, Aden J, Ryan K, Blackbourne LH. Tranexamic acid for trauma patients: a critical review of the literature. J Trauma. 2011;71(1 Suppl):S9–14.
58. Morrison JJ, Dubose JJ, Rasmussen TE, Midwinter MJ. Military application of tranexamic acid in trauma emergency resuscitation (MATTERs) study. Arch Surg. 2012;147(2):113–9.
59. Eckert MJ, Wertin TM, Tyner SD, Nelson DW, Izenberg S, Martin MJ. Tranexamic acid administration to pediatric trauma patients in a combat setting: the pediatric trauma and tranexamic acid study (PED-TRAX). J Trauma Acute Care Surg 2014;77(6):852–8; discussion 8.
60. Valle EJ, Allen CJ, Van Haren RM, Jouria JM, Li H, Livingstone AS, et al. Do all trauma patients benefit from tranexamic acid? J Trauma Acute Care Surg. 2014;76(6):1373–8.
61. Cole E, Davenport R, Willett K, Brohi K. Tranexamic acid use in severely injured civilian patients and the effects on outcomes: a prospective cohort study. Ann Surg. 2015;261(2):390–4.
62. Harvin JA, Peirce CA, Mims MM, Hudson JA, Podbielski JM, Wade CE, et al. The impact of tranexamic acid on mortality in injured patients with hyperfibrinolysis. J Trauma Acute Care Surg. 2015;78(5):905–9; discussion 9–11.
63. Roberts I. Fibrinolytic shutdown: fascinating theory but randomized controlled trial data are needed. Transfusion. 2016;56(Suppl 2):S115–8.
64. Aedo-Martin D, Garcia-Canas R, Navarro-Suay R, Martinez-Roldan M, Banos-Turza R, Tamburri-Bariain R. Use of tranexamic acid in combat casualties. Experience of the Spanish medical corps. Clinical series and literature review. Rev Esp Cir Ortop Traumatol. 2016;60(3):200–5.
65. Jawa RS, Singer A, McCormack JE, Huang EC, Rutigliano DN, Vosswinkel JA. Tranexamic acid use in United States Trauma Centers: a national survey. Am Surg. 2016;82(5):439–47.
66. Advanced trauma life support (ATLS(R)): the ninth edition. J Trauma Acute Care Surg. 2013;74(5):1363–6.
67. Pikoulis E, Delis S, Psalidas N, Leppaniemi A, Derlopas K, Pavlakis E, et al. Presentation of blunt small intestinal and mesenteric injuries. Ann R Coll Surg Engl. 2000;82(2):103–6.
68. Kemmeter PR, Senagore AJ, Smith D, Oostendorp L. Dilemmas in the diagnosis of blunt enteric trauma. Am Surg. 1998;64(8):750–4.
69. Chandler CF, Lane JS, Waxman KS. Seatbelt sign following blunt trauma is associated with increased incidence of abdominal injury. Am Surg. 1997;63(10):885–8.
70. Levine H, Simon RJ, Smith TR, Ivatury R, Stahl W. Guaiac testing in the diagnosis of rectal trauma: what is its value? J Trauma. 1992;32(2):210–2.
71. Morley JE. Dehydration, hypernatremia, and hyponatremia. Clin Geriatr Med. 2015;31(3):389–99.
72. Rittenhouse KJ, To T, Rogers A, Wu D, Horst M, Edavettal M, et al. Hyponatremia as a fall predictor in a geriatric trauma population. Injury. 2015;46(1):119–23.
73. Cumming K, Soiza RL. Hyponatraemia after fracture is often caused by hypovolaemia, not SIADH. Adv Orthop. 2015;2015:959213.
74. Zauner A, Cabot JR, Bassaganyas R. Ultrasonics in traumatology. Rev Esp Reum Enferm Osteoartic. 1953;5(3):127–31.
75. Seewald K. Ultrasonics in accident surgery. Monatsschr Unfallheilkd Versicherungsmed. 1955;58(10):312–5.
76. Woeber K, Seewald K. Ultrasonic in accident surgery. Monatsschr Unfallheilkd Versicherungsmed. 1957;60(1):28–9.
77. Ramirez AA, Ramirez L, De Leon F. Ultrasonics in traumatic injuries. J Philipp Med Assoc. 1958;34(2):111–6.
78. Rozycki GS, Ochsner MG, Schmidt JA, Frankel HL, Davis TP, Wang D, et al. A prospective study of surgeon-performed ultrasound as the primary adjuvant modality for injured patient assessment. J Trauma Acute Care Surg. 1995;39(3):492–500.
79. Han DC, Rozycki GS, Schmidt JA, Feliciano DV. Ultrasound training during ATLS: an early start for surgical interns. J Trauma Acute Care Surg. 1996;41(2):208–13.
80. Scalea TM, Rodriguez A, Chiu WC, Brenneman FD, Fallon WF, Kato K, et al. Focused assessment with sonography for trauma (FAST): results from an international consensus conference. J Trauma Acute Care Surg. 1999;46(3):466–72.
81. Kirkpatrick AW, Sirois M, Laupland KB, Liu D, Rowan K, Ball CG, et al. Hand-held thoracic sonography for detecting post-traumatic pneumothoraces: the extended focused assessment with sonography for trauma (EFAST). J Trauma. 2004;57(2):288–95.
82. Soult MC, Weireter LJ, Britt RC, Collins JN, Novosel TJ, Reed SF, et al. Can routine trauma bay chest x-ray be bypassed with an extended focused

assessment with sonography for trauma examination? Am Surg. 2015;81(4):336–40.
83. Root HD, Hauser CW, McKinley CR, Lafave JW, Mendiola RP Jr. Diagnostic peritoneal lavage. Surgery. 1965;57:633–7.
84. Gumbert JL, Froderman SE, Mercho JP. Diagnostic peritoneal lavage in blunt abdominal trauma. Ann Surg. 1967;165(1):70–2.
85. Natarajan B, Gupta PK, Cemaj S, Sorensen M, Hatzoudis GI, Forse RA. FAST scan: is it worth doing in hemodynamically stable blunt trauma patients? Surgery. 2010;148(4):695–700.
86. Talari H, Moussavi N, Abedzadeh-Kalahroudi M, Atoof F, Abedini A. Correlation between intra-abdominal free fluid and solid organ injury in blunt abdominal trauma. Arch Trauma Res. 2015;4(3):e29184.
87. Holmes G, Romero J, Waxman K, Diaz G. FAST enough? A validation study for focused assessment with sonography for trauma ultrasounds in a Level II trauma center. Am Surg. 2012;78(10):1038–40.
88. McKenney M, Lentz K, Nunez D, Sosa JL, Sleeman D, Axelrad A, et al. Can ultrasound replace diagnostic peritoneal lavage in the assessment of blunt trauma? J Trauma. 1994;37(3):439–41.
89. Lee MJ, Sperry JL, Rosengart MR. Evaluating for acute mesenteric ischemia in critically ill patients: diagnostic peritoneal lavage is associated with reduced operative intervention and mortality. J Trauma Acute Care Surg. 2014;77(3):441–7.
90. Chereau N, Wagner M, Tresallet C, Lucidarme O, Raux M, Menegaux F. CT scan and diagnostic peritoneal lavage: towards a better diagnosis in the area of nonoperative management of blunt abdominal trauma. Injury. 2016;47:2006–11.
91. Cue JI, Miller FB, Cryer HM 3rd, Malangoni MA, Richardson JD. A prospective, randomized comparison between open and closed peritoneal lavage techniques. J Trauma. 1990;30(7):880–3.
92. Lopez-Viego MA, Mickel TJ, Weigelt JA. Open versus closed diagnostic peritoneal lavage in the evaluation of abdominal trauma. Am J Surg 1990;160(6):594–6; discussion 6–7.
93. Whitehouse JS, Weigelt JA. Diagnostic peritoneal lavage: a review of indications, technique, and interpretation. Scand J Trauma Resusc Emerg Med. 2009;17:13.
94. Thal ER. Evaluation of peritoneal lavage and local exploration in lower chest and abdominal stab wounds. J Trauma. 1977;17(8):642–8.
95. Fischer RP, Beverlin BC, Engrav LH, Benjamin CI, Perry JF Jr. Diagnostic peritoneal lavage: fourteen years and 2,586 patients later. Am J Surg. 1978;136(6):701–4.
96. Ivatury RR, Cayten CG, Society RH. The textbook of penetrating trauma. Philadelphia: Williams & Wilkins; 1996.
97. Nagy KK, Roberts RR, Joseph KT, Smith RF, An GC, Bokhari F, et al. Experience with over 2500 diagnostic peritoneal lavages. Injury. 2000;31(7):479–82.
98. Livingston DH, Lavery RF, Passannante MR, Skurnick JH, Fabian TC, Fry DE, et al. Admission or observation is not necessary after a negative abdominal computed tomographic scan in patients with suspected blunt abdominal trauma: results of a prospective, multi-institutional trial. J Trauma Acute Care Surg. 1998;44(2):273–82.
99. Ozmen V, NE MS Jr, Nichols RL, Smith J, Flint LM. Autotransfusion of potentially culture-positive blood (CPB) in abdominal trauma: preliminary data from a prospective study. J Trauma. 1992;32(1):36–9.
100. Schwieger IM, Gallagher CJ, Finlayson DC, Daly WL, Maher KL. Incidence of cell-saver contamination during cardiopulmonary bypass. Ann Thorac Surg. 1989;48(1):51–3.
101. Caliste XA, McArthur KA, Sava JA. Autotransfusion in emergent operative trauma resuscitation. Eur J Trauma Emerg Surg. 2014;40(5):541–5.
102. Li J, Sun SL, Tian JH, Yang K, Liu R, Li J. Cell salvage in emergency trauma surgery. Cochrane Database Syst Rev. 2015;1
103. Rhee P, Inaba K, Pandit V, Khalil M, Siboni S, Vercruysse G, et al. Early autologous fresh whole blood transfusion leads to less allogeneic transfusions and is safe. J Trauma Acute Care Surg. 2015;78(4):729–34.
104. Fischer PE, Fabian TC, Magnotti LJ, Schroeppel TJ, Bee TK, Maish GOI, et al. A ten-year review of Enterocutaneous fistulas after laparotomy for trauma. J Trauma Acute Care Surg. 2009;67(5):924–8.
105. Hahler B, Schassberger D, Novakovic R, Lang S. Managing complex, high-output, enterocutaneous fistulas: a case study. Ostomy Wound Manage. 2009;55(10):30–42.
106. Tong CY, Lim LL, Brody RA. High output enterocutaneous fistula: a literature review and a case study. Asia Pac J Clin Nutr. 2012;21(3):464–9.
107. Lucas CE, Ledgerwood AM. Prospective evaluation of hemostatic techniques for liver injuries. J Trauma. 1976;16(6):442–51.
108. Pachter HL, Spencer FC. Recent concepts in the treatment of hepatic trauma: facts and fallacies. Ann Surg. 1979;190(4):423–9.
109. Fabian TC, Stone HH. Arrest of severe liver hemorrhage by an omental pack. South Med J. 1980;73(11):1487–90.
110. Carmona RH, Peck DZ, Lim RC Jr. The role of packing and planned reoperation in severe hepatic trauma. J Trauma. 1984;24(9):779–84.
111. Myrhoj T, Moller P. Liver packing and planned reoperation in the management of severe hepatic trauma. Ann Chir Gynaecol. 1987;76(4):215–7.
112. Aprahamian C, Wittmann DH, Bergstein JM, Quebbeman EJ. Temporary abdominal closure (TAC) for planned relaparotomy (etappenlavage) in trauma. J Trauma. 1990;30(6):719–23.
113. Burch JM, Ortiz VB, Richardson RJ, Martin RR, Mattox KL, Jordan GL Jr. Abbreviated laparotomy and planned reoperation for critically injured patients. Ann Surg. 1992;215(5):476–83. discussion 83–4

114. Roberts DJ, Ball CG, Feliciano DV, Moore EE, Ivatury RR, Lucas CE, et al. History of the innovation of damage control for management of trauma patients: 1902–2016. Ann Surg. 2017;265:1034–44.
115. Pommerening MJ, DuBose JJ, Zielinski MD, Phelan HA, Scalea TM, Inaba K, et al. Time to first take-back operation predicts successful primary fascial closure in patients undergoing damage control laparotomy. Surgery. 2014;156(2):431–8.
116. Burlew CC, Moore EE, Cuschieri J, Jurkovich GJ, Codner P, Crowell K, et al. Sew it up! A Western Trauma Association multi-institutional study of enteric injury management in the postinjury open abdomen. J Trauma Acute Care Surg. 2011;70(2):273–7.
117. Ordonez C, Garcia A, Parra MW, Scavo D, Pino LF, Millan M, et al. Complex penetrating duodenal injuries: less is better. J Trauma Acute Care Surg. 2014;76(5):1177–83.
118. Bradley M, Galvagno S, Dhanda A, Rodriguez C, Lauerman M, DuBose J, et al. Damage control resuscitation protocol and the management of open abdomens in trauma patients. Am Surg. 2014;80(8):768–75.
119. Glaser J, Vasquez M, Cardarelli C, Dunne J, Elster E, Hathaway E, et al. Ratio-driven resuscitation predicts early fascial closure in the combat wounded. J Trauma Acute Care Surg. 2015;79(4 Suppl 2):S188–92.
120. Cheatham ML. Nonoperative management of intraabdominal hypertension and abdominal compartment syndrome. World J Surg. 2009;33(6):1116–22.
121. Kirkpatrick AW, Roberts DJ, De Waele J, Jaeschke R, Malbrain ML, De Keulenaer B, et al. Intra-abdominal hypertension and the abdominal compartment syndrome: updated consensus definitions and clinical practice guidelines from the World Society of the Abdominal Compartment Syndrome. Intensive Care Med. 2013;39(7):1190–206.
122. Kirkpatrick AW, Roberts DJ, Jaeschke R, De Waele JJ, De Keulenaer BL, Duchesne J, et al. Methodological background and strategy for the 2012–2013 updated consensus definitions and clinical practice guidelines from the abdominal compartment society. Anaesthesiol Intensive Ther. 2015;47 Spec No:s63–77.
123. Bjorck M, Kirkpatrick AW, Cheatham M, Kaplan M, Leppaniemi A, De Waele JJ. Amended classification of the open abdomen. Scand J Surg. 2016;105(1):5–10.
124. Senn EJ. Traumatic intestinal rupture, with special reference to indirect applied force. Am J Med Sci. 1904;127:965–77.
125. M'Ardle JS. Enterectomy and enterorrhaphy. Dublin J Med Sci. 1888;85(2):123–37.
126. Croft J. Croft's case of rupture of the small intestine. Trans Med Soc Lond 1890:141–9.
127. Cope VZ. The early diagnosis and treatment of ruptured intestine. Proc R Soc Med. 1914;7(Surg Sect):86–107.
128. Moore EE, Moore FA. American Association for the Surgery of Trauma Organ Injury Scaling: 50th anniversary review article of the Journal of Trauma. J Trauma. 2010(1529-8809 (Electronic)).
129. Iinuma Y, Hirayama Y, Yokoyama N, Otani T, Nitta K, Hashidate H, et al. Intraoperative near-infrared indocyanine green fluorescence angiography (NIR-ICG AG) can predict delayed small bowel stricture after ischemic intestinal injury: report of a case. J Pediatr Surg. 2013;48(5):1123–8.
130. Boni L, David G, Mangano A, Dionigi G, Rausei S, Spampatti S, et al. Clinical applications of indocyanine green (ICG) enhanced fluorescence in laparoscopic surgery. Surg Endosc. 2015;29(7):2046–55.
131. Jafari MD, Wexner SD, Martz JE, EC ML, Margolin DA, Sherwinter DA, et al. Perfusion assessment in laparoscopic left-sided/anterior resection (PILLAR II): a multi-institutional study. J Am Coll Surg. 2015;220(1):82–92e1.
132. McKenney MG, Nir I, Levi DM, Martin L. Evaluation of minor penetrating duodenal injuries. Am Surg. 1996;62(11):952–5.
133. Piper CC, Yeo CJ, Cowan SW. Roscoe Reid Graham (1890 to 1948): a Canadian pioneer in general surgery. Am Surg. 2014;80(5):431–3.
134. Mouly C, Chati R, Scotte M, Regimbeau JM. Therapeutic management of perforated gastro-duodenal ulcer: literature review. J Visc Surg. 2013;150(5):333–40.
135. Tanaka R, Kosugi S, Sakamoto K, Yajima K, Ishikawa T, Kanda T, et al. Treatment for perforated gastric ulcer: a multi-institutional retrospective review. J Gastrointest Surg. 2013;17(12):2074–81.
136. Vaughan GD III, Frazier OH, Graham DY, Mattox KL, Petmecky FF, Jordan GL Jr. The use of pyloric exclusion in the management of severe duodenal injuries. Am J Surg. 1977;134(6):785–90.
137. Martin TD, Feliciano DV, Mattox KL, Jordan GL Jr. Severe duodenal injuries. Treatment with pyloric exclusion and gastrojejunostomy. Arch Surg. 1983;118(5):631–5.
138. Feliciano DV, Martin TD, Cruse PA, Graham JM, Burch JM, Mattox KL, et al. Management of combined pancreatoduodenal injuries. Ann Surg. 1987;205(6):673–80.
139. Cogbill TH, Moore EE, Feliciano DV, Hoyt DB, Jurkovich GJ, Morris JA, et al. Conservative management of duodenal trauma: a multicenter perspective. J Trauma. 1990;30(12):1469–75.
140. Nassoura ZE, Ivatury RR, Simon RJ, Kihtir T, Stahl WM. A prospective reappraisal of primary repair of penetrating duodenal injuries. Am Surg. 1994;60(1):35–9.
141. Ivatury RR, Malhotra AK, Aboutanos MB, Duane TM. Duodenal Injuries: A Review. Eur J Trauma Emerg Surg. 2007;33(3):231–7.
142. Schroeppel TJ, Saleem K, Sharpe JP, Magnotti LJ, Weinberg JA, Fischer PE, et al. Penetrating duodenal trauma: a 19-year experience. J Trauma Acute Care Surg. 2016;80(3):461–5.

143. Lind T, Cederberg C, Olausson M, Olbe L. 24-Hour intragastric acidity and plasma gastrin after omeprazole treatment and after proximal gastric vagotomy in duodenal ulcer patients. Gastroenterology. 1990;99(6):1593–8.
144. Lagoo J, Pappas TN, Perez A. A relic or still relevant: the narrowing role for vagotomy in the treatment of peptic ulcer disease. Am J Surg. 2014;207(1):120–6.
145. Berne CJ, Donovan AJ, White EJ, Yellin AE. Duodenal "diverticulization" for duodenal and pancreatic injury. Am J Surg. 1974;127(5):503–7.
146. Cruz RJ Jr, Vincenzi R. Modified duodenal diverticulization technique for the management of duodenal fistulas. Am J Surg. 2010;199(2):17.
147. Delcore R, Stauffer JS, Thomas JH, Pierce GE. The role of pancreatogastrostomy following pancreatoduodenectomy for trauma. J Trauma. 1994;37(3):395–400.
148. Maret G, Delore X. Cephalic duodenopancreatectomy for closed abdominal injury. Lyon Chir. 1965;61:122–4.
149. Brawley RK, Cameron JL, Zuidema GD. Severe upper abdominal injuries treated by pancreaticoduodenectomy. Surg Gynecol Obstet. 1968;126(3):516–22.
150. Foley WJ, Gaines RD, Fry WJ. Pancreaticoduodenectomy for severe trauma to the head of the pancreas and the associated structures: report of three cases. Ann Surg. 1969;170(5):759–65.
151. Krige JE, Kotze UK, Setshedi M, Nicol AJ, Navsaria PH. Surgical management and outcomes of combined pancreaticoduodenal injuries: analysis of 75 consecutive cases. J Am Coll Surg. 2016;222(5):737–49.
152. Yeo CJ, Cameron JL, Maher MM, Sauter PK, Zahurak ML, Talamini MA, et al. A prospective randomized trial of pancreaticogastrostomy versus pancreaticojejunostomy after pancreaticoduodenectomy. Ann Surg. 1995;222(4):580–92.
153. Duffas J-P, Suc B, Msika S, Fourtanier G, Muscari F, Hay JM, et al. A controlled randomized multicenter trial of pancreatogastrostomy or pancreatojejunostomy after pancreatoduodenectomy. Am J Surg. 2005;189(6):720–9.
154. Crippa S, Cirocchi R, Randolph J, Partelli S, Belfiori G, Piccioli A, et al. Pancreaticojejunostomy is comparable to pancreaticogastrostomy after pancreaticoduodenectomy: an updated meta-analysis of randomized controlled trials. Langenbeck's Arch Surg. 2016:1–11.
155. Keck T, Wellner UF, Bahra M, Klein F, Sick O, Niedergethmann M, et al. Pancreatogastrostomy versus pancreatojejunostomy for RECOnstruction after PANCreatoduodenectomy (RECOPANC, DRKS 00000767): perioperative and long-term results of a multicenter randomized controlled trial. Ann Surg. 2016;263(3):440–9.
156. Kurisu A, Kobayashi H, Kawashima K. Pancreaticogastrostomy after pancreaticoduodenectomy: a rational approach to severe combined pancreaticoduodenal injury. J Trauma. 1999;46(5):970–2.
157. Martín GM, Morillas PJ, Pino JCR, Canis JMM, Argenté FXG. Reconstruction after pancreatic trauma by pancreaticogastrostomy. Int J Surg Case Rep. 2015;9:92–4.
158. Kurosaki I, Hatakeyama K, Kobayashi T, Nihei KE. Pancreaticogastrostomy: unreliable long-term pancreatic duct patency. Hepato-Gastroenterology. 2003;50(50):545–9.
159. Rault A, SaCunha A, Klopfenstein D, Larroudé D, Epoy FND, Collet D, et al. Pancreaticojejunal anastomosis is preferable to Pancreaticogastrostomy after Pancreaticoduodenectomy for Longterm outcomes of pancreatic exocrine function. J Am Coll Surg. 2005;201(2):239–44.
160. Murrell ZA, Stamos MJ. Reoperation for anastomotic failure. Clin Colon Rectal Surg. 2006;19(4):213–6.
161. Miller PR, Fabian TC, Croce MA, Magnotti LJ, Elizabeth Pritchard F, Minard G, et al. Improving outcomes following penetrating colon wounds: application of a clinical pathway. Ann Surg. 2002;235(6):775–81.
162. Jenkinson LR, Houghton PW, Steele KV, Donaldson LA, Crumplin MK. The Biethium bridge—an advance in stoma care. Ann R Coll Surg Engl. 1984;66(6):420–2.
163. Sarmiento JM, Yugueros P, Garcia AF, Wolff BG. Bullets and their role in sepsis after colon wounds. World J Surg. 1997;21(6):648–52.
164. Golub R, Golub RW, Cantu R Jr, Stein HD. A multivariate analysis of factors contributing to leakage of intestinal anastomoses. J Am Coll Surg. 1997;184(4):364–72.
165. Alves A, Panis Y, Trancart D, Regimbeau JM, Pocard M, Valleur P. Factors associated with clinically significant anastomotic leakage after large bowel resection: multivariate analysis of 707 patients. World J Surg. 2002;26(4):499–502.
166. Tan WP, Talbott VA, Leong QQ, Isenberg GA, Goldstein SD. American Society of Anesthesiologists class and Charlson's comorbidity index as predictors of postoperative colorectal anastomotic leak: a single-institution experience. J Surg Res. 2013;184(1):115–9.
167. Rosoff L, Berne CJ. Oliguria in surgical patients. Calif Med. 1961;95:1–5.
168. Tang IY, Murray PT. Prevention of perioperative acute renal failure: what works? Best Pract Res Clin Anaesthesiol. 2004;18(1):91–111.
169. Dunser MW, Takala J, Ulmer H, Mayr VD, Luckner G, Jochberger S, et al. Arterial blood pressure during early sepsis and outcome. Intensive Care Med. 2009;35(7):1225–33.
170. Leone M, Asfar P, Radermacher P, Vincent JL, Martin C. Optimizing mean arterial pressure in septic shock: a critical reappraisal of the literature. Crit Care. 2015;19:101.
171. Salottolo KM, Mains CW, Offner PJ, Bourg PW, Bar-Or D. A retrospective analysis of geriatric trauma patients: venous lactate is a better predictor of mortality than traditional vital signs. Scand J Trauma Resusc Emerg Med. 2013;21:7.

172. Pandit V, Rhee P, Hashmi A, Kulvatunyou N, Tang A, Khalil M, et al. Shock index predicts mortality in geriatric trauma patients: an analysis of the National Trauma Data Bank. J Trauma Acute Care Surg. 2014;76(4):1111–5.
173. Lappas DG, Powell WM Jr, Daggett WM. Cardiac dysfunction in the perioperative period: pathophysiology, diagnosis, and treatment. Anesthesiology. 1977;47(2):117–37.
174. Hebert PC, Wells G, Martin C, Tweeddale M, Marshall J, Blajchman M, et al. Variation in red cell transfusion practice in the intensive care unit: a multicentre cohort study. Crit Care. 1999;3(2):57–63.
175. Spinella PC. Warm fresh whole blood transfusion for severe hemorrhage: U.S. military and potential civilian applications. Crit Care Med. 2008;36(7 Suppl):S340–5.
176. Napolitano LM, Kurek S, Luchette FA, Corwin HL, Barie PS, Tisherman SA, et al. Clinical practice guideline: red blood cell transfusion in adult trauma and critical care. Crit Care Med. 2009;37(12):3124–57.
177. January CT, Wann LS, Alpert JS, Calkins H, Cigarroa JE, Cleveland JC Jr, et al. 2014 AHA/ACC/HRS guideline for the management of patients with atrial fibrillation: a report of the American College of Cardiology/American Heart Association task force on practice guidelines and the Heart Rhythm Society. Circulation. 2014;130(23):e199–267.
178. Holmes JHI, Brundage SI, P-c Y, Hall RA, Maier RV, Jurkovich GJ. Complications of surgical feeding jejunostomy in trauma patients. J Trauma Acute Care Surg. 1999;47(6):1009.
179. Miranda LE, Sabat BD, Carvalho EA. A low-output colocutaneous fistula healed by Surgisis anal plug. Tech Coloproctol. 2009;13(4):315–6.
180. Lai JM, Chuang TY, Francisco GE, Strayer JR. Diversion colitis: a cause of abdominal discomfort in spinal cord injury patients with colostomy. Arch Phys Med Rehabil. 1997;78(6):670–1.
181. Del Pino A, Cintron JR, Orsay CP, Pearl RK, Tan A, Abcarian H. Enterostomal complications: are emergently created enterostomas at greater risk? Am Surg. 1997;63(7):653–6.
182. Jimenez-Perez J, Casellas J, Garcia-Cano J, Vandervoort J, Garcia-Escribano OR, Barcenilla J, et al. Colonic stenting as a bridge to surgery in malignant large-bowel obstruction: a report from two large multinational registries. Am J Gastroenterol. 2011;106(12):2174–80.
183. Lee CM, Huh JW, Park YA, Cho YB, Kim HC, Yun SH, et al. Risk factors of permanent stomas in patients with rectal cancer after low anterior resection with temporary stomas. Yonsei Med J. 2015;56(2):447–53.
184. Mehta N, Babu S, Venugopal K. An experience with blunt abdominal trauma: evaluation. Clin Pract. 2014;4(2):599.
185. Torba M, Gjata A, Buci S, Bushi G, Zenelaj A, Kajo I, et al. The influence of the risk factor on the abdominal complications in colon injury management. G Chir. 2015;36(2):57–62.
186. Pittman DM, Smith LE. Complications of colostomy closure. Dis Colon Rectum. 1985;28(11):836–43.
187. Schnuriger B, Inaba K, Eberle BM, Wu T, Talving P, Bukur M, et al. Microbiological profile and antimicrobial susceptibility in surgical site infections following hollow viscus injury. J Gastrointest Surg. 2010;14(8):1304–10.
188. Benjamin E, Siboni S, Haltmeier T, Inaba K, Lam L, Demetriades D. Deep organ space infection after emergency bowel resection and anastomosis: the anatomic site does not matter. J Trauma Acute Care Surg. 2015;79(5):805–11.
189. Chavarria-Aguilar M, Cockerham WT, Barker DE, Ciraulo DL, Richart CM, Maxwell RA. Management of destructive bowel injury in the open abdomen. J Trauma Acute Care Surg. 2004;56(3):560–4.
190. Wilmore DW, Robinson MK. Short bowel syndrome. World J Surg. 2000;24(12):1486–92.
191. Dabney A, Thompson J, DiBaise J, Sudan D, McBride C. Short bowel syndrome after trauma. Am J Surg. 2004;188(6):792–5.
192. Banerjee A, Warwicker P. Acute renal failure and metabolic disturbances in the short bowel syndrome. QJM. 2002;95(1):37–40.
193. Wilmore DW, Dudrick SJ. Growth and development of an infant receiving all nutrients exclusively by vein. JAMA. 1968;203(10):860–4.
194. Dudrick a SJ, J M Long I. Applications and hazards of intravenous hyperalimentation. Annu Rev Med. 1977;28(1):517–26.
195. Pironi L, Arends J, Bozzetti F, Cuerda C, Gillanders L, Jeppesen PB, et al. ESPEN guidelines on chronic intestinal failure in adults. Clin Nutr. 2016;35(2):247–307.
196. Wall EA. An overview of short bowel syndrome management: adherence, adaptation, and practical recommendations. J Acad Nutr Diet. 2013;113(9):1200–8.
197. Guo M, Li Y, Li J. Effect of growth hormone, glutamine, and enteral nutrition on intestinal adaptation in patients with short bowel syndrome. Turk J Gastroenterol. 2013;24(6):463–8.
198. Tappenden KA. Intestinal adaptation following resection. J Parenter Enter Nutr. 2014;38(1 suppl):23S–31S.
199. Jeppesen PB, Sanguinetti EL, Buchman A, Howard L, Scolapio JS, Ziegler TR, et al. Teduglutide (ALX-0600), a dipeptidyl peptidase IV resistant glucagon-like peptide 2 analogue, improves intestinal function in short bowel syndrome patients. Gut. 2005;54(9):1224–31.
200. Vipperla K, O'Keefe SJ. Targeted therapy of short-bowel syndrome with teduglutide: the new kid on the block. Clin Exp Gastroenterol. 2014;7:489–95.
201. Reilly PM, Rotondo MF, Carpenter JP, Sherr SA, Schwab CW. Temporary vascular continuity during damage control: intraluminal shunting for proximal superior mesenteric artery injury. J Trauma Acute Care Surg. 1995;39(4):757–60.

202. Aydin U, Unalp OV, Yazici P, Guler A. Success of microvascular surgery; repair mesenteric injury and prevent short bowel syndrome: a case report. BMC Emerg Med. 2007;7:11.
203. Ceulemans LJ, Monbaliu D, De Roover A, Detry O, Troisi RI, Rogiers X, et al. Belgian multicenter experience with intestinal transplantation. Transpl Int. 2015;28(12):1362–70.
204. Smith JM, Skeans MA, Horslen SP, Edwards EB, Harper AM, Snyder JJ, et al. OPTN/SRTR 2013 annual data report: intestine. Am J Transplant. 2015;15(S2):1–16.
205. Onwubiko C, Mooney DP. The value of official reinterpretation of trauma computed tomography scans from referring hospitals. J Pediatr Surg. 2016;51(3):486–9.
206. Leeper CM, Lin E, Hoffman M, Fombona A, Zhou T, Kutcher M, et al. Computed tomography abbreviated assessment of sarcopenia following trauma: the CAAST measurement predicts 6-month mortality in older adult trauma patients. J Trauma Acute Care Surg. 2016;80(5):805–11.
207. Allen GS, Moore FA, Cox CS, Mehall JR, Duke JH. Delayed diagnosis of blunt duodenal injury. J Am Coll Surg. 1998;187

22 Management of Pancreatic Injury in the Geriatric Patient

Charles E. Lucas and Anna M. Ledgerwood

Surgeons always like to perform their magic on young adults who are in training in some athletic event for the upcoming Olympics. Unfortunately, our society continues to age so that more and more operations are performed in the elderly. The challenges of surgery in the geriatric population relate to the adverse events that aging has on both physical well-being and mental acumen [1–3]. The extent of physical derangement is often referred to by the popular term "frailty" whereas the progressive mental deterioration often falls under the name of "Alzheimer's disease [3]." Although aging, per se, is not the cause of fragility or reduced acumen, the trend is for both to become progressively worse each year. Clearly, the effect of fragility and decreased cognitive function impair successful surgical treatment [1, 4]. This is true not only for elective surgery but especially for emergency operations after injury.

Many papers have emphasized that the compromised elderly patient can tolerate a major operative procedure but cannot tolerate major complication [1]. This principle applies even more to the geriatric trauma patient. Consequently, the surgeon must focus on providing an efficient and prompt diagnosis of organ injury in order to make timely intervention before the ravages of an untreated major injury lead to complications and death. Prompt diagnosis as a means of optimizing efficient therapy is more difficult in the geriatric patient with pancreatic injury. Few geriatric patients with pancreatic injury have been stabbed or shot. Less than 1% of the patients treated at an inner-city trauma center for stab wound or gunshot wound to the abdomen will be a senior citizen [5]. Consequently, these patients will be victims of blunt trauma due to a motor vehicle collision (MVC), a same-level fall, a fall from a height, or an assault. Even in the elderly, alcohol is often a cofactor associated with blunt pancreatic injury.

Blunt Abdominal Trauma: Historical Vignettes

During the midportion of the twentieth century, making a diagnosis of a blunt retroperitoneal organ injury depended upon a careful physical examination followed by frequent reexamination [6]. A patient who is not under the influence of alcohol typically has early pain and tenderness in the epigastrium with stable vital signs. This discomfort, or pain, becomes more pronounced by

C.E. Lucas, M.D., F.A.C.S. (✉)
Michael and Marian Ilitch Department of Surgery, Wayne State University School of Medicine, 4201 St. Antoine Avenue, Detroit, MI 48201, USA
e-mail: clucas@med.wayne.edu

A.M. Ledgerwood, M.D.
Wayne State University School of Medicine, Detroit, MI, USA

A. Rodriguez et al. (eds.), *Geriatric Trauma and Acute Care Surgery*, https://doi.org/10.1007/978-3-319-57403-5_22

6 h by which time there will often be a rise in the serum amylase compared to the serum amylase drawn on admission [7–9]. The progression of pain and tenderness leads to exploratory laparotomy where all organs, especially the retroperitoneal pancreas, are carefully examined. The onset of diagnostic peritoneal lavage (DPL) allowed for the early diagnosis of hemoperitoneum or peritoneal contamination from an intraperitoneal hollow viscus injury; subsequent laparotomy would allow the unsuspected pancreatic injury to be discovered [10]. Unfortunately, the DPL is negative when there is an isolated pancreatic injury. The advent of ultrasonography (FAST) allowed for earlier diagnosis of hemoperitoneum but provided marginal help for making an early diagnosis of blunt retroperitoneal injury [10]. Consequently, the contrast CT scan is the most sensitive test for the early identification of blunt pancreatic injury. Cirillo and coworkers assessed a number of imaging studies in trying to identify the optimal test for diagnosing blunt pancreatic injury [11]. They confirmed that the enhanced CT scan, despite a number of false negatives, is the best first-line examination. When question exists about ductal injury, an MRI cholangiopancreatogram may be helpful. The "gold standard" for identifying ductal injury continues to be the ERCP [11–13].

Bokhari and coworkers summarized the Eastern Association for the Surgery of Trauma (EAST) guidelines for making an early diagnosis of blunt pancreatic injury. These authors pointed out that the initial amylase may not be helpful but that a rise in amylase or an elevated amylase at 6 h suggests pancreatic injury [14]. Takishina and coworkers identified that a significant rise in amylase at 3 h after admission is very sensitive in predicting blunt pancreatic injury [9]. This rise in serum amylase at 6 h after injury has been observed by the authors [7]. The EAST guidelines also point out the significant false-negative exams with the enhanced CT scan and the lack of specificity regarding leukocytosis. When the patient is undergoing laparotomy for other reasons, the performance of an intraoperative ERCP may be helpful in identifying whether there is a ductal injury [13].

Emergent ERCP for Blunt Pancreatic Injury

The role of urgent ERCP for assessing pancreatic ductal integrity is outlined in the following case summary [12]. This 23-year-old man was driving a car when he collided with a truck; his upper torso bent the steering wheel. Despite momentary loss of consciousness, he was wide awake when he arrived in the emergency department at an outlying hospital, had stable vital signs, and had multiple facial abrasions. He had an obvious closed right femur fracture. Abdominal examination showed hypoactive bowel sounds and mild upper abdominal tenderness particularly in the left upper quadrant. His initial amylase was 50 units/L and rose to 240 units/L by 2 h. A DPL was negative. The CT revealed a probable transverse fracture of the distal pancreas (Fig. 22.1). He, therefore, was transferred to our Level I trauma center for abdominal exploration; upon arrival 5 h after injury, he was stable and had minimal left upper quadrant tenderness although the amylase had risen to 478 u/L. Two hours following arrival, he had an ERCP which demonstrated a normal pancreatic duct without extravasation (Fig. 22.2). Consequently, he was treated nonoperatively with nasal gastric suction until the pain ceased after which, on day 8, he had ORIF of the femur fracture, was started on diet on

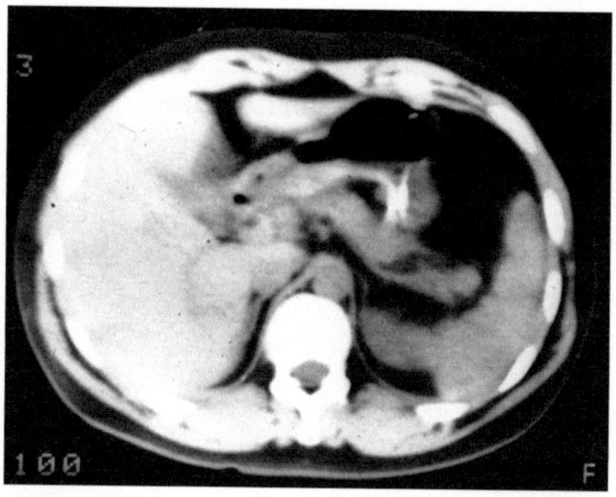

Fig. 22.1 Grade 2 pancreatic tail injury after MVC. This patient was transferred for laparotomy to repair a pancreatic body transection. Because his abdominal findings did not suggest major pancreatic injury, he underwent an emergency ERCP

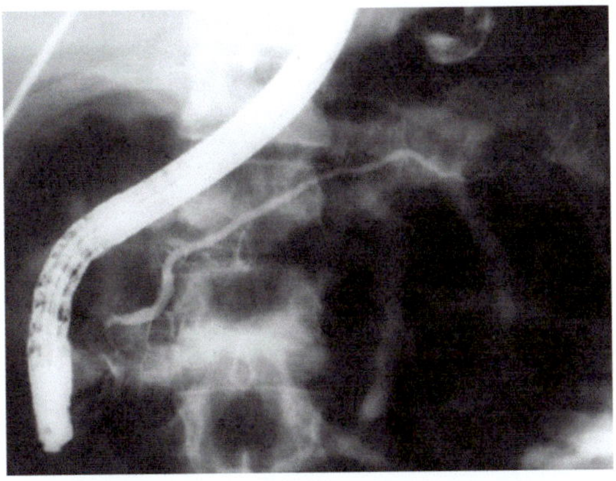

Fig. 22.2 Emergency ERCP for blunt pancreatic injury. The above patient had emergent ERCP 12 h after injury; this showed no ductal disruption or extravasation, thereby leading to successful nonoperative therapy

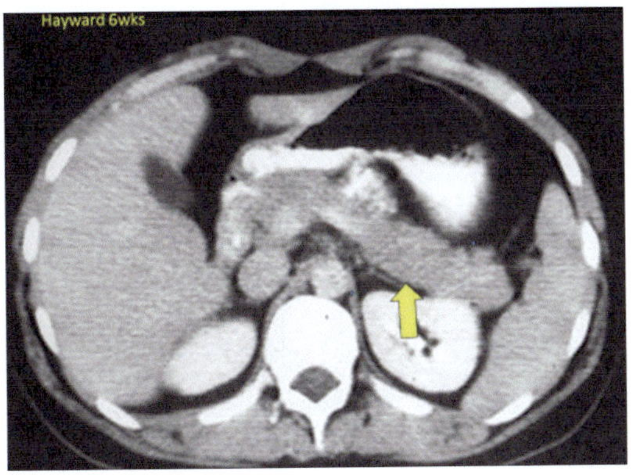

Fig. 22.3 The pancreatic body, in the above patient, was thickened at 2 months that the patient was asymptomatic

day 9, and was discharged home on day 10. Subsequent outpatient ERCP and serum amylase levels were normal. The CT scan, at 2 months, showed thickening of the pancreatic body; he was asymptomatic (Fig. 22.3). Although this injury occurred in a young, healthy patient, the principles of diagnosis and management apply to the elderly, particularly when frailty is a comorbidity. ERCP is helpful when there is question of ductal injury [13].

Nonoperative Management (NOM) for Blunt Pancreatic Injury

The past decade has seen a remarkable change in the surgical approach to blunt intraperitoneal solid organ injuries, particularly the liver and the spleen [15, 16]. Since the first study on NOM for blunt splenic injuries was prospectively initiated by Tom and coworkers in 1978 and published in 1985, the shift from NOM for blunt splenic injury has increased from less than 5% to almost 90% [16, 17]. A similar pattern has been seen for patients with blunt liver injury [15]. The experience gained from the NOM of blunt liver and splenic injuries has slowly transferred to the pancreas [18]. Most authors now recommend NOM for grade 1 and grade 2 blunt pancreatic injuries which can be successfully treated with percutaneous drains when there is evidence of a peripancreatic fluid collection [18, 19]. Some of these patients actually improve and have successful NOM without the addition of percutaneous drains [18]. Takishina and coworkers recommended NOM for all patients with minor (grade 1–2) blunt pancreatic injury [9]. The treatment of grade 3 blunt pancreatic injury has become more controversial. Leppanimi and coworkers recommend exploration with distal resection from the point of the pancreatic ductal injury [19]. Bokhari and coworkers identify a higher incidence of pancreaticocutaneous fistulae in patients with grade 3 injury treated without distal pancreatectomy [14]. Hamidian-Jahromi and coworkers noted that the nonsurgical treatment of patients with grade 3 pancreatic ductal injury was associated with a longer duration of pancreaticocutaneous fistula compared to the operative group (Fig. 22.4) [18].

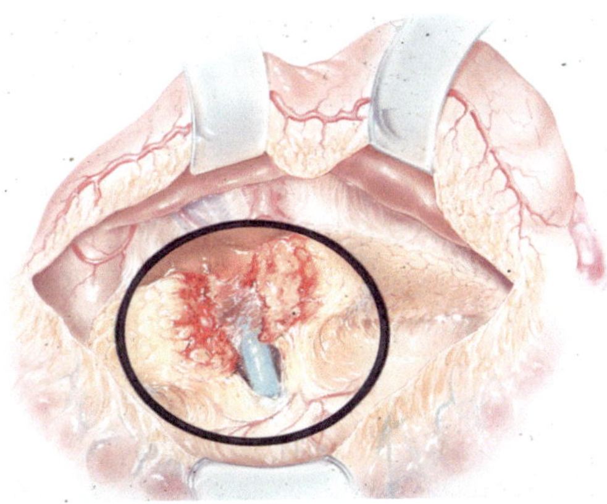

Fig. 22.4 Typical grade 3 pancreatic transection. Patients with pancreatic injury following MVC often have a transection over or to the left of the superior mesenteric vein. This is best treated, in the elderly patient undergoing laparotomy, with distal pancreatectomy with splenectomy

The long-term complication rate, however, was similar between the two groups. On the basis of a retrospective review, these patients required longer total parenteral nutrition, had a longer duration of a pancreaticocutaneous fistula, and had an increased length of stay but the overall mortality was comparable to those treated with laparotomy and definitive treatment of the pancreatic injury [18]. When a pancreatic fistula ensues, the value of octreotide therapy to close the fistula must be considered [20, 21]. Bokhari and coworkers support the work of others that there is a decrease in secretion volume from the fistula but that cure of the fistula typically does not occur [14]. The natural history of a pancreatic fistula without proximal ductal obstruction is a gradual closure. Many years ago, the authors treated a number of patients who had post-injury pancreatic fistulae with intermittent octreotide which would be given for 10 days, discontinued for 10 days, given for 10 days, with this sequence continued until closure [22]. The volume of the fistula drainage progressively decreased during each 10 day interval independent of octreotide therapy, until closure.

The blunt grade 4 pancreatic injury with partial or complete transection across the head of the pancreas without associated duodenal injury will almost always be diagnosed early with significant changes seen on the CT scan [11]. The nonoperative treatment of a grade 4 pancreatic injury which is isolated has a much greater morbidity and mortality than definitive operative therapy [18]. The immediate challenge following early exploration will be to assure hemostasis and then identify the optimal procedure depending upon both findings and patient comorbidities [7]. When the head of the pancreas is transected, this usually occurs at the point where the third portion of the common bile duct passes through the pancreas (Fig. 22.5). In the stable patient this may be treated by over-sewing and hemostasis of the remnant of the pancreas attached to the medial wall of the duodenum followed by a Roux-en-Y drainage of the remaining pancreas with the end of the pancreas being sewed to the side of the Roux-en-Y jejunal loop (Fig. 22.6). When this is technically not possible, the treatment may consist of a 90% pancreatectomy with splenectomy which would be a highly morbid

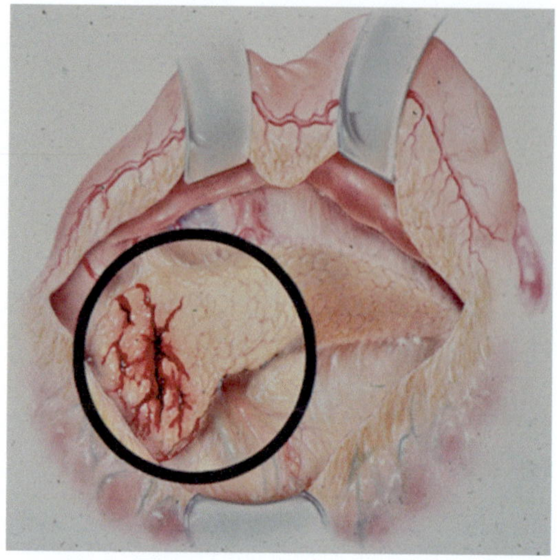

Fig. 22.5 Grade 4 pancreatic head laceration. The grade 4 pancreatic injury is associated with complete or partial transection of the head of the pancreas, often with ductal injury, but without duodenal injury

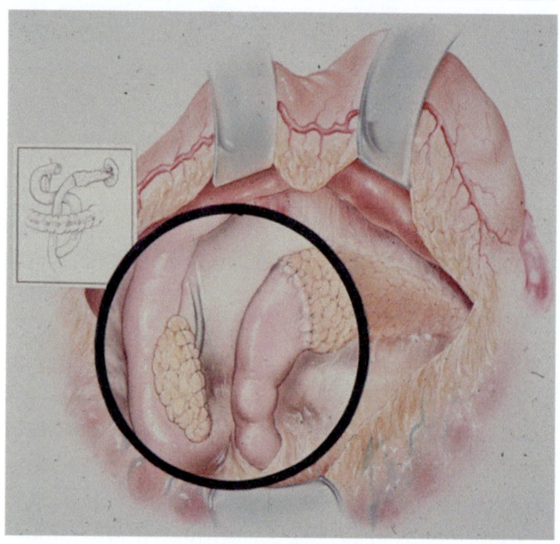

Fig. 22.6 Non-resectional therapy for grade 4 pancreatic injury. When the transection extends through the pancreas, the duodenal side of the pancreas may be made hemostatic with simple interrupted sutures, whereas the distal pancreas is drained into a Roux-en-Y jejunal limb

procedure to be performed in an elderly patient with significant comorbidities. When the extent of frailty is significant, wide drainage of the area may be all that can be achieved over the short term with the expectation that one would have to deal with the subsequent pancreaticocutaneous fistula at a later date when, hopefully, the patient is more stable. This is best achieved with closed suction drainage [23].

The grade 5 pancreatic injury has either extensive disruption with vascular embarrassment of the head of the pancreas or has a large laceration of the head of the pancreas in association with a duodenal rupture [7]. When this complex injury occurs in a young healthy stable patient, the definitive procedure would be a pancreaticoduodenectomy [24]. This operation, however, would have a prohibitive morbidity and mortality rate in the elderly patient with extensive comorbidities associated with the hemorrhagic shock insult associated with this injury [1, 4]. The Whipple operation typically takes 5–7 h in stable patients being operated upon electively and is much more prolonged in the unstable patient with severe injury with hemorrhage, and hematoma in the area of tissue dissection. Consequently, one may rely on the staged Whipple operation where the pancreaticoduodenectomy is performed in order to provide hemostasis and removal of the ruptured duodenum followed by damage control packing with plans to come back in 1–3 days in order to complete the operation after the patient has been stabilized. When this grade 5 injury involves severe laceration of the head of the pancreas with duodenal rupture, a lesser procedure may be indicated in the elderly patient. The traditional options in this setting have included the duodenal diverticulization procedure (Fig. 22.7), the pyloric exclusion procedure (Fig. 22.8), or the triple-intraluminal drain procedure with decompressive gastrostomy, decompressive retrograde jejunostomy, and feeding anterior jejunostomy [7, 25]. The authors prefer the duodenal diverticulization which consists of primary duodenal repair, antrectomy with gastrojejunostomy, and wide drainage [7].

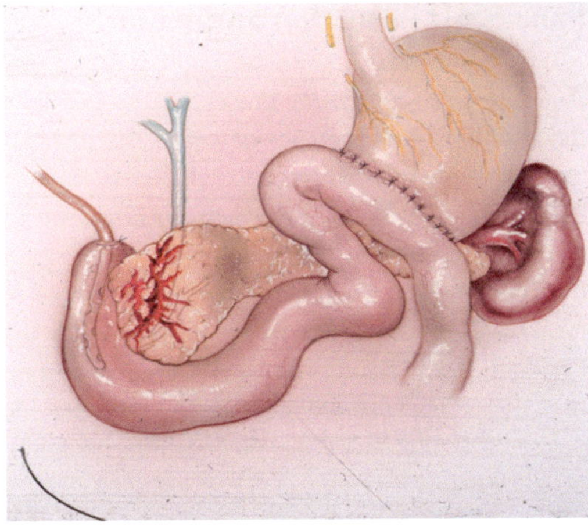

Fig. 22.7 Duodenal diverticulization for grade 5 pancreatic injury. With grade 5 pancreatic injury, the associated duodenal perforation must be closed and the food stream may be diverted away from the duodenum with the duodenal diverticulization procedure consisting of antrectomy and end-to-side gastrojejunostomy

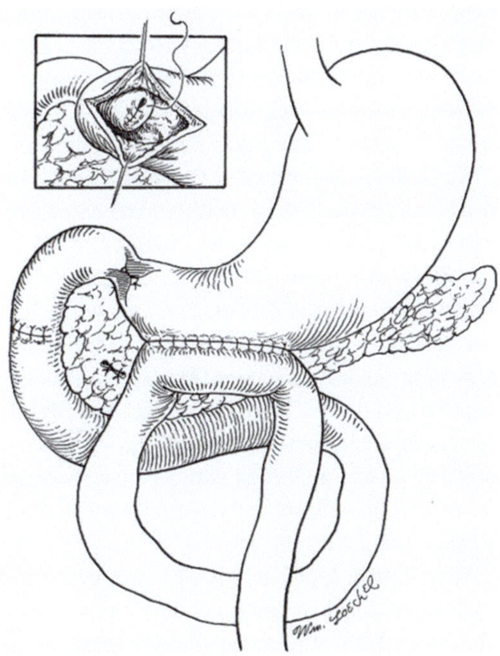

Fig. 22.8 Duodenal exclusion procedure. Grade 5 pancreatic injuries with transection or deep lacerations of the head of the pancreas in association with duodenal rupture can be treated by the pyloric exclusion procedure consisting of primary repair of the duodenum, inferior gastrojejunostomy, oversewing of the pylorus, and wide drainage of the pancreatic injury

Pancreatic Resection and Frailty

Augustin and coworkers presented an excellent report on how frailty affects outcome after pancreatic resection for malignancy [1]. These authors developed a Frailty Index which consisted of 15 comorbidities and the current functional status of their patients [1]. Their Frailty Index is simple to measure, is objective, and has been validated in the National Surgical Quality Initiative Program (NSQIP). They utilized a score to measure the degree of frailty; this score ranged from no frailty (0) to a low level of frailty (1, 2), moderate frailty (3, 4), or severe frailty (5 or greater). They evaluated 13,492 elective pancreatic operations in elderly patients of whom 8830 had pancreaticoduodenectomy, 4382 underwent distal pancreatectomy with splenectomy, and 280 had total pancreatectomy [1]. They showed that the factors that contributed most to frailty and a bad outcome were age, BMI, female gender, recent weight loss, preoperative infection, and hypoalbuminemia. They looked at the effect of the Frailty Index on recovery following pancreaticoduodenectomy, distal pancreatectomy with splenectomy, or total pancreatectomy for malignancy. Their findings demonstrated that the likelihood of death or a Clavien level 4 morbidity increased from 7.5% in patients with no frailty to 40.7% ($p \leq 0.0001$) in patients with frailty as defined by a Frailty Index score of 5 or greater. Following distal pancreatectomy the likelihood of death or a level 4 Clavien complication ranged from 3.6% in patients without frailty to 27.8% in patients with frailty. Finally, after total pancreatectomy, the incidence of death or a level 4 Clavien complication increased from 5.2% in patients without frailty to 31.2% in patients with frailty [1].

The Frailty Index is not only a predictor of in-hospital death or major complication but is also a predictor of post-discharge morbidity and mortality. Maxwell and coworkers looked at a group of injured patients who were over 65 years of age and were treated at a Level I trauma center during an 18-month period [3]. The mean age was 77 years and the median injury severity score was 10. Utilizing well-established systems for assessing pre-injury cognitive impairment and physical frailty, both were predictive of subsequent mortality 1 year after discharge. Age was also a predictor of mortality by 1 year after discharge [3]. Consequently, the physician caring for patients with blunt pancreatic injury has to make decisions based upon these preinjury conditions.

Surgical Exposure of the Injured Pancreas

Since almost all geriatric patients with pancreatic injury will have sustained blunt trauma, the typical exposure to the pancreas is made through an upper midline incision. Sometimes the patient may be a candidate for diagnostic laparoscopic examination which, if positive, will be followed by an upper midline incision in most circumstances. Definitive laparoscopic repair of blunt pancreatic injury in the elderly is probably being performed but the authors have no experience with this approach. The anatomic principles, however, would remain the same in that the same technical steps need to be performed in order to provide both access and definitive treatment of the pancreas.

Once the abdomen is opened, the approach to the pancreas is best provided by dividing the greater omentum outside the arcades of the right and left gastroepiploic vessels (Fig. 22.9). This provides

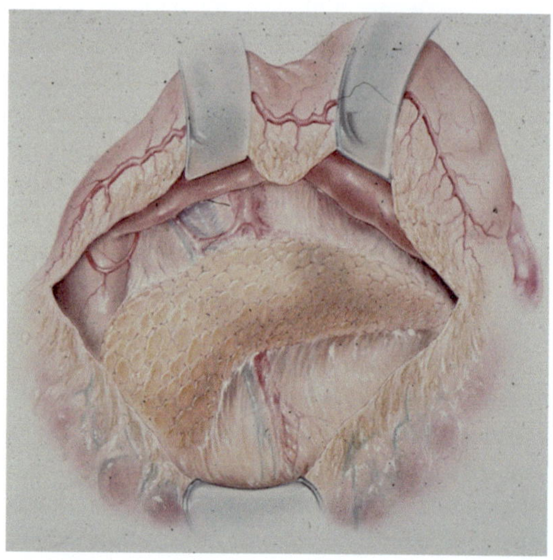

Fig. 22.9 Pancreatic exposure within the lesser sac. The anterior portion of the pancreas can be widely exposed by entering the lesser sac through the greater omentum just outside the arcades of the gastroepiploic vessels

excellent exposure to the full length of the pancreas on the anterior surface. Examination of the interior border of the pancreas is made possible by dividing the inferior attachments of the superior leaf of the transverse colonic mesentery from the inferior border of the pancreas; this division should be done right at the border of the inferior border of the pancreas which is avascular. The superior border of the pancreas can be exposed by dividing the posterior leaf of the lesser omentum from the superior border of the pancreas; again, this division should be at the border of the pancreas which is avascular. By this time, the operating surgeon will have identified whether there are any injuries to the pancreas with the exception of the posterior surface.

The posterior surface of the body and tail of the pancreas is best exposed by freeing up the spleen from its attachments, then gently dissecting the plane posterior to the spleen and the pancreas, and lifting the pancreas anteriorly and medially. The spleen will accompany the pancreas and should not be pulled less there be an avulsion of the splenic hilar vessels or a capsular tear (Fig. 22.10). The posterior portion of the head of the pancreas is best exposed by the performance of an extended Kocher maneuver which can be carried out to the level of the superior mesenteric artery (Fig. 22.11). These maneuvers will provide complete exposure to all of the pancreas.

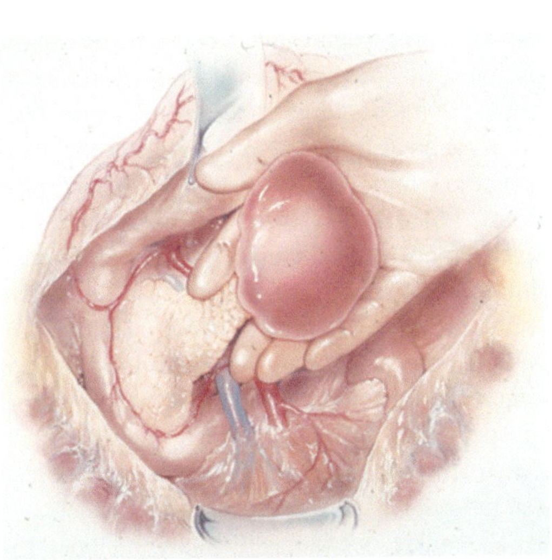

Fig. 22.10 Exposure of the posterior body and tail of the pancreas. Excellent visualization of the posterior body and tail of the pancreas can be achieved by rotating the pancreas with spleen anteriorly and medially

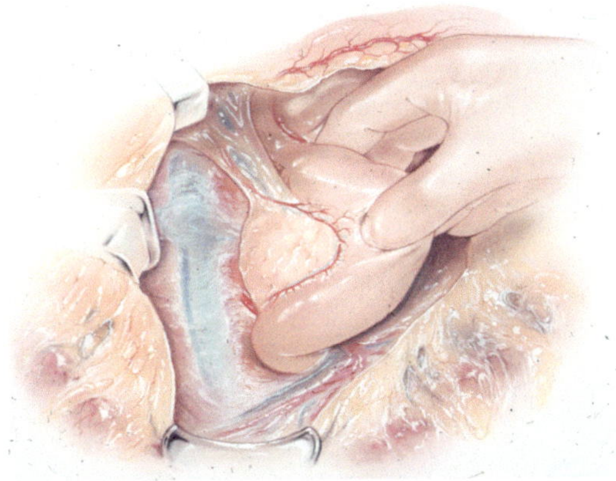

Fig. 22.11 Exposure of the posterior pancreatic head. Complete exposure of the posterior pancreatic head can be provided by an extended Kocher maneuver with the head of the pancreas rotated anteriorly and medially to the extent of the superior mesenteric artery

Abbreviated Injury Severity and Treatment

The optimal surgical treatment of blunt pancreatic injury correlates with injury severity [7]. The abbreviated injury severity (AIS) score provides excellent guidelines for therapeutic decisions (Table 22.1). A pancreatic grade 1 injury includes a small hematoma less than 2 cm, a small (less than 2 cm) peripheral laceration, or a small contusion. Grade 1 injuries may not be apparent on imaging studies so that one has to rely on serial clinical examination and serial amylase levels or an exploratory laparotomy performed for other injuries. If left untreated, a grade 1 injury may cause adynamic ileus and a possible pancreatic infection leading to a lesser sac abscess [9]. When diagnosed at laparotomy performed for other reasons, the laceration, if bleeding, should be made hemostatic with electrocoagulation; the hematoma should be unroofed followed by careful hemostasis, and the small contusion should be left alone. External drainage with a Jackson-Pratt drain is indicated for all of these conditions. If diagnosed after nonoperative management of blunt injury in the elderly, percutaneous drainage of the peripancreatic area will usually suffice [9].

A grade 2 pancreatic injury includes a parenchymal hematoma greater than 3 cm or a peripheral laceration more than 2 cm. When diagnosed at the time of laparotomy performed for another

Table 22.1 Pancreatic abbreviated injury severity

Grade	
1	Small hematoma; contusion; shallow laceration <2 cm
2	Parenchymal hematoma >3 cm; peripheral laceration >2 cm without major ductal injury
3	Transection distal pancreas; deep laceration with ductal injury
4	Deep laceration or transection pancreatic head
5	Severe combined pancreatic head transection with duodenal rupture

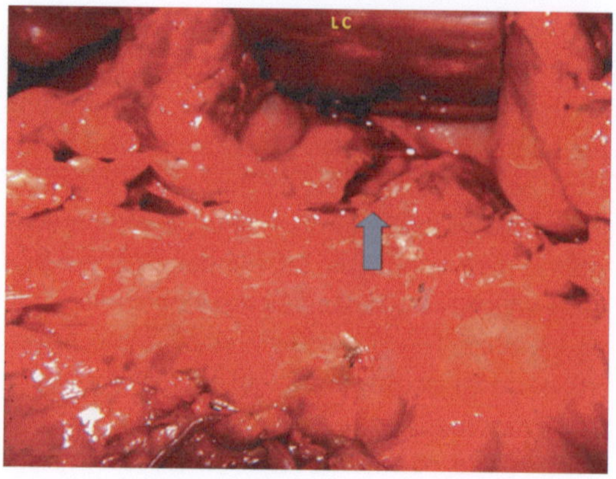

Fig. 22.12 Grade 3 pancreatic transection overlying superior mesenteric vein. This patient had transection of the pancreas (*arrow*) overlying the superior mesenteric vein

injury, they should be managed in the same way as a grade 1 injury. The contrast CT is more likely to show peripancreatic fluid or evidence of pancreatic edema with grade 2 injury compared to a grade 1 injury. Care should be taken, however, to make sure that the hematoma or laceration does not extend into the major pancreatic duct. A pancreatic drain, placed at laparotomy done for other injuries or for a peripancreatic fluid collected in patients being observed will often yield a fluid with an elevated amylase level which will gradually decrease over the 2–14 days. Drainage beyond that time is an indication for an ERCP to identify whether there is a major ductal laceration or more proximal ductal obstruction.

A classic grade 3 pancreatic injury after blunt trauma typically is a transection of the body of the pancreas just to the left of the superior mesenteric vein. This transection will often overlie the vertebral column (Fig. 22.12). The patient, typically, has epigastric pain and tenderness. The contrast CT will demonstrate lesser sac fluid and the laceration in the body or tail of the pancreas. Typically, this is a transverse laceration (Fig. 22.1). The optimal procedure for the geriatric patient with a grade 3 transection of the pancreatic body is distal pancreatectomy with splenectomy. Although distal pancreatectomy with splenic salvage has been used in selective circumstances, the serious complications of this procedure, including ischemic necrosis of the lower pole of the spleen, would be an excessive risk for the elderly patient [26]. As previously indicated, the elderly patient can tolerate a major operation but cannot tolerate a major complication. When the patient has a partial transection of the pancreas which comes in proximity to the main pancreatic duct, simple drainage may be all that is indicated if the patient is frail and has major comorbidities [27]. Likewise, when the patient with a suspected grade 3 injury seen on CT scan has minimal symptoms and is frail, non-operative management with later percutaneous drainage of the lesser sac may be safest [18, 23].

A grade 4 blunt pancreatic injury includes a deep laceration with ductal disruption to the head of the pancreas or a complete transection of the head of the pancreas (Fig. 22.5). Treatment options in this setting might include wide external drainage, pancreaticoduodenectomy in the presence of complete transection, simple oversewing of the proximal duodenal side of the fractured pancreas followed by drainage of the distal pancreas into a Roux-en-Y jejunal limb (Fig. 22.6), or a 90% distal pancreatectomy with splenectomy. All of these injuries require wide drainage. When comorbidities and excessive frailty preclude this type of major operative procedure, wide drainage of the lesser sac and peripancreatic area is mandatory with the hope that the patient will slowly improve as the leaking pancreatic fluid develops into a pseudocyst which can more safely be treated in the frail patient.

The grade 5 pancreatic injury includes the combination of a severe deep injury to the head of the pancreas in association with a duodenal rupture [7]. Sometimes these injuries are so massive that anything less than a pancreaticoduodenectomy will be associated with failure despite the fact that the Whipple operation would have a high death rate in the elderly patient [1, 19]. Lesser operations could include the duodenal diverticulization procedure (Fig. 22.7), the pyloric exclusion procedure (Fig. 22.8), or the combination of decompressive tube gastrostomy, decompressive retrograde tube jejunostomy, and an antegrade feeding tube jejunostomy [7, 24]. Geriatric patients with severe frailty are unlikely to survive any complicated pancreatic resection or pancreatic diversion. Following repair of the duodenal injury which is mandatory, the patient may be a candidate for extensive external drainage with the hopes that nutrition can be maintained by the intravenous route while the pancreatic tissues eventually heal and ductal continuity is reestablished. This decision would only be made because it is clear to the operating surgeon that the elderly, frail patient would not tolerate the more ideal but more extensive procedure [1]. Even patients with minimum frailty in the geriatric age group are unlikely to survive an emergency pancreaticoduodenectomy [1]. Clearly, the decision to perform the Whipple operation in this setting would reflect the surgeon's judgment that frailty is not an issue.

Much debate exists regarding the ideal nonresectional therapy for a patient with a grade 5 pancreatic injury. Following repair of the duodenal injury, which is mandatory, the patient could be treated by one of the three procedures as described above. The authors prefer duodenal diverticulization, whereby the food is permanently diverted away from the duodenal pancreatic complex (Fig. 22.7).

The Missed Injury

Occasionally, patients with blunt abdominal trauma have a pancreatic injury which is missed on the initial evaluation, thereby resulting in delayed therapy. This is more likely to occur in the body or tail of the pancreas (Fig. 22.13). When laparotomy is delayed because of a missed injury, there will often be extensive inflammation within the lesser sac with or without a pancreatic pseudocyst. When the patient is compromised, as might occur in the elderly, simple external drainage of the peripancreatic fluid may be enough to improve the patient's overall condition until one can identify the specific anatomy by an ERCP or a pancreaticocutaneous fistulogram (Fig. 22.14).

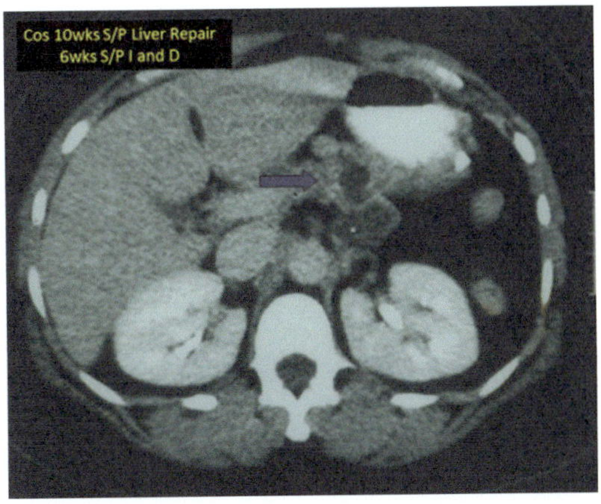

Fig. 22.13 ERCP for posttraumatic pancreatic pseudocyst formation. This 73-year-old man had a liver injury following an MVC. This was repaired primarily but an associated pancreatic injury was missed. When transferred back to Michigan, he had open drainage of the lesser sac which led to a refractory pancreaticocutaneous fistula associated with a pseudocyst (*arrow*)

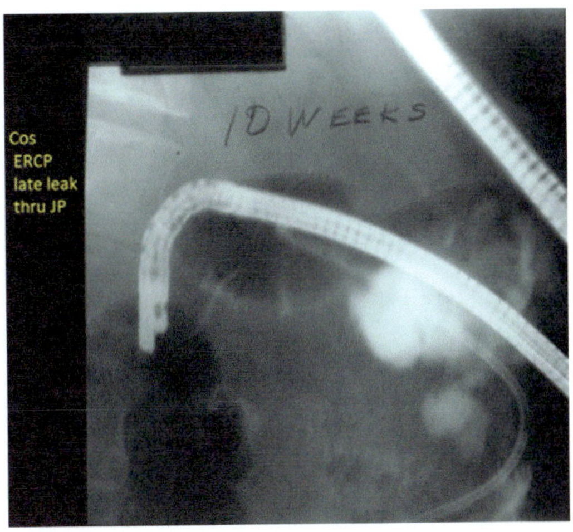

Fig. 22.14 ERCP on the above patient demonstrated leakage from the main pancreatic duct into the fistula tract. Although there was no obstruction between the pseudocyst and the ampulla, the fistula was refractory for 3 months to nonoperative therapy. Cystogastrostomy resulted in prompt fistula closure

When a subsequent pseudocyst develops in association with a pancreaticocutaneous fistula, one needs to be certain that the pancreatic duct between the ampulla and the fistula, or pseudocyst, is not obstructed. When the duct is unobstructed, a cystogastrostomy by the endoscopic or open approach, depending upon the circumstances, will allow the pancreaticocutaneous fistula to close as the pancreatic juice is diverted into the low-pressure stomach. This is often better tolerated than doing a distal pancreatectomy and splenectomy, especially in the elderly.

Sometimes, the missed injury is recognized within the first 72 h after injury. The patient depicted in Fig. 22.15 was involved in an MVC and sustained a grade 2 liver injury which was treated nonoperatively. By 36 h after injury, she had pain and tenderness in the left upper quadrant associated with fever, leukocytosis, and tachycardia. Review of the previous scan identified the grade 2 pancreatic injury and the repeat scan on post-injury day 2 (Fig. 22.15) showed peripancreatic edema and a crack across the tail of the pancreas. Operation revealed that the pancreatic injury extended to the main duct and was, at this time, associated with peripancreatic inflammation and fat necrosis. She was treated by distal pancreatectomy with splenectomy and recovered uneventfully. Percutaneous treatment of this injury would likely have failed because she had already developed major signs of inflammation including tachycardia.

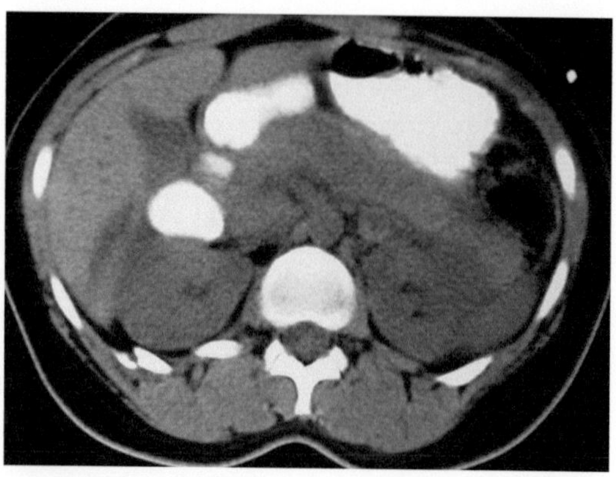

Fig. 22.15 Missed pancreatic tail injury. This patient was a victim of an MVC/pedestrian mishap and was found to have a grade 1 liver injury in the right lobe. He also had a grade 1 pancreatic tail injury which was not appreciated on the initial CT scan. Progressive abdominal tenderness led to a repeat CT on day 2 (*above*) which showed peripancreatic phlegmon; laparotomy on post-injury day 2 revealed a type 2 pancreatic injury with extensive inflammation and peripancreatic fat necrosis within the lesser sac which was treated by distal pancreatectomy with splenectomy

Post-distal Pancreatectomy Fistula

Whenever a patient has a distal pancreatectomy with or without splenectomy there are a number of ways of closing the resected pancreatic margin. Ligation of the exposed pancreatic duct is recommended but often the duct is of such small size that it cannot be readily visualized within the adjacent pancreatic parenchyma. For many years the authors recommended that the pancreatic stump be closed in a fish mouth manner with interrupted sutures to bring the inferior margin to the superior margin after which closed suction drains are placed. The results of using a GIA stapler to divide the pancreas and bring about definitive closure have also been used with great success in patients having distal pancreatectomy as part of the debulking procedure for malignancy. Regardless of which technique is used, there often will be some drainage of pancreatic fluid as evidenced by a high amylase. This drainage typically decreases quickly and seldom extends beyond 1 week. When one has continued drainage, a more proximal pancreatic ductal obstruction should be resected or else a portion of injured pancreas has been left behind.

Whenever a patient has a distal pancreatectomy with splenectomy for blunt pancreatic injury but continues to have persistent pancreatic fluid drainage as evidenced by a very high amylase, one should anticipate that not all of the injured pancreas was resected. Such patients need an ERCP which will identify the site of leakage (Fig. 22.16). This patient needs to be stabilized and reexplored with the objective to identify the injured segment of the pancreatic stump which was not removed at the time of the first operation (Fig. 22.16). This will be a very difficult operation since the continued leakage of pancreatic juice adjacent to the pancreatic fistula will cause an extensive inflammation which will mandate that the operation be performed in a

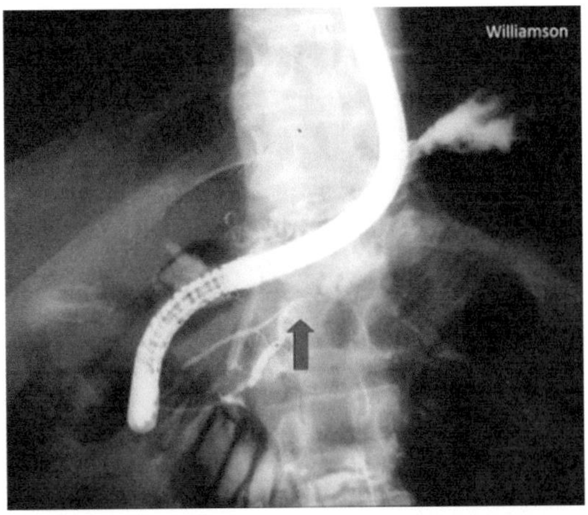

Fig. 22.16 Post-distal pancreatectomy fistula. This 67-year-old patient had a distal pancreatectomy with splenectomy after falling on a table while hanging tree lights. He had persistent drainage as part of a long-term pancreaticocutaneous fistula. ERCP demonstrated a second injury in the remaining pancreas necessitating a more proximal pancreatectomy

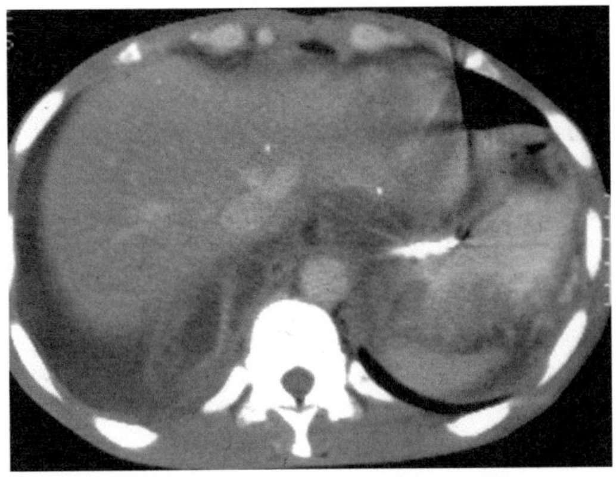

Fig. 22.17 Pancreatic ascites. This patient had both abdominal ascites and pleural effusion which persisted for about 12 weeks after he was treated for blunt thoracic trauma and multiple rib fractures. Thoracentesis identified a right pleural effusion which had a high amylase whereas the abdominal CT scan demonstrated ascites and a small cyst near the pancreas

very slow and deliberate manner. Once the injury is identified, the inflamed sclerotic pancreatic stump needs to be freed up for either a re-resection with closure of the stump or a decompression into a Roux-en-Y jejunal loop.

Pancreatic Ascites or Empyema

A missed pancreatic injury following blunt trauma may also lead to pancreatic ascites which can easily be confused with liver ascites when there is a history of significant alcohol use. When the leaking pancreatic juice is not walled off by the lesser sac tissues in the development of a peripancreatic pseudocyst, the fluid in the drain throughout the peritoneal cavity can lead to pancreatic ascites. The small communications between the chest and abdomen allow for this pancreatic ascites, when extensive, to accumulate within the chest as a pleural effusion (Fig. 22.17). Although this can happen on either side, most patients with pancreatic ascites and associated pleural effusion have the effusion located in the right chest. Confirmation that the ascites or pleural effusion is of pancreatic origin can be made by measuring amylase levels of the pericentesis or thoracentesis aspirate. Once identified as being pancreatic fluid, the patient should have an ERCP which will pinpoint the source of the pancreatic leak (Fig. 22.18). Definitive surgery even in the geriatric patient is best achieved by a lateral Roux-en-Y side-to-side pancreaticojejunostomy incorporating the site of the fistula into the anastomosis.

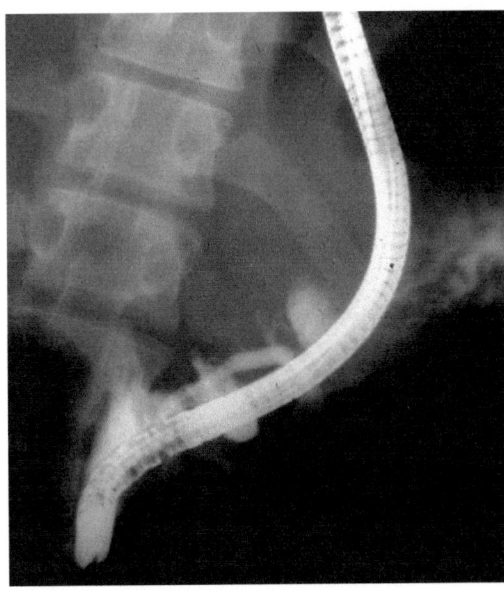

Fig. 22.18 Origin of pancreatic ascites. ERCP in the above patient showed a leak from the main pancreatic duct in the midportion of the body of the pancreas. He was successfully treated with a lateral Roux-en-Y pancreaticojejunostomy

References

1. Augustin T, Chalikonda S, Wey J, Burstein M, Merrig-Stiff G, Walsh N. Frailty predicts risk of life threatening complications and mortality after pancreatic resections. Surg 2016;160(4):987–996.
2. Callcut RA, Wakam G, Conroy AS, Kornbligh L, Howard BM, Campion EM, Nelson MF, Mell MW, Cohen MJ. Discovering the truth about life after discharge: long-term trauma-related mortality. J Trauma Acute Care Surg. 2016;80:210–7.
3. Maxwell CA, Mion LC, Mukherjee K, Dietrich MS, Minnick A, Addison M, Miller RS. Preinjury physical frailty and cognitive impairment among geriatric trauma patients determine postinjury functional recovery and survival. J Trauma Acute Care Surg. 2016;80:195–203.
4. Cook AC, Bellal J, Kenji I, Nakonezny PA, Bruns BR, Kerby JD, Brasel KJ, Wolf SE, Cuschieri J, Paulk ME, Rhodes RL, Brakenridge SC, Phelan HA. Multicenter external validation of the Geriatric Trauma Outcome Score: A study by the Prognostic Assessment of Life and Limitations after Trauma in the Elderly (PALLIATE) consortium. J Trauma Acute Care Surg. 2016;80:204–9.
5. Lucas CE. Injury severity scoring after gunshot wounds treated at an inner-city trauma center. (Submitted).
6. Lucas CE, Ledgerwood AM. Injuries to the stomach, duodenum, pancreas, small bowel, colon and rectum. In: Wilmore C, Harken H, Soper M, editors. ACS Surgery Principles and Practice 2003. New York, NY: webMD Inc; 2003. p. 420–31.
7. Lucas CE. Diagnosis and treatment of pancreatic and duodenal injury. Surg Clin North Am. 1977;57(1):49–65.
8. Mayer JM, Tomczak R, Rau B, Gebhard F, Beger HG. Pancreatic injury in severe trauma: early diagnosis and therapy improves the outcome. Dig Surg. 2002;19:291–7.
9. Takishina T, Sugimoto K, Hirata M, Asari Y, Ohwada T, Kakita A. Serum amylase level on admission in the diagnosis of blunt injury to the pancreas: its significance and limitations. Ann Surg. 1997;226:70–6.
10. Lucas CE. Abdominal organ injury: diagnosis, treatment, and education. Second annual WR Ghent lecture on trauma. Can J Surg. 1990;33(3):189–95.
11. Cirillo RL, Koniaris LG. Detecting blunt pancreatic injuries. J Gastrointest Surg. 2002;6:587–98.
12. Hayward SR, Lucas CE, Sugawa C, Ledgerwood AM. Emergency endoscopic retrograde cholangiopancreatography. (Brief clinical note). Arch Surg. 1989;124(6):745–6.
13. Wind P, Tiret E, Cunningham C, Frileux P, Cugnenc PH, Parc R. Contribution of endoscopic retrograde pancreatography in management of complications following distal pancreatic trauma. Am Surg. 1999; 65:777–83.
14. Bokhari F, Phelan H, Holevar M, Brautigam R, Collier B, Como JJ, Clancy K, Cumming JK, Cullinane D, Smith L. Diagnosis and management of pancreatic trauma. East Practice Management Guidelines. 2009. https://www.east.org/education/practice-management-guidelines/pancreatic-trauma-diagnosis-and-management-of.
15. Lucas CE, Ledgerwood AM. The academic challenge of teaching psychomotor skills for hemostasis of solid organ injury. J Trauma. 2009;66(3):636–40.
16. Tom WW, Howells GA, Bree RL, Schwab R, Lucas RJ. A nonoperative approach to the adult ruptured spleen sustained from blunt trauma. Am Surg. 1985;51:367–71.
17. Meguid AA, Bair HA, Howell GA, Bendick PJ, Kerr HH, Villalba MR. Prospective evaluation of criteria for the nonoperative management of blunt splenic trauma. Am Surg. 2003;69(3):238–43.
18. Hamidian-Jahromi AH, D'Agostino HR, Zibari GB, Chu QD, Clark C, Shokouh-Amiri H. Surgical versus nonsurgical management of traumatic major pancreatic duct transection: institutional experience and review of the literature. Pancreas. 2013;42:76–87.
19. Leppanimi AK, Haapiainen RK. Pancreatic trauma with proximal duct injury. Ann Chir Gynaecol. 1954;83:191–5.
20. Amirata E, Livingston DH, Elcavage J. Octreotide acetate decreases pancreatic complications after pancreatic trauma. Am J Surg. 1994;168(4):345–7.
21. Nwariaku FE, Terricina A, Myleski WJ, Minei JP, Carrico CJI. Octreotide beneficial following pancreatic injury? Am J Surg. 1995;170:582–5.
22. Lucas CE, Ledgerwood AM. Ongoing unpublished personal data.
23. Fabian TC, Kudsk KA, Croce MA, Payne LW, Mangiante EC, Voeller GR, Britt LG. Superiority of closed suction drainage for pancreatic trauma: a randomized, prospective study. Ann Surg. 1990;211:724–30.
24. Asensio JA, Petrone P, Roldan G, Kuncir E, Demetriades D. Pancreatiocoduodenectomy: a rare procedure for the management of complex pancreaticoduodenal injuries. J Am Coll Surg. 2003;197:937–42.
25. Schroeppel TJ, Saleem K, Sharpe JP, Magnotti LJ, Weinberg JA, Riter E, Croce MA, Fabian TC. Penetrating duodenal trauma: a 19 year experience. J Trauma Acute Care Surg. 2016;80(3):461–5.
26. Patcher JL, Hofstetter SR, Liang HG, Hoballah J. Traumatic injuries to the pancreas: the role of distal pancreatectomy with splenic preservation. J Trauma. 1989;29:1352–5.
27. Patton JH Jr, Lyden SP, Croce MA, Pritchard FE, Minard G, Kudsk KA, Fabian TC. Pancreatic trauma: a simplified management guideline. J Trauma. 1997;43:234–41.

Part X

Vascular Injury

Geriatric Cerebrovascular Injury

23

Peter B. Letarte

Introduction

The incidence and prevalence of cerebrovascular disease increase with age. Acute care surgeons are sure to encounter this set of diseases when treating the emergently sick and injured in this age group. Cerebrovascular disease often presents in isolation, with elderly patient who awakens with a new set of neuro-deficits or presents after a collapse with new associated neuro-deficits. Often these presentations are masked by other entities, such as the patient who suffers from spontaneous intracerebral hemorrhage while driving or the patient who has a stroke and falls while intoxicated. The acute care surgeon must be able to discern the presence of cerebrovascular disease within the patient's presenting symptom complex and then rapidly incorporate the oftentimes limited care the patient requires into the patient's care plan.

Ischemic Strokes

While ischemic stroke is the usual purview of neurologists and neurointensivist, the acute care surgeon will encounter patients who are experiencing an acute stroke, either as a cause of or as a sequela of their presenting traumatic complaint. This is especially likely in the geriatric age group.

Stroke is ranked fifth in causes of death in the United States. There have been recent significant declines in the stroke rate in those older than 65 years old, although these declines have not been enjoyed by all ethnic groups uniformly.

Stroke patients over 85 years old make up 17% of all stroke patients. These patients have a higher risk-adjusted mortality, greater disability, and longer hospitalizations; receive less evidence-based care; and are less likely to be discharged to their original place of residence. Over the last few years, men over the age of 84 are the only group who have not enjoyed a decline in death from stroke. From 2010 to 2050, the number of incident strokes is expected to more than double with the majority of the increase occurring in those over 75 years of age and among minorities. These trends increase the imperative for all acute care providers to identify stroke in the elderly and to institute standard protocols in a timely fashion [1].

Stroke Management

The goal of treatment is to rapidly remove reverse cerebral ischemia by removing the offending vessel's obstruction. The American Heart Association has standard protocols for stroke management.

P.B. Letarte, M.D., F.A.A.N.S., F.A.C.S.
Neurosurgeon, Premier Health,
Dayton, OH, USA
e-mail: Letartefamily@comcast.net

A. Rodriguez et al. (eds.), *Geriatric Trauma and Acute Care Surgery*,
https://doi.org/10.1007/978-3-319-57403-5_23

As stated in the 2015 updates for these guidelines "Rapid administration of intravenous recombinant tissue-type plasminogen activator (r-tPA) to appropriate patients remains the mainstay of early treatment of acute ischemic stroke" [2]. The key goal for any stroke care system is the reperfusion of the brain, soon enough to minimize ischemic damage of the brain and to avoid the follow-on hemorrhage which can occur if reperfusion occurs too late, after ischemic injury has started to compromise the integrity of the cerebral vascular endothelium. Two classes of treatment can be used to achieve this goal. The first is intravenous fibrinolysis, such as r-TPA. The second class of treatments are endovascular, intra-arterial techniques such as intra-arterial thrombolysis, and mechanical embolectomy [3].

The goal then is to get the patient, with certain exceptions, to r-tPA within 3 h of onset of symptoms and within 60 min of arrival in the emergency room, or, in acute care situations, within 60 min of identification of the stroke. The rate-limiting steps in this process are diagnosis of stroke and decision making. To address this, the AHA has set time frames for the interim steps. Acute care surgeons should be proficient in these steps since it is likely that at some point in the workup of an emergent geriatric patient, the presence of a stroke may be suspected.

The first step is identification of the presence of stroke. As soon as stroke is suspect by the team, immediate contact with a stroke team should be made, either by activating the stroke team within the institution providing care or contacting a supporting hospital that provides stroke services. The likely outcome of attempting to improvise stroke care will be the failure to meet treatment deadlines and the denial of access to reperfusion services for the patient. This is especially true in the elderly.

The suspicion of stroke can be solidified by the use of either the Cincinnati Prehospital Stroke Scale or the Los Angeles Prehospital Stroke Screen. Once the diagnosis is established, the stroke team can be assisted by assuring that the early pieces of the stroke protocol are done. It should be ascertained that the time of onset of the symptoms and the time of arrival to the ED or, in an inpatient setting the time the problem was identified, are well documented in the chart. Adequate oxygenation of the patient should be assured. A complete blood count, coagulation studies, electrolytes, and serum glucose should be obtained but only the results of the serum glucose are needed to start fibrinolytic therapy. Starting fibrinolytic therapy should not be delayed awaiting lab results other than glucose. A rapid serum glucose in some form is the best option. AHA protocol also requires that non-contrasted CT of the brain be obtained and interpreted within 45 min of presentation. This is a key rate-limiting step and obtaining such a scan is an emergent priority and should be instituted immediately. An EKG and chest X-ray may be obtained but also should not delay the administration of fibrinolytic therapy in any way. If intra-arterial techniques are to be considered, some form of vascular imaging, either a CT angiogram of the head and neck, an MRA, or a standard cerebral angiogram, will be required. It is important to remember that these images are not required for intravenous fibrinolytic therapy and obtaining them should not delay the start of this therapy. Emergently, only the non-contrasted CT of the brain will be required. The last piece of information the stroke team will require is a National Institute of Health Stroke Score. This is a useful tool but requires brief training to use due to the need for consistency between providers administering it. Initiating all these measures quickly will save the stroke team a great deal of time.

The expertise of the stroke team will be needed as these results are obtained. The interpretation of the clinical examination, the non-contrast CT, and the patient's labs require specialized decision making and expertise, and must be done rapidly to meet the 60-min "door-to-needle" goal. This process includes in a discussion of the risks and benefits with the patient and in many cases the administration of a fibrinolytic agent.

The process also includes a checklist with absolute and relative contraindications to fibrinolytic therapy on them. Surgeons can assist the stroke team by alerting the stroke team if some of these contraindications are present. Some contraindications of which the surgeon may have a special knowledge are a history of head trauma in the previous 3 months, a clinical presentation suggestive of subarachnoid hemorrhage, a history of previous intracranial hemorrhage, a history of an arterial puncture within the last 7 days in a non-compressible site, the presence of active bleeding, or the presence of a bleeding diathesis, including those caused by anticoagulants. Relative contraindications for therapy including major surgery or serious trauma in the last 14 days or seizure at the onset of symptoms, all things of which the surgeon may have special knowledge.

Lastly, some patients may have fibrinolytic therapy out to 4.5 h from the onset of symptoms. In the geriatric age group an absolute contraindication for therapy over 3 h is age greater than 80 or being on any anticoagulant.

A key determinant of whether fibrinolytic therapy can be given is whether hemorrhage is present on the CT scan. Strokes are either ischemic or hemorrhagic and a hemorrhagic stroke is an absolute contraindication to the administration of fibrinolytic. For the acute care surgeon, the presence of hemorrhagic stroke should be considered in elderly trauma patients who present with intraparenchymal hemorrhage. The possibility of a hemorrhagic stroke causing a motor vehicle accident or a fall needs to be considered and the appropriate changes in the treatment paradigm considered. It is likely in these cases that the possibility of stroke will not be considered until the trauma head CT is obtained.

The key metrics for this system include onset to treatment time and "door-to-needle" time. To accomplish this, these guidelines emphasize the need for stroke to be cared for within a system of care. This system is comprised of primary stroke centers which are organized and equipped to provide specialized emergency stroke care and which are closely associated with a comprehensive stroke center which can provide more advanced stroke services such as neurointervention and neurocritical care. Many hospitals that do not have stroke teams have telemedicine arrangements with supporting institutions, allowing stroke experts to perform this decision and administer fibrinolytic prior to transporting the patient.

For the acute care surgeon, the goal is to identify a patient who may be having a stroke and to assure that the patient's stroke care is rapidly assumed by certified stroke system of care.

Guidelines for early stroke care are covered in the Advanced Cardiac Life Support course. These guidelines emphasize the early identification of stroke and then the previously mentioned rapid administration of rTPA to those appropriate to receive it [3].

Transient Ischemic Attack

On occasion, presenting stroke symptoms will clear, in the emergency department or prior to arrival in the emergency department. These patients should receive a non-contrast CT scan to survey for areas of hypodensity. A significant number of patients with transient symptoms will have findings on CT. Patients whose symptoms have cleared should have the NIHSS or Canadian Stroke Scales administered to assure that no microdefect is present. Once this is confirmed, no fibrinolytic therapy should be offered. Should patients with stroke scores of 0 have hypodensities on CT, fibrinolytics are contraindicated, both due to the increased risk of breakthrough hemorrhage at the site of infarction and due to the absence of treatable symptoms [3].

Previous definitions of TIA which defined TIA as symptoms lasting less than 24 h are less operative under current guidelines. Therapeutic decision making is now based on the immediate stroke scale and emergent imaging.

Patients with TIAs are generally admitted for workup of the causes of their TIA. Causes for TIA can include intra- or extracranial atherosclerosis and cardiac diseases such as atrial fibrillation, myocardial infarction or left ventricular thrombus, cardiomyopathy, and valvular heart disease. An EKG is appropriated in the early workup and follow-up echocardiography will be ordered by the managing team.

Progressive Stroke

One stroke scenario may require rapid decision making by the acute care surgeon and that is stroke in progression or crescendo TIA. Patients with steadily progressing stroke symptoms or worsening TIA need an emergent non-contrast head CT. If hemorrhage is not visualized, a CT angiogram or MRA should be obtained to look for severe stenosis or occlusion of the intracranial, carotid, or vertebral arteries. Emergent carotid endarterectomy has historically been considered in these patients. More commonly now, endovascular thrombolysis and stenting are considered, though, as of 2015, the efficacy of these methods was still being evaluated with ongoing trials. Of note, many of the these studies will not include patients over 70 years of age since it appears that they can expect a much less robust recovery from stoke, thereby reducing the utility of these high-risk procedures in the elderly [2, 3].

Spontaneous Intracerebral Hemorrhage

As noted above, obtaining a CT scan very early in the care of a patient suspected of stroke is essential. A key reason to obtain this scan is to identify patients who are suffering from a hemorrhagic stroke versus an ischemic stroke. Spontaneous intracerebral hemorrhages or hypertensive strokes have multiple etiologies, one of which is poorly controlled hypertension. They usually occur in the white matter of the brain, often in the basal ganglia.

Fibrinolytic therapy has no utility in hemorrhagic stroke and in fact is dangerous in these patients, making the presence of hemorrhagic strokes an absolute contraindications to the therapy.

Once a hemorrhagic stroke is identified, the patient should have a thorough history taken, focusing on time and pattern of onset of the symptoms, and the patient's history of hypertension, diabetes, elevated cholesterol, and smoking. Recent surgery, especially carotid surgery or stenting, should be noted. Any history of substance abuse, particularly cocaine use, should be noted as should any history of liver disease.

Complete vital signs should be obtained. Fever is associated with early neurologic deterioration in this patient group. The initial blood pressure is important; its management is discussed below. A thorough neurological examination is critical and should include some measure of level of consciousness, such as the Glasgow Coma Score. Complete blood count, coagulation studies, and electrolytes should be obtained as should toxicology studies to screen for cocaine and other sympathomimetic.

A principal concern in patients with ICH is hematoma expansion, which often leads to clinical deterioration. One factor often suspected on contributing to hematoma expansion is coagulopathy, often from oral anticoagulants or platelet abnormalities.

Patients with coagulopathy due to warfarin should have their INR reversed with PCC and vitamin K. PCC acts to lower INR significantly faster than vitamin K alone. Vitamin K can require hours to reverse coagulopathy and so should be used as an adjunct to more rapid reversal agents.

FFP has been used as a reversal agent in the past and studies have not demonstrated superiority in the outcome for PCC over FFP. However, PPC reverses the INR more rapidly than FFP and complications from fluid overload with FFP are well documented [4].

Recombinant factor VIIa does not restore all the vitamin K-dependent factors and so may not restore thrombin generation as well as PCC. rFVIIa has been studied in non-coagulopathic patients with ICH and has been found to limit enlargement of the hematoma but not to affect clinical outcome. These patients also had increased thromboembolic events resulting in a recommendation against rFVIIa in non-coagulopathic patients [5].

Other anticoagulants are now commonly seen in patients presenting with ICH. These new anticoagulants include factor II and factor Xa inhibitors. Antidotes to many of these new agents are now becoming available but their impact on limiting the expansion, morbidity, and mortality of ICH in patients taking these agents is unknown.

A second immediate concern in patients presenting with ICH is blood pressure management. Many patients have extremely high blood pressure after ICH. The concern in these patients is the perceived conflict between leaving the blood pressure elevated, risking expansion of the hematoma, and lowering the blood pressure too far, risking cerebral ischemia. Many practitioners feel that the injured brain requires a higher-than-normal pressure to stay perfused and so picking a target blood pressure for the ICH patient becomes important. There is evidence that lowering the SBP to 140 mmHg in patients presenting with an SBP of 150–220 mmHg is probably safe. AHA guidelines, however, recommend that in patients presenting with an SBP >180 or a MAP >150, and who do not have evidence of elevated ICP, lowering the SBP to around 160 mmHg or a MAP of 110 mmHg should be the goal. If the patient has clinical evidence of elevated ICP (pupillary asymmetry, asymmetric examination, declining GCS), then an ICP monitor should be placed and the blood pressure lowered while maintaining a CPP of 60 mmHg. Patients presenting with an SBP >200 mmHg or a MAP >150 mmHg should have their BP lowered immediately, irrespective of ICP, to 180 mmHg and then the previous guideline can be followed [4, 6].

The role of surgery in the management of ICH is uncertain. The tension is between the desire to reduce the mass effect of the clot as well as the toxicity of the hematoma to the surrounding brain and the morbidity of the procedure to remove it. In the supratentorial space, several large studies have failed to demonstrate that a surgery improves outcome. It has been pointed out frequently that the data in many of these studies may be corrupted by the failure to randomize patients who presented with "clearly surgical" lesions, who instead are taken to the OR outside of the study [4, 7, 8].

Patients with cerebellar lesions >3 cm in diameter, who are symptomatic, need surgery. The AHA guideline authors have made this a recommendation while stating that a study on this group is unlikely to be done. They caution against using a ventriculostomy as a temporizing measure in these patients. In the supratentorial space, however, there is no evidence that surgery improves outcome [4]. Patient with lesions larger than 30 cm^3, within 1 cm of the surface of the brain, may be appropriate candidates for evacuation but these patients did not reach statistical significance in the STITCH II trial [8]. In the thalamus and basal ganglia, where many of these bleeds occur, few consider evacuation of these clots, with the concordant severe morbidity, advisable. Decision making in the elderly is particularly difficult since they tolerate neither the clot nor the surgery well. The hazard of severe disability as an outcome is particularly high in the elderly, usually increased by surgery. It is the authors' practice to be particularly judicious with surgery in this age group.

Since clinical trials for surgery have failed to demonstrate a statistical benefit from surgery, trials to establish the optimum timing of surgery for ICH have also been inconclusive. Surgery from 4 to 96 h after presentation has been studied with no firm conclusion reached [4].

Acute care surgeons who find themselves managing an ICH should obtain the best history possible, reverse coagulation abnormalities, control the patient's blood pressure, and arrange to transfer care to a facility with neurosurgical and neurocritical care capabilities.

The emergent cerebrovascular imaging priorities for the elderly patient will be addressed by a head CT without contrast. In fact, it is important not to delay care, such as fibrinolytic therapy for ischemic stroke, for other studies. Follow-on studies, CT angiography, or MRI/MRA or MRV are often obtained. These studies are not needed for initial care but may be quickly needed for follow-on care. In the case of ischemic stroke for example, CT angiography or MRA will be needed if endovascular therapy is contemplated, either with intravenous fibrinolytic therapy or in lieu of it. In the case of spontaneous intracerebral hemorrhage, CT angiography and contrast-enhanced CT can show contrast extravasation from the hematoma, which is felt to be a predictor of hematoma expansion. In any case, follow-on noninvasive vascular imaging will often reveal several new pathologies of which the acute care surgeon should be aware.

Vascular Malformations

AVMs are malformations that allow arterial blood to flow directly into the venous system without the usual interposed capillary system. They enlarge with age and can progress from low-flow lesions in childhood to medium- to high-flow lesions in adulthood.

The peak age for hemorrhage of AVM is 15–20 years of age [9]. The average age of diagnosis for AVMs is 33 years old and 64% are diagnosed prior to age 40 [10]. There is, however, still an incidence into the later years.

AVM can occur in the dura, in the brain parenchyma, or as a combination of both. In the parenchyma, they can occur in the pial surface of the brain, subcortically, periventricularly, or as a combination of these.

Fifty percent of AVMs present as hemorrhage, and on noninvasive vascular imaging or a contrasted head CT, an AVM will be discovered as the source of the bleed [11]. Dural AVMs may appear as a large hemorrhage originating from a point on the dural surface usually near a dural venous sinus and usually the transverse sinus, the confluence of the transverse and sigmoid sinus or the tentorium.

Periventricular AVMs will hemorrhage at the wall of the ventricle, often hemorrhaging into the ventricle.

Subcortical and pial AVMs will appear as large hemorrhages with large complexes of blood vessels near or within them becoming apparent with noninvasive vascular imaging or contrast administration.

All AVMs will require a four-vessel angiogram and emergent neurosurgical consultation.

Aneurysmal Subarachnoid Hemorrhage

The most common cause of diffuse subarachnoid blood on CT is trauma. The finding, however, is usually associated with a ruptured aneurysm and this diagnosis should not be overlooked in elderly patients presenting emergently. The common conundrum in trauma is to determine if the SAH is due to the trauma or if the trauma was caused by a rupturing aneurysm.

The peak age for aneurysmal rupture is 55–60 years old, making it more of a geriatric diagnosis [12]. Patients over 70 tend to present with a greater degree of neurological impairment [13].

The greatest threat to a patient presenting with a ruptured aneurysm is rebleeding. Securing the aneurysm to prevent this is a critical priority early in presentation. Obtaining neurosurgical and neurointerventional services for this purpose, quickly, is crucial.

In elderly patients presenting with SAH, the index of suspicion for a ruptured aneurysm should be high, even in those presenting with a trauma history. After the patient is stabilized, noninvasive imaging should be used to rule out an aneurysm.

Once an aneurysm is identified, there are three priorities to the patient's care. First, blood pressure must be scrupulously controlled. As with spontaneous intracerebral hemorrhage, the goal is to lower the blood pressure enough to lower the risk of rerupture but not enough to create new cerebral ischemia. Each practitioner will have their own guideline but maintaining the SBP in the 120–150 range, depending on the patient's baseline blood pressure, is usual.

Second, arrangements must be made to secure the aneurysm. The greatest threat to a patient presenting with a ruptured aneurysm is rerupture. Four percent of secured aneurysms will rebleed within the first day. Fifteen to twenty percent will rebleed within the first 14 days [14]. Making rapid arrangements to secure the aneurysm will mitigate this risk. These arrangements must include prompt neurosurgical and neurointerventional consults and arrangement for a four-vessel angiogram.

This angiogram should be performed by a neurointerventionist, allowing the aneurysm to be secured at the same time, if possible, and avoiding the additional risk and delay of a second angiogram. In the vast majority of centers, the interventional radiologist and the neurosurgeon work closely together and will decide together which aneurysms should be coiled and which should be clipped. There is little utility in four-vessel angiograms obtained outside of the institution that will do the final treatment. Obtaining these angiograms adds unneeded risk and delays the transfer of the patient to definitive care.

Third, subarachnoid blood can occlude the outflow of cerebral spinal fluid from the brain causing hydrocephalous. Patients with aneurysmal rupture can develop hydrocephalous rapidly. Early placement of an EVD is needed. This also requires the early involvement of a neurosurgeon.

A fourth threat to these patients is vasospasm. If this is to occur, it usually occurs 7–14 days after the hemorrhage. Strategies for treating or limiting vasospasm include keeping the patient slightly hypervolemic and allowing the blood pressure to rise, permissive hypertension. These will not be concerns of the acute care surgeon since the patient will have been transferred to more specialized care during this period. It is mentioned here only to emphasize that neither of the strategies is appropriate until the aneurysm has been secured.

In a similar fashion, hyponatremia, usually due to cerebral salt wasting, may occur later in the patient's course and is addressed with volume resuscitation and some salt replacement. Once again, aggressive fluid resuscitation should be avoided until the aneurysm has been secured.

Cerebral Vein Thrombosis

A wide variety of conditions have been associated with cerebral venous thrombosis, including pregnancy, birth control pills, sickle cell disease, dehydration, infections, malignancy, hypercoagulable states, and trauma.

The most commonly involved sinuses are the superior sagittal sinus and the left transverse sinus.

Blockage of these vessels impedes cerebral blood flow creating ischemia. The presentation of deep cerebral vein thrombosis is highly variable. Some clues that it may be present are bilateral, white matter infarctions on the CT scan. The patients commonly have a headache in addition to other less common symptoms. Papilledema is an unusual finding that is commonly found in deep cerebral vein thrombosis and may provide a clue to its presence. The definitive diagnosis can be made with noninvasive imaging, CT angiography, or MRA.

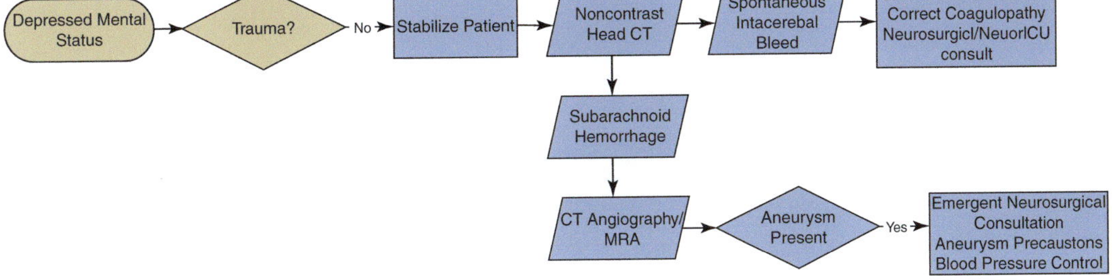

References

1. Mozaffarian D, Benjamin EJ, Go AS, Arnett DK. Heart disease and stroke statistics-2016 update: a report from the American Heart Association. Circulation. 2016;133(4):e38–60.
2. Powers WJ, Derdeyn CP, Biller J, Coffey CS, Hoh BL, Jauch EC, Johnston KC, Johnston SC, Khalessi AA, Kidwell CS, Meschia JF, Ovbiagele B, Yavagal DR. 2015 American Heart Association/American Stroke Association focused update of the 2013 guidelines for the early management of patients with acute ischemic stroke regarding endovascular treatment: a guideline for healthcare professionals from the American Heart Association/American Stroke Association. Stroke. 2015;46(10):3020–35.
3. Jauch EC, Saver JL, Adams HP Jr, Bruno A, Connors JJ, Demaerschalk BM, Khatri P, McMullan PW Jr, Qureshi AI, Rosenfield K, Scott PA, Summers DR, Wang DZ, Wintermark M, Yonas H. Guidelines for the early management of patients with acute ischemic stroke: a guideline for healthcare professionals from the American Heart Association/American Stroke Association. Stroke. 2013;44(3):870–947.
4. Morgenstern LB, Hemphill JC 3rd, Anderson C, Becker K, Broderick JP, Connolly ES Jr, Greenberg SM, Huang JN, MacDonald RL, Messe SR, Mitchell PH, Selim M, Tamargo RJ. Guidelines for the management of spontaneous intracerebral hemorrhage: a guideline for healthcare professionals from the American Heart Association/American Stroke Association. Stroke. 2010;41(9):2108–29.
5. Mayer SA, Brun NC, Begtrup K, Broderick J, Davis S, Diringer MN, Skolnick BE, Steiner T. Efficacy and safety of recombinant activated factor VII for acute intracerebral hemorrhage. N Engl J Med. 2008;358(20):2127–37.
6. Anderson CS, Huang Y, Wang JG, Arima H, Neal B, Peng B, Heeley E, Skulina C, Parsons MW, Kim JS, Tao QL, Li YC, Jiang JD, Tai LW, Zhang JL, Xu E, Cheng Y, Heritier S, Morgenstern LB, Chalmers J. Intensive blood pressure reduction in acute cerebral haemorrhage trial (INTERACT): a randomised pilot trial. Lancet Neurol. 2008;7(5):391–9.
7. Mendelow AD, Gregson BA, Fernandes HM, Murray GD, Teasdale GM, Hope DT, Karimi A, Shaw MD, Barer DH. Early surgery versus initial conservative treatment in patients with spontaneous supratentorial intracerebral haematomas in the International Surgical Trial in Intracerebral Haemorrhage (STICH): a randomised trial. Lancet. 2005;365(9457):387–97.
8. Mendelow AD, Gregson BA, Rowan EN, Murray GD, Gholkar A, Mitchell PM. Early surgery versus initial conservative treatment in patients with spontaneous supratentorial lobar intracerebral haematomas (STICH II): a randomised trial. Lancet. 2013;382(9890):397–408.
9. Perret G, Nishioka H. Report on the cooperative study of intracranial aneurysms and subarachnoid hemorrhage. Section VI. Arteriovenous malformations. An analysis of 545 cases of cranio-cerebral arteriovenous malformations and fistulae reported to the cooperative study. J Neurosurg. 1966;25(4):467–90.
10. Ondra SL, Troupp H, George ED, Schwab K. The natural history of symptomatic arteriovenous malformations of the brain: a 24-year follow-up assessment. J Neurosurg. 1990;73(3):387–91.
11. Drake CG. Cerebral arteriovenous malformations: considerations for and experience with surgical treatment in 166 cases. Clin Neurosurg. 1979;26:145–208.
12. Biller J, Toffol GJ, Kassell NF, Adams HP Jr, Beck DW, Boarini DJ. Spontaneous subarachnoid hemorrhage in young adults. Neurosurgery. 1987;21(5):664–7.
13. Yamashita K, Kashiwagi S, Kato S, Takasago T, Ito H. Cerebral aneurysms in the elderly in Yamaguchi, Japan. Analysis of the Yamaguchi Data Bank of Cerebral Aneurysm from 1985 to 1995. Stroke. 1997;28(10):1926–31.
14. Winn HR, Richardson AE, Jane JA. The long-term prognosis in untreated cerebral aneurysms: I. The incidence of late hemorrhage in cerebral aneurysm: a 10-year evaluation of 364 patients. Ann Neurol. 1977;1(4):358–70.

24 Geriatric Vascular Trauma and Vascular emergencies

Justin Boccardo

Peripheral Vascular Injuries

Justin Boccardo, M.D., F.A.C.S.
Department of Vascular Surgery,
Bayfront Punta Gorda,
700 East Marion Ave,
Punta Gorda, FL, 33950, USA
justinboccardo@hotmail.com

Abstract
We review the epidemiology, diagnosis, and management of vascular injuries to the extremities in this chapter. For the purpose of practical learning we define the extremities as upper anything distal to the intrathoracic subclavian artery, and lower as anything distal to the common iliac arteries. We present any injuries resulting from blunt and penetrating noniatrogenic trauma.

Keywords
Peripheral trauma; Vascular injuries; Geriatric vascular trauma

J. Boccardo, M.D., F.A.C.S.
Department of Vascular Surgery, Bayfront Punta Gorda, 700 East Marion Ave, Punta Gorda, FL 33950, USA
e-mail: justinboccardo@hotmail.com

Introduction

Any injury to a peripheral vessel could result in major morbidity and limb loss and even lead to death if not diagnosed and treated promptly. This is particularly important when dealing with the geriatric population.

Great improvements and evolution of technology have occurred in the diagnosis and treatment of peripheral vascular diseases in the last decades. We will show how endovascular interventions can aide and sometimes even replace the traditional open techniques to treat these injuries. In the geriatric population these minimally invasive alternatives can reduce blood loss and cardiovascular events.

Epidemiology

Vascular trauma is rare in the geriatric patient population. These injuries are predominantly blunt, with the thoracic aorta being the most commonly injured vessel. Peripheral injuries occur mostly from penetrating trauma or associated with major orthopedic trauma. Although vascular injuries occur less frequently than in the nongeriatric cohort, in the geriatric patient, vascular injury is associated with a fourfold increase in adjusted mortality [1].

A. Rodriguez et al. (eds.), *Geriatric Trauma and Acute Care Surgery*,
https://doi.org/10.1007/978-3-319-57403-5_24

Diagnosis

Taking into consideration the care of the patient holistically, here we focus on the vascular injuries themselves.

Many times patients arrive to the hospital with tourniquets or manual/digital pressure to the affected limb. However, peripheral injuries are not always easy to identify and may lead to difficult resuscitation efforts, limb loss, or even death if not identified and treated promptly.

The classic assessment of "hard" and "soft" signs can become very helpful to determine the next step in management (Table 24.1). These signs require basic physical exam skills and are for the most part self-explanatory. The soft signs, though, will most of the times require additional diagnostic modalities, many times leading to catheter angiography for not only diagnosis but also treatment of these injuries.

During the examination of the patient, ankle brachial index (ABI) and wrist brachial index (WBI) are a very useful, simple, quick, and noninvasive way of identifying perfusion anomalies. It is performed by measuring the pressure which results in the loss of Doppler signals after compressing proximally with a pressure cuff. The index is calculated by dividing the ankle value to the brachial one for ABI and the wrist value to the brachial one for WBI. Anything below 0.9 is abnormal (Figs. 24.1 and 24.2) [2].

Table 24.1 Hard signs and Soft signs in vascular trauma

Clinical signs of extremity arterial injury
Hard signs
• Absent distal pulse
• Palpable thrill or audible bruit
• Actively expanding hematoma
• Active pulsatile bleeding
Soft signs
• Diminished distal pulse
• History of significant hemorrhage
• Neurologic deficit
• Proximity of wound to named vessel

Computer tomographic angiography (CTA) is widely used in trauma patients. It is very helpful in localizing vessel injuries and other associated injuries around the blood vessels. It has reduced the number of catheter angiographies performed as well as ultrasounds for vessel injuries.

Treatment Options

Observation

Surgical therapy is not required in all cases of vessel injury. This is particularly important when dealing with geriatric population, with limited reserve, common coronary, and renal disease, that would make any invasive procedure high risk.

Some reports have shown that nonoperative management is acceptable in some instances [3]. Small, non-flow-limiting dissections, small extravasations, and arteriovenous fistulas can all be observed for resolution or progression of limb threat.

Endovascular Treatment

Reports of endovascular therapy have shown equal results to open in terms of limb salvage and bleeding control [4]. Since its low invasiveness compared to open revascularization, it reduces morbidity in situation where there are multi-organ trauma and multiple comorbidities present.

Endovascular techniques are diagnostic and therapeutic. But in many instances they can help in bleeding control until access and control to the vessel by open surgery is achieved (Fig. 24.3).

If the guidewire can pass through the affected site, a covered stent should strongly be considered as definitive treatment for a transection or an occlusive injury (Fig. 24.4).

The main issue with endovascular treatments is the presence of thrombosis distal to the injured site. Percutaneous thrombectomy catheters may

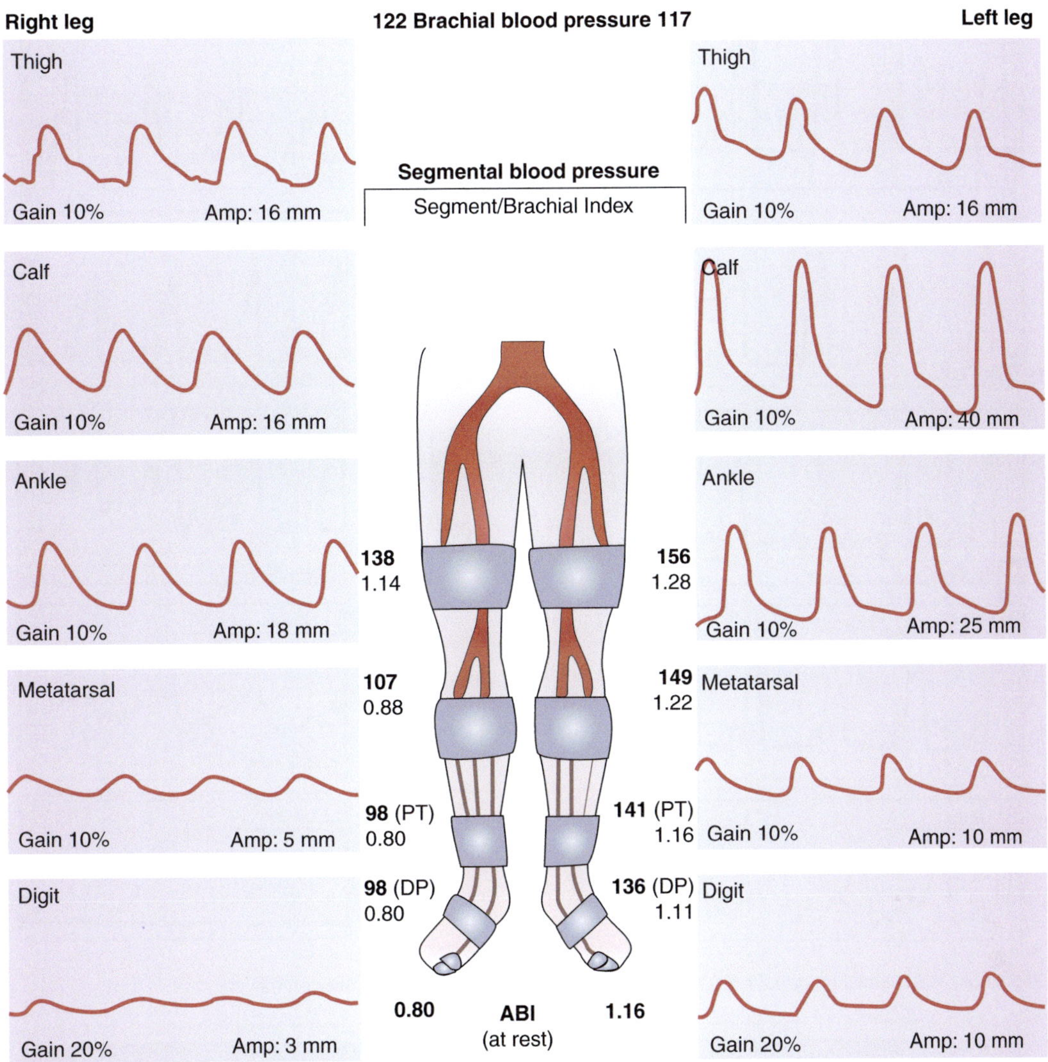

Fig. 24.1 ABI showing normal values for the left lower extremity and abnormal values on the right

be ineffective to completely restore flow to the limb. However, hybrid interventions where the repair of the injured artery can be performed with a stent graft and the thrombectomy to open the vessel distally, are becoming more common and very successful. This way of thinking unfolds one very complex situation into a few simpler ones dealt with separately.

Open Treatment

Even though open control and repair are still considered "standard of care" for traumatic vessel injuries, in today's technologically ever-evolving world, it must be considered one more tool and not more or less important than other techniques. When considering open revascularization, the surgical bed should be

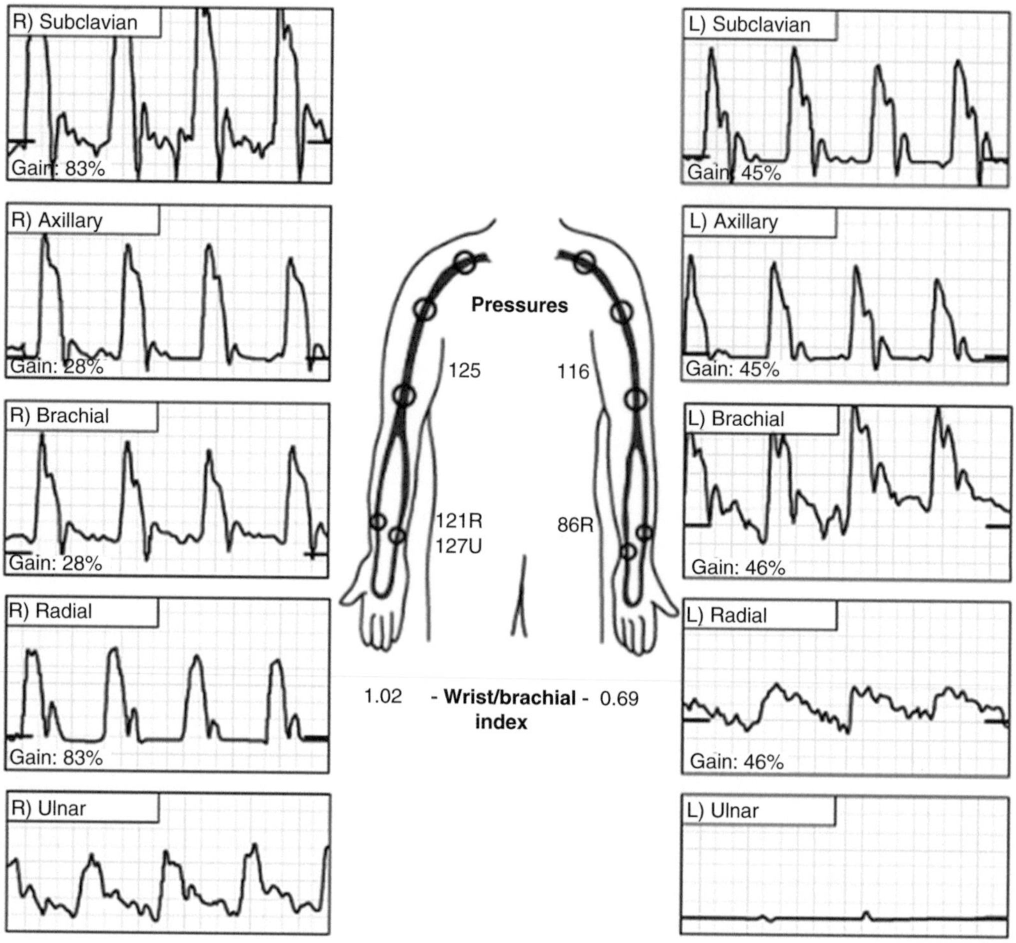

Fig. 24.2 WBI showing normal right upper extremity values and abnormal values on the left

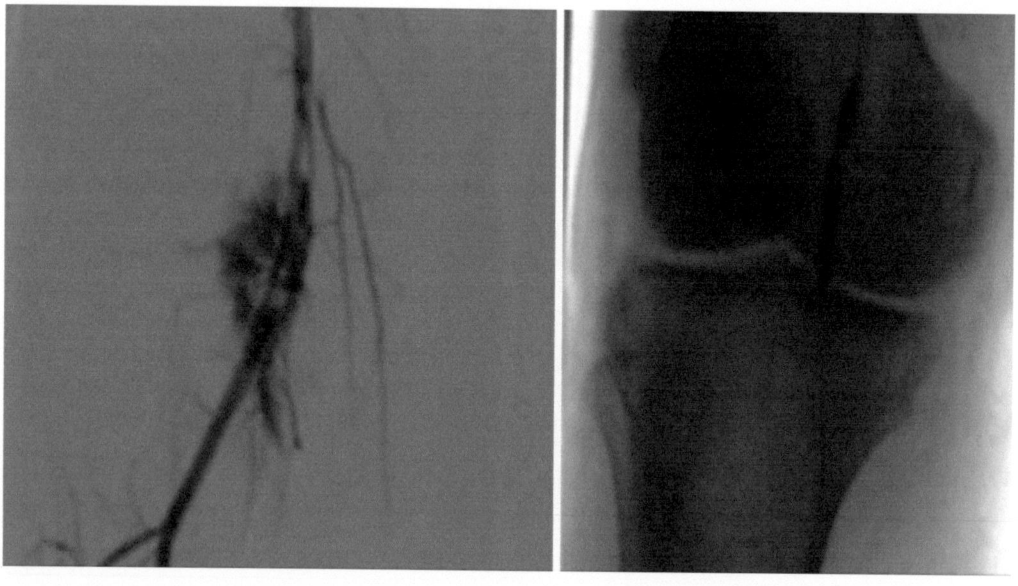

Fig. 24.3 Extravasation of popliteal artery injury controlled with intra-arterial balloon

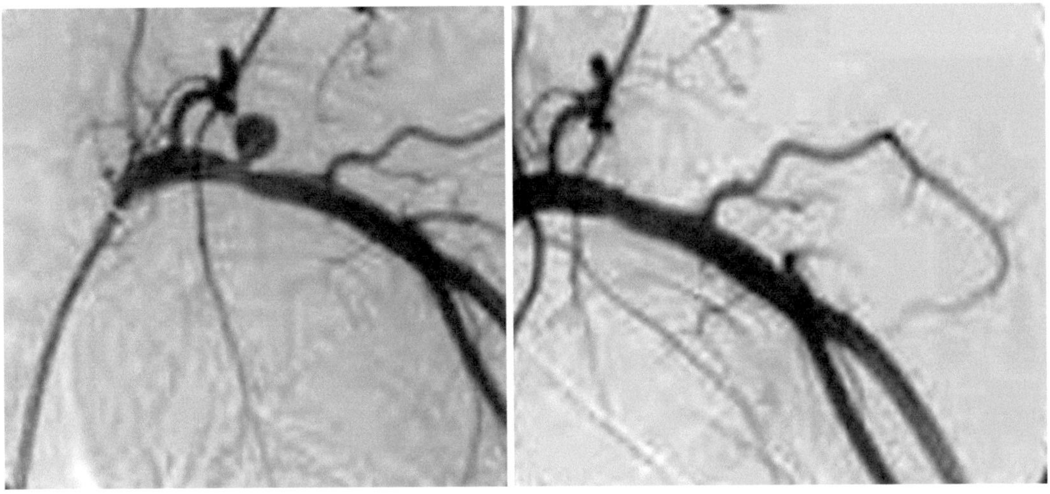

Fig. 24.4 Left subclavian artery injury after stab to shoulder repaired with covered stent graft

radiolucent and the team should be prepared to add endovascular instrumentation at any time during the case.

When conduit for revascularization is needed, using the greater saphenous vein (GSV) from the injured or affected limb is common practice. No data supports this way of practice, but creating more trauma to an otherwise functional limb may delay recovery and cause increased morbidity.

Proximal and distal control should be obtained, and in areas where this may be hindered by tissue trauma or orthopedic elements, endovascular proximal control is preferred.

Vascular repair is intended to control bleeding and restore in-line flow to the affected limb. Many times the latter is not possible because of hemodynamic instability or extensive tissue loss. The geriatric population does not appear to have higher amputation rates than other trauma demographics. They do, however, have higher postoperative mortality and morbidity rates as previously noted.

The possible repairs are direct repair with end-to-end anastomosis by spatulated ends, bypass, or patch angioplasty. Autologous vein should be used in the last two if possible. Prosthetic materials carry a higher risk of infection and lower patency rates [5].

Early fasciotomy should be considered in all patients with revascularization of an extremity after ischemia resulting from trauma. Fasciotomies make wound management complex.

Postoperative Care

Standard intensive care monitoring of critically ill geriatric trauma patients is described elsewhere. However, pulse and Doppler signal exams are performed hourly in conjunction with vital signs. The location and quality of the pulse (present, absent, weak) or the Doppler signal are documented by nursing and surgical team. Change in the vascular examination or signs of bleeding warrant immediate communication with the surgeon.

Mechanical thromboprophylaxis in the form of pneumatic compression devices is initiated along with subcutaneous prophylactic dosing of heparin or low-molecular-weight heparin if the risk of bleeding is sufficiently low. When a venous injury was treated with ligation, the leg should be elevated and wrapped from the toes to the groin with compression with openings to monitor the arterial pulse or the Doppler signal. Compartment syndrome should always be evaluated even if a fasciotomy has been performed.

Conclusion

Vascular trauma in the geriatric population is uncommon, but if not treated promptly it has a high limb loss rate. Initial hemorrhage control including the use of tourniquets and direct or manual pressure with or without hemostatic agents is part of the treatment algorithm.

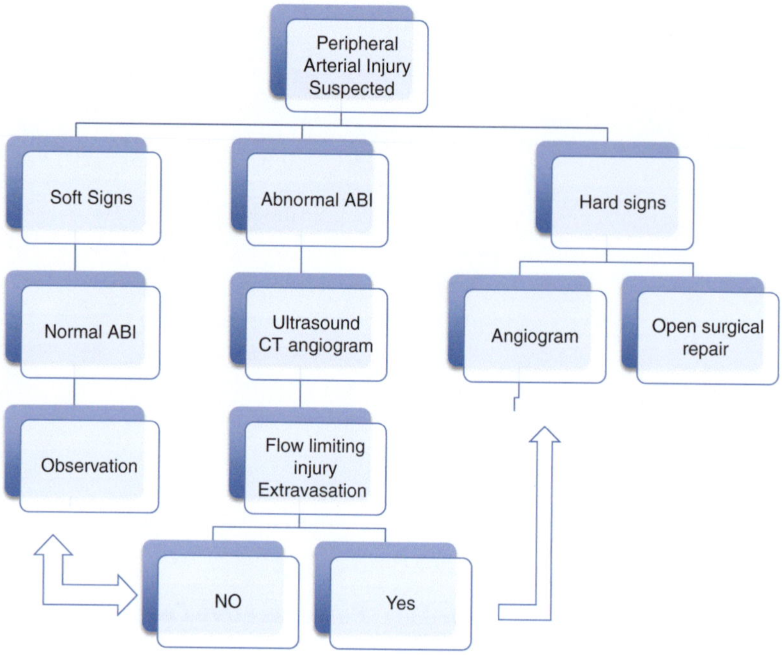

With hemorrhage control, the management sequence is:

1. Evaluation and diagnosis of injury level
2. Restoration of perfusion by open or endovascular techniques
3. Close postoperative monitoring

The choice of management depends on the anatomic location of the extremity vascular injury, the physiologic status of the patient, and the ability of the surgical team to incorporate endovascular tools to the treatment.

A multidisciplinary approach is imperative in these cases. The low functional reserve seen in some of these geriatric patients makes endovascular revascularization very appealing in spite of its lower patency rates.

Abdominal Aortic Aneurysm Rupture Repair in the Geriatric Population

Justin Boccardo, M.D., F.A.C.S.
Department of Vascular Surgery,
Bayfront Punta Gorda,
700 East Marion Ave, Punta Gorda,
FL, 33950, USA
justinboccardo@hotmail.com

Abstract

AAA is relatively common in the elderly. EVAR in this population is efficient with a success rate exceeding 90% in all cases. Since open repair has extensively being reported and studied, we focus on endovascular repair of this pathology in this chapter.

Introduction

The prevalence of abdominal aortic aneurysm (AAA) is difficult to report; however it is diagnosed in 5–10% of men above the age of 65 [6]. Endovascular abdominal aortic aneurysm repair (EVAR) has been well tested and it has become the primary means of repair for elective patients. The large EVAR trials have shown that it is associated with less operating time and blood loss and better perioperative morbidity than open repair [7]. EVAR is more than an alternative to open repair for the elderly, who have significantly more comorbidities and less reserve.

EVAR is safe in octogenarians and it is superior to open repair across various age spectrums in terms of postoperative early and medium-term morbidity [8–11].

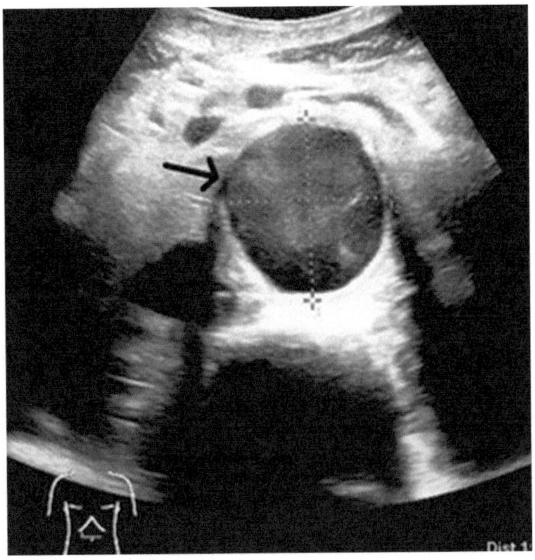

Fig. 24.5 Ultrasound of the abdomen showing an abdominal aortic aneurysm. Note the iliac veins pushed to the side in front of the aneurysm

Diagnosis and Treatment

The classic presentation of ruptured AAA is hypotension, abdominal pain, and a pulsatile abdominal mass. However, this triad is found in less than half of cases. Hypotension might be transient and could have resolved if the bleeding is retroperitoneal and has tamponaded, temporarily. Rupture can also present with isolated back rather than abdominal pain [12].

Extreme caution must be taken when examining an elderly individual with new renal colic, musculoskeletal back pain, or even syncope without considering ruptured AAA. In these workups, AAA should be in the differential diagnosis list.

Once the diagnosis of AAA is entertained, a bedside ultrasound is fast and very useful to aid in the diagnosis (Fig. 24.5).

CT is the preferred imaging study for any patient being considered for EVAR. Not only will it diagnose the AA and its rupture, but it also provides crucial information for landing zones, graft sizes, and conduits (Fig. 24.6) in preparation for repair.

Permissive hypotension (SBP of 80–100 mm Hg) during this diagnostic phase is of utmost importance since aggressive resuscitation might create pressures in the arterial system that could cause rebleeding in an otherwise contained rupture. This is aided by adequate pain control and beta-blockers.

Once the decision is made to take the patient to the operating room, induction of anesthesia should not be initiated until the field has been prepped and draped for both open and endovascular repair.

In the operating room, bilateral groin cut downs for vessel control is our access of choice. However, there have been reports of percutaneous access as well [13].

An intra-aortic occlusive balloon can be placed in the suprarenal position to control

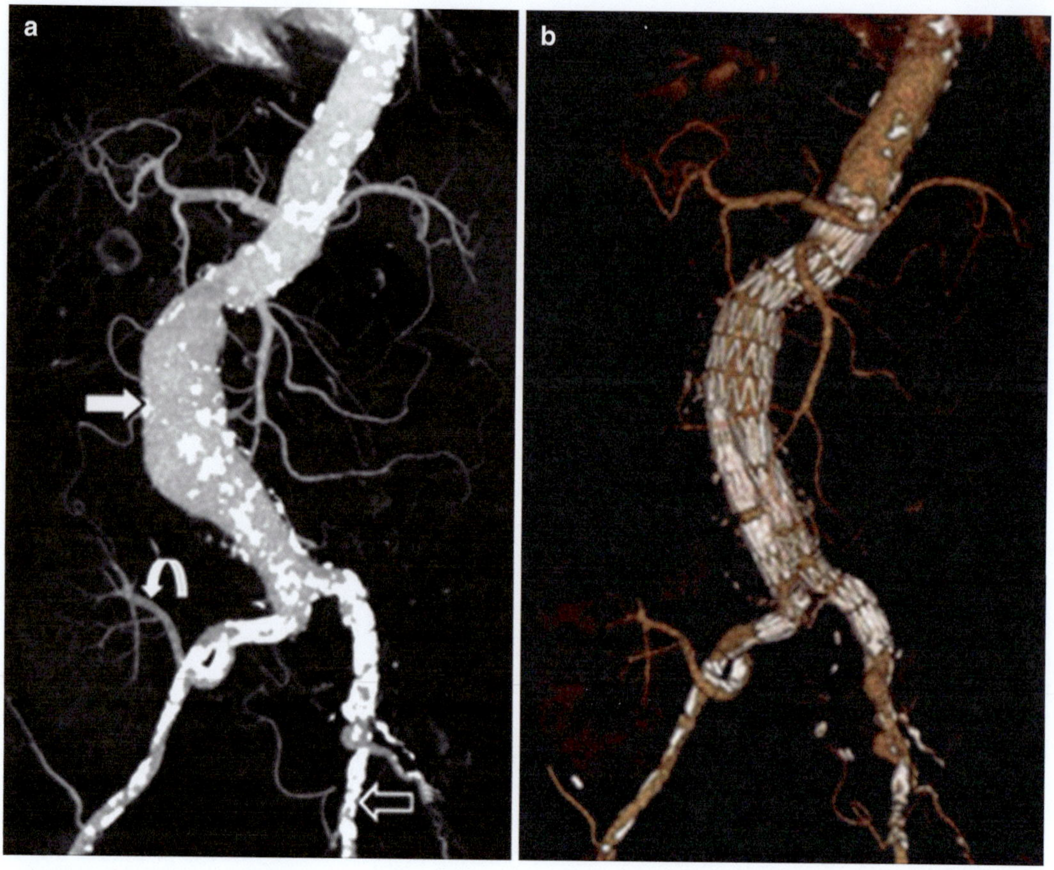

Fig. 24.6 (**a**) CTA reconstruction showing an infrareanl aneurysm with the exact position of the renal, internal, and external iliac arteries with their measurements. (**b**) EVAR completion with the stent graft in place excluding the arterial flow away from the aneurysm

bleeding in the unstable patient. Otherwise, one can proceed with the deployment of the endografts. Once no threatening endoleaks are present, we start with full resuscitation measures as needed, including blood transfusions and coagulopathy treatment.

It is very important to have a rupture AAA protocol in place at the institution for minimal time wasting and graft availability (Fig. 24.7) [15, 16].

Overview

The National Hospital Discharge Survey results showed a mortality rate for repair of ruptured AAAs of 48% (95% CI 46–50%) in 2002 [17].

Any improvement in these results is welcomed. EVAR appears to provide many answers to this complex issue.

There are seven retrospective studies analyzing non-ruptured EVAR results in an elderly population. A recent meta-analysis by Biancari et al. [18] included six of these studies [19–24]. They found significantly higher perioperative mortality after open repair (pooled mortality rates: 8.6% vs. 2.3%; risk ratio: 3.87; 95% CI: 3.19–4.68).

Several randomized trials have compared open repair versus EVAR in patients with ruptured AAA [14, 16, 25–34]. The Dutch trial randomly assigned 132 patients who were anatomically suitable for either repair similarly and found no difference in 30-day mortality between EVAR and OR (25 versus 21%).

Overall, EVAR is better in terms of early- and medium-term mortality and morbidity in both elective and ruptured geriatric patients.

EVAR is now employed as a first-line procedure for the treatment of a non-ruptured AAA in anatomically suitable candidates. Randomized

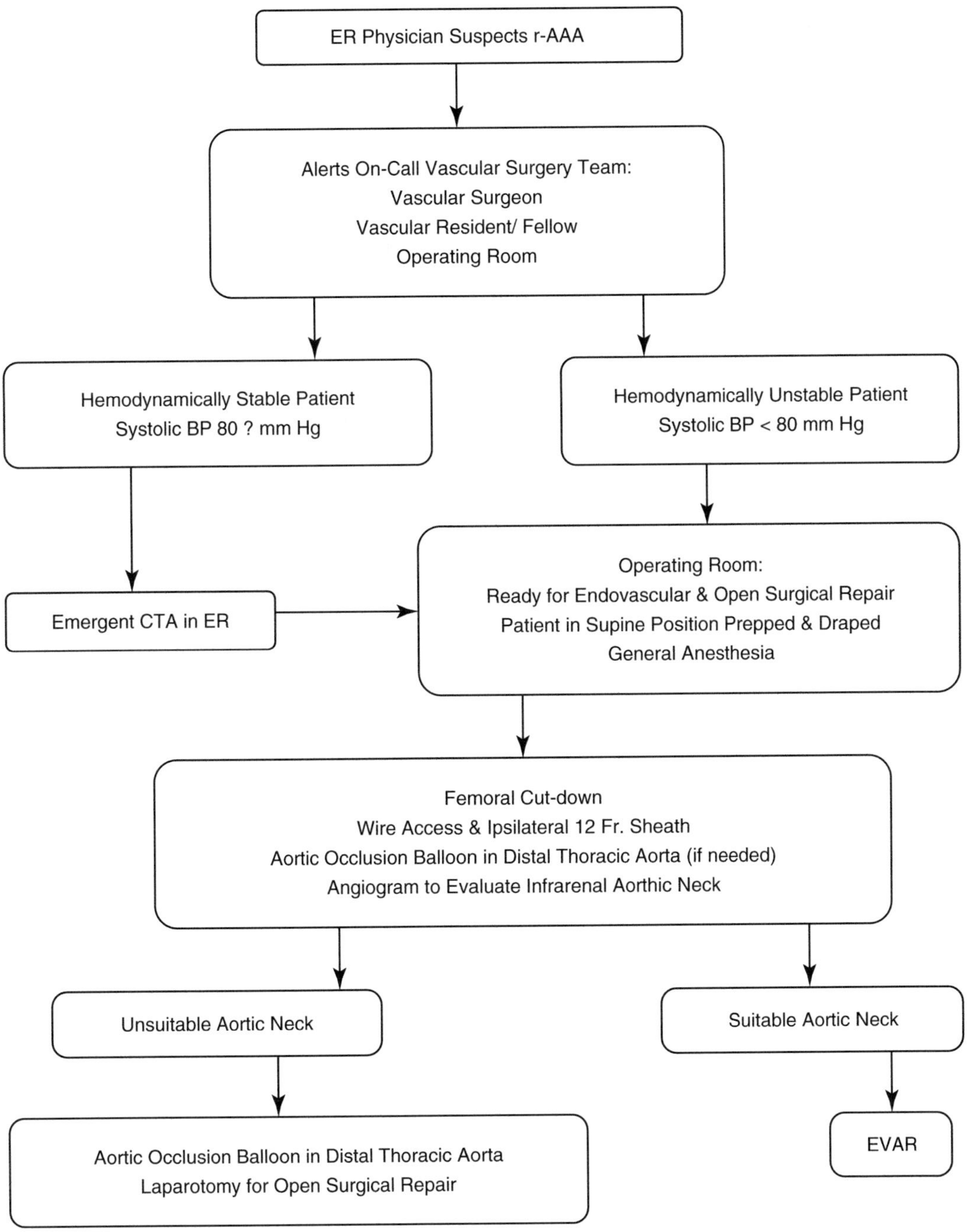

Fig. 24.7 Ruptured AAA protocol guiding care [14]

controlled trials and large prospective registries disclosed a clear early mortality and morbidity benefit over open repair and similar medium- and long-term results for the general population, even with the high re-intervention rates. Brinkman et al. reported a 68% survival (Kaplan-Meier analysis) 3 years after EVAR in octogenarians and Fonseca et al. a 95% survival rate after 5 years.

Re-intervention is the main drawback of EVAR, as evidenced in randomized studies and other multicenter reports. Even using the latest generation devices in a relatively healthy population, such as in the ACE trial, re-intervention among those undergoing EVAR remains as high as 16% over a period of 3 years (2.4% vs. 16%, $P < 0.0001$).

An interesting observation is the fact that EVAR seems to benefit this old population the most, in terms of preventing morbidity and mortality, at least over the short term. In the large analysis by Schwarze et al. including all hospital discharges for EVAR and open aneurysm repair over a 5-year period, patients above the age of 85 had the greatest benefit in terms of early mortality, cardiovascular complications, pulmonary complications, hospital stay, and acute renal failure compared to the younger cohorts. Schermerhorn et al. found that the perioperative EVAR survival benefit was strongly related to age, with those above the age of 85 having an absolute reduction in mortality of 8.5%, which was maintained at 3 years.

Overall, we suggest that EVAR is the preferred method of treating an AAA in the elderly, both elective and ruptured. The currently available data confirm its superiority in terms of early morbidity and mortality among the general population, and the fact that it performs similar to open repair in the medium term. All registries and studies comparing EVAR and open repair in those above the age of 80 have disclosed superior performance in the early-term and 5-year survival rates can be as high as 95%. This practically means that EVAR should be the procedure of choice in the geriatric population, when anatomical criteria are met.

Acute Mesenteric Ischemia

Justin Boccardo, M.D., F.A.C.S.
Department of Vascular Surgery,
Bayfront Punta Gorda,
700 East Marion Ave, Punta Gorda,
FL, 33950, USA
justinboccardo@hotmail.com

Abstract
The diagnosis and management of patients with acute mesenteric arterial ischemia (AMI) are challenging. This chapter reviews the etiology, clinical presentation, diagnosis, and treatment for patients with AMI. The information in this chapter is based on our experience, as well as selected data that we have analyzed from the literature.

Introduction

Acute mesenteric ischemia (AMI) is a life-threatening condition and many times treatment is not initiated due to missed diagnoses. Operative superior mesenteric artery (SMA) embolectomy for AMI is the mainstay of treatment. Angiography, vasodilators, and technological improvements have reduced the mortality to approximately 50% [35, 36].

Endovascular or hybrid endovascular-surgical treatments for all forms of AMI are increasing in their use and results are equal or better than historical reports.

Epidemiology

Most patients are 60–70 years old. Women are affected three times as frequently as men are [37, 38].

Patients with a history of atrial fibrillation or flutter, recent myocardial infarction, congestive heart failure, or peripheral arterial emboli are at risk for an SMA embolus. In contrast, a careful history may reveal postprandial abdominal pain, weight loss, and food intolerance, all of which clearly raise the suspicion of an acute SMA thrombotic occlusion.

The most common risk factors are smoking and hypertension. Two-thirds of patients have had symptomatic disease in the coronary, cerebrovascular, renal, or peripheral circulation [39, 40].

A national database review identified that patients undergoing angioplasty and stenting for AMI had higher rates of comorbidities than those undergoing open surgical repair, including hypertension, peripheral vascular disease, coronary artery disease, atrial fibrillation or flutter, and chronic renal failure [41].

Diagnosis

The patients have a history of severe abdominal pain out of proportion to their physical examination findings. Delays in diagnosis and treatment remain the greatest challenge to reducing morbidity and mortality for all forms of AMI [42].

High clinical suspicion is very important and the diagnosis should be confirmed by an imaging study such as CTA, MRA, or angiography. Ultrasound is helpful in limited cases due to the extreme pain and limited imagines obtained due to the patient's poor compliance in these situations [43].

Laboratory results may be inconclusive depending on the stage of the disease process. The most common laboratory abnormalities are hemoconcentration, leukocytosis, high anion gap, and possibly lactic acidosis in more advanced cases. Lactic acid is an indirect marker of tissue injury. It is usually elevated in AMI patients. However, it is seldom elevated early and specifically enough in the serum to diagnose acute mesenteric ischemia [44]. High amylase, aspartate aminotransferase, and lactate dehydrogenase can also be observed [45] (Fig. 24.8).

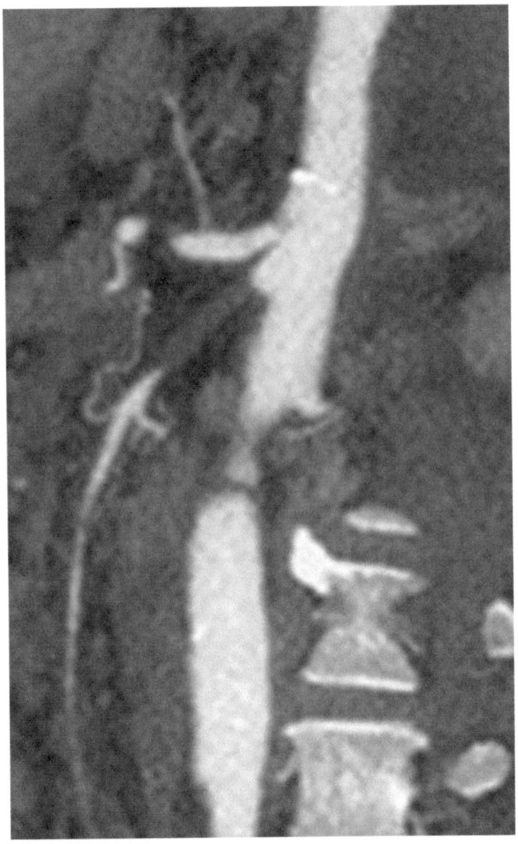

Fig. 24.8 CTA showing SMA thrombosis with reconstitution past the occlusion

Superior mesenteric vein (SMV) thrombosis, often caused by a hypercoagulable state, is present in 5–15% of cases of AMI. It is rare in the geriatric population. There is usually a personal or family history of venous thromboembolism.

Non-occlusive mesenteric ischemia (NOMI) develops as the result of a low-flow state with vasospasm of the branches of the SMA, rather than acute occlusion. NOMI can develop in patients who are hypotensive, on vasopressors, severely volume depleted, or on dialysis. Generally more common in critically ill patients, it may occur acutely in situations such as trauma or cocaine abuse. NOMI has a very high mortality rate, likely due to the combination of comorbidities and difficulty in making this diagnosis [46].

Treatment

AMI is a surgical emergency. Patients presenting with anything suggestive of AMI should undergo arteriography or CTA before operation if there is no evidence of peritonitis or shock. Patients with rebound tenderness, abdominal rigidity, severe acidosis, or shock should undergo immediate operation [35, 36].

Fluid resuscitation should begin immediately with isotonic crystalloid solution and continue with blood, if necessary. Electrolyte imbalances (hyperkalemia) should be monitored and corrected along with broad-spectrum antibiotics. If there are no contraindications, intravenous heparin for full anticoagulation should be initiated.

In our experience, we make sure that intravascular volume has been maximized before initiating vasopressors.

Endovascular Intervention

Thrombolysis followed by balloon angioplasty or stent placement of the stenotic artery at the time of arteriography is a reasonable option if diagnosis is made early, the patient is hemodynamically stable, there are no signs of peritonitis, and the thrombus burden is small [47]. This allows for revascularization without the need for a laparotomy in an already compromised individual. Failure of thrombolytic therapy or a worsening clinical status warrants operation.

Laparoscopy has become more useful for "quick look" even after successful endovascular revascularization in patients that remain intubated or with altered mental status that makes their exam unreliable.

The goals of therapy are always restoration of SMA blood flow and resection of nonviable bowel.

Open Revascularization

If the patient has peritoneal signs, or the endovascular instruments are not available, laparotomy with open thrombectomy has excellent results as well [37].

The SMA is isolated at the base of the mesentery with the transverse colon retracted superiorly and the small intestine retracted toward the right side except for the distal duodenum or proximal jejunum.

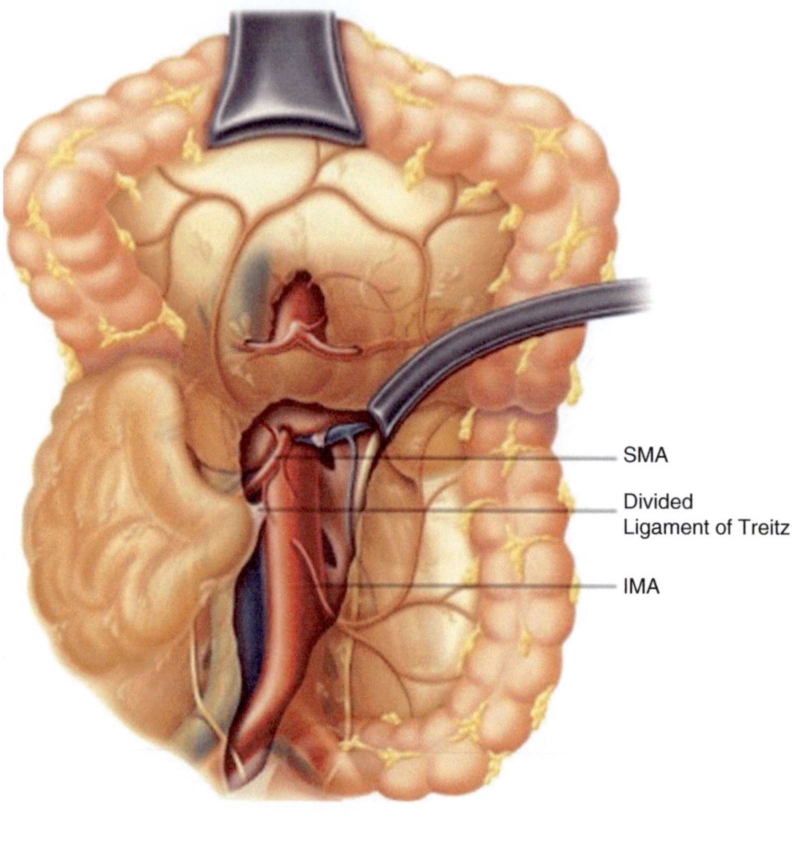

Table 24.2 Outcomes after open and endovascular revascularization for acute superior mesenteric artery occlusion *n* (%)

References	Publication year	Population	Study period	Endovascular or hybrid therapy/all cases	Bowel resection	30-d or in-hospital mortality
Schermerhorn et al. [22]	2009	United States	2000–2006	1875 (35)	2138 (41)	1615 (31)
Block et al. [18]	2010	Sweden	1999–2006	42 (26)	80 (51)[a]	61 (37)
Arthurs et al. [23]	2011	Cleveland, OH, United States	1999–2008	56 (80)	60 (80)	29 (41)
Ryer et al. [24]	2012	Rochester, MI, United States	1990–2010	11 (12)	38 (41)	20 (22)

[a]Incomplete data in six patients

If the artery is soft, it is opened transversely. Embolectomy catheters (3 and 4) are passed proximally and distally in the artery to extract the embolic material and thrombus. Primary closure is performed.

The artery should be opened longitudinally if clinical findings or the arteriogram suggests in situ thrombosis or if atherosclerotic disease is palpable in the SMA. Closure can be done with saphenous vein, bovine pericardium, or prosthetic if excellent inflow is achieved.

Outcomes

There are four retrospective studies (Table 24.2) reporting outcomes after open vascular and endovascular surgery for acute SMA occlusion [48–51].

There are a lot of potential conflicts and biases when comparing the two. Sicker patients or in extremis tend to undergo open revascularization, whereas more stable ones endovascular treatments.

There seems to be lower bowel morbidity and lower mortality after endovascular therapy for acute thrombotic occlusion compared with open vascular surgery. One important aspect of the endovascular or hybrid approach compared with open vascular surgery, which may influence outcome, is that angiographic monitoring is part of the procedure after endovascular surgery, whereas there is room for much improvement in the percentage and quality of monitoring after open vascular surgery [48].

Morbidity and mortality are directly related to the need for bowel resection, length of intubation, and open revascularization [50].

Overall, this catastrophe carries an over 50% mortality rate and multiple comorbid complications for those who survive it.

References

1. Konstantinidis A, Inaba K, Dubose J, Barmparas G, Lam L, Plurad D, Branco BC, Demetriades D. Vascular trauma in geriatric patients: a national trauma databank review. J Trauma. 2011;71(4):909–16.
2. Weaver FA, et al. Is arterial proximity a valid indication for arteriography in penetrating extremity trauma? A prospective analysis. Arch Surg. 1990;125:1256–60.
3. Stain SC, Yellin AE, Weaver FA, Pentecost MJ. Selective management of nonocclusive arterial injuries. Arch Surg. 1989;124(10):1136–41.
4. Worni M, et al. Use of endovascular therapy for peripheral arterial lesions: an analysis of the National Trauma Data Bank from 2007 to 2009. Ann Vasc Surg. 2013;27:299–305.
5. Feliciano DV, et al. Five-year experience with PTFE grafts in vascular wounds. J Trauma. 1985;25:71–82.
6. Cosford PA, Leng GC. Screening for abdominal aortic aneurysm. Cochrane Database Syst Rev. 2007;CD002945.
7. Lovegrove RE, Javid M, Magee TR, et al. A meta-analysis of 21,178 patients undergoing open or endovascular repair of abdominal aortic aneurysm. Br J Surg. 2008;95:677–84.
8. Greenhalgh RM, Brown LC, Kwong GP, et al. Comparison of endovascular aneurysm repair with open repair in patients with abdominal aortic aneurysm (EVAR trial 1), 30-day opera- tive mortality results: randomised controlled trial. Lancet. 2004;364:843–8.

9. Greenhalgh RM. Commentary: impact of EVAR and DREAM trials on clinical practice. J Endovasc Ther. 2007;14:541–3.
10. De Bruin JL, Baas AF, Buth J, et al. Long-term outcome of open or endovascular repair of abdominal aortic aneurysm. N Engl J Med. 2010;362:1881–9.
11. Prinssen M, Verhoeven EL, Buth J, et al. A randomized trial comparing conventional and endovascular repair of abdominal aortic aneurysms. N Engl J Med. 2004;351:1607–18.
12. Banerjee A. Atypical manifestations of ruptured abdominal aortic aneurysms. Postgrad Med J. 1993;69:6–11. https://doi.org/10.1136/pgmj.69.807.6.
13. Smith TA, Ramirez DE. Awake, percutaneous repair of a ruptured abdominal aortic aneurysm. Ochsner J. 2013;13(2):248–51.
14. Mehta M, Taggert J, Clement Darling III R, Chang BB, Kreienberg PB, Paty PSK, Roddy SP, Sternbach Y, Ozsvath KJ, Shah DM. Establishing a protocol for endovascular treatment of ruptured abdominal aortic aneurysms: outcomes of a prospective analysis. J Vasc Surg 2006;44(1):1–8; discussion 8.
15. Starnes BW, Quiroga E, Hutter C, Tran NT, Hatsukami T, Meissner M, Tang G, Kohler T. Management of ruptured abdominal aortic aneurysm in the endovascular era. J Vasc Surg. 2010;51(1):9–17; discussion 17–8. doi:https://doi.org/10.1016/j.jvs.2009.08.038.
16. Wallace GA, Starnes BW, Hatsukami TS, et al. Favorable discharge disposition and survival after successful endovascular repair of ruptured abdominal aortic aneurysm. J Vasc Surg. 2013;57:1495.
17. Bown MJ, Sutton AJ, Bell PRF, et al. A meta-analysis of 50 years of ruptured abdominal aortic aneurysm repair. Br J Surg. 2002;89:714.
18. Biancari F, Catania A, D'Andrea V. Elective endovascular vs. open repair for abdominal aortic aneurysm in patients aged 80 years and older: systematic review and meta-analysis. Eur J Vasc Endovasc Surg. 2011;42:571–6.
19. Raval MV, Eskandari MK. Outcomes of elective abdominal aortic aneurysm repair among the elderly: endovascular versus open repair. Surgery. 2012;151:245–60.
20. Schermerhorn ML, O'Malley AJ, Jhaveri A, et al. Endovascular vs. open repair of abdominal aortic aneurysms in the Medicare population. N Engl J Med. 2008;358:464–74.
21. Sicard GA, Rubin BG, Sanchez LA, et al. Endoluminal graft repair for abdominal aortic aneurysms in high-risk patients and octogenarians: is it better than open repair? Ann Surg. 2001;234:427–435; discussion 435–437.
22. Leon LR Jr, Labropoulos N, Laredo J, et al. To what extent has endovascular aneurysm repair influenced abdominal aortic aneurysm management in the state of Illinois? J Vasc Surg. 2005;41:568–74.
23. Paolini D, Chahwan S, Wojnarowski D, et al. Elective endovascular and open repair of abdominal aortic aneurysms in octogenarians. J Vasc Surg. 2008;47:924–7.
24. de Donato G, Setacci C, Chisci E, et al. Abdominal aortic aneurysm repair in octogenarians: myth or reality? J Cardiovasc Surg. 2007;48:697–703.
25. IMPROVE Trial Investigators. Endovascular strategy or open repair for ruptured abdominal aortic aneurysm: one-year outcomes from the IMPROVE randomized trial. Eur Heart J. 2015;36:2061.
26. IMPROVE Trial Investigators, Powell JT, Hinchliffe RJ, et al. Observations from the IMPROVE trial concerning the clinical care of patients with ruptured abdominal aortic aneurysm. Br J Surg. 2014;101:216.
27. Hinchliffe RJ, Bruijstens L, MacSweeney ST, Braithwaite BD. A randomised trial of endovascular and open surgery for ruptured abdominal aortic aneurysm - results of a pilot study and lessons learned for future studies. Eur J Vasc Endovasc Surg. 2006;32:506.
28. Reimerink JJ, Hoornweg LL, Vahl AC, et al. Endovascular repair versus open repair of ruptured abdominal aortic aneurysms: a multicenter randomized controlled trial. Ann Surg. 2013;258:248.
29. Desgranges P, Kobeiter H, Katsahian S, et al. Editor's choice - ECAR (Endovasculaire ou Chirurgie dans les Anévrysmes aorto-iliaques Rompus): a French randomized controlled trial of endovascular versus open surgical repair of ruptured Aorto-iliac aneurysms. Eur J Vasc Endovasc Surg. 2015;50:303.
30. Hoornweg LL, Wisselink W, Vahl A, et al. The Amsterdam acute aneurysm trial: suitability and application rate for endovascular repair of ruptured abdominal aortic aneurysms. Eur J Vasc Endovasc Surg. 2007;33:679.
31. Sweeting MJ, Ulug P, Powell JT, et al. Ruptured aneurysm trials: the importance of longer-term outcomes and meta-analysis for 1-year mortality. Eur J Vasc Endovasc Surg. 2015;50:297.
32. Antoniou GA, Georgiadis GS, Antoniou SA, et al. Endovascular repair for ruptured abdominal aortic aneurysm confers an early survival benefit over open repair. J Vasc Surg. 2013;58:1091.
33. von Meijenfeldt GC, Ultee KH, Eefting D, et al. Differences in mortality, risk factors, and complications after open and endovascular repair of ruptured abdominal aortic aneurysms. Eur J Vasc Endovasc Surg. 2014;47:479.
34. Prinssen M, Verhoeven EL, Buth J, et al. A randomized trial comparing conventional and endovascular repair of abdominal aortic aneurysms. N Engl J Med. 2004;351:1607.
35. Kassahun WT, et al. Unchanged high mortality rates from acute occlusive intestinal ischemia: six year review. Langenbeck's Arch Surg. 2008;393:163–71.
36. Oldenburg WA, et al. Acute mesenteric ischemia: a clinical review. Arch Intern Med. 2004;164:1054–62.
37. Taylor LM, Moneta GL, Porter JM. Treatment of acute intestinal ischemia caused by arterial occlusions. Rutherford Vascular surgery. 5th ed. Philadelphia: WB Saunders; 2000. p. 1512–8.
38. Park WM, Gloviczki P, Cherry KJ, et al. Contemporary management of acute mesenteric isch-

emia: factors associated with survival. J Vasc Surg. 2002;35:445–52.
39. Taylor LM, Moenta GL, Porter JM. Treatment of chronic visceral ischemia. Rutherford Vascular surgery. 5th ed. Philadelphia: WB Saunders; 2000. p. 1532–41.
40. Wilson DB, Mostafavi K, Craven TE, et al. Clinical course of mesenteric artery stenosis in elderly Americans. Arch Intern Med. 2006;166(19):2095–100.
41. Schermerhorn ML, et al. Mesenteric revascularization: management and outcomes in the United States, 1988–2006. J Vasc Surg. 2009;50:341–8.
42. Kougias P, et al. Determinants of mortality and treatment outcome following surgical interventions for acute mesenteric ischemia. J Vasc Surg. 2007;46:467–74.
43. Moneta GL. Diagnosis of intestinal ischemia. Rutherford Vascular surgery. 5th ed. Philadelphia: WB Saunders; 2000. p. 1501–10.
44. Demir IE, Ceyhan GO, Friess H. Beyond lactate: is there a role for serum lactate measurement in diagnosing acute mesenteric ischemia? Dig Surg. 2012;29(3):226–35.
45. Kolkman JJ, et al. Occlusive and non-occlusive gastrointestinal ischaemia: a clinical review with special emphasis on the diagnostic value of tonometry. Scand J Gastroenterol Suppl. 1998;225:3–12.
46. Spangler R, Van Pham T, Khoujah D, Martinez JP. Abdominal emergencies in the geriatric patient. Int J Emerg Med. 2014;7:43.
47. Gallego AM, Ramirez P, Rodriquez JM, et al. Role of urokinase in the superior mesenteric artery embolism. Surgery. 1996;120:111–3.
48. Block TA, Acosta S, Björck M. Endovascular and open surgery for acute occlusion of the superior mesenteric artery. J Vasc Surg. 2010;52:959–66.
49. Schermerhorn ML, Giles KA, Hamdan AD, Wyers MC, Pomposelli FB. Mesenteric revascularization: management and outcomes in the United States, 1988–2006. J Vasc Surg. 2009;50:341–8. e1
50. Arthurs ZM, Titus J, Bannazadeh M, Eagleton MJ, Srivastava S, Sarac TP, Clair DG. A comparison of endovascular revascularization with traditional therapy for the treatment of acute mesenteric ischemia. J Vasc Surg. 2011;53:698–704; discussion 704–705.
51. Ryer EJ, Kalra M, Oderich GS, Duncan AA, Gloviczki P, Cha S, Bower TC. Revascularization for acute mesenteric ischemia. J Vasc Surg. 2012;55:1682–9.

Part XI

Urologic Injury

25 Geriatric Urologic Trauma

Gregory P. Murphy, Jack W. McAninch, and Benjamin N. Breyer

Introduction

Geriatric trauma is becoming an increasing problem as the largest segment of the population ages over 65 years [1–3]. Trauma is the ninth leading cause of death in the geriatric population [2]. The most common mechanism of injury sustained by the elderly is blunt trauma, specifically falls and motor vehicle collisions, while penetrating trauma is rare [1, 4]. Urologic injuries represent 9% of the total injuries to older patients [5].

While the diagnosis and management of geriatric urologic trauma patients is quite similar to younger adults, the outcomes tend to be worse. This is likely due to increasing comorbidities and decreasing physiologic reserve [1–5]. The best outcomes are seen in level 1 trauma centers with lower complication and death rates compared to less experienced centers [6]. Centers that utilized geriatric consult teams had lower rates of delirium [1, 2]. This highlights the need for appropriate triage to centers capable of managing geriatric trauma patients.

G.P. Murphy, M.D. (✉) • J.W. McAninch, M.D.
B.N. Breyer, M.D.
University of California - San Francisco Urology Department, San Francisco General Hospital, 1001 Potrero Avenue, Suite 3A20, San Francisco, CA 94110, USA
e-mail: Gregory.murphy@ucsf.edu; Jack.mcaninch@ucsf.edu; Benjamin.breyer@ucsf.edu

Renal Trauma

Renal trauma is the most common genitourinary (GU) injury in all trauma patients as well as the elderly [1–5]. Computed tomography (CT) scan with IV contrast including immediate and delayed imaging is the ideal diagnostic modality for renal injuries (see Fig. 25.1). Patients with gross hematuria, microscopic hematuria, and shock or a mechanism of injury causing a high index of suspicion for renal injury should undergo a CT scan [7]. Studies have shown that there is a higher rate of acute kidney injury (AKI) in elderly trauma patients [8, 9]. This has raised concerns that using iodinated contrast may lead to higher

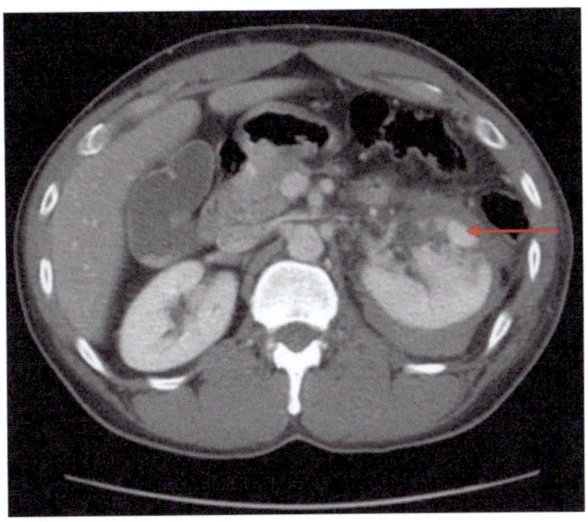

Fig. 25.1 Grade 3 left renal laceration after blunt trauma

A. Rodriguez et al. (eds.), *Geriatric Trauma and Acute Care Surgery*, https://doi.org/10.1007/978-3-319-57403-5_25

rates of AKI and worse outcomes. One study reviewed the risks factors for AKI and did not find IV contrast to be a significant risk. Their conclusion was that IV contrast was safe to use in the elderly trauma patient [8].

Staging of renal trauma is based on the American Association for the Surgery of Trauma (AAST) system. Grades ranging from grade 1 to 5 are described in Table 25.1 [2, 10]. Though the AAST grading system is predictive of the need for nephrectomy and the risk of mortality, it has not however been specifically validated in the geriatric population [1, 2, 11].

There has been a major paradigm shift in the management of renal injuries over the last few decades. Conservative management with observation has replaced surgery as the mainstay of treatment for the patient who is hemodynamically stable [7]. Some grade 4 and 5 injuries may require angioembolization by interventional radiology or operative exploration if there is hemodynamic instability [7, 12]. Angioembolization has been less successful in the elderly, requiring repeat procedures [13]. Rates of operative intervention are not significantly different in the elderly in blunt or penetrating trauma [5]. However, when operative exploration is undertaken, there is a higher rate of nephrectomy and higher rate of mortality [5].

Table 25.1 American Association for the Surgery of Trauma Organ Injury Severity Scale for the Kidney

Grade	Type	Description
I	Contusion	Microscopic or gross hematuria, urological studies normal
	Hematoma	Subcapsular, nonexpanding without parenchymal laceration
II	Hematoma	Nonexpanding perirenal hematoma confined to renal retroperitoneum
	Laceration	<1 cm parenchymal depth of renal cortex without urinary extravasation
III	Laceration	>1 cm depth of renal cortex, without collecting system rupture or urinary extravasation
IV	Laceration	Parenchymal laceration extending through the renal cortex, medulla, and collecting system
	Vascular	Main renal artery or vein injury with contained hemorrhage
V	Laceration	Completely shattered kidney

Ureteral Trauma

Ureteral injury is rare in trauma patients of all ages as well as the geriatric population [1, 14]. The most common mechanism for injury is a penetrating trauma, specifically gun-shot wounds [15]. Rates in general population were 2.6% versus 1.7% in the geriatric population [5]. Ureteral trauma is often associated with multiple other injuries to the bowel or vasculature so a multidisciplinary approach is beneficial. Furthermore, a high index of suspicion is required to diagnose these injuries as there is no foolproof laboratory or radiologic test [1, 2]. Delays in diagnosis can lead to further morbidity and worse outcomes [2]. If the patient is stable, a CT with delayed images or a retrograde pyelogram under anesthesia may help delineate an injury [7]. However, operative exploration may be necessary to rule out an injury in patients undergoing laparotomy who do not have preoperative imaging [7].

If a ureteral contusion is seen, ureteral stenting or surgical repair is recommended [7]. If a laceration to the ureter is seen, principles of repair include debridement of devitalized tissue, followed by a tension-free repair and watertight anastomosis [2, 16]. If the patient has life-threatening injuries, the ureter can be tied off and a nephrostomy tube placed until a more prudent time for repair [2, 7]. Ureteral repair requires a large armamentarium of surgical options. If the injury is to a distal segment of the ureter, a ureteral reimplant can be undertaken. If there is a larger segment of distal ureter injured, a psoas hitch or Boari flap may be required to bridge the gap [2, 7, 16]. The most common type of traumatic ureteral injury is a short segment of the midureter which can often be managed by a ureteroureterostomy [17]. Rarely a transureterostomy, ileal ureter, or autotransplant may be required electively if a significant portion of the ureter is damaged. These repairs have significant downsides so should only be used as a last resort [2, 7, 16]. To minimize the risk of complications, a ureteral stent and a retroperitoneal drain should be left in place after the ureter is repaired. Typically, the drain is removed prior to discharge if the output is low and the creatinine is consistent with serum. Ureteral stents are kept for 4–8 weeks [2, 16].

Bladder Trauma

Bladder injury is most commonly associated with pelvic fractures. Eighty percent of bladder injuries occur in patients with pelvic fractures while 5.7% of pelvic fracture patients have associated bladder injuries [18]. In younger patients, a significant force is required to cause a pelvic fracture so the most common mechanism of injury is motor vehicle crash or crush injuries. In the elderly, presumably due to osteoporosis, there is a higher incidence of pelvic fractures from lesser impact injuries such as falls [2, 19].

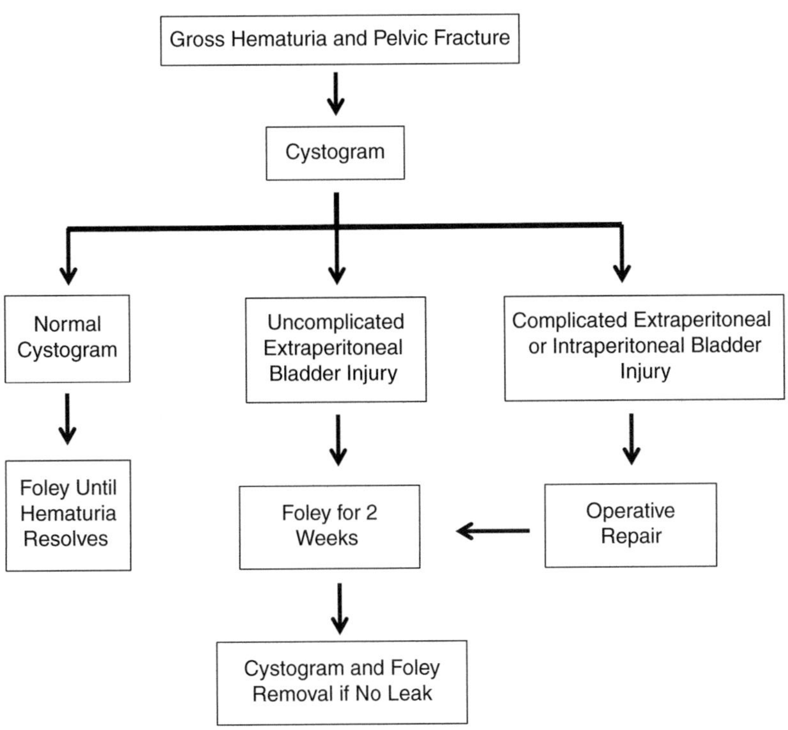

Algorithm for Bladder Trauma

Pelvic fractures are associated with significant morbidity and mortality in the elderly [2, 20]. Concomitant bladder injuries were more common in the elderly compared to the general population. But these injuries were less likely to require operative intervention [5]. This retrospective review of the National Trauma Data Bank did not specify location of bladder injury so the authors speculate that the reason for less operative intervention may be due to differing location of the injury [5].

The bladder sits deep in the pelvis where it is well protected from injury. When a fracture occurs, the bladder can be torn at its fascial attachments causing a laceration. A blow to the abdomen with a full bladder can lead to rupture at the dome. Less commonly, a bony spicule can lacerate the bladder [18].

Diagnosis of bladder injury is by cystogram (plain film or CT). The absolute indication for a cystogram is a patient with a pelvic fracture and gross hematuria. Relative indications include gross hematuria with a mechanism of injury concerning for bladder injury or a pelvic fracture with indicators of bladder rupture such as inability to void, abdominal distention, and pain [6].

Management of bladder injuries depends on whether the injury is intraperitoneal or extraperitoneal. Intraperitoneal injuries typically occur when there is rupture of a full bladder at the dome or from penetrating injuries. A two-layer closure with absorbable suture is recommended to repair intraperitoneal injuries. Uncomplicated extraperitoneal injuries can be managed conservatively with extended catheter drainage alone. Complicated extraperitoneal injuries such as those with bony spicules in the bladder, heavy hematuria, concomitant vaginal or rectal injuries, or bladder neck injuries should be managed operatively [7]. Extraperitoneal injuries should be explored and closed from within the bladder so as not to disrupt a pelvic hematoma [2]. Urethral catheter drainage alone is typically sufficient and patients often do not require suprapubic tube drainage after surgery [7]. The catheter can be left in for 7–10 days after surgery and a cystogram prior to removal will confirm that there is no extravasation [2].

Urethral Trauma

Urethral injuries are much more common in males than females [1]. The male urethra can be divided into anterior and posterior segments [2]. Posterior urethral injuries occur during pelvic fractures in about 5% of cases [21]. Essentially the prostate and membranous urethra tear away from the bulbar urethra creating a distraction defect. Posterior urethral injuries can be suspected when there is blood at the meatus or if there is a high-riding prostate on rectal exam. Diagnosis is by retrograde urethrogram which should be performed with oblique views to better evaluate the length of the urethra [2]. Primary realignment can be attempted in the stable patient but close follow-up is needed as many patients will develop a stenosis. Suprapubic drainage is another primary option with a delayed posterior urethroplasty after the patient has recovered. Immediate urethroplasty is not recommended for the majority of urethral injuries due to the extent of tissue damage and poor outcomes [2].

Anterior urethral injuries most commonly occur from straddle injuries (see Fig. 25.2). In this case, the bulbar urethra is compressed by the pubic bone. Similarly, patients present with blood at the meatus and a retrograde urethrogram will be diagnostic. A catheter may be gently attempted, but if this is unsuccessful, suprapubic drainage will be required and likely a urethroplasty at a later date [2]. Contrary to posterior urethral injuries, uncomplicated penetrating injuries to the anterior urethra can be repaired promptly with urethroplasty [6].

Genital Trauma

Injuries to the scrotum, testes, and penis occur less frequently in the elderly population [5]. Mechanisms of injury include sexual intercourse for penile fractures, sports injury, and blunt trauma for testicular rupture, burns, and machine accidents for genital skin loss. These activities and injuries lend themselves to a younger patient population [1].

Our group reviewed the National Electronic Injury Surveillance System which provides a sample of emergency department presentations in the United States excluding those from MVC and acts of violence. The majority of GU injuries were to external genitalia. The elderly were more likely to sustain injuries from falls often in bathroom or shower. In this cohort, as patient age

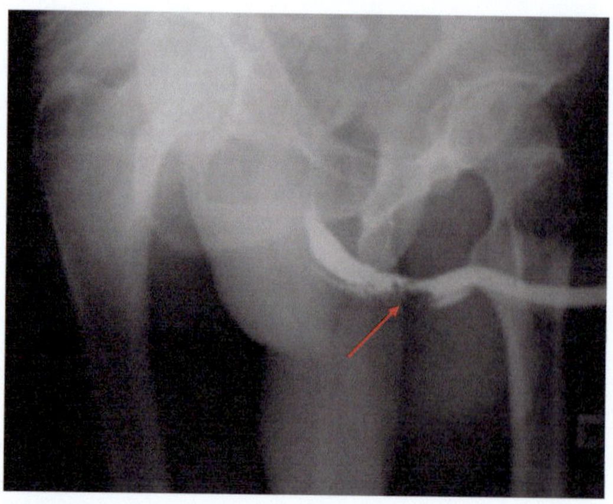

Fig. 25.2 RUG after straddle injury

increased, there was a higher rate of inpatient admission [22].

Penile fractures can be suspected if a pop is felt followed by immediate detumescence during intercourse. An eggplant deformity has been described and requires operative exploration and corporal repair if an injury is found (see Fig. 25.3). Concomitant urethral injury should be suspected if the patient has blood at the meatus [2] (see Fig. 25.4). Some studies have discussed ultrasound or MRI as a possible diagnostic modality but neither is very accurate and a missed injury can lead to chronic problems with curvature so operative exploration is recommended in most cases [2, 7].

Testicular injury is rare but most present with scrotal swelling and hematoma. When testicular rupture is suspected from blunt trauma, operative exploration is required. Similarly, penetrating scrotal wounds should be explored when testicular injury is suspect. In equivocal cases, ultrasound can be used to assess testicular viability but surgery should not be delayed. During exploration, nonviable tissue should be debrided and the tunica closed if salvageable. If there is no viable tissue remaining, an orchiectomy is needed [2, 7].

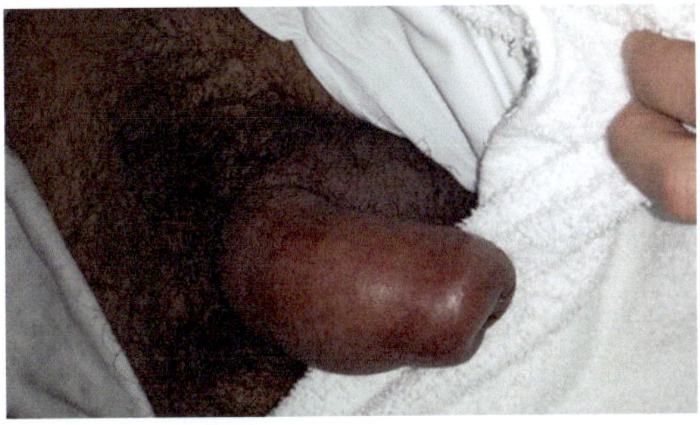

Fig. 25.3 Eggplant deformity after penile fracture

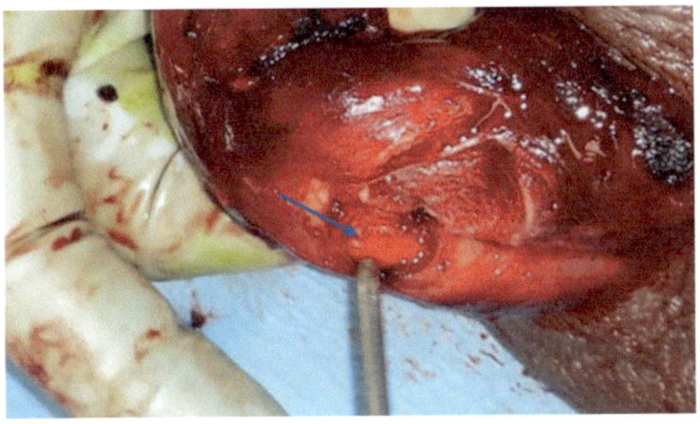

Fig. 25.4 Operative exploration of penile fracture with urethral injury. *Arrow* shows catheter across the urethral injury below the corporal rupture

Genital skin loss injuries require minimal debridement and local wound care only in most cases. If less than 50% of the scrotal skin is damaged, the defect can often be closed primarily. If greater than 50% of the scrotal skin is involved, skin grafting is recommended [1, 7].

Conclusion

Overall, more research is needed into the differences between the adult and geriatric urologic trauma patients. As a rule, geriatric trauma injuries are managed in a similar fashion to their younger cohort. Despite this, the elderly, being more frail and with more comorbidities, generally have worse outcomes and therefore require a level of expertise to manage. These patients should be transferred to an appropriate trauma center with specialists in the fields of trauma, urology, and geriatrics to provide a multidisciplinary approach and comprehensive care.

References

1. Metcalf MR, Broghammer J. Genitourinary trauma in geriatric patients. Curr Opin Urol. 2016;26:165–70.
2. Broghammer JA, Windsperger AP, Elliott SP. Genitourinary trauma in geriatric patients. In: Griebling TL, editor. Geriatric urology. New York: Springer; 2014. p. 417–41.
3. Bonne S, Schuerer DJ. Trauma in the older adult: epidemiology and evolving geriatric trauma principles. Clin Geriatr Med. 2013;29(1):137–50.
4. Labib N, Nouh T, Winocour S, et al. Severely injured geriatric population: morbidity, mortality, and risk factors. J Trauma. 2011;71(6):1908–14.
5. Bjurlin MA, Goble SM, Fantus RJ, Hollowell CM. Outcomes in geriatric genitourinary trauma. J Am Coll Surg. 2011;213(3):415–21.
6. Garwe T, Roberts ZV, Albrecht RM, et al. Direct transport of geriatric trauma patients with pelvic fractures to a Level I trauma center within an organized trauma system: impact on two-week incidence of in-hospital complications. Am J Surg. 2012;204:921–5.
7. Morey AF, Brandes S, Dugi DD 3rd, et al. Urotrauma: AUA guideline. J Urol. 2014;192(2):327–35.

8. Kim DY, Kobayashi L, Costantini TW, et al. Is contrast exposure safe among the highest risk trauma patients? J Trauma Acute Care Surg. 2012;72(1):61–6; discussion 66–7.
9. Vivino G, Antonelli M, Moro ML, et al. Risk factors for acute renal failure in trauma patients. Intensive Care Med. 1998;24(8):808–14.
10. Moore EE, Shackford SR, Pachter HL, et al. Organ injury scaling: spleen, liver, and kidney. J Trauma. 1989;29(12):1664–6.
11. Santucci RA, McAninch JW, Safir M, Mario LA, Service S, Segal MR. Validation of the American Association for the Surgery of Trauma organ injury severity scale for the kidney. J Trauma. 2001;50(2):195–200.
12. Breyer BN, McAninch JW, Elliott SP, Master VA. Minimally invasive endovascular techniques to treat acute renal hemorrhage. J Urol. 2008;179(6):2248–52.
13. Hotaling JM, Sorensen MD, Smith TG 3rd, Rivara FP, Wessells H, Voelzke BB. Analysis of diagnostic angiography and angioembolization in the acute management of renal trauma using a national data set. J Urol. 2011;185(4):1316–20.
14. Santucci RA, Hunter CB. Ureteral Trauma. 2014. http://emedicine.medscape.com/article/440933-overview. Accessed 9 Oct 2015.
15. Siram SM, Gerald SZ, Greene WR, et al. Ureteral trauma: patterns and mechanisms of injury of an uncommon condition. Am J Surg. 2010;199(4):566–70.
16. Serafetinides E, Kitrey ND, Djakovic N, et al. Review of the current management of upper urinary tract injuries by the EAU Trauma Guidelines Panel. Eur Urol. 2015;67(5):930–6.
17. Elliott SP, McAninch JW. Ureteral injuries from external violence: the 25-year experience at San Francisco General Hospital. J Urol. 2003;170(4 Pt 1):1213–6.
18. Gomez RG, Cabellos L, Coburn M, et al. Consensus statement on bladder injuries. BJU Int. 2004;94(1):27–32.
19. Nanninga GL, de Leur K, Panneman MJ, van der Elst M, Hartholt KA. Increasing rates of pelvic fractures among older adults: The Netherlands, 1986-2011. Age Ageing. Sep 2014;43(5):648–53.
20. Prieto-Alhambra D, Aviles FF, Judge A, et al. Burden of pelvis fracture: a population-based study of incidence, hospitalisation and mortality. Osteoporos Int. 2012;23(12):2797–803.
21. Figler BD, Hoffler CE, Reisman W, et al. Multidisciplinary update on pelvic fracture associated bladder and urethral injuries. Injury. 2012;43(8):1242–9.
22. Breyer BN, et al. Product related adult genitourinary injuries treated at emergency departments in the United States from 2002 to 2010. J Urol. 2013;189(4):1362–8.

Part XII

Plastics/Skin and Soft Tissue Injury

26 Plastics/Skin and Soft-Tissue Injury Trauma

Sharline Z. Aboutanos

Introduction

Aging affects every layer of the skin. The epidermis becomes thinner with age and the junction between the epidermis and the dermis flattens [1]. This age-related change can lead to an increased tendency for shearing injury, which is commonly seen in the elderly trauma population. A reduction in hair follicles and decreased lubrication of the skin are also noted. These changes can make the skin drier and more prone to cracking. While these intrinsic skin changes occur as one ages, the addition of extrinsic factors, such as ultraviolet light, and disease progression, such as diabetes and peripheral vascular disease, can further complicate healing of the skin and soft tissue after injury in the geriatric age group.

Age-related changes of the bone have also been documented. These changes include bone becoming more porous and a decrease in osteoblast activity [2]. Therefore, with increasing age, bone strength decreases, which may lead to an increased propensity for fracture. Specifically in cranial bone, there is an increased risk for loss of bone mineral content in women more than men. Also, the risk for osteoporotic fracture in the mandible is higher in edentulous individuals [2]. This background knowledge is important for surgeons faced with the challenge of treating an elderly patient with skin and soft-tissue injury and facial fractures.

S.Z. Aboutanos, M.D., F.A.A.P., F.A.C.S.
Richmond Plastic Surgeons, 1630 Wilkes Ridge Parkway, Suite 201, Richmond, VA 23233, USA
e-mail: sharlinezaboutanos@gmail.com

Initial Consultation

There are several key facts one must elicit at the time of initial plastic surgery consultation surrounding the injury of the elderly trauma patient with skin and soft-tissue injury and/or facial fracture. This information includes history of present illness (location, time of injury, and mechanism of injury), past medical history (coexisting illnesses), medications, and social history.

Most injuries in the elderly occur at home [3, 4]. Typical mechanisms of injury include walking, ground-level falls, assault, and motor vehicle crashes. When walking, furniture, carpet, steps, and pets can play a role in injury. Time of injury is pertinent because delay in treatment of skin lacerations and open wounds can lead to increased infection rate [5]. Additionally, increased swelling in the initial post-injury period can increase tension on laceration repair, therefore increasing the chance of unfavorable scarring and dehiscence.

In the elderly population, facial fractures after falls occur more commonly in women compared to men [6, 7]. The most common facial fractures

A. Rodriguez et al. (eds.), *Geriatric Trauma and Acute Care Surgery*,
https://doi.org/10.1007/978-3-319-57403-5_26

reported in the elderly are malar and orbital [6–8]. There are reports that elderly patients with facial fractures are more severely injured, and have a higher mortality and a higher rate of brain injury when compared to younger patients [8]. Other reports conclude that elderly patients suffer from less severe facial fractures and can be treated conservatively for the majority of cases [7].

Past medical history also plays an important role in geriatric injury, especially dementia, diabetes mellitus, poor vision, venous stasis disease, peripheral vascular disease, stroke, malnutrition, depression, osteoporosis, and congestive heart failure. Medications, such as anticoagulants, antiplatelet medications, steroids, and sleep aids, can also affect injury severity. A history of alcohol use in the elderly patient must also be determined. History of tobacco abuse can affect healing of skin and soft-tissue injuries, especially in crush injuries and/or vascularly compromised tissue. Social history to determine the patient's living arrangements and history of interpersonal domestic violence is also important and relevant to patient discharge arrangements and outpatient treatment plans [4, 9].

Physical Exam

Initial management of the injured patient focuses on the advanced trauma life support (ATLS) protocol and stabilization of the patient. During the initial evaluation, one can identify facial fractures and soft-tissue injury. Facial fractures can have associated injuries, which include airway compromise, hemorrhage, brain and spinal injury, trauma to the orbital globe and blindness, and dental injury or tooth loss.

Airway compromise can be associated with bleeding from upper airway as well as aspiration of foreign bodies. Emergent airway management by the trauma team may include endotracheal intubation, cricothyroidotomy, or tracheotomy. Most upper airway bleeding can be managed by applying direct pressure; however, in cases of severe hemorrhagic injury, nasal packing may be necessary. If these measures fail, angiographic embolization may be utilized for severe bleeding.

Neurologic or spinal injury must be ruled out prior to pursuing repair of facial fractures to avoid exacerbating these injuries during surgical manipulation of the facial bones. Cervical spine precautions are required until negative clinical and radiological exam is determined. An altered mental status may prevent clinical clearance; therefore one may consider obtaining computed tomography (CT) of the neck or magnetic resonance imaging for definitive evaluation.

After ABCDE survey, a detailed head exam may be performed. Routine and methodical examination of the patient's head from a superior to inferior direction allows one to avoid missing an injury. Skin, soft tissue, neurovascular structures, and bones should be evaluated. Swelling may impair accurate examination of the underlying structures; therefore repeat examination after the initial 48 h post-injury may be warranted. However, high-velocity mechanism of injury, bony instability, crepitus, step-offs, and malocclusion could indicate underlying bony injury. In addition to the nasal bones, careful assessment of the nasal septum and the presence of a nasal septal hematoma must be documented and addressed. Trigeminal and facial nerve function must be tested in addition to changes in sensation in the upper, mid, and lower face. Injuries of the facial nerve can be associated with parotid duct injuries. Visual disturbances or ocular injury warrant expedited ophthalmologic consultation. Dental occlusion and injury to the tongue, gums, and teeth must also be noted.

Imaging

Computed tomography (CT) scan is the most effective radiologic examination ordered to evaluate the facial bones. Typically, a maxillofacial CT, which can be ordered in conjunction with a head CT, obtained at 3 mm intervals or less is adequate to rule out injuries of the skull and facial bones (Figs. 26.1 and 26.2). In cases of

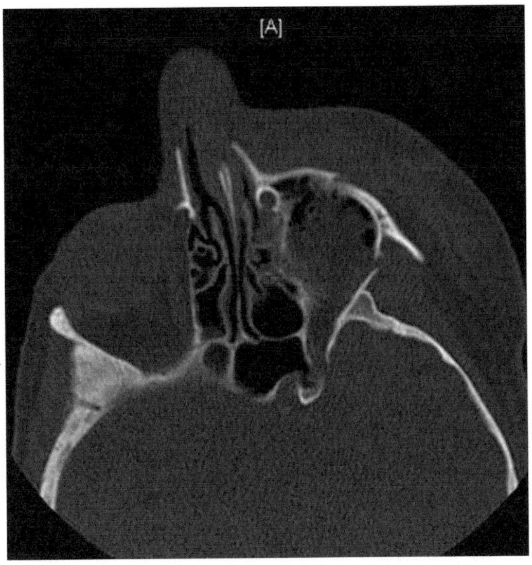

Fig. 26.1 Axial image of maxillofacial CT scan of a 74-year-old woman who sustained facial fractures after falling 13 steps at her home. Images demonstrate soft-tissue swelling in left periorbital area with subcutaneous air, fracture of the left maxillary sinus, and fracture of the left orbital floor

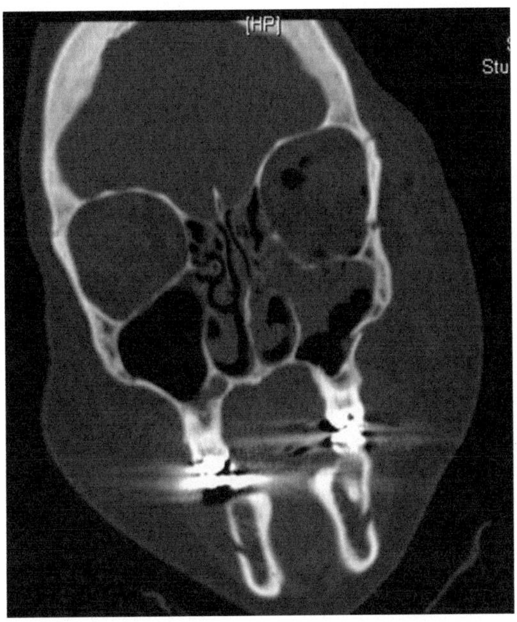

Fig. 26.2 Coronal image of maxillofacial CT scan of the same patient in Fig. 26.1

complex craniofacial trauma, a three-dimensional reconstruction of the facial skeleton can aid in surgical planning. Other helpful radiologic exams include a panoramic radiograph (Panorex) to evaluate the mandible, notably the condyles, and teeth. Additionally, CT angiogram may be necessary to rule out associated injuries to the cerebrovascular structures of the head and neck [10].

Treatment

Soft-Tissue Injuries

Treatment of soft-tissue injuries begins with avoiding infection and closing open wounds within the first 24 h after injury. Irrigation with saline and/or chlorhexidine soap brush can be performed after the patient is admitted to the emergency department under local anesthesia. Typically, 1% lidocaine with epinephrine is used. For more severely contaminated wounds, washout and debridement should occur in the operating room with anesthesia to properly cleanse the wounds of debris while the patient is comfortable and cooperative.

Linear or stellate injuries can be repaired after proper cleansing of the wound. Devitalized tissue can be debrided sharply to create clean, viable edges for repair. Both dermal and epidermal layers should be repaired to promote optimal scar formation by lessening tension on the closure. Location of the injury dictates the size and type of suture used. Typically, carefully placed interrupted sutures are utilized to accurately approximate the edges of the wound. Sutures in the face should be removed in 5–7 days to decrease suture tracking. Because of the effects of aging and the thinner quality of skin seen in the elderly, additional challenges are faced during laceration repair. A technique to facilitate closure in this population has been reported and is performed by placing sutures through Steri-Strips. The Steri-Strips prevent the suture material from cutting through the skin and prevent shearing of the thin skin to keep it in place after suture removal [11].

Crush injury, contusions, and vascular compromise can result in poorer healing and scar outcomes. In these instances, wound care, rather than laceration repair, may be warranted (Fig. 26.3). Depending on the patient's drug allergies, wound care with bacitracin or silver sulfadiazine ointment can provide moisture to the wound while promoting an antibacterial environment. Wound care dressings should be applied in such a manner so as to limit maceration and injury to the surrounding peri-wound skin edges and avoid pain with future dressing changes. Eventual delineation of nonviable tissue over the next 24–48 h can lead to accurate surgical debridement of these areas in the operating room (Fig. 26.4). Small areas of stable, dry, clean scab can remain to function as a biologic dressing during the wound healing process. Reconstruction of a resultant defect to restore appearance and function depends on the size and location of the defect. The reconstructive ladder must be considered in each case. Options include wound healing by secondary intention, skin grafting, or flap repair. In circumstances where the patient has limited mobility, pressure relief and frequent turns during the patient's hospital stay are crucial to avoid deep tissue injury and formation of pressure ulcers in pressure-sensitive areas.

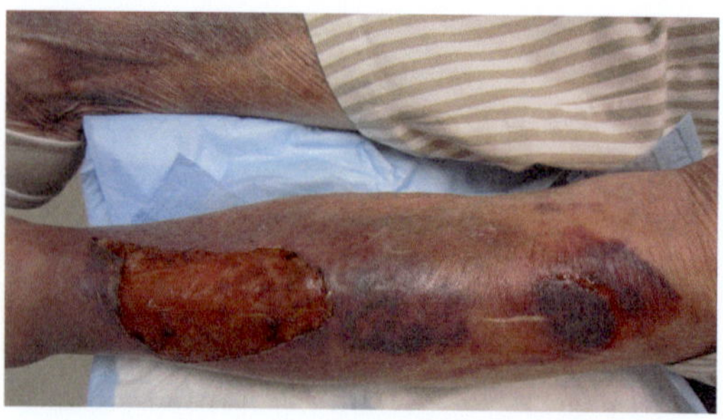

Fig. 26.3 83-year-old woman sustained left anterior leg wounds status post-fall during the night and hitting the corner of a table. Her wounds are significant for ecchymosis, laceration, and full-thickness skin loss. She also has a history of tobacco use. Her findings are consistent with skin and soft-tissue injuries sustained by the elderly population

Large hematomas should be evacuated to avoid pressure on underlying structures and infection. In areas of the face, hematomas of the ear and nasal septum must be evacuated as soon as possible to avoid deformity to the underlying cartilage.

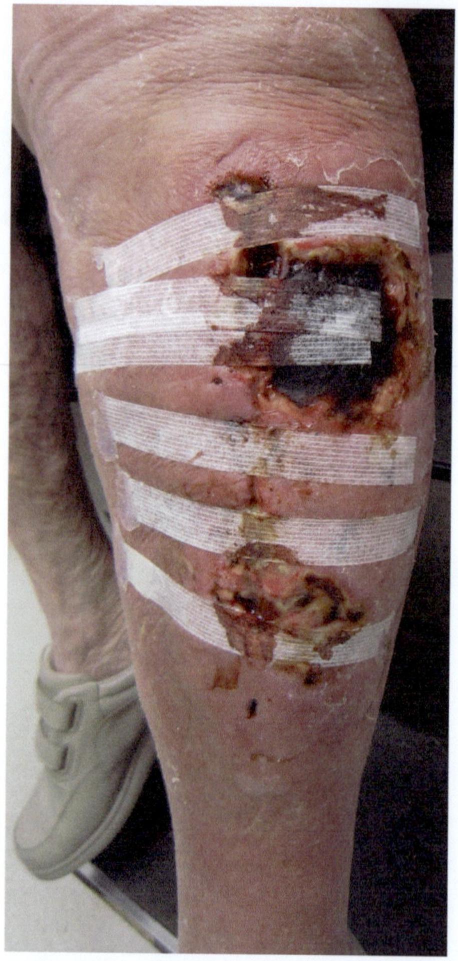

Fig. 26.4 70-year-old woman sustained left anterior leg wounds status post-motor vehicle crash 3 weeks prior. She reports being admitted to the intensive care unit for rib fractures and chest pain. She was subsequently discharged with home health follow-up of her leg wounds. After this visit, she was taken to the operating room for debridement and washout of the infected areas and placement on intravenous antibiotics

Facial Fractures

Indications for facial fracture repair oftentimes depend on the facial bone involved, the angle of the fracture, the degree of comminution, and other associated injuries. For the most part, facial fracture repair in the elderly is similar to patients of other ages. It is worth noting that in the elderly population there is a higher incidence of edentulous mandible and this condition may complicate mandibular fracture repair. Mandibulomaxillary fixation (MMF) in this group of patients is difficult to achieve with the patient's dentures, if present. Additionally, there is increased difficulty with eating and maintaining proper nutrition postoperatively. Patients with atrophic mandibles benefit from open reduction and internal fixation using a rigid reconstruction plate. Placing more screws on either side of the fracture may be necessary in the atrophic mandible. Other acceptable alternatives include external fixation.

Patients with facial fractures are often placed on a soft diet to prevent further trauma to facial bones and limit pain with mastication. Nutrition consultation is useful in this scenario to help identify foods specific to this diet that deliver adequate caloric needs during periods of healing and high energy demand.

Interdisciplinary care of geriatric trauma patients is vital to increasing survival and improving outcomes after injury. This team includes, but is not limited to, trauma and critical care specialists, emergency room physicians and nurses, geriatricians, pharmacists, wound care nurses, nutritionists, chaplains, and other surgical specialists. Injury and trauma prevention targeted toward the elderly population may also be useful.

References

1. Greenhalgh DG. Management of the skin and soft tissue in the geriatric surgical patient. Surg Clin N Am. 2015;95:103–14.
2. Kloss F, Gassen R. Bone and aging: effects on the maxillofacial skeleton. Exp Gerontol. 2006;41(2):123–9.
3. Hwang K, Huan F, Hwang PJ. Comparison of facial trauma in late middle age (55–65 years) and old age (older than 65 years). J Craniofac Surg. 2013;24:909–13.
4. Chalya P, Mabula JB, Ngayomela I, Mbelenge N, Dass RM, Mchembe M, Ngallaba SE, Gilyoma JM. Geriatric injuries among patients attending a regional hospital in Shinyanga Tanzania. Tanzan J Health Res. 2012;14(1):15–20.
5. Waseem M, Lakdawala V, Patel R, Kapoor R, Leber M, Sun X. Is there a relationship between wound infection and laceration closure times? Int J Emerg Med. 2012 Jul;5(1):32–8.
6. Clavijo-Alvarez JA, Deleyiannis FW, Peitzman AB, Zenati MS. Risk factors for death in elderly patients with facial fractures secondary to falls. J Craniofac Surg. 2012;23(2):494–8.
7. Atisha DM, van Rensselaer BT, Allori AC, Puscas L, Erdmann D, Marcus JR. Facial fractures in the aging population. Plast Reconstr Surg. 2016;137(2):587–93.
8. Toivari M, Suominen AL, Lindqvist C, Thoren H. Among patients with facial fractures, geriatric patients have an increased risk for associated injuries. J Oral Maxillofac Surg. 2016;17:1–7.
9. Hackenberg EAM, Salinen V, Koljonen V, Handolin L. Severe intimate partner violence affecting both young and elderly patients of both sexes. Eur J Trauma Emerg Surg [Internet]. 2016. Available from Medline: http://www-ncbi-nlm-nih-gov.proxy.library.vcu.edu/pubmed/26936195.
10. Biffl WL, Moore EE, Offner PJ, Brega KE, Francio RJ, Elliott JP, Burch JM. Optimizing screening for blunt cerebrovascular injuries. Am J Surg. 1999;178(6):512–22.
11. Davis M, Nakhdjevani A, Lidder S. Suture/Steristrip combination for the management of lacerations in thin-skinned individuals. J Emerg Med. 2011;40(3):322–3.

27 Soft Tissue Infections in the Elderly

Margaret H. Lauerman and Sharon Henry

Introduction

Necrotizing soft-tissue infection (NSTI) is a morbid and potentially mortal diagnosis in a patient of any age (Fig. 27.1). Extensive soft-tissue debridement leaves large, potentially disfiguring wounds in patients who survive (Fig. 27.2). Sepsis and organ dysfunction are frequent occurrences in patients with NSTI requiring intensive care unit (ICU) admission. Successful care of patients with NSTI involves coordinating operation for early source control and critical care management for support of organ dysfunction. Preexisting medical comorbidities more commonly present in the elderly can make management of NSTI even more problematic. As a result the challenges in the diagnosis and treatment of NSTI are more acute in elderly patients.

Epidemiology

Skin and soft-tissue infections (SSTI) are a common problem. Annually there are 867,777 cases of SSTI diagnosed in the United States. Approximately 6000 patients yearly develop a NSTI, accounting for only 0.7% of SSTIs [1]. It is estimated Group A streptococcus infection (GAS) specifically accounts for 650–800 of the NSTI cases per year [2]. Overall NSTI represents a small portion of surgical pathology, with only 0.1% of surgical cases performed for treatment of a NSTI [3]. Therefore, surgeons typically may see only a handful of these cases in their careers. The elderly comprise a significant portion of

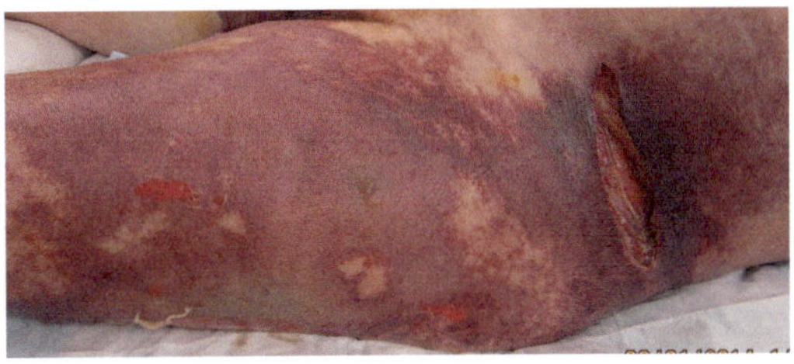

Fig. 27.1 NSTI involving the flank, leg, and perineum in a 76-year-old prior to debridement. He has multiple medical comorbidities including coronary artery disease, hypertension, prostate cancer, rheumatoid arthritis, and chronic hip pain. He was brought to his community emergency room with complaints of worsening of his chronic hip pain and not feeling himself for 5 days. His family noted him to be short of breath and unable to ambulate. In the emergency room he was hypotensive and desaturating. He was intubated and resuscitated. A non-contrast CT scan (he had acute kidney injury on presentation) documented extensive air in hip and thigh. Incisions were made under local in the ED and he was transferred to a tertiary referral center for further management where he underwent wide debridement but continued to require pressors; after discussion with the family he was transitioned to comfort care and he expired with 48 h of admission.

M.H. Lauerman, M.D. • S. Henry, M.D. (✉)
Program in Trauma University of Maryland School of Medicine, University of Maryland Medical Center R A Cowley Shock Trauma Center,
22 South Greene Street, Baltimore, MD 21201, USA
e-mail: mlauerman@umm.edu; shenry@umm.edu

A. Rodriguez et al. (eds.), *Geriatric Trauma and Acute Care Surgery*,
https://doi.org/10.1007/978-3-319-57403-5_27

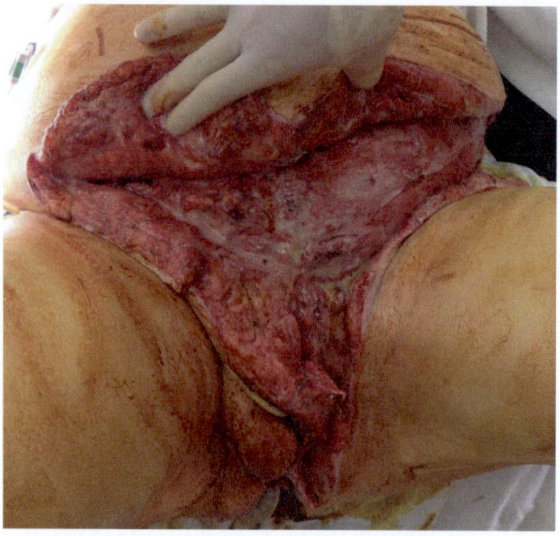

Fig. 27.2 Large residual perineal and abdominal wall wound after NSTI debridement in an elderly patient

patients with NSTI, with over one-quarter of patients with NSTI over the age of 60 [4].

Types of Necrotizing Soft-Tissue Infection

NSTIs are classified into subgroups by bacteria type (Table 27.1) [5], and type I NSTI is thought to target patients with poor health and medical comorbidities [6], and is the most common type of NSTI in the United States [5]. The elderly may be more susceptible to type I NSTI given their higher rates of comorbidities, such as diabetes mellitus and malignancies [7, 8]. Type II NSTI, which includes GAS infection, is thought to be precipitated by minor local trauma, allowing bacterial entry into the underlying tissues [6]. GAS infections increase with age [9]. Type III NSTI is also seen in patients >65 years despite the association with environmental exposure [10].

Etiology of Necrotizing Soft-Tissue Infections

The list of potential causes of NSTI in geriatric patients is long and (Table 27.2) includes gastrointestinal, gynecologic, integumentary, genitourinary, and traumatic pathology. Prevalence of many etiologies of NSTI increases with age. Rates of malignancy, chronic wounds, traumatic injury, and decubitus ulcers are higher in the elderly, making geriatric patients an at-risk population for NSTI [8, 12–14].

Clinical Presentation

Differentiating NSTI from cellulitis can be difficult in any patient. Erythema, warmth, and tenderness, the most common clinical exam findings of NSTI [4], are also present in uncomplicated SSTIs. The presence of skin necrosis, bullae, skin discoloration, crepitus, and discharge [4] is more specific for NSTIs but these are not universally present. The elderly have some specific conditions which can make the clinical diagnosis of NSTI more difficult. Evaluation of geriatric patients can be confounded by the higher prevalence of chronic edema, chronic wounds, skin discoloration, and hematoma formation from anticoagulation for conditions such as atrial fibrillation [13, 16, 17].

Given the overlap in clinical exam findings with NSTI and uncomplicated SSTI, scoring systems have been developed to differentiate NSTI from uncomplicated SSTI, such as the Laboratory Risk Indicator for Necrotizing Fasciitis (LRINEC) score [18, 19]. However, this NSTI prediction score is imperfect, particularly in the elderly. The LRINEC score utilizes laboratory values such as hemoglobin, sodium, and creatinine [18] that in the elderly are more likely to be abnormal at baseline [20–22]. The ability to distinguish a NSTI from an uncomplicated SSTI in an elderly patient remains difficult even when this score is utilized.

Radiologic imaging is another potential tool for differentiating NSTI from SSTI. Plain X-ray, computerized tomography (CT), and magnetic resonance imaging (MRI) are all potential imaging options. Both X-ray and CT can detect subcutaneous emphysema, the hallmark of a NSTI. Air within the subcutaneous tissues or tracking along the fascia on imaging is diagnostic of NSTI and

Table 27.1 Types of NASTI and the bacterial burden associated with the NSTI types [5, 11]

NSTI type	Bacteria	Clinical characteristics
Type I	Infection can include anaerobic and aerobic bacteria. Bacterial load is polymicrobial	Most common type of NSTI. Local spread of disease is less aggressive
Type II	Can be monomicrobial or combined with staph. Most commonly GAS. Can be MRSA alone	Aggressive local spread of disease
Type III	Monomicrobial infection with gram-negative bacteria	Often with exposure to warm, costal water
Type IV	Fungal infection	Often associated with immunocompromised patients

Table 27.2 Etiologies of NSTI in geriatric patients [4, 15]

Etiologies of NSTI
Chronic wound
Trauma
Injection (medications)
Intravenous drug use
Integumentary
Perianal abscess
Postoperative infection
Bartholin's abscess
Perforated genitourinary tract
Decubitus ulcer
Perforated rectal/anal cancer
Perforated viscus
Strangulated hernia
Burns
Self-induced (i.e.: Munchausen's syndrome)
Idiopathic

should prompt operative exploration. However, the absence of these findings does not exclude NSTI [23]. Thus, the addition of imaging does not guarantee that the correct diagnosis will be made. Interpretation of the finding of subcutaneous emphysema may be influenced by the presence of a chronic wound, which is not an uncommon finding in the elderly [13]. The limitations of radiographic imaging in NSTI apply to both younger and geriatric patients. Additionally geriatric patients are more likely to have chronic renal disease which limits the use of intravenous contrast [22]. Changes related to tissue enhancement will be missed without contrast; however subcutaneous air can still be detected. CT may still provide useful information in this circumstance when interpreted in combination with the clinical presentation.

Medical comorbidities are frequently present in patients with NSTI. Patients with NSTI have higher rates of diabetes mellitus (47%), hypertension (51%), respiratory disease (31%), neurologic disease (23%), cardiac disease (17%), and peripheral vascular disease (17%) than the overall surgical patient population [3]. Some studies suggest that not only are rates of comorbidities higher in NSTI, but the presence of these comorbidities is associated with a higher mortality [3, 4]. Heart failure, chronic obstructive pulmonary disease, and renal disease increase with age, placing elderly patients at higher risk of mortality in NSTI due to their preexisting medical conditions [24–26].

Additionally, patients with NSTI commonly present with physiologic derangements. Eighty percent of patients with NSTI have a sepsis spectrum diagnosis at admission. Twenty-six percent of patients with NSTI present in septic shock [3]. The presence of sepsis on admission is associated with higher mortality in patients with NSTI. Elderly patients treated for infection are more likely to present with sepsis and more frequently die due to sepsis than their younger counterparts [27]. The elderly with NSTI are likely at increased risk of mortality given their susceptibility to sepsis.

A diagnosis of NSTI may be delayed in geriatric patients, as infections are common in the elderly. Greater than 54% of infections occur in patients over 65 years, with the two most common infectious etiologies being urinary tract infection (UTI) and pneumonia [28]. Geriatric patients are often treated empirically for sepsis when a source of the infection remains unknown, during which an unidentified NSTI may be progressing. Even though non-NSTI sources are far more frequent causes of infection in the elderly, the index of suspicion must be high for NSTI when an elderly patient presents with sepsis, particularly when the source is not determined.

Treatment

Early debridement is of great importance in NSTI. Multiple studies correlate time to debridement with survival; survival decreases linearly with time to debridement [4, 11, 29, 30]. Much of the benefit of early debridement may result from the removal of the nidus for the patient's systemic illness by obtaining local source control.

With progression of illness and subsequent organ failure, an association is seen between mortality and number of organs failed. As the number of organs failed increases, mortality increases in a stepwise fashion [4]. Patients presenting with organ dysfunction in sepsis are more often older [31]. While organ dysfunction is a serious event in any patient with NSTI, in the elderly it carries a far more grave prognosis.

Elderly patients have well-documented barriers to medical care which often delay medical attention, allowing their underlying NSTI to progress untreated. Older patients are more likely to report barriers to medical care, such as transportation limitations and concern over medical bills [32]. With 1.4 million adults living in a nursing home, a large proportion of the geriatric population does not directly control their ability to access medical care [33]. Elderly patients with cognitive decline may be unable to convey their symptoms, further delaying their presentation to medical care.

Outcomes

Mortality is high overall in NSTI, ranging from 6 to 76%, with many reviews reporting mortality greater than 20% [11]. Increasing age is associated with a higher mortality rate in NSTI; patients over the age of 60 years have a 28% absolute increase in mortality compared with younger patients [4]. Even after controlling for comorbidities, demographic variables, and preoperative sepsis, age remains an independent predictor of mortality in NSTI [3, 4]. Long-term mortality is also a consideration in those patients with NSTI who survive their initial hospitalization. After discharge, patients with a previous NSTI have an excess mortality when compared to the general population that increases with age [34].

Beyond mortality, many other in-hospital complications often occur in patients with NSTI [4, 35] (Table 27.3). These complications compound the effect of a NSTI in the elderly and contribute to the higher mortality found in elderly patients [36].

Limb loss is particularly devastating in geriatric patients with extremity NSTI. While age does not predict limb loss in NSTI [15], the ability to achieve a good functional outcome after amputation declines with age [37]. Elderly patients often have preexisting mobility limitations such as decreased walking speed [38] and underlying balance, strength, and coordination problems already account for a majority of falls in older adults [39]. At baseline, 24% of elderly patients rely on a mobility device such as a cane to ambulate

Table 27.3 Rates of in-hospital complications in patients with NSTI [4, 35]

Complication	Frequency (%)
Acute renal failure	7–32
Hepatic failure	0–6
ARDS	24–29
MOF	21
Stroke	2.5
Heart failure	2.0
Clostridium difficile colitis	9
Other infections	27

[40]. An amputation in an elderly patient can further impair previously limited mobility.

Level of amputation for geriatric patients can be crucial for regaining independence, as the amount of energy required to ambulate increases from a partial foot to below-knee (BKA) to above-knee amputation (AKA). BKA requires a 40–60% increase in energy expenditure, while AKA requires a 90–120% increase in energy expenditure. In the elderly, up to 80% of patients with a BKA are recommended for prosthesis training, and up to 90% of those patients are able to utilize the prosthesis; however, only 30% of patients with a AKA or higher are recommended for prosthesis training, and only 40% of those patients ultimately are able to utilize their prosthesis [41].

Preexisting medical comorbidities often impede recovery from an amputation in geriatric patients. Concurrent arthritis may limit mobility, vision loss may exacerbate loss of proprioception with a prosthesis, and cardiovascular disease may impair the ability to participate in rehabilitation or to even propel a wheelchair in those not eligible for a prosthesis [41]. These patient comorbidities are associated with the inability to achieve independence in activities of daily living after amputation [42]. However, the importance of rehabilitation after amputation must be stressed as the ability to perform activities of daily living increases over time [41, 42].

Patients with NSTI have persistent, long-term difficulties after leaving the hospital. Patients report a moderate level of distress overall and distress about their NSTI operative site specifically. Most patients report pain and physical limitations. While the level of distress does not increase in older patients, elderly patients report more pain and physical limitations, although these improve with time from discharge [43].

Social functioning is decreased to a greater extent in elderly patients with NSTI. While overall patients report a moderately good quality of life after debridement of NSTI, older patients report a lower quality of life. Specifically geriatric patients report worse fatigue which may impact postoperative social functioning [43]. Patients with NSTI report depression, post-traumatic stress disorder (PTSD), fear of further infection, changes in family dynamic, sexual difficulty, and loss of employment, to which the elderly are not immune [44].

Conclusions

NSTI is a morbid and mortal condition. Older age is associated with an increased mortality, and the comorbid conditions and complications often associated with NSTI also have a higher mortality in the elderly. Barriers to care in the elderly may delay presentation for medical attention and debridement. Elderly patients with an amputation face difficulty in returning to independence given their underlying comorbidities and increased energy requirements. The risks of NSTI do not end with discharge, as after discharge elderly patients have worse physical and social function. The elderly are a high-risk group among patients with NSTI.

References

1. Edelsberg J, Taneja C, Zervos M, Haque N, Moore C, Reyes K, et al. Trends in US hospital admissions for skin and soft tissue infections. Emerg Infect Dis. 2009;15(9):1516–8.
2. Necrotizing fasciitis: a rare disease, especially for the healthy. 2015. http://www.cdc.gov/features/necrotizingfasciitis/. Accessed 7 Mar 2016.
3. Mills MK, Faraklas I, Davis C, Stoddard GJ, Saffle J. Outcomes from treatment of necrotizing soft-tissue infections: results from the National Surgical Quality Improvement Program database. Am J Surg. 2010;200(6):790–6; discussion 796–7.
4. Elliott DC, Kufera JA, Myers RA. Necrotizing soft tissue infections. Risk factors for mortality and strategies for management. Ann Surg. 1996;224(5):672–83.
5. Morgan MS. Diagnosis and management of necrotising fasciitis: a multiparametric approach. J Hosp Infect. 2010;75(4):249–57.
6. Shiroff AM, Herlitz GN, Gracias VH. Necrotizing soft tissue infections. J Intensive Care Med. 2014;29(3):138–44.
7. Incidence of diagnosed diabetes per 1,000 population aged 18–79 years, by sex and age, United States, 1997–2014. 2015. http://www.cdc.gov/diabetes/statistics/incidence/fig5.htm. Accessed 7 Mar 2016.
8. SEER incidence and U.S. death rates, age-adjusted and age-specific rates, by race and sex. http://seer.

cancer.gov/csr/1975_2012/browse_csr.php?sectionSEL=2&pageSEL=sect_02_table.07.html. Accessed 7 Mar 2016.

9. Active Bacterial Core Surveillance (ABCs) report emerging infections program network group A streptococcus, provisional—2014. 2015. http://www.cdc.gov/abcs/reports-findings/survreports/gas14.pdf. Accessed 24 Mar 2016.
10. Kuo YL, Shieh SJ, Chiu HY, Lee JW. Necrotizing fasciitis caused by Vibrio vulnificus: epidemiology, clinical findings, treatment and prevention. Eur J Clin Microbiol Infect Dis. 2007;26(11):785–92.
11. McHenry CR, Piotrowski JJ, Petrinic D, Malangoni MA. Determinants of mortality for necrotizing soft-tissue infections. Ann Surg. 1995;221(5):558–63; discussion 563–5.
12. Coleman S, Gorecki C, Nelson EA, Closs SJ, Defloor T, Halfens R, et al. Patient risk factors for pressure ulcer development: systematic review. Int J Nurs Stud. 2013;50(7):974–1003.
13. Gould L, Abadir P, Brem H, Carter M, Conner-Kerr T, Davidson J, et al. Chronic wound repair and healing in older adults: current status and future research. Wound Repair Regen. 2015;23(1):1–13.
14. Rates of TBI-related Emergency Department Visits by Age Group—United States, 2001–2010. 2016. http://www.cdc.gov/traumaticbraininjury/data/rates_ed_byage.html. Accessed 7 Mar 2016.
15. Anaya DA, McMahon K, Nathens AB, Sullivan SR, Foy H, Bulger E. Predictors of mortality and limb loss in necrotizing soft tissue infections. Arch Surg. 2005;140(2):151–7; discussion 158.
16. Feinberg WM, Blackshear JL, Laupacis A, Kronmal R, Hart RG. Prevalence, age distribution, and gender of patients with atrial fibrillation. Analysis and implications. Arch Intern Med. 1995;155(5):469–73.
17. Beebe-Dimmer JL, Pfeifer JR, Engle JS, Schottenfeld D. The epidemiology of chronic venous insufficiency and varicose veins. Ann Epidemiol. 2005;15(3):175–84.
18. Wong CH, Khin LW, Heng KS, Tan KC, Low CO. The LRINEC (Laboratory Risk Indicator for Necrotizing Fasciitis) score: a tool for distinguishing necrotizing fasciitis from other soft tissue infections. Crit Care Med. 2004;32(7):1535–41.
19. Wall DB, Klein SR, Black S, de Virgilio C. A simple model to help distinguish necrotizing fasciitis from nonnecrotizing soft tissue infection. J Am Coll Surg. 2000;191(3):227–31.
20. Patel KV. Epidemiology of anemia in older adults. Semin Hematol. 2008;45(4):210–7.
21. Mohan S, Gu S, Parikh A, Radhakrishnan J. Prevalence of hyponatremia and association with mortality: results from NHANES. Am J Med. 2013;126(12):1127–37. e1
22. Tiao JY, Semmens JB, Masarei JR, Lawrence-Brown MM. The effect of age on serum creatinine levels an aging population: relevance to vascular surgery. Cardiovasc Surg. 2002;10(5):445–51.
23. Wysoki MG, Santora TA, Shah RM, Friedman AC. Necrotizing fasciitis: CT characteristics. Radiology. 1997;203(3):859–63.
24. Bui AL, Horwich TB, Fonarow GC. Epidemiology and risk profile of heart failure. Nat Rev Cardiol. 2011;8(1):30–41.
25. Akinbami L, Liu X. Chronic obstructive pulmonary disease among adults aged 18 and over in the United States, 1998–2009. 2015. http://www.cdc.gov/nchs/data/databriefs/db63.htm. Accessed 7 Mar 2015.
26. Kidney Disease Statistics for the United States. http://www.niddk.nih.gov/health-information/health-statistics/Pages/kidney-disease-statistics-united-states.aspx#3. Accessed 7 Mar 2016.
27. Martin GS, Mannino DM, Moss M. The effect of age on the development and outcome of adult sepsis. Crit Care Med. 2006;34(1):15–21.
28. Emori TG, Banerjee SN, Culver DH, Gaynes RP, Horan TC, Edwards JR, et al. Nosocomial infections in elderly patients in the United States, 1986–1990. National Nosocomial Infections Surveillance System. Am J Med. 1991;91(3B):289S–93S.
29. Freischlag JA, Ajalat G, Busuttil RW. Treatment of necrotizing soft tissue infections. The need for a new approach. Am J Surg. 1985;149(6):751–5.
30. Wong CH, Chang HC, Pasupathy S, Khin LW, Tan JL, Low CO. Necrotizing fasciitis: clinical presentation, microbiology, and determinants of mortality. J Bone Joint Surg Am. 2003;85-A(8):1454–60.
31. Neveu H, Kleinknecht D, Brivet F, Loirat P, Landais P. Prognostic factors in acute renal failure due to sepsis. Results of a prospective multicentre study. The French Study Group on Acute Renal Failure. Nephrol Dial Transplant. 1996;11(2):293–9.
32. Fitzpatrick AL, Powe NR, Cooper LS, Ives DG, Robbins JA. Barriers to health care access among the elderly and who perceives them. Am J Public Health. 2004;94(10):1788–94.
33. Nursing Home Care. 2015. http://www.cdc.gov/nchs/fastats/nursing-home-care.htm. Accessed 7 Mar 2016.
34. Light TD, Choi KC, Thomsen TA, Skeete DA, Latenser BA, Born JM, et al. Long-term outcomes of patients with necrotizing fasciitis. J Burn Care Res. 2010;31(1):93–9.
35. Bulger EM, Maier RV, Sperry J, Joshi M, Henry S, Moore FA, et al. A novel drug for treatment of necrotizing soft-tissue infections: a randomized clinical trial. JAMA Surg. 2014;149(6):528–36.
36. Xu J, Murphy S, Kochanek K, Bastian B. Deaths: final data for 2013. 2016. http://www.cdc.gov/nchs/data/nvsr/nvsr64/nvsr64_02.pdf. Accessed 7 Mar 2016.
37. Helm P, Engel T, Holm A, Kristiansen VB, Rosendahl S. Function after lower limb amputation. Acta Orthop Scand. 1986;57(2):154–7.
38. Purser JL, Weinberger M, Cohen HJ, Pieper CF, Morey MC, Li T, et al. Walking speed predicts health status and hospital costs for frail elderly male veterans. J Rehabil Res Dev. 2005;42(4):535–46.

39. Robinovitch SN, Feldman F, Yang Y, Schonnop R, Leung PM, Sarraf T, et al. Video capture of the circumstances of falls in elderly people residing in long-term care: an observational study. Lancet. 2013;381(9860):47–54.
40. Gell NM, Wallace RB, LaCroix AZ, Mroz TM, Patel KV. Mobility device use in older adults and incidence of falls and worry about falling: findings from the 2011–2012 national health and aging trends study. J Am Geriatr Soc. 2015;63(5):853–9.
41. Coletta EM. Care of the elderly patient with lower extremity amputation. J Am Board Fam Pract. 2000;13(1):23–34.
42. Vogel TR, Petroski GF, Kruse RL. Impact of amputation level and comorbidities on functional status of nursing home residents after lower extremity amputation. J Vasc Surg. 2014;59(5):1323–30. e1
43. Pikturnaite J, Soldin M. Impact of necrotising fasciitis on quality of life: a qualitative analysis. Burns. 2014;40(5):848–51.
44. Hakkarainen TW, Burkette Ikebata N, Bulger E, Evans HL. Moving beyond survival as a measure of success: understanding the patient experience of necrotizing soft-tissue infections. J Surg Res. 2014;192(1):143–9.

Part XIII

Thermal Injury

Thermal Injury

28

Gabriel Hundeshagen, David N. Herndon, and Jong O. Lee

The Geriatric Burn Patient

Epidemiology

In 2015, approximately 200,000 burn injuries occurred in individuals over the age of 60 years in the United States, representing 13.4% of all burn injuries during that year [1]. In this elderly burn population, flame burns represent over half (55%) of all cases, with scald burns accounting for about one-quarter of cases (23%) [1]. A relatively large percentage of burn injuries are related to cooking accidents in this age group. Figures 28.1 and 28.2 depict typical second- and third degree burns. In contrast to the overrepresentation of males in younger burn patients, the male-to-female proportion decreases steadily with increasing age [1]. A small, yet considerable and likely underreported percentage of elderly thermal injury is related to self-neglect and elder abuse [2]. Both conditions should be taken into consideration when assessing the etiology of geriatric burn injuries. Measures that can be taken to avoid recurrence include the activation of adult protective services (APS) [3].

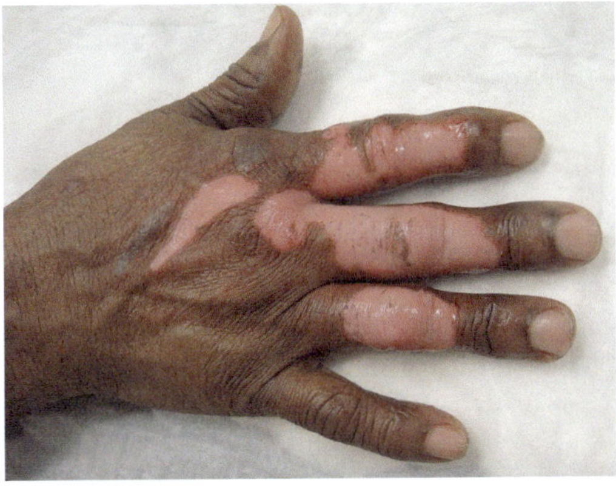

Fig. 28.1 Seventy-two-year-old woman with second-degree grease burn to the dorsum of right hand

G. Hundeshagen, M.D.
Department of Surgery, University of Texas Medical Branch (UTMB), 301 University Blvd, Galveston, TX 77550, USA

Department of Hand, Plastic and Reconstructive Surgery, Burn Trauma Center, BG Trauma Center Ludwigshafen, University of Heidelberg, Ludwig-Guttmann-Str. 13, Ludwigshafen 67071, Germany
e-mail: gabrielhundeshagen@gmail.com

D.N. Herndon, M.D., F.A.C.S. (✉)
Department of Surgery, University of Texas Medical Branch (UTMB), 301 University Blvd, Galveston, TX 77550, USA

Department of Surgery, Shriners Hospitals for Children®—Galveston (SHC-G), 815 Market Street, Galveston, TX 77550, USA
e-mail: dherndon@utmb.edu

J.O. Lee, M.D.
Department of Surgery, University of Texas Medical Branch (UTMB), 301 University Blvd, Galveston, TX 77550, USA
e-mail: jolee@utmb.edu

A. Rodriguez et al. (eds.), *Geriatric Trauma and Acute Care Surgery*, https://doi.org/10.1007/978-3-319-57403-5_28

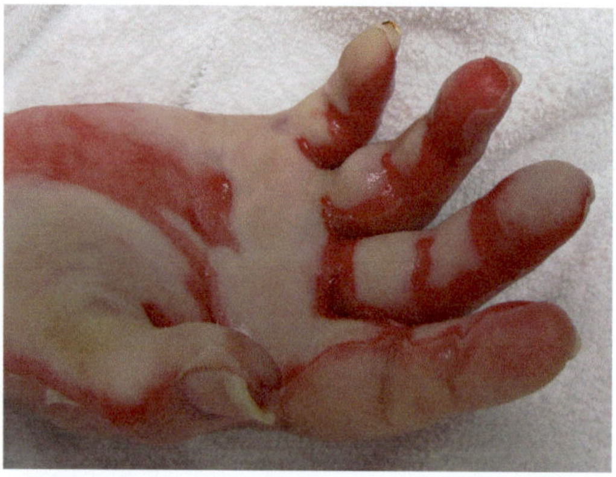

Fig. 28.2 Seventy-nine-year-old woman with third-degree contact burn to right hand

Outcome

Although mortality has decreased in all age groups in recent decades, overall outcomes of thermal injury are worse for the very young and the very old [1]. For example, a 60% overall mortality rate is seen with a 45–55% total body surface area (TBSA) burn at the age of 60–69 years, with this rate also being seen in burns covering only 20–29% of the TBSA at ages over 80 years. Mortality rates due to thermal injury increase steadily with age, averaging 7.4% for patients older than 60 years, 12.9% for those older than 70 years, and 21% for those older than 80 years [1]. During their hospitalization, the elderly are more prone to complications such as pneumonia, urinary tract infections, and respiratory failure [4]. A recent study of a large database of elderly burn patients was not able to determine a defined "cutoff age" at which an outcome worsens significantly, but it reinforced the notion that even small burn injuries can be life threatening despite access to standardized modern burn care [5].

Risk Factors

Elderly patients with thermal injury have various risk factors that are unique to their age group, complicate treatment, and worsen outcomes. Reduced cardiopulmonary reserve may lead to earlier pulmonary and cardiac failure, while atherosclerosis and coronary artery disease with or without previous infarction further strain the heart during post-burn stress [6]. Malnutrition is common in the elderly and can be strongly exacerbated by the burn-induced hypermetabolic and hypercatabolic response [7]. The resulting massive loss in lean body mass that occurs over a short time impairs wound healing, increases immune deficiency, decreases anabolic compensation, and prolongs overall recovery time [8, 9]. The aging skin progressively thins due to decreased epidermal turnover rates as well as a reduction in dermal cells, vascularity, and extracellular matrix proteins [10]. These phenomena put the elderly at significantly higher risk of full-thickness burns and impair regenerative capacity [11].

Treatment

The overall principles of treating geriatric burn patients are identical to those for younger patients. Individual differences in treatment commonly result from comorbidities and adverse conditions arising during patient management.

Initial Assessment

The Advanced Burn Life Support (ABLS) guidelines issued by the American Burn Association provide a valuable overview of the initial steps in treating a burn patient. A primary assessment of any burn patient should address a secure airway, breathing, circulation, neurological disabilities, and environmental factors contributing to the injury and should quickly resolve all related problems as soon as possible. Intubation should be performed liberally when inhalation injury or worsening of the patient's airway and breathing is suspected, as progressing burn- and resuscitation-induced edema can make later attempts difficult or impossible. A secondary assessment should be directed towards a full-body physical examination and obtaining a detailed history including specifics about the injury, comorbidities, allergies, and medications being taken by the patient. Tetanus vaccination status should be evaluated and updated as necessary. The patient's body temperature should be maintained meticulously with blankets and/or heating devices, as loss of body temperature due to the impaired skin barrier is a frequent complication of burn injury. The extent and severity of second- and third-degree TBSA burns should be assessed using either the rule of nines (Fig. 28.3) or the 1% rule (patient's palm and digits represent 1% TBSA). Resuscitation should be initiated accordingly, and a Foley catheter should be considered for precise monitoring of urinary output in patients with burns larger than 15% TBSA. A nasogastric tube can be placed to counter nausea and vomiting. Wounds should not be treated with creams or special dressings. Rather, they should be covered with sterile dry dressings until they can be evaluated by a burn physician.

Admission and Referral

After initial assessment of burn severity, initiation of resuscitation, and stabilization of the patient, referral to a burn center should be initiated for the following cases:

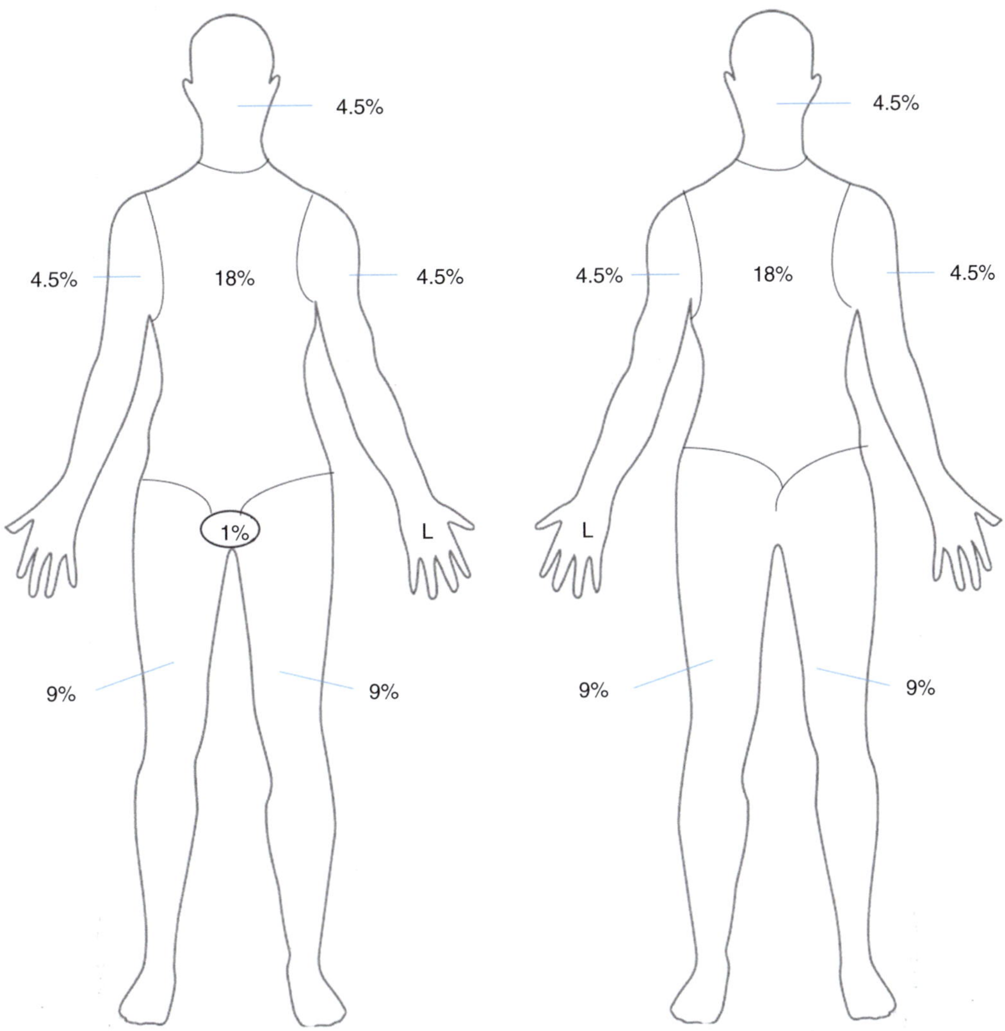

Fig. 28.3 Rule of nine to estimate burn size as percent total body surface area (TBSA) burned. Various body parts are representing their surface area as multiples of 9

- Partial-thickness burns exceeding 10% TBSA
- Any burns of face, hands, feet, genitalia, perineum, or major joints
- Any full-thickness burn
- Pediatric burns, if the hospital is not equipped or staffed to treat children
- Inhalation injury
- Chemical burns
- Electrical burns, including lightning injury
- Patients who are expected to require special psychological or rehabilitative intervention [12]

Combination of Trauma and Burns

Patients with burns and concomitant trauma should be assessed to determine which injury poses the greatest risk for morbidity and mortality. Joint physician judgment in concordance with regional medical center plans and triage protocols is essential. Fractures may be initially stabilized in a trauma center before referral to a burn center while mindfully minimizing delay of burn care as much as reasonably possible. Ideally, any burn patient should reach a burn center within 72 h of injury.

Initial Resuscitation

Next to general intensive care measures to stabilize a patient after burn injury, resuscitation plays a key role in post-burn treatment. Fluid requirement is dependent on burn size, depth, and onset of resuscitation [13]. Due to decreased resistance to edema formation and fluid accumulation, higher resuscitation volumes can be needed to avoid hypovolemia in the elderly [14]. However, impaired cardiac function may demand cautious volume therapy to avoid congestive heart failure. While successful resuscitation should be monitored primarily through measures of hemodynamic stability, vital signs, and urinary output, the Parkland formula can be used to calculate the fluid requirement during the first 24 h. ABSL guidelines and the Brooke formula suggest more restrictive fluid management to avoid over-resuscitation. Benicke's formula, which includes other variables, is more tailored to the elderly patient population and provides age-adjusted estimates of initial fluid demand during the first 24 h post-burn [15, 16].

Parkland formula:

$$\text{Predicted volume}(\text{mL}) = \text{weight in kg} \times \text{TBSA } 2^{\text{nd}} \& 3^{\text{rd}} \times \mathbf{4mL}$$

Modified Brooke formula:

$$\text{Predicted volume}(\text{mL}) = \text{weight in kg} \times \text{TBSA } 2^{\text{nd}} \& 3^{\text{rd}} \times \mathbf{2mL}$$

Benicke's formula:

$$\text{Predicted volume}(\text{mL}) = (50 \times \text{weight in kg}) + \left(300 \times \text{TBSA } 2^{\text{nd}} \& 3^{\text{rd}}\right) + (3500 \times \text{IHI}) + (4000 \times \text{BAL}) - (3500 \times \text{age} \geq 65 \text{ years})^{*}$$

**First 24 h; IHI: Inhalation injury present: yes = 1, no = 0; BAL: blood alcohol level, <0.1% = 0, ≥0.1 = 1*

The first half of the calculated volume should be given during the first 8 h after the burn as Ringer's lactate, and the other half should be given over the next 16 h. Infusion therapy is monitored and adjusted according to vital signs, circulatory stability, and hourly urinary output measures.

Wound Management

Partial-Thickness Burns

Superficial and deep partial-thickness burn wounds should undergo initial cleaning and removal of blisters and nonviable tissue. They should then be covered with a dressing that enables re-epithelialization of the affected area without painful adherence during dressing changes. Dressing options include hydrocolloids, polyurethane film dressings, silicone-coated nylon dressings, reabsorbable polylactic acid compounds, or foam dressings with or without antimicrobial silver coating. Full re-epithelialization can normally be expected after 10–14 days but can be delayed due to comorbidities as described above.

Full-Thickness Burns

As early burn wound excision and wound closure are paramount to survival and decreasing morbidity, the clinician should not be tempted by a patient's advanced age to take less aggressive therapeutic approaches [17]. Burn eschars of a full-thickness defect should be excised tangentially, and the resulting wound should ideally be covered with autologous split-thickness skin graft (STSG). The prospect of multiple surgical grafting procedures in large burns necessitates special considerations in the elderly. For example, donor-site healing may be impaired due to the aforementioned thinning of regenerative dermal layers. Likewise, donor-site morbidity may increase due to comorbidities complicating wound healing in general. The use of thinner STSG is warranted to ameliorate these problems [11]. Whenever full closure of burn wounds cannot be achieved, temporal coverage with alloplastic dermal substitutes is necessary until sufficient STSG is available for definitive wound closure.

Perioperative Optimization

Several interventions are available to counter burn-induced pathophysiological changes with the goal of optimizing patient recovery. Elderly patients experience a substantial proinflammatory, hypermetabolic, and hypercatabolic response to thermal injury [5]. High energy demand is met with increased protein turnover and degradation, which in turn necessitates a compensatory protein intake of up to 1.5–2 g/(kg/day) [18, 19] and supplementation of micronutrients [9, 20]. Hypercatabolism can be further ameliorated through the adjunctive use of anabolic agents. Insulin, when infused continuously for intensive euglycemic control, can promote muscle anabolism [21], reduce resting energy expenditure, restore insulin sensitivity [22], and reduce mortality and complications due to infection [23]. The orally available testosterone analogue oxandrolone aids in the restoration of lost lean body mass and can improve wound healing in malnourished adults, independent of age [24, 25]. Hypermetabolism in acute burn patients can be countered by β-adrenergic blockade with propranolol. When dosed to lower heart rate by 15–20%, propranolol can effectively optimize cardiac work and energy expenditure, increase muscle-protein balance, and reduce the degree of fatty infiltration of the liver [18, 25, 26]. As the aging cardiovascular system is less responsive to β-receptor stimulation and more prone to adverse cardiac outcomes due to preexisting comorbidities such as coronary artery disease, clinicians should stratify elderly patients according to their individual risk to identify those in need of additional evaluation [27]. Accordingly cautious use of β-blockers may be necessary to avoid intraoperative complications. Pain is often undertreated in elderly burn patients and can further increase catecholamine-induced stress; lead to post-traumatic stress disorder, depression, and delirium; and delay rehabilitative activity [28, 29]. At the same time, reduced clearance rates of certain therapeutic agents may necessitate individual dosing approaches to ensure that symptoms are alleviated while drug concentrations are maintained in a safe range. Combination therapies including various analgesic agents, patient-controlled analgesia, adjunct psychotherapy, and appropriate sedation when necessary can alleviate stress, reduce morbidity, and improve outcomes of burn injury [30].

Rehabilitation

Rehabilitation enables elderly burn patients to regain their physical activity level and psychological abilities after an often devastating injury. Specialized physical and occupational therapy has to begin as early as possible after the injury as any loss of function, strength, or independence is difficult to recover in this population. Therefore, aggressive rehabilitation management is indicated and should include sufficient wound healing, scar prevention, splinting, casting, pressure therapy, pharmacological therapy, exercise, and psychological support [31].

Conclusion

Despite therapeutic improvements and overall reduction in morbidity and mortality, the growing geriatric burn population and their pathophysiological risk profile pose a major challenge to the burn surgeon. While physiological age, comorbidities, and pre-injury functional status should influence surgical decision making, age alone should not determine whether an elderly patient should be aggressively treated surgically. Nonetheless, therapeutic goals can shift from purely expanding life span to maintaining the greatest possible amount of independence and quality of life or merely ameliorating suffering, as directed by the patient and their family.

References

1. American Burn Association. ABA annual burn repository [internet]. 2015. [Cited 18 Apr 2016]. http://www.ameriburn.org/NBR.php.
2. Bird PE, Harrington DT, Barillo DJ, McSweeney A, Shirani KZ, Goodwin CW. Elder abuse: a call to action. J Burn Care Rehabil. 1998;19(6):522–7.
3. National Adult Protective Services Association | National Adult Protective Services Association [Internet]. [Cited 27 Apr 2016]. http://www.napsa-now.org/.
4. 2015NBRAnnualReport.pdf [Internet]. [Cited 2016 Apr 18]. http://www.ameriburn.org/2015NBRAnnualReport.pdf.
5. Jeschke MG, Pinto R, Costford SR, Amini-Nik S. Threshold age and burn size associated with poor outcomes in the elderly after burn injury. Burns. 2016;42(2):276–81.
6. Koupil J, Brychta P, Říhová H, Kincová S. Special features of burn injuries in elderly patients. Acta Chir Plast. 2001;43(2):57–60.
7. Demling RH. The incidence and impact of pre-existing protein energy malnutrition on outcome in the elderly burn patient population. J Burn Care Rehabil. 2005;26(1):94–100.
8. Darby E, Anawalt DBD. Male hypogonadism. Treat Endocrinol. 2012;4(5):293–309.
9. Kagansky N, Berner Y, Koren-Morag N, Perelman L, Knobler H, Levy S. Poor nutritional habits are predictors of poor outcome in very old hospitalized patients. Am J Clin Nutr. 2005;82(4):784–91.
10. Waller JM, Maibach HI. Age and skin structure and function, a quantitative approach (II): protein, glycosaminoglycan, water, and lipid content and structure. Skin Res Technol. 2006;12(3):145–54.
11. Gosain A, DiPietro LA. Aging and wound healing. World J Surg. 2004;28(3):321–6.
12. American Burn Association. American Burn Association advanced burn life support provider manual 2011. Chicago, IL: American Burn Association.
13. Greenhalgh DG. Burn resuscitation. J Burn Care Res. 2007;28(4):555–65.
14. Bowser-Wallace BH, Cone JB, Caldwell FT. Hypertonic lactated saline resuscitation of severely burned patients over 60 years of age. J Trauma. 1985;25(1):22–6.
15. Benicke M, Perbix W, Lefering R, Knam F, Ipaktchi KR, Tannapfel A, et al. New multifactorial burn resuscitation formula offers superior predictive reliability in comparison to established algorithms. Burns 2009;35(1):30–5.
16. Warden GD. Burn shock resuscitation. World J Surg. 1992;16(1):16–23.
17. Burdge JJ, Katz B, Edwards R, Ruberg R. Surgical treatment of burns in elderly patients. J Trauma. 1988;28(2):214–7.
18. Williams FN, Herndon DN, Jeschke MG. The hypermetabolic response to burn injury and interventions to modify this response. Clin Plast Surg. 2009;36(4):583–96.
19. Wolfe RR. Herman Award Lecture, 1996: relation of metabolic studies to clinical nutrition—the example of burn injury. Am J Clin Nutr. 1996;64(5):800–8.
20. Forbes GB. Influence of nutrition. In: Human body composition. New York: Springer; 1987. p. 209–47.
21. Ferrando AA, Chinkes DL, Wolf SE, Matin S, Herndon DN, Wolfe RR. A submaximal dose of insulin promotes net skeletal muscle protein synthesis in patients with severe burns. Ann Surg. 1999;229(1):11–8.
22. Fram RY, Cree MG, Wolfe RR, Mlcak RP, Qian T, Chinkes DL, et al. Intensive insulin therapy improves insulin sensitivity and mitochondrial function in severely burned children. Crit Care Med. 2010;38(6):1475–83.
23. Jeschke MG, Kulp GA, Kraft R, Finnerty CC, Mlcak R, Lee JO, et al. Intensive insulin therapy in severely burned pediatric patients: a prospective randomized trial. Am J Respir Crit Care Med. 2010;182(3):351–9.
24. Demling RH, DeSanti L. The rate of restoration of body weight after burn injury, using the anabolic agent oxandrolone, is not age dependent. Burns. 2001;27(1):46–51.
25. Miller JT, Btaiche IF. Oxandrolone treatment in adults with severe thermal injury. Pharmacotherapy. 2009;29(2):213–26.

26. Herndon DN, Hart DW, Wolf SE, Chinkes DL, Wolfe RR. Reversal of catabolism by beta-blockade after severe burns. N Engl J Med. 2001;345(17):1223–9.
27. Lee TH, Marcantonio ER, Mangione CM, Thomas EJ, Polanczyk CA, Cook EF, et al. Derivation and prospective validation of a simple index for prediction of cardiac risk of major noncardiac surgery. Circulation. 1999;100(10):1043–9.
28. Ferrell BA. Assessing pain in the elderly. Consult Pharm J Am Soc Consult Pharm. 2010;25 Suppl A:5–10.
29. Gregoretti C, Decaroli D, Piacevoli Q, Mistretta A, Barzaghi N, Luxardo N, et al. Analgo-sedation of patients with burns outside the operating room. Drugs. 2008;68(17):2427–43.
30. Murphy KD, Lee JO, Herndon DN. Current pharmacotherapy for the treatment of severe burns. Expert Opin Pharmacother. 2003;4(3):369–84.
31. Frontera WR, Meredith CN, O'Reilly KP, Knuttgen HG, Evans WJ. Strength conditioning in older men: skeletal muscle hypertrophy and improved function. J Appl Physiol (1985). 1988;64(3):1038–44.

Part XIV

Acute Care Surgery Introduction: Common Abdominal Emergencies

System Impact and Demographics of Abdominal Surgical Emergencies

29

Laura S. Buchanan and Jose J. Diaz

Introduction

A 75-year-old woman presents to her local emergency department with 2 days of abdominal pain, is found to have appendicitis, and undergoes appendectomy. Nearing discharge on postoperative day 2, she develops volume overload from a congestive heart failure exacerbation, and then acute renal failure induced by her diuresis. She then develops atrial fibrillation with rapid response after her rate control failed to be resumed postoperatively. On hospital day 6 she is recommended for subacute rehab placement due to deconditioning. While awaiting placement she aspirates and is transferred to intensive care with pneumonitis. She proceeds to develop delirium, and respiratory failure. After 2 weeks she finally leaves the acute hospital to spend an additional 30 days in skilled nursing. Perhaps we should tell her that she is lucky for avoiding a postoperative heart attack, urinary tract infection, intra-abdominal abscess, malnutrition, and pressure ulcers. Modifications in her care could have decreased risk for each of her complications. Addressing each complication individually becomes analogous to putting out a series of fires while ignoring a group of dedicated arsonists. The most effective way to care for a geriatric patient is to create a system of care addressing the complex physiology and decreased reserve of this population.

L.S. Buchanan, M.D.
J.J. Diaz, C.N.S., F.A.C.S., F.C.C.M (✉)
R Adams Cowley Shock Trauma Center, University of Maryland Medical Center, Baltimore, MD, USA
e-mail: lbuchanan@umm.edu; jdiaz@umm.edu

Aging Populations in Acute Care Surgery

The most fundamental and in some ways most difficult part of discussing acute care surgery in the elderly is to define who is old. Medicare starts at 65; Social Security benefits start at 62, and AARP eligibility at age 50. Most social science literature, census data, and retirement benefits start at age 65. The World Health Organization struggles with these definitions across populations. If the average life expectancy is lower, should the definition of elderly also be lower? If so, then how do we compare elderly across populations? The American College of Surgeons (ACS) defines optimal preoperative assessment of the geriatric surgical patient, but does not specify an age at which the assessment should be implemented. The chronologic age is a nonspecific indicator of an individual's physiologic age; however, in most developed countries 65 is used as a cutoff in data collection and population description.

Regardless of the cutoff selected, the population of older Americans is increasing and not expected to peak until 2030. Heavily contributing

A. Rodriguez et al. (eds.), *Geriatric Trauma and Acute Care Surgery*,
https://doi.org/10.1007/978-3-319-57403-5_29

to this expansion, the baby-boomer generation started reaching age 65 in 2011. To view this expansion overtime, in 1970 only 9.8% of the population was age 65 and older. In 2010 it had increased to 13%. The total number of individuals over age 65 will continue to increase to the anticipated peak of 20% by 2030. This population trend is reflected in trauma and emergency surgery patient populations. At our center annual trauma admissions over age 60 doubled from 2001 to 2010 (700–1400, or an increase from 12 to 21%). As the population ages, healthcare needs increase. Model-based predictions of future healthcare needs project that by the year 2025 there will be an 8–12% increase in outpatient and ER visits, a 19% increase in inpatient days, and a 17% increase in demand for general surgeons [1].

Equally important to note is the increased resource utilization observed by this population. In 2002 the average annual healthcare cost for an older adult was $11,000 compared to $3000 for a younger adult. Fifty-two percent of Medicare costs are incurred in the last 60 days of life. Despite increased utilization compared to younger adults, there is evidence that individual utilization is decreasing. Expenditures in the last 6 months of life for Medicare beneficiaries decreased from $15,300 (1999) to $13,400 (2013) and end-of-life hospitalization decreased from 131 per 100 deaths to 103 over the same time period [2]. In addition to the challenges of a geriatric population, acute care surgery has been associated with increased resource utilization and cost compared to elective populations [3].

Emergency general surgery makes up 7–25% of all hospital admissions [4, 5]. As many as 30–44% of acute care surgery admissions went on to require surgery [4, 6]. In a 2014 retrospective review Deiner compared younger adults (<65) to older adults (≥65), evaluating surgical characteristics and 48-h outcomes [7]. A third of all surgeries were in the older population. The majority of older patient surgeries occurred at community hospitals. Mortality at 48 h increased with age over 70, and doubled for patients over age 90. Complications such as hemodynamic instability, respiratory complication, and resuscitation increased with increasing age. Perioperative mortality after emergency general surgery is 15–20% but increases as high as 50% for individuals aged 80 and above [8]. The increased mortality by age is demonstrated well by examining a single disease such as appendicitis where the risk of death is increased sevenfold for patients over age 70 [9]. Complications after laparotomy in elderly are associated with threefold increase in mortality [8]. A significant number of elderly patients can undergo emergent surgery, but it is the complications which are not well tolerated. If they occur decisions to intervene early must be essential. The discussion becomes more complicated when one must balance survival vs. long-term functional status.

Goals of Care: Healthcare Team Versus the Patient

Clinicians and patients often have different goals of care. Health performance measures describe mortality and length of stay, while patients want estimates of return to home and independence. Research in patient-centered outcomes is lacking. Our perceptions of limited functional recovery may be inaccurate. Seventy-nine percent of older adults return to preadmission residential status by 6 months after nonelective abdominal surgery [10]. However, functional deficit and recovery after emergency general surgery are not described. In elective surgical populations some function and independence are lost with a delay in recovery compared to younger adults. Presumably the acuity of illness requiring emergency surgery and inability to perform preoperative optimization only exacerbate and prolong the functional impact of emergency surgery.

Additional research on quality of life, activities of daily living, and return to activity is desperately needed in this field. A patient-centered outcome framework for acutely ill elderly identified several surgery-related areas for research including monitoring postoperative patient-centered outcomes, identifying perioperative strategies to optimize care, and utility of frailty assessment in preoperative evaluation [10].

Recognizing that our field has not yet described the impact on quality of life, goals of interventions must account for quality of life. While age is not a contraindication to surgery, the risk of prolonged dependency at the end of life may be significant. Preservation of function may take precedence over extension of life. Patients and caregivers should be included in decisions and given realistic expectations of anticipated outcomes.

Prediction of Outcome

While common sense tells us that older, sicker patients have worse outcomes than young healthy counterparts, it is difficult to predict the outcome for a single individual. The concept of frailty is gaining utility in surgical populations as a tool to predict outcome and to individualize preoperative counseling. ACS defines frailty as "a syndrome of decreased physiologic reserve and resistance to stressors, which leaves patient more vulnerable to poor health outcomes" [11]. Frailty is clinically distinct from disability or comorbidity. A frail patient is one who lacks reserve to compensate for physiologic challenge. Measures of frailty include cognitive function, nutritional status, walking speed, grip strength, and recent falls among others and can be tested in an elective setting but can be difficult to measure during acute illness. Multiple frailty scales and measures have been developed with varying utility in the acute care emergency surgery population. All need additional validation in elderly, emergency surgery populations. Ozban and colleges performed a retrospective review of 112 emergency general surgery patients and compared expected mortality with that predicted by several major models. In this analysis APACHE II scores had the best correlation with predicted mortality [12]. The Charlson Age-Co-morbidity Index (CACI) has been shown to correlate with mortality and ICU admission after emergency surgery, but has not yet been evaluated in older patients [13]. Both of these remain difficult to apply to emergency populations due to the high number of variables and difficulty with bedside application. A modified frailty index (Emergency General Surgery Frailty Index or EGSFI) was recently published utilizing only 15 measures and accurately predicting risk for complication in an initial small population [14]. Significant work remains to be done to establish and validate the best tool for measuring frailty and predicting outcome in the geriatric emergency surgery population.

System Design and Optimization of Care

Elderly, acute care surgery patients challenge both community hospitals and referral centers. Experience with trauma care in the elderly suggests that there may be benefit in treatment on an acute care surgery service. In injury there is established benefit for treatment of elderly at designated trauma centers. Similarly, there is established benefit in length of stay and complication rates for patients managed with certified acute care surgery programs [15]. The combination of improved care for emergency surgery diagnoses and complexity of elderly patients suggests that transfer to a certified acute care surgery program should be considered when available, and when transfer will not cause a delay in care.

The specialized needs of this population extend beyond the surgical team. Specialized anesthesia, pharmacy, rehabilitation services, and nursing can all benefit the elderly patient. To best meet the needs of an elderly acute care surgery population, the healthcare system must become involved in the patient care. From presentation to after rehabilitation, additional resources and alternative management strategies will improve patient care.

System Goals and Design

In establishing expertise in the care of this patient it is vital to design a system meeting current patient care guidelines. The ACS and American Geriatric Society (AGS) have complied and published detailed Best Practice Guidelines for Perioperative Management of the Geriatric

Patient [16]. Implementation requires multidisciplinary participation including anesthesia, pharmacy, nursing, and infrastructure support.

Despite increased perioperative risk in this population, and many unanswered research questions, the ACS best practice guidelines can assist in developing institutional and individual practice patterns, including preoperative management, intraoperative management, postoperative management, and care transitions [12]. These are in addition to previously published ACS guidelines for elective preoperative optimization of the geriatric patient [17]. Because of the emergent nature of acute care surgery, the preoperative optimization recommendations are not addressed in this discussion. Implementation of a comprehensive geriatric care program as outlined in these guidelines cannot effectively be done on an individual basis, but by institutional and cultural changes in the care of hospitalized elderly.

Implementation of a dedicated geriatric care model will facilitate cultural improvement in geriatric care. Four examples of geriatric care models are discussed in the ACS/AGS Best Practice Guidelines and are reviewed here. A *Geriatric Consultation Service* model utilizes a geriatrician, nurse specialist, or interdisciplinary team to perform a comprehensive geriatric assessment and evaluate specific complications and situations. Benefits of this system are difficult to measure, but include diagnosis and treatment of medical conditions, and educated review of medications and risk. An *Acute Care for Elders* (ACE) model utilizes dedicated hospital wards combined with daily multidisciplinary rounds, and nursing expertise. An ACE unit has carpeted floors, universal handrails, uncluttered hallways, family visiting space, and raised toilet seats and door handles. On admission, staff and patients focus on return to home with early discharge planning and needs assessment. Medication reviews and risk assessment for complications are protocoled and implemented routinely. ACE models are associated with lower cost, shorter length of stay, and decreased functional decline. *Hospital Elder Life Program* (HELP) focuses on cognitive and sensory functioning. An orientation board is provided with caregiver names, schedules, and orienting information. Therapeutic activities are incorporated into caregiver interactions including discussion of current events and word games. Sleep deprivation is minimized. Early and frequent mobilization is utilized. HELP models also focus on visual and hearing aids and early recognition of dehydration and inadequate nutrition. HELP care models do not require a dedicated unit and have limited physical changes compared to the standard hospital room and are associated with reduction in sedative medication, reduction in delirium, and prevention of cognitive and functional decline. *Nurses Improving Care for Healthsystem Elderly* (NICHE) utilizes nursing-based interventions often in combination with an ACE model unit. Staff nurses have specialized training and autonomy to initiate geriatric protocols. NICHE models improve compliance with protocols and improve clinical outcomes.

The *immediate preoperative care* of an elderly patient can be improved by ensuring that appropriate advance directive and goals of care issues are discussed. A healthcare proxy should be established. Consider shortening fluid fast to decrease dehydration and electrolyte imbalances. Carefully review medications to ensure that necessary medications are continued perioperatively and appropriate medications have been held. Preexisting DNR directives should undergo reconsideration and discussion. It is not appropriate to routinely set aside the patient preference, or to uphold the order without discussion of specific perioperative risks and benefits of resuscitation. Take care to use appropriate perioperative antibiotic dosing. Recognize elderly who are at increased risk of venous thromboembolism and make sure that they receive appropriate prophylaxis. Even routine preoperative medication for anxiety/analgesia should be reconsidered in the elderly acute care surgery patient. The routine use of benzodiazepines may contribute to postoperative delirium.

Intraoperative management includes consideration of regional anesthesia to avoid postoperative complications. Perioperative analgesia should include multi-modal, or opioid-sparing techniques (Table 29.1). Postoperative nausea should be risk stratified and avoided with prophylactic

Table 29.1 Strategies for management of analgesia and nausea in the perioperative period

Common analgesics and anxiolytics to avoid	Preferred analgesic techniques	Nausea treatment to avoid	Preferred nausea treatment and avoidance
Barbiturates	Perioperative acetaminophen	Transdermal scopolamine	5-HT3 receptor antagonists (ondansetron)
Benzodiazepines	Scheduled acetaminophen	Metoclopramide (unless gastroparesis)	Avoid volatile anesthetics
Nonbenzodiazepine hypnotics	Regional techniques	Promethazine	Avoid nitrous oxide
Pentazocine		Prochlorperazine	Incorporation of regional anesthesia
Meperidine			
Skeletal muscle relaxants			
Non-Cox NSAIDS			

interventions and risk mitigation. System norms should include strategies to avoid pressure ulcers and nerve damage from positioning. Perioperative fluid management can be tenuous and may require hemodynamic monitoring and continuation of cardiac medications. Pulmonary complications can be reduced with epidural, avoidance on intermediate and long-acting neuromuscular blocking agents, and utilization of laparoscopic approaches when feasible.

The *postoperative management* includes prevention and treatment strategies regarding delirium, pulmonary complications, falls, malnutrition, urinary tract infection (UTI), pressure ulcers, and functional decline. Effective management of these complications is best done by provider education and institutional protocols incorporating best practice.

Postoperative delirium occurs in 9–44% of patients. Routine delirium screening with a validated tool such as the confusion assessment method (CAM) may result in misdiagnosis and overtreatment; however it is appropriate in high-risk populations. When delirium is identified, evaluate for uncontrolled pain, hypoxia, pneumonia, infection, electrolyte disturbance, urinary retention, fecal impaction, medications, and hypoglycemia. After addressing such underlying causes, utilize established multidisciplinary nonpharmacologic interventions such as elimination of restraints, restore vision and hearing aids, and frequent reorientation. Pharmacologic therapy is second line, and the preferred agent is low-dose Haldol, followed by atypical antipsychotics such as risperidone and olanzapine. Benzodiazepines should not be used.

Prevention of pulmonary complications is accomplished by minimizing aspiration risk, and maximizing mobilization and pulmonary toilet. Establishing nursing-based norms for activity such as out of bed at mealtimes, and clearly labeled distance markers in hallways can help create a culture encouraging postoperative activity.

Early mobilization must be balanced with fall prevention. Universal fall screening should be performed. Restoration of vision and hearing aids, and assistive walking devices, are instrumental. Scheduled toileting and minimization of tethers can decrease fall incidence and are easily incorporated into unit protocols.

While most surgeons recognize the importance of adequate nutrition, a significant barrier for elderly is often overlooked. Dentures should be available and in use during PO meals. Absence of dentures makes many regular diet menu items inedible. Oral nutritional supplementation should be added liberally to geriatric patients, especially in those who are undernourished, frail, demented, and/or following orthopedic procedures. Oral supplementation with high protein can reduce pressure ulcers.

UTI prevention is vital and should follow catheter-associated UTI strategies implemented at the institution. Maintain clinical concern for urinary retention and evaluate. Indwelling catheters should not be used as a treatment for incontinence or frequent urination.

Functional decline is experienced by a third of elderly patients undergoing acute medical hospitalization and often persists to 12 months following discharge. Surgery adds additional risk for functional decline. Prevention of and recovery from this complication require a multimodal, multidisciplinary, system-wide approach spanning transitions in care. Interventions require a dedicated geriatric care model, structural modification (handrails, large clocks, uncluttered hallways), frequent staff education, daily targeted rounds, and bridging rehabilitation and therapy strategies after discharge throughout recovery.

The majority of pressure ulcers develop during acute hospitalizations and within 2 weeks of admission. Two-thirds of pressure ulcers are in patients over age 70. Institutional adaptation of a validated risk-scoring system with graded intervention is more effective than clinical judgement alone. A nurse-led wound team is often instrumental in monitoring and implementing cultural changes.

Care Transitions refers to establishment of continuity as a patient moves though healthcare settings and home. Often caregiver and patient education are inadequate. As many as 20% of Medicare recipients will have a 30-day hospital readmission. An effective transitional care coordinator meets the patient before discharge, follows up with phone calls and discussion, and reengages the patient during clinic follow-up. The coordinator also works to ensure a smooth transition from rehab to home in patients. Many elderly postoperative patients would benefit from a transitional care program but special attention should be paid for open wounds, new ostomies, prolonged hospitalization, and those with poor social support.

Even with knowledge of care goals, implementation can be problematic. A single-institution review of elderly patients undergoing elective abdominal operations found only a 46% compliance with NSQIP guidelines including subscores of 0% for delirium screening, 13% for documentation of oral intake, and 35% pressure ulcer risk assessment [18]. Clearly, significant change must be implemented at a system level with monitoring, maintenance, and education to improve care, decrease complications, and maximize postoperative quality of life in this at risk population.

Facilitating Research in System Design

Additional research can have direct impact on outcomes and quality of life for elderly after emergency surgery. System design and implementation should incorporate a prospective database including relevant variables. If starting or expanding an existing system, review the National Institute of Health Toolbox. The NIH has developed and validated a set of measures for ages 3–85 evaluating cognitive, emotional, motor, and sensory function and can be useful for describing function. The lack of data on functional outcome also makes this a field that would benefit from patient-centered outcome research.

Conclusion: Critical Components to Provide Geriatric Emergency General Surgery Care

Optimal care of geriatric patients must include a systematic approach to improving care. Preoperative evaluation must include comprehensive evaluation including frailty assessment, medical optimization, and consideration of goals of treatment. Goals of treatment should not be excluded to treatment limitations, but should include expectations of functional status with treatment options. Care throughout the perioperative period must include consideration of issues unique to the geriatric patient. Attention should include prevention of delirium, appropriate medication selection, and dosing. Treatment should include a multidisciplinary team with surgery, medicine or geriatrics, anesthesia, pharmacy, nursing, and rehabilitation services with collaboration with patients, family, and caregivers. Patient care areas should facilitate early mobilization and provide reorientation cues. Future research focus should include patient-centered and functional outcomes. Systematic and multidisciplinary changes can improve care and outcomes for elderly emergency general surgery patients.

References

1. Dall TM, Gallo PD, Chakrabarti R, West T, Semilla AP, Storm MV. The care span: an aging population and growing disease burden will require a large and specialized health care workforce by 2025. Health Aff. 2013;32(11):2013–20.
2. Krumholz HM, Nuti SV, Downing NS, Normand S-T, Wang Y. Mortality, hospitalizations, and expenditures for the medicare population aged 65 years or older, 1999–2013. JAMA. 2015;314(4):355–65.
3. Lissauer ME, Galvagno SM, Rock P, Narayan M, Shah P, Spencer H, et al. Increased ICU resource needs for an academic emergency general surgery service. Crit Care Med. 2014;42(4):910–7.
4. Gale SC, Shafi S, Dombrovskiy VY, Arumugam D, Crystal JS. The public health burden of emergency general surgery in the United States: a 10-year analysis of the Nationwide Inpatient Sample—2001 to 2010. J Trauma Acute Care Surg. 2014;77(2):202–8.
5. Bruns BR, Tesoriero R, Narayan M, Klyushnenkova EN, Chen H, Scalea TM, et al. Emergency general surgery: defining burden of disease in the State of Maryland. Am Surg. 2015;81(8):829–34.
6. Narayan M, Tesoriero R, Bruns BR, Klyushnenkova EN, Chen H, Diaz JJ. Acute care surgery: defining the economic burden of emergency general surgery. J Am Coll Surg. 2016;222(4):691–9.
7. Deiner S, Westlake B, Dutton RP. Patterns of surgical care and complications in elderly adults. J Am Geriatr Soc. 2014;62(5):829–35.
8. Desserud KF, Veen T, Søreide K. Emergency general surgery in the geriatric patient. Br J Surg. 2016;103(2):e52–61.
9. Andersson RE. Short and long-term mortality after appendectomy in Sweden 1987 to 2006. Influence of appendectomy diagnosis, sex, age, co-morbidity, surgical method, hospital volume, and time period. A national population-based cohort study. World J Surg. 2013;37(5):974–81.
10. Davis PJB, Bailey JG, Molinari M, Hayden J, Johnson PM. The impact of nonelective abdominal surger y on the residential status of older adult patients. Ann Surg. 2016;263(2):274–9.
11. Chow WB, Rosenthal RA, Merkow RP, Ko CY, Esnaola NF. Optimal preoperative assessment of the geriatric surgical patient: a best practices guideline from the American College of Surgeons National Surgical Quality Improvement Program and the American Geriatrics Society. J Am Coll Surg. 2012;215(4):453–66.
12. Özban M, Birsen O, Senel M, Özden A, Kabay B. The analysis of scoring systems predicting mortality in geriatric emergency abdominal surgery. Ulus Travma Acil Cerrahi Derg. 2015;21(3):182–6.
13. St-Louis E, Iqbal S, Feldman LS, Sudarshan M, Deckelbaum DL, Razek TS, et al. Using the age-adjusted Charlson comorbidity index to predict outcomes in emergency general surgery. J Trauma Acute Care Surg. 2014;78(2):318–23.
14. Jokar TO, Ibraheem K, Rhee P, Kulavatunyou N, Haider A, Phelan HA, et al. Emergency general surgery specific frailty index: a validation study. J Trauma Acute Care Surg. 2016;81(2):254–60.
15. Khalil M, Pandit V, Rhee P, Kulvatunyou N, Orouji T, Tang A, et al. Certified acute care surgery programs improve outcomes in patients undergoing emergency surgery: a nationwide analysis. J Trauma Acute Care Surg. 2015;79(1):60–4.
16. Mohanty S, Rosenthal RA, Russell MM, Neuman MD, Ko CY, Esnaola NF. Optimal perioperative management of the geriatric patient: a best practices guideline from the American College of Surgeons NSQIP and the American Geriatrics Society. J Am Coll Surg. 2016;222(5):930–47.
17. Chow WB, Rosenthal RA, Merkow RP, Ko CY, Esnaola NF. Optimal preoperative assessment of the geriatric surgical patient: a best practices guideline from the American College of Surgeons National Surgical Quality Improvement Program and the American Geriatrics Society. J Am Coll Surg. 2012;215(4):453–66.
18. Bergman S, Martelli V, Monette M, Sourial N, Deban M, Hamadani F, et al. Identification of quality of care deficiencies in elderly surgical patients by measuring adherence to process-based quality indicators. J Am Coll Surg. 2013;217(5):858–66.

Clostridium difficile Infection: Considerations in the Geriatric Population

30

Molly Flanagan and Paula Ferrada

Introduction

Clostridium difficile infection (CDI) in the elderly is an increasingly significant problem in industrialized countries [1]. Diarrhea in elderly patients causes significant morbidity, ranging from incontinence and isolation to dehydration, hospitalization, and death [2]. The complicated interplay of host and environmental risk factors creates a setting in which elderly patients are particularly susceptible to CDI [3–7].

Risk Factors

Host factors that increase susceptibility to CDI include age greater than 65 and age-related factors such as decline in immune function, renal dysfunction, multiple comorbidities, and alteration in intestinal microbiota [3, 6]. Environmental age-related factors include increased exposure to antibiotics and increased exposure to healthcare facilities [8, 9]. Acid-suppression medications, including histamine-2 blockers and proton pump inhibitors, have been implicated in the development of CDI. It has been proposed that normal gastric pH provides defense against *C. difficile* spores [5]. Older patients are also at greater risk for recurrent CDI [4, 10].

Microbiology

C. difficile is a spore-forming anaerobic gram-positive rod that is spread via the fecal-oral route. Patients are infected with either the vegetative form of the bacillus or with spores from their environment. The spores provide an effective reservoir in the healthcare setting for reinfection and transmission [3, 11, 12]. The virulence of *C. difficile* is toxin mediated, with toxin A and B as the causative agents for infection. They lead to colonocyte disruption and death via activation of Rho GTPases [12, 13]. Strains of *C. difficile* that are non-toxin producing do not cause diarrheal illness [8, 14–16].

Epidemiology

The incidence of CDI has increased over the past two decades especially among the elderly, with emergence of a more virulent strain during an epidemic in Quebec from 2002 to 2004 [17, 18]. The North American PFGE type 1 and PCR ribotype 027 (NAP1/027) strain of the Quebec

M. Flanagan, M.D. • P. Ferrada, M.D., F.A.C.S. (✉)
VCU Surgery Trauma, Critical Care and Emergency Surgery, PO Box 980454, Richmond, VA 23298-0454, USA
e-mail: pferrada@mcvh-vcu.edu

A. Rodriguez et al. (eds.), *Geriatric Trauma and Acute Care Surgery*,
https://doi.org/10.1007/978-3-319-57403-5_30

epidemic had a high case-fatality rate and its hypervirulence was suggested to be from increased toxin production [19, 20]. While the spectrum of disease caused by this strain is broad, from asymptomatic to fulminant complicated CDI, it continues to be associated with a higher overall mortality [14, 15].

Long-Term Care Facilities

With the ageing of the baby-boomer generation, increasing numbers of patients are requiring extended care and long-term care facilities [18, 21]. Long-term acute care hospitals have emerged as a common choice for patients requiring skilled care for patients who have multiple comorbidities and an acute illness that has a reasonable chance of recovery. A study of a long-term care facility showed that *C. difficile* infection is endemic in the long-term care facility population, with an infection rate of 0.97 cases per 1000 resident-days. The incidence of CDI was highest in the patients in the subacute ward, where the sickest patients had been recently discharged from an acute hospitalization. Patients in the nursing home unit had the lowest incidence of CDI, suggesting that the source of CDI was from inpatient hospitalization rather than among the long-term nursing home residents [7, 22].

Prevention

Prevention of healthcare-acquired CDI in the elderly population starts with antibiotic stewardship. A study examining the effect of restricting the use of ceftriaxone and ciprofloxacin showed a significant decrease in the incidence of CDI [23]. Strict hand washing with soap and water by healthcare providers is also essential, as well as enforcing hand washing with visitors and families. Contact precautions, including private rooms or cohorts, gowns, and gloves, should be worn by providers from the time that CDI is suspected until 48 h after the patient again has formed stools. For cleaning the patient's environment, sodium hypochlorite solution is effective at killing *C. difficile* spores. Ultraviolet-C emitter lamps can enhance spore killing after traditional cleaning, particularly in difficult-to-clean areas [11, 24–28].

Diagnosis

CDI most commonly presents with watery diarrhea, abdominal cramping, leukocytosis, and fever; however severe complicated CDI can also present with ileus. Stool studies should be sent on patients with diarrhea who have had recent antibiotic use or hospitalization. The gold standard test is culture of toxigenic *C. difficile* on anaerobic culture medium for 24–48 h and then cell cytotoxicity assay looking for toxins A and B. These tests are relatively time consuming and difficult to perform, however. Current recommendations are to perform nucleic acid amplification tests (NAAT) or glutamate dehydrogenase screening tests for *C. difficile* organisms and then enzyme immunoassay (EIA) for toxin A/B [8, 27, 29].

Medical Therapy

Discontinuation of offending antibiotics is the first step in treatment of CDI. While any antibiotic has the potential to disrupt the patient's normal intestinal flora, the medications most commonly associated with CDI are cephalosporins, clindamycin, and fluoroquinolones [5, 9, 16, 19, 20, 30, 31].

Mild-to-Moderate Disease

Mild-to-moderate disease is associated with diarrhea and abdominal cramping, but without significant systemic symptoms. Oral metronidazole 500 mg three times per day for 10–14 days is the first line agent for the first episode of mild-moderate CDI. Early trials examining PO vancomycin versus metronidazole revealed no difference in outcomes for mild disease. Metronidazole is absorbed completely, and the 6–15% concentration in stool is attributed to secretion. The mean concentration of metronidazole in liquid stool is 9.3 mcg/g and decreases to 1.2 mcg/g in solid stool and is undetectable in asymptomatic patients. Therefore there is little rationale to continue therapy beyond 10–14 days if no diarrhea is present. In patients that do not respond to metronidazole, oral vancomycin may be used instead. Oral vancomycin is not routinely recommended by the CDC for mild disease to prevent the selection of vancomycin-resistant enterococcus [5, 6, 8, 29, 32].

Severe Disease

Severe CDI is characterized by abdominal pain, diarrhea, fever >38.5 C, hypoalbuminemia <2.5 mg/dL, serum creatinine >1.5× baseline, or WBC >15 × 109 cells/mm^3. Oral vancomycin 125 mg four times per day for 10–14 days is recommended for severe CDAD [33]. Vancomycin is poorly absorbed and fecal concentrations of the drug can reach very high levels, up to 3300 mcg/g in patients receiving 2 g per day [16, 34]. Given that the MIC of vancomycin is usually 1.0–2.0 and never more than 16, resistance is a low concern (Cohen). Because it is poorly absorbed, there are few systemic effects and it is well tolerated [5, 6, 8, 29, 32].

Severe Complicated Disease

Severe complicated CDI includes patients with hypotension, ileus, need for ICU admission, WBC >35 × 109 cells/mm^3 or less than 2 × 109 cells/mm^3, or presence of end-organ dysfunction. In cases of complicated CDI where ileus may prevent oral agents from reaching the colon, the recommended therapy is oral vancomycin 500 mg four times daily plus addition of intravenous metronidazole 500 mg three times daily, and vancomycin enemas. Kim et al. showed that 33 of 47 patients (70%) with severe complicated CDI responded to intracolonic vancomycin flushes with complete response and no need for surgery [35]. Multivariate analysis suggested that advanced age and hypoalbuminemia were risk factors for medical treatment failure and that these patients should be considered for early surgical intervention [5, 6, 8, 16, 29, 32].

Recurrent Disease

Recurrence occurs in up to 25% of patients successfully treated for CDI, and this risk increases to 50% in some series for patients aged greater than 65 [10]. Pepin et al. showed that there is no difference in rate of recurrence whether metronidazole or vancomycin was used for the initial episode of CDI. Recurrent disease may be treated with the same agent as for the initial episode, and selection of an agent should be based on the severity of the recurrence. Metronidazole should not be used for the second recurrence because of risk for neurotoxicity (Cohen) [5, 6, 8, 29, 36].

Fidaxomicin is a relatively narrow-spectrum macrolide that is bactericidal against *C. difficile*. It can be substituted for oral vancomycin in recurrent CDI, especially in older adults who are at high risk for future recurrences (advanced age, ongoing need for antibiotics) [37]. Like oral vancomycin, it is poorly absorbed in the oral form and achieves high fecal concentration. However, its narrow spectrum may allow for less suppression of normal intestinal flora compared to other agents [38]. Louie et al. showed that fidaxomicin had equivalent efficacy to oral vancomycin for CDI with a lower risk of recurrence [6, 8, 29, 39, 40].

Fecal Microbiota Transplantation

Fecal microbiota transplantation (FMT) is another promising therapy for recurrent CDI. CDI results from suppression of the patients normal gut flora with overgrowth of the *C. difficile* bacteria [41]. The principle behind FMT is to infuse normal gut flora from a healthy donor and the normal gut microbiome will prevent recurrence of CDI. Overall resolution of symptoms occurs in about 90% of patients based on meta-analysis of several case series and one randomized controlled trial. Methods of delivery include delivery of slurry via nasogastric or nasointestinal tube, delivery by colonoscope, enema, and encapsulated and frozen forms. Colonoscopic delivery may lead to the highest rate of resolution [6, 29, 37, 42–48]. Use of FMT on the large scale is currently limited by perceived concerns for safety and acceptability by patients. However, qualitative analyses indicate that up to 94% of patients would be amenable to FMT if proposed by their physicians [49].

Surgical Intervention

Surgical mortality for CDI ranges from 19 to 80%. However, early surgical intervention is associated with decreased mortality [50]. Seder et al. showed a decrease in mortality when surgery was performed prior to need for vasopressors [51]. Development of complicated disease, including perforation and peritonitis, was similarly associated with higher mortality. While the exact timing of surgery to gain this benefit remains difficult to elucidate, several studies suggest decrease in mortality within 3–5 days from diagnosis or if the patient clinically worsens. Awaiting hemodynamic instability as a trigger to operate is associated with an increase in mortality, and clinicians should avoid allowing patients to progress to shock and multiorgan system failure prior to surgical intervention. Early surgical consultation is advisable for patients with severe CDI [50, 52–56].

Total abdominal colectomy (TAC) remains the recommended procedure for severe/complicated CDI requiring surgery. Lipsett et al. showed that partial colectomy for CDI carried a mortality of 100%, while TAC only had mortality of 14% [57]. Again, peritonitis was associated with higher mortality [52–56].

A promising study by Neal et al. described an innovative procedure designed to preserve colon. An ileostomy is created and anterograde colonic washing with vancomycin flushes is performed. They showed a decrease in mortality compared to historical controls (from 50 to 19% surgical mortality). While this procedure has the clear theoretical benefit of preserving colon with low mortality, several questions remain, including reproducibility in other institutions and incidence of recurrent CDI after ileostomy reversal [50, 58].

Conclusion

CDI is a significant cause of morbidity and mortality in the elderly population, particularly in patients with frequent exposure to the healthcare industry. Judicious use of antibiotics and strict hygiene in hospitals and long-term care facilities are mandatory for prevention of CDI. Maintaining a high index of suspicion in elderly patients with diarrhea allows for early treatment if CDI is confirmed, and early surgery can be lifesaving in severe, refractory CDI.

References

1. Centers for disease control and prevention. QuickStats: Rates of Clostridium difficile infection among hospitalized patients aged C65 years,* by age group—National Hospital Discharge Survey, United States, 1996–2009. http://www.cdc.gov/mmwr/preview/mmwrhtml/mm6034a7.htm?s_cid=mm6034a7_w.
2. Trinh C, Prabhakar K. Diarrheal diseases in the elderly. Clin Geriatr Med. 2007;23(4):833–56. https://doi.org/10.1016/j.cger.2007.06.005.
3. Britton RA, Young VB. Role of the intestinal microbiota in resistance to colonization by Clostridium difficile. Gastroenterology. 2014;146(6):1547–53. https://doi.org/10.1053/j.gastro.2014.01.059.
4. Eaton SR, Mazuski JE. Overview of severe Clostridium difficile infection. Crit Care Clin. 2013;29(4):827–39. https://doi.org/10.1016/j.ccc.2013.06.004.
5. Mizusawa M, Doron S, Gorbach S. Clostridium difficile diarrhea in the elderly: current issues and management options. Drugs Aging. 2015;32(8):639–47. https://doi.org/10.1007/s40266-015-0289-2.
6. Cohen SH, Gerding DN, Johnson S, et al. Clinical practice guidelines for Clostridium difficile infection in adults: 2010 update by the society for healthcare epidemiology of America (SHEA) and the infectious diseases society of America (IDSA). Infect Control Hosp Epidemiol. 2010;31:431–55.

7. Zacharioudakis IM, Zervou FN, Pliakos EE, Ziakas PD, Mylonakis E. Colonization with toxinogenic C. difficile upon hospital admission, and risk of infection: a systematic review and meta-analysis. Am J Gastroenterol. 2015;110(3):381–90; quiz 391. doi:https://doi.org/10.1038/ajg.2015.22.
8. Sartelli M, Malangoni MA, Abu-Zidan FM, et al. WSES guidelines for management of Clostridium difficile infection in surgical patients. World J Emerg Surg. 2015;10:38.
9. Bauer MP, Notermans DW, van Benthem BH, et al. Clostridium difficile infection in europe: a hospital-based survey. Lancet. 2011;377(9759):63–73. https://doi.org/10.1016/S0140-6736(10)61266-4.
10. Garey KW, Sethi S, Yadav Y, DuPont HL. Meta-analysis to assess risk factors for recurrent Clostridium difficile infection. J Hosp Infect. 2008;70(4):298–304. https://doi.org/10.1016/j.jhin.2008.08.012.
11. Rodriguez C, Korsak N, Taminiau B, et al. Clostridium difficile infection in elderly nursing home residents. Anaerobe. 2014;30:184–7. https://doi.org/10.1016/j.anaerobe.2014.08.007.
12. Denève C, Janoir C, Poilane I, Fantinato C, Collignon A. New trends in Clostridium difficile virulence and pathogenesis. Int J Antimicrob Agents. 2009;33(Suppl 1):S24–8. https://doi.org/10.1016/S0924-8579(09)70012-3.
13. Awad MM, Johanesen PA, Carter GP, Rose E, Lyras D. Clostridium difficile virulence factors: insights into an anaerobic spore-forming pathogen. Gut Microbes. 2014;5(5):579–93. https://doi.org/10.4161/19490976.2014.969632.
14. Kuehne SA, Cartman ST, Heap JT, Kelly ML, Cockayne A, Minton NP. The role of toxin A and toxin B in Clostridium difficile infection. Nature. 2010;467(7316):711–3. https://doi.org/10.1038/nature09397.
15. Kuehne SA, Collery MM, Kelly ML, Cartman ST, Cockayne A, Minton NP. Importance of toxin A, toxin B, and CDT in virulence of an epidemic Clostridium difficile strain. J Infect Dis. 2014;209(1):83–6. https://doi.org/10.1093/infdis/jit426.
16. Aslam S, Hamill RJ, Musher DM. Treatment of Clostridium difficile-associated disease: old therapies and new strategies. Lancet Infect Dis. 2005;5(9):549–57. https://doi.org/10.1016/S1473-3099(05)70215-2.
17. Clements AC, Magalhães RJ, Tatem AJ, Paterson DL, Riley TV. Clostridium difficile PCR ribotype 027: assessing the risks of further worldwide spread. Lancet Infect Dis. 2010;10(6):395–404. https://doi.org/10.1016/S1473-3099(10)70080-3.
18. Crogan NL, Evans BC. Clostridium difficile: an emerging epidemic in nursing homes. Geriatr Nurs. 2007;28(3):161–4. https://doi.org/10.1016/j.gerinurse.2007.04.005.
19. Pépin J, Routhier S, Gagnon S, Brazeau I. Management and outcomes of a first recurrence of Clostridium difficile-associated disease in Quebec, Canada. Clin Infect Dis. 2006;42(6):758–64. https://doi.org/10.1086/501126.
20. Pépin J, Saheb N, Coulombe M, et al. Emergence of fluoroquinolones as the predominant risk factor for Clostridium difficile-associated diarrhea: a cohort study during an epidemic in Quebec. Clin Infect Dis. 2005;41(9):1254–60. https://doi.org/10.1086/496986.
21. Chopra T, Goldstein EJC. Clostridium difficile infection in long-term care facilities: a call to action for antimicrobial stewardship. Clin Infect Dis. 2015;60(Suppl 2):S72–6. https://doi.org/10.1093/cid/civ053.
22. Laffan AM, Bellantoni MF, Greenough WB, Zenilman JM. Burden of Clostridium difficile-associated diarrhea in a long-term care facility. J Am Geriatr Soc. 2006;54(7):1068–73. http://proxy.library.vcu.edu/login?url=http://search.ebscohost.com/login.aspx?direct=true&AuthType=ip,url,cookie,uid&db=ccm&AN=106336610&site=ehost-live&scope=site. doi: https://doi.org/10.1111/j.1532%E2%80%935415.2006.00768.x
23. Dancer SJ, Kirkpatrick P, Corcoran DS, Christison F, Farmer D, Robertson C. Approaching zero: temporal effects of a restrictive antibiotic policy on hospital-acquired Clostridium difficile, extended-spectrum β-lactamase-producing coliforms and meticillin-resistant *Staphylococcus aureus*. Int J Antimicrob Agents. 2013;41(2):137–42. https://doi.org/10.1016/j.ijantimicag.2012.10.013.
24. Anderson DJ, Gergen MF, Smathers E, et al. Decontamination of targeted pathogens from patient rooms using an automated ultraviolet-C-emitting device. Infect Control Hosp Epidemiol. 2013;34(5):466–71. https://doi.org/10.1086/670215.
25. Vonberg R, Kuijper EJ, Wilcox MH, et al. Infection control measures to limit the spread of Clostridium difficile. Clin Microbiol Infect. 2008;14(Suppl 5):2–20. https://doi.org/10.1111/j.1469-0691.2008.01992.x.
26. Khanafer N, Voirin N, Barbut F, Kuijper E, Vanhems P. Hospital management of Clostridium difficile infection: a review of the literature. J Hosp Infect. 2015;90(2):91–101. https://doi.org/10.1016/j.jhin.2015.02.015.
27. Luciano JA, Zuckerbraun BS. Clostridium difficile infection: prevention, treatment, and surgical management. Surg Clin N Am. 2014;94(6):1335–49. https://doi.org/10.1016/j.suc.2014.08.006.
28. Thomas C, Stevenson M, Riley TV. Antibiotics and hospital-acquired Clostridium difficile-associated diarrhoea: a systematic review. J Antimicrob Chemother. 2003;51(6):1339–50. https://doi.org/10.1093/jac/dkg254.
29. Bagdasarian N, Rao K, Malani PN. Diagnosis and treatment of Clostridium difficile in adults: a systematic review. JAMA. 2015;313(4):398–408. https://doi.org/10.1001/jama.2014.17103.

30. Feazel LM, Malhotra A, Perencevich EN, Kaboli P, Diekema DJ, Schweizer ML. Effect of antibiotic stewardship programmes on Clostridium difficile incidence: a systematic review and meta-analysis. J Antimicrob Chemother. 2014;69(7):1748–54. https://doi.org/10.1093/jac/dku046.
31. Slimings C, Riley TV. Antibiotics and hospital-acquired Clostridium difficile infection: update of systematic review and meta-analysis. J Antimicrob Chemother. 2014;69(4):881–91. https://doi.org/10.1093/jac/dkt477.
32. Nelson RL, Kelsey P, Leeman H, et al. Antibiotic treatment for Clostridium difficile-associated diarrhea in adults. Cochrane Database Syst Rev. https://doi.org/10.1002/14651858.CD004610.pub4.
33. Zar FA, Bakkanagari SR, Moorthi KM, Davis MB. A comparison of vancomycin and metronidazole for the treatment of Clostridium difficile-associated diarrhea, stratified by disease severity. Clin Infect Dis. 2007;45(3):302–7. https://doi.org/10.1086/519265.
34. Johnson SH, Bettin SR, Quick KM, Clabots JN, Peterson CR, Gerding LR, Dale N. Treatment of asymptomatic Clostridium difficile carriers (fecal excretors) with vancomycin or metronidazole. A randomized, placebo-controlled trial. Ann Intern Med. 1992;117:297–302.
35. Kim JH, Muder RR. Clostridium difficile enteritis: a review and pooled analysis of the cases. Anaerobe. 2011;17(2):52–5. https://doi.org/10.1016/j.anaerobe.2011.02.002.
36. O'Horo JC, Jindai K, Kunzer B, Safdar N. Treatment of recurrent Clostridium difficile infection: a systematic review. Infection. 2014;42(1):43–59.
37. Goldberg EJ, Bhalodia S, Jacob S, et al. Clostridium difficile infection: a brief update on emerging therapies. Am J Health Syst Pharm. 2015;72(12):1007–12. https://doi.org/10.2146/ajhp140645.
38. Cornely OA, Miller MA, Louie TJ, Crook DW, Gorbach SL. Treatment of first recurrence of Clostridium difficile infection: fidaxomicin versus vancomycin. Clin Infect Dis. 2012;55(Suppl 2):S154–61. https://doi.org/10.1093/cid/cis462.
39. Louie TJ, Miller MA, Mullane KM, et al. Fidaxomicin versus vancomycin for Clostridium difficile infection. N Engl J Med. 2011;364(5):422–31. https://doi.org/10.1056/NEJMoa0910812.
40. Chahine EB, Sucher AJ, Mantei K. Fidaxomicin: a novel macrolide antibiotic for Clostridium difficile infection. Consult Pharm. 2014;29(9):614–24. https://doi.org/10.4140/TCP.n.2014.614.
41. Zanella Terrier MC, Simonet ML, Bichard P, Frossard JL. Recurrent Clostridium difficile infections: the importance of the intestinal microbiota. World J Gastroenterol. 2014;20(23):7416–23. https://doi.org/10.3748/wjg.v20.i23.7416.
42. Cammarota G, Ianiro G, Gasbarrini A. Fecal microbiota transplantation for the treatment of Clostridium difficile infection: a systematic review. J Clin Gastroenterol. 2014;48(8):693–702. https://doi.org/10.1097/MCG.0000000000000046.
43. Gough E, Shaikh H, Manges AR. Systematic review of intestinal microbiota transplantation (fecal bacteriotherapy) for recurrent Clostridium difficile infection. Clin Infect Dis. 2011;53(10):994–1002. https://doi.org/10.1093/cid/cir632.
44. Kassam Z, Lee CH, Yuan Y, Hunt RH. Fecal microbiota transplantation for Clostridium difficile infection: systematic review and meta-analysis. Am J Gastroenterol. 2013;108(4):500–8. https://doi.org/10.1038/ajg.2013.59.
45. Li YT, Cai HF, Wang ZH, Xu J, Fang JY. Systematic review with meta-analysis: long-term outcomes of faecal microbiota transplantation for Clostridium difficile infection. Aliment Pharmacol Ther. 2016;43(4):445–57. https://doi.org/10.1111/apt.13492.
46. Petrof EO, Khoruts A. From stool transplants to next-generation microbiota therapeutics. Gastroenterology. 2014;146(6):1573–82. https://doi.org/10.1053/j.gastro.2014.01.004.
47. Rao K, Young VB. Fecal microbiota transplantation for the management of Clostridium difficile infection. Infect Dis Clin N Am. 2015;29(1):109–22. https://doi.org/10.1016/j.idc.2014.11.009.
48. van Nood E, Vrieze A, Nieuwdorp M, et al. Duodenal infusion of donor feces for recurrent Clostridium difficile. N Engl J Med. 2013;368(5):407–15. https://doi.org/10.1056/NEJMoa1205037.
49. Pakyz AL, Moczygemba LR, VanderWielen LM, Edmond MB. Fecal microbiota transplantation for recurrent Clostridium difficile infection: the patient experience. Am J Infect Control. 2016;44(5):554–9. https://doi.org/10.1016/j.ajic.2016.01.018.
50. Ferrada P, Velopulos CG, Sultan S, et al. Timing and type of surgical treatment of Clostridium difficile-associated disease: a practice management guideline from the eastern association for the surgery of trauma. J Trauma Acute Care Surg. 2014;76(6):1484–93. https://doi.org/10.1097/TA.0000000000000232.
51. Seder CW, Villalba MR, Robbins J, Ivascu FA, Carpenter CF, Dietrich M. Early colectomy may be associated with improved survival in fulminant Clostridium difficile colitis: an 8-year experience. Am J Surg. 2009;197(3):302–7. https://doi.org/10.1016/j.amjsurg.2008.11.001.

52. Halabi WJ, Nguyen VQ, Carmichael JC, Pigazzi A, Stamos MJ, Mills S. Clostridium difficile colitis in the united states: a decade of trends, outcomes, risk factors for colectomy, and mortality after colectomy. J Am Coll Surg. 2013;217(5):802–12. https://doi.org/10.1016/j.jamcollsurg.2013.05.028.
53. Sailhamer EA, Carson K, Chang Y, et al. Fulminant Clostridium difficile colitis: Patterns of care and predictors of mortality. Arch Surg. 2009;144(5):433–9; discussion 439. doi: https://doi.org/10.1001/archsurg.2009.51.
54. Ali SO, Welch JP, Dring RJ. Early surgical intervention for fulminant pseudomembranous colitis. Am Surg. 2008;74(1):20–6.
55. Longo WE, Mazuski JE, Virgo KS, Lee P, Bahadursingh AN, Johnson FE. Outcome after colectomy for Clostridium difficile colitis. Dis Colon Rectum. 2004;47(10):1620–6.
56. Hall JF, Berger D. Outcome of colectomy for Clostridium difficile colitis: a plea for early surgical management. Am J Surg. 2008;196(3):384–8. https://doi.org/10.1016/j.amjsurg.2007.11.017.
57. Lipsett PA, Samantaray DK, Tam ML, Bartlett JG, Lillemoe KD. Pseudomembranous colitis: a surgical disease? Surgery. 1994;116(3):491–6.
58. Neal MD, Alverdy JC, Hall DE, Simmons RL, Zuckerbraun BS. Diverting loop ileostomy and colonic lavage: an alternative to total abdominal colectomy for the treatment of severe, complicated Clostridium difficile associated disease. Ann Surg. 2011;254(3):423–7; discussion 427. doi: https://doi.org/10.1097/SLA.0b013e31822ade48.

31 Acute Diverticulitis

Manuel Lorenzo and Vanessa Shifflette

Epidemiology and Pathogenesis

A colonic diverticulum is an acquired condition that results from the herniation of mucosa through defects in the muscle layer, causing sac-like protrusions. Diverticulosis and diverticular disease are terms used to describe the presence of diverticula without associated inflammation. When inflammation accompanies the diverticulum, the term "diverticulitis" is used and indicates a microscopic versus macroscopic perforation [1].

Diverticulosis is an extremely common condition in Western countries, with prevalence increasing with age. Diverticular disease is estimated to be present in greater than 65% of patients over the age of 65 [2]. The most common site for diverticulosis is the left colon in the Western nations while in Asian nations diverticula occur primarily in the right colon [3, 4]. Diverticular disease is complicated by infection in about 10–25% of patients [5].

The formation of diverticula is a multifactorial process that may include diets low in fiber, changes in colonic motility and pressure, and structural changes within the colonic wall. The latter factors are associated with the aging process [6]. The colonic wall develops areas of weakness located at points of penetration by the vasa recta. The diverticula may occur in response to increased intraluminal pressure at these areas of weakness.

Diverticulitis is the presence of inflammation or infection surrounding a diverticulum. The usual presentation for patients is left-sided abdominal pain, low-grade fever, and possible leukocytosis. As 99% of diverticula involve the sigmoid colon [7], left lower quadrant pain is the most common presentation. Geriatric patients are known to have redundant sigmoid colons and may therefore present with right lower quadrant abdominal pain. Other symptoms seen in these patients include failure to thrive, anorexia, abdominal distention, dehydration, and altered mental status. Most patients are classified as either uncomplicated or complicated diverticulitis. Uncomplicated diverticulitis is a result of simple inflammation around the diverticulum and limited to the colonic wall or adjacent tissues. Patients presenting with uncomplicated diverticulitis may not warrant hospital admission. However, features of complicated diverticulitis include abscess formation, diverticular perforation, fistula formation, or abdominal obstruction, and will warrant hospital admission. Severe cases may present with hemodynamic instability, sepsis, and peritonitis.

M. Lorenzo, M.D. (✉) • V. Shifflette, M.D.
Associates in Surgical Acute Care,
221 W. Colorado Blvd, Pavilion 2, Suite 425,
Dallas, TX 75208, USA
e-mail: drmanuellorenzo@yahoo.com;
vkshifflette@gmail.com

A. Rodriguez et al. (eds.), *Geriatric Trauma and Acute Care Surgery*,
https://doi.org/10.1007/978-3-319-57403-5_31

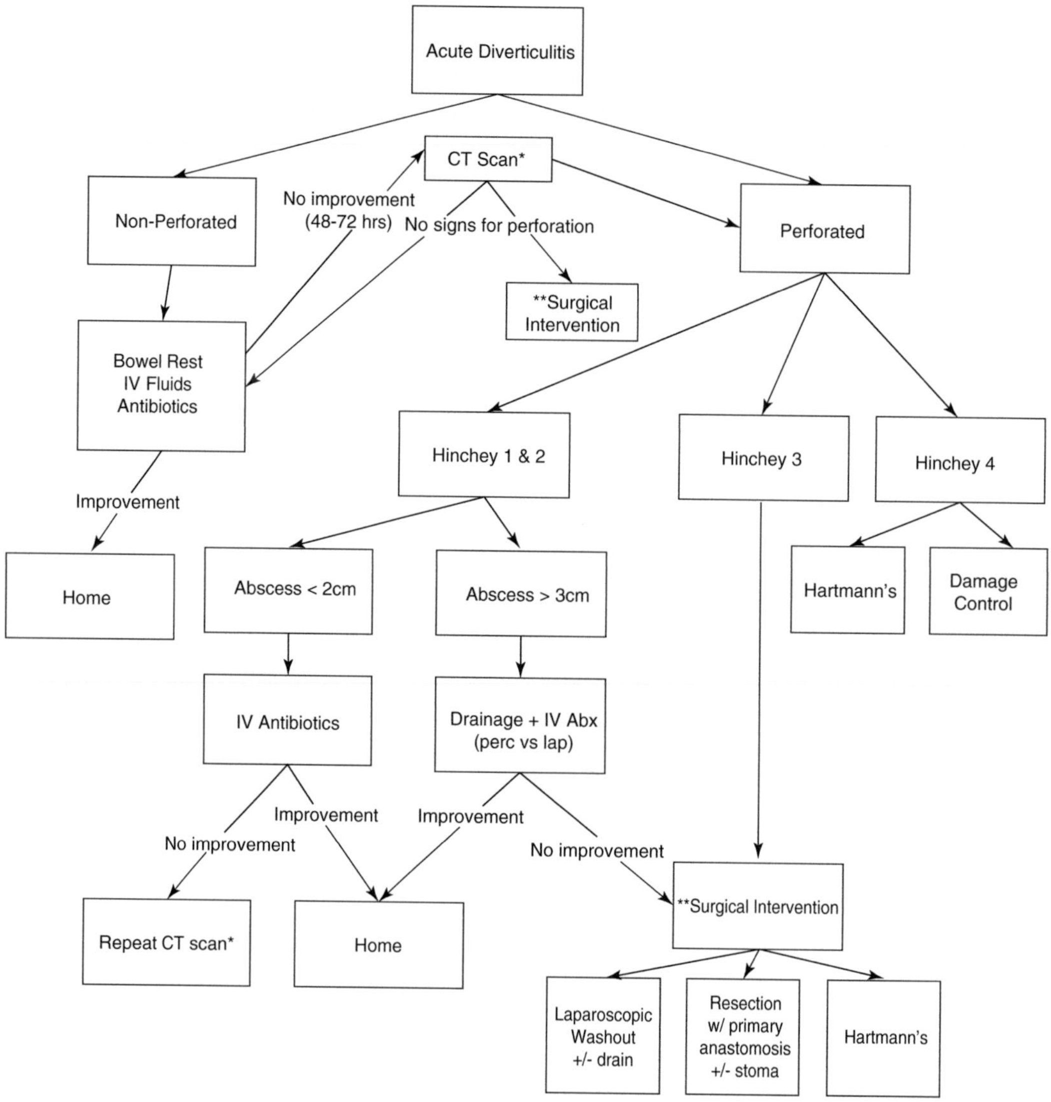

Fig. 31.1 Acute diverticulitis treatment algorithm

Computed tomography (CT) imaging is a necessary part of the algorithm in diagnosing and classifying patients as having uncomplicated versus complicated diverticulitis (Fig. 31.1). Classifying these patients helps guide the management and treatment, thereby influencing overall outcomes. In 1978, Hinchey popularized a classification created to further categorize complicated diverticulitis (Table 31.1) [8]. The risk for death associated with the Hinchey classification was found to be 5% for stage 1 and 2, 13% for stage 3, and 43% for stage 4 [9].

Table 31.1 Classification for complicated diverticulitis

	Hinchey classification (1978)
Stage 1	Pericolic or intramesenteric abscess
Stage 2	Walled-off pelvic abscess
Stage 3	Generalized purulent peritonitis
Stage 4	Generalized feculent peritonitis

Management and Treatment

The main goal in the management of acute diverticular disease in the geriatric patient is the return of the patient to the same level of premorbid physical and mental function. Geriatric patients are at a higher risk of developing complications and mortality as compared to a younger cohort presenting the same type and level of disease [10]. The surgeon has to not only promptly manage the primary surgical disease of the patient, but also aggressively optimize their chronic medical conditions. It has been shown that early intervention to address medical and surgical problems of the geriatric patient results in a decrease in morbidity and mortality among this population [11, 12]. Elderly patients should be admitted to an area, ideally under the care of nurses with experience in geriatrics, that can provide continuous cardiopulmonary monitoring, aggressive pulmonary care, prompt identification of clinical deterioration, and ability to perform immediate medical interventions.

In general, most geriatric patients with diverticulitis will respond to conservative (nonoperative) treatment, with only 10% of the patients requiring surgical intervention during the same hospitalization. A high index of suspicion is required by the healthcare professional, as clinical symptoms in many geriatric patients do not adequately reflect the gravity of their condition upon initial evaluation. These patients could generate an inadequate response to physiological stress (normal WBC count, minimal abdominal pain, no tachycardia, etc.) due to poor physiological reserve, medications, and/or immunologic compromise. Geriatric patients with uncomplicated diverticulitis should be promptly triaged and started on medical management consisting of intravenous broad-spectrum antibiotics, fluid resuscitation, and bowel rest (clear liquid diet or nothing per mouth) (Fig. 31.2). Clinical findings suggestive of improvement include resolution of abdominal pain, leukocytosis, ileus, and fever. The group of geriatric patients that respond to medical management are discharged home with a regimen of oral antibiotics with aerobic and anaerobic coverage for 10–14 days and instructions to follow a low-residue diet with a generous intake of oral fluids. Otherwise, hemodynamically stable geriatric patients without generalized peritonitis and no significant clinical deterioration, but without signs of improvement after 48–72 h of initiation of medical treatment, warrant a repeat CT scan (Fig. 31.3). Complications of diverticulitis include abscess formation (16%), perforation (10%), obstruction (5%), and fistula formation (2%) [13, 14].

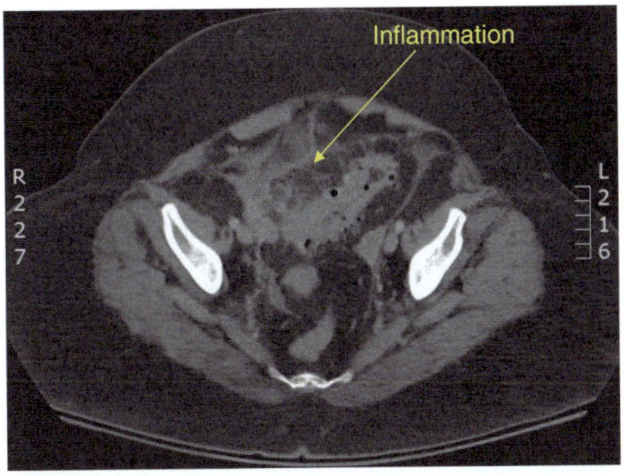

Fig. 31.2 Uncomplicated diverticulitis

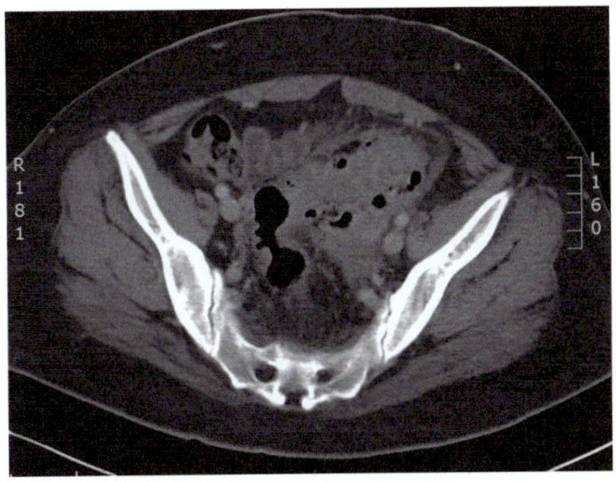

Fig. 31.3 Diverticulitis with no improvement

Complicated Diverticulitis

Geriatric patients that present with an intra-abdominal or retroperitoneal abscess or those who develop an abscess during hospitalization are candidates for percutaneous drainage as an adjunct to their medical management (Fig. 31.4). These patients are classified as Hinchey stage 1 and 2 (Table 31.1). Abscesses less than 2 cm in size will usually respond to conservative management without other intervention. In general, at our institution, CT-guided percutaneous drainage

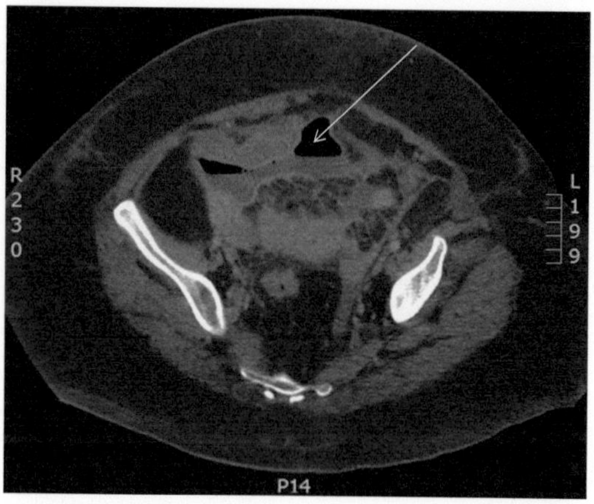

Fig. 31.4 Complicated diverticulitis with pelvic abscess (*arrow*)

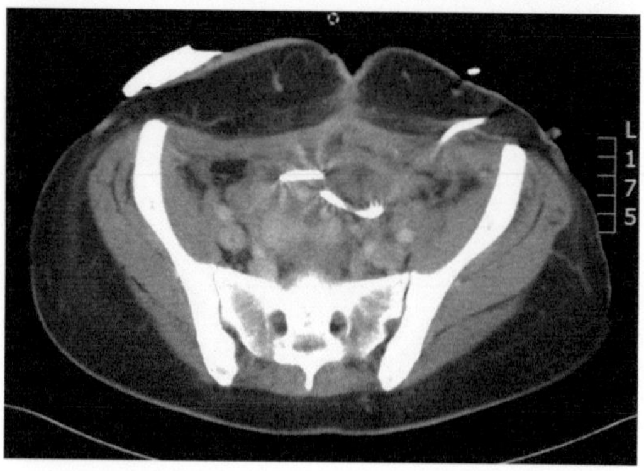

Fig. 31.5 Percutaneous drainage of pelvic abscess

is readily employed in abscesses greater than 3 cm in size (Fig. 31.5). Durmishi et al. showed that drainage of Hinchey 2 diverticulitis guided by computed tomography was successful in two-thirds of the cases, and 35% of the patients eventually underwent a safe elective sigmoid resection with primary anastomosis [15]. Brandt et al. reported a drainage failure rate of 15–30% with a recurrence rate of 40–50% with combined treatment of antibiotics with percutaneous drainage [16]. The high recurrence rate in these patients is thought to reflect the more severe degree of involvement at the time of presentation in those patients with abscess. For geriatric patients with abscesses inappropriate for percutaneous drainage (location precludes percutaneous access or multiloculated abscesses), laparoscopic drain placement has proven to be an acceptable option. In our institution, geriatric patients with an inaccessible abscess are taken to the operating room for laparoscopic drainage of the abscess or abscesses, irrigation of the infected area, and placement of a drain. Follow-up drain management includes surveillance of the amount and characteristics of its output. Diminishing output with resolution of symptoms and return of bowel function would be indications for removal of the drain. Persistent purulent or feculent output should warrant further radiological imaging to evaluate for fistula formation.

Laparoscopic peritoneal lavage with drain placement should also be considered for Hinchey stage 3 geriatric patients with localized peritonitis and hemodynamic stability [17].

This approach can be considered a "bridge" surgical step to avoid a Hartmann's procedure and perform an elective laparoscopic or open sigmoidectomy [18]. Toorenvliet et al. showed that patients with Hinchey stage 3 purulent peritonitis and sepsis were successfully controlled in 95.7% of patients with an overall mortality of 1.7% and a morbidity of 10.4% and only four (1.7%) patients received a colostomy [19].

A key consideration on this type of management is the assiduous evaluation for a colonic perforation. Vennix et al. concluded that lavage is feasible in the majority of patients, but that patient selection and rigorous assessment for occult perforations are imperative [20, 21]. The SCANDIV Randomized Clinical Trial compared study patients with perforation treated with lavage only vs. resection, showing no difference in mortality between the two groups (13.9% vs. 11.5%, respectively). At 12 months post-presentation, four patients had died after lavage and six patients had died after sigmoidectomy ($p = 0{\cdot}43$). The lavage-only group however had a higher incidence of complications such as formation of intra-abdominal abscess and development of secondary peritonitis [22].

Patients that present with Hinchey stage 4 and patients of all Hinchey stages who fail to show clinical response to treatment will need surgical intervention. Indications for early surgical intervention are generalized peritonitis, uncontained pneumoperitoneum, uncontrolled sepsis, and hemodynamic

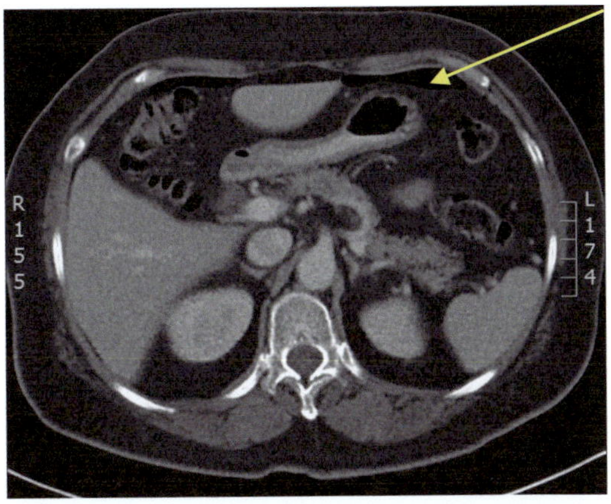

Fig. 31.6 Free perforation with pneumoperitoneum (*arrow*)

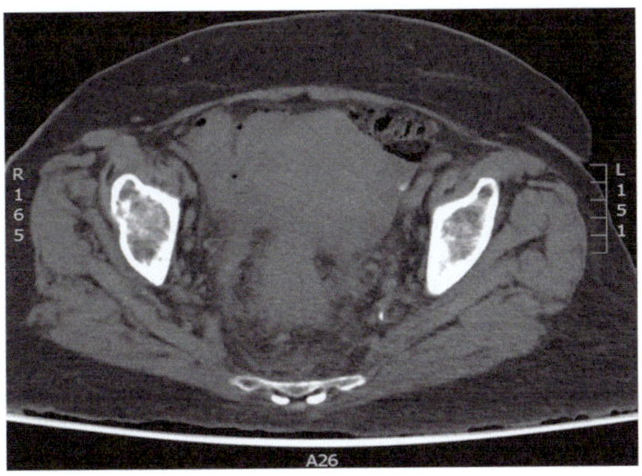

Fig. 31.7 Feculent peritonitis with pneumoperitoneum

instability (Figs. 31.6, and 31.7). Hartmann's procedure should be strongly considered for Hinchey stage 4 geriatric patients, as they are unlikely to tolerate the secondary insult of an anastomotic leak. Damage control procedures with spillage restraint while minimizing operative time are the best options for geriatric patients with severe abdominal sepsis. Resection of the perforated colonic segment, extensive irrigation, and application of an abdominal negative pressure wound therapy system are safe interventions given the improved outcomes in patients with abdominal sepsis [23, 24]. In our institution, geriatric patients who undergo this technique with a second abdominal irrigation and stoma creation have shown significantly better outcomes. While closure of the abdominal fascia is most commonly complicated by wound infection (24%), this problem is negligible with the use of a negative-pressure device on the open wound. Fukuda et al. found that the most common causes of death in the elderly patients suffering from diverticulitis were sepsis related to peritonitis (5.3%) and postoperative pneumonia (4.3%) [25]. Several studies have compared resection with primary anastomosis with or without a defunctioning stoma and nonrestorative resection with no difference in mortality found between the two groups. Retrospective studies by Salem et al. and Shilling et al. showed primary anastomosis with a defunctioning stoma to be the procedure of choice among select high-risk patients [26, 27]. However, these studies did not show age-stratified data among the analyzed populations. As a basic rule, the most fundamental principle in the management of geriatric patients with diverticulitis is to perform the safest management and/or procedure with the lowest risk for morbidity and mortality.

Fistula Formation

The incidence of fistula formation with diverticular disease varies widely in the literature. Comparato et al. demonstrated that 10% of the patients with peridiverticular abscesses progressed to form fistulas between the colon and surrounding structures [14]. Woods et al. found that up to 20% of the patients surgically treated for diverticular disease formed fistulas. The type of fistulas formed were colovesical (65%), colovaginal (25%), coloenteric (6.5%), and colouterine (3%) [28].

Symptoms suggestive of colovesical fistula include pneumaturia, dysuria, or fecaluria. Physical exam is usually benign, and a urinalysis is typically nonspecific with bacteria. A CT scan or barium enema may be helpful with diagnosis (Fig. 31.8). Imaging may show a thickened bladder wall with adjacent colonic thickening concerning for the colovesical fistula. Air within the bladder, without history of prior instrumentation, would further suggest the abnormal communication. Endoscopy and cystoscopy are other adjuncts, which may aid with the diagnosis. Once the fistula anatomy has been delineated, treatment remains operative resection of the affected colon with simple repair of the involved organ [5].

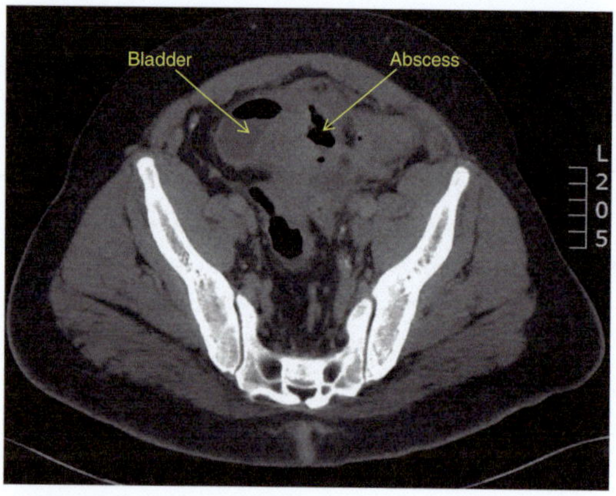

Fig. 31.8 Colovesical fistula

Obstruction

Colonic obstruction can be seen acutely with inflammatory diverticulitis, or more commonly as a late complication secondary to fibrosis and stricture formation as a result from previous attacks. These patients can be found presenting to the emergency room with nausea, vomiting, and abdominal distention. Most of these patients will respond to medical management that will allow elective resection later. Patients with no response may require operative management such as a Hartmann's procedure or primary resection with anastomosis and protective stoma [29]. There is literature describing the successful use of self-expanding metallic stents in relieving colonic obstruction due to diverticular disease [30, 31]. These stents may be used as a bridge to surgery [30] to allow optimization of the patient's condition for a definitive colonic resection, but may come with a higher incidence of complications [31]. The use of colonic stents during the acute phase of the disease is controversial due to the risk of perforation or exacerbation of the disease. Given the lack of evidence, colonic stents for the acute phase of diverticular disease cannot yet be recommended.

Hemorrhage

Diverticular disease is also known to cause massive lower gastrointestinal bleeding. This is usually associated with diverticulosis and not diverticulitis, as a result of erosion into the perforating vasa recta vessels. The majority of bleeding associated with diverticulosis will spontaneously stop in about 80% of patients [5]. Surgical resection is reserved for patients with persistent or recurrent diverticular hemorrhage.

References

1. Jacobs DO. Clinical practice. Diverticulitis. N Engl J Med. 2007;357(20):2057–66.
2. West AB. The pathology of diverticulitis. J Clin Gastroenterol. 2008;42(10):1137–8.
3. Vermeulen J, Van der Harst E, Lange JF. Pathophysiology and prevention of diverticulitis and perforation. Neth J Med. 2010;68(10):303–9.
4. Ryan P. Changing concepts in diverticular disease. Dis Colon Rectum. 1983;26:12–8.
5. Bullard KM, Rothenberger DA. Colon, rectum, anus. In: Brunicardi CF, Andersen DK, Billiar TR, et al., editors. Schwartz's principles of surgery. 8th ed. New York: McGraw-Hill; 2005. p. 1082–4.
6. Heise CP. Epidemiology and pathogenesis of diverticular disease. J Gastrointest Surg. 2008;12(8):1309–11.
7. Hughes LE. Postmortem survey of diverticular disease of the colon. II. The muscular abnormality of the sigmoid colon. Gut. 1969;10(5):344–51.
8. Hinchey EJ, Schaal PG, Richard GK. Treatment of perforated diverticular disease of the colon. Adv Surg. 1978;12:85–109.
9. Schlesinger WH, Page CP, Gaskell HV III, et al. Operative management of diverticular emergencies: strategies and outcomes. Arch Surg. 2000;135(5):558–62. discussion 62–3
10. Shifflette VK, Lorenzo M, Mangram AJ, Truitt MS, Amos JD, Dunn EL. Should age be a factor to change from a level II to a level I trauma activation? J Trauma. 2010;69(1):88–92.
11. Mangram AJ, Mitchell CD, Shifflette VK, Lorenzo M, Truitt MS, Goel A, Lyons MA, Nichols DJ, Dunn EL. Geriatric trauma service: a one-year experience. J Trauma Acute Care Surg. 2012;72(1):119–22.
12. Lorenzo M, Barba C. Will patient outcomes improve if we admit and manage geriatric patients in a specialized unit in the trauma center? Abstract presentation. Jackson Hole, Wyoming: Western Trauma Association; 2005.
13. Gearhart SL. Diverticular disease of colon. In: Cameron JL, Cameron AM, editors. Current surgical therapy. 10th ed. Philadelphia: Elsevier Saunders; 2011. p. 133.
14. Comparato G, Pilotto A, et al. Diverticular disease in the elderly. Dig Dis. 2007;25:151–9.
15. Durmishi Y, Gervaz P, Brandt D, Bucher P, Platon A, Morel P, Poletti PA. Results from percutaneous drainage of Hinchey stage II diverticulitis guided

by computed tomography scan. Surg Endosc. 2006;20(7):1129–33. Epub 2006 Jun 3
16. Brandt D, Gervaz P, et al. Percutaneous CT scan – guided drainage vs. antibiotherapy alone for Hinchey II diverticulitis: a case control study. Dis Colon Rectum. 2006;49:1533–8.
17. Sorrentino M, Brizzolari M, Scarpa E, Malisan D, Bruschi F, Bertozzi S, Bernardi S, Petri R. Laparoscopic peritoneal lavage for perforated colonic diverticulitis: a definitive treatment? Retrospective analysis of 63 cases. Tech Coloproctol. 2015;19(2):105–10. https://doi.org/10.1007/s10151-014-1258-1. Epub 2014 Dec 31
18. Cirocchi R, et al. Laparoscopic peritoneal lavage: a definitive treatment for diverticular peritonitis or a "bridge" to elective laparoscopic sigmoidectomy?: a systematic review. Medicine (Baltimore). 2015;94(1):e334.
19. Toorenvliet BR, Swank H, et al. Laparoscopic peritoneal lavage for perforated colonic diverticulitis: a systematic review. Color Dis. 2010;12(9):862–7.
20. McDermott FD, Collins D, et al. Minimally invasive and surgical management strategies tailored to the severity of acute diverticulitis. Br J Surg. 2014;101:e90–9.
21. Vennix S, et al. Laparoscopic peritoneal lavage or sigmoidectomy for perforated diverticulitis with purulent peritonitis: a multicentre, parallel-group, randomised, open-label trial. Lancet. 2015;386(10000):1269–77. https://doi.org/10.1016/S0140-6736(15)61168-0. Epub 2015 Jul 22
22. Schultz JK, Yaqub S, Wallon C, Blecic L, Forsmo HM, Folkesson J, Buchwald P, Körner H, Dahl FA, Øresland T. SCANDIV laparoscopic lavage vs primary resection for acute perforated diverticulitis: the SCANDIV Randomized clinical trial. JAMA. 2015;314(13):1364–75.
23. Cheatham M, Demetriades D, et al. Prospective study examining clinical outcomes associated with a negative pressure wound therapy system and Baker's vacuum packing technique. World J Surg. 2013;77(9):2018–30.
24. Kirkpatrick AW, Roberts DJ, et al. Active negative pressure peritoneal therapy after abbreviated laparotomy: the intra peritoneal vacuum randomized controlled trial. Ann Surg. 2015;262(1):38–46.
25. Fukuda N, Wada J, et al. Factors predicting mortality in emergency abdominal surgery in the elderly. World J Emerg Surg. 2012;7:12.
26. Schilling MK, Maurer CA, et al. Primary vs secondary anastomosis after sigmoid colon resection for perforated diverticulitis (Hinchey stage III and IV); a prospective outcome and cost analysis. Dis Colon Rectum. 2001;44:699–703.
27. Salem I, Flum DR. Primary anastomosis or Hartman's procedure for patients with diverticular peritonitis? A systematic review. Dis Colon Rectum. 2004;47:1953–64.
28. Woods RJ, Lavery IC, Fazio VW, et al. Internal fistulas in diverticular disease. Dis Colon Rectum. 1988;31:591–6.
29. Thorson AG, Goldberg SM. Benign colon: diverticular disease. In: Wolff BG, Fleshman JW, Beck DE, et al., editors. The ASCRS textbook of colon and rectal surgery. New York: Springer; 2007. p. 274.
30. Small AJ, Young-Fadok TM, Baron TH. Expandable metal stent placement for benign colorectal obstruction: outcomes for 23 cases. Surg Endosc. 2008;22(2):454–62.
31. Forshaw MJ, Sankararajah D, Stewart M, et al. Self-expanding metallic stents in the treatment of benign colorectal disease: indications and outcomes. Color Dis. 2006;8(2):102–11.

Cholecystitis

32

Syed Nabeel Zafar and Edward E Cornwell III

Introduction

Gallstone disease represents one of the most common causes of abdominal pain and should always be considered in the differential diagnosis. Acute cholecystitis specifically may account for up to 15% of diagnoses among elderly patients presenting with acute abdominal pain [1]. In this chapter, we discuss the acute presentation, diagnostic workup, and management of both acute calculous cholecystitis (ACC) and acute acalculous cholecystitis (AAC).

Acute Calculous Cholecystitis

The most common cause of cholecystitis is cholelithiasis. Approximately 10–20% [2] of Americans have gallstones; however only 1–2% of them per year develop symptoms or complications [3, 4]. These complications include biliary colic, cholecystitis (acute or chronic), choledocholithiasis, cholangitis, gallstone pancreatitis, and gallstone ileus. Typically symptoms are intermittent with spontaneous resolution before major complications occur; therefore surgery for asymptomatic cholelithiasis is generally unnecessary.

Pathophysiology

The inciting event leading to acute cholecystitis is obstruction at the neck of the gallbladder. Most commonly a gallstone lodges at the Hartmann's pouch leading to increased intraluminal pressure, venous congestion, and mucosal ischemia. This releases an inflammatory reaction with infiltration of neutrophils. Eventually, the ischemia and subsequent vasculitis may lead to mucosal ulcerations, gangrene, and necrosis of the gallbladder wall. In up to 50% of cases there may also be secondary bacterial infection with accumulation of empyema which can eventually perforate and cause systemic sepsis or intra-abdominal abscesses. The most common organisms responsible for this secondary infection include gram-negative bacilli—*Escherichia coli*, Klebsiella species, Enterobacter species, and anaerobes including Bacteroides and Clostridia species.

The pathophysiology in patients presenting with biliary colic or symptomatic gallstone disease that falls short of ACC is similar. The obstruction is however relieved in minutes to hours and subsequent distention and increased intraluminal pressure do not occur.

S.N. Zafar, M.D., M.P.H. • E.E. Cornwell III, M.D., F.A.C.S., F.C.C.M., F.W.A.C.S. (✉)
Department of Surgery, Howard University Hospital, 2041 Georgia Ave NW, Washington, DC 20060, USA
e-mail: syed.zafar@howard.edu; ecornwell@howard.edu

A. Rodriguez et al. (eds.), *Geriatric Trauma and Acute Care Surgery*,
https://doi.org/10.1007/978-3-319-57403-5_32

Clinical Presentation

Patients generally present with right upper quadrant or epigastric pain which is typically constant and often increases in severity over the course of several hours to even days. They often have a history of similar shorter episodes in the past (biliary colic). The pain is frequently brought on by eating, particularly fatty meals. Patients often display signs of systemic inflammation such as tachycardia, fever, and leukocytosis. On physical exam right upper quadrant or epigastric tenderness may be present. A Murphy's sign may also be elicited—this is the abrupt cessation of deep inspiration with the examiner's hand firmly palpating the area of the gallbladder fossa. A thorough history and physical examination must also include investigation regarding the signs and symptoms of biliary obstruction such as icterus and clay-colored stools.

Laboratory investigations include a complete blood cell count and serum chemistries including liver panels. Usually, there will be leukocytosis with a left shift. The bilirubin, alkaline phosphatase, transaminases, and amylase may be slightly elevated. However, a high or rising level of total bilirubin or serum alkaline phosphatase should be concerning for choledocholithiasis while a very high level of amylase and lipase would be suspicious for gallstone pancreatitis.

Radiological Investigation

While ultrasound confirmation of cholelithiasis and assessment of common duct size provide the final clue to the precise diagnosis, there should be a strong clinical suspicion by the time this study is obtained. Specifically, a thorough history and physical exam, an assessment of the WBC, alkaline phosphate, bilirubin, and amylase should give a strong clinical impression of the patient's place in the spectrum of disease from asymptomatic cholelithiasis to symptomatic gallstone disease (acute cholecystitis, choledocholithiasis, gallstone pancreatitis, and cholangitis).

Ultrasound examination of the right upper quadrant is very sensitive and specific for the diagnosis of acute cholecystitis and is often the only radiological test that needs to be ordered. Radiological findings favoring the diagnosis of ACC include demonstration of gallstones or sludge, gallbladder wall thickening (≥4 mm), gallbladder distension, or pericholecystic fluid. Ultrasonographic measurement of the common bile duct (CBD) is also very informative to the diagnosis of choledocholithiasis. In elderly patients the CBD is often normally dilated (>7 mm); however, a size in mm greater than one-tenth of the patient's age should raise concerns.

Cholescintigraphy also known as hepatobiliary iminodiacetic acid (HIDA) scanning is a nuclear imaging procedure used to evaluate the uptake and excretion of radioactive tracers from the gallbladder. It has a sensitivity of 97% and specificity of 94% for the diagnosis of acute cholecystitis [5]. However, its accuracy is severely diminished with prolonged fasting, resulting in many false positives. If the gallbladder is not visualized within 1 h of injection and the radioactive tracer is visualized in the duodenum, the HIDA scan is considered positive and signifies obstruction at the cystic duct and a diagnosis of cholecystitis can be made. Cholescintigraphy is time consuming and costly and is never the first test in the diagnostic workup of gallbladder disease. In fact it is unnecessary in most instances of ACC as the clinical picture and ultrasound imaging is diagnostic in the great majority of cases. The HIDA scan has a role when there is diagnostic ambiguity.

Management

Often patients presenting with cholecystitis have had poor to nil intake for several hours. Management begins with intravenous fluid resuscitation, correction of electrolytes, keeping the patient NPO, analgesia, and IV antibiotics. Even though infection is not the primary inciting event, bacterial overgrowth and secondary infection can occur in up to 50% of patients. It is difficult to determine clinically which patient has or will develop secondary infection and therefore it is prudent to initiate broad-spectrum antibiotics in all patients with a diagnosis of acute cholecystitis.

The definitive treatment is early laparoscopic cholecystectomy. Elderly patients, immunocompromised patients, and diabetic patients may present in a delayed manner and are more likely to suffer from complications and therefore urgent laparoscopic cholecystectomy is recommended. (See chapter on perioperative management.) Laparoscopic cholecystectomy within the first 24–48 h of presentation yields lower complications, hospital length of stay, and healthcare cost [6].

Other Clinical Conditions

A few disease entities are worth special mention. Cholelithiasis may become complicated by one of several disease conditions which require specific management strategies; these are briefly mentioned here. *Choledocholithiasis* occurs when a gallstone is lodged in the common bile duct. Besides the usual presentation described above the patient will often have an elevated bilirubin and alkaline phosphatase level, and a dilated common bile duct upon ultrasound. Often an endoscopic retrograde cholangiogram confirms the diagnosis and facilitates papillotomy and retrieval of the lodged CBD stone, prior to a laparoscopic cholecystectomy. Other techniques of CBD exploration exist; however they are beyond the scope of this chapter. The biliary tree can also become secondarily infected after an obstructing gallstone and *ascending cholangitis* can occur. This is manifested by Charcot's triad of jaundice, right upper quadrant pain, and fever/chills or Reynolds pentad with the addition of hypotension and altered mental status. Ascending cholangitis is a surgical emergency and the biliary tree must be decompressed by endoscopic or percutaneous transhepatic cholangiography and drainage. Patients will require laparoscopic cholecystectomy once stabilized. *Gallstone pancreatitis* is another related disease entity in which a small gallstone passing into the distal common bile duct triggers activation of pancreatic autolytic enzymes resulting in acute pancreatitis. The pancreatitis is managed appropriately and the patient should receive a laparoscopic cholecystectomy prior to discharge.

Gallstone ileus is a disease process more commonly seen in elderly patients. A large impacting gallstone at the Hartmann's pouch causing cholecystitis goes untreated and eventually erodes in through the wall of the gallbladder and adjacent duodenum causing a cholecystoduodenal fistula. This gallstone may get lodged in the distal small bowel resulting in small bowel obstruction. The patient typically presents with signs and symptoms of small bowel obstruction. Upon plain-film abdominal radiograph the classic findings known as Rigler's triad including pneumobilia, sign of small bowel obstruction, and presence of radiolucent gallstones may be present [7]. This mechanical small bowel obstruction must be treated emergently with intravenous fluid resuscitation, nasogastric decompression, and surgery once the patient is adequately resuscitated. The operation typically involves an enterotomy just over the stone to facilitate its removal. It is critical to examine the remainder of the small bowel for other gallstones which may be present in up to 16% of cases. These patients are usually elderly and frail, and attempts at cholecystectomy are avoided. The cholecystoduodenal fistula has frequently spontaneously closed by the time patients undergo surgery.

Acute Acalculous Cholecystitis

Acute inflammation of the gallbladder in the absence of gallstones accounts for up to 5% of all patients with acute cholecystitis [8]. AAC includes risk factors that are often present in critical illness and therefore complicates the clinical outcome of patients who are already physiologically compromised. Effective prophylaxis against AAC has not been established. It is imperative for surgical intensivists to maintain a high index of suspicion of this infrequently occurring disease to make an early diagnosis.

Pathophysiology

The development of acute gallbladder wall inflammation in the absence of gallstones involves three major pathophysiologic mechanisms: (a) gallbladder ischemia, (b) biliary stasis, and (c) Hageman factor XII activation. Unfortunately, the clinical conditions that correspond to these mechanisms are found in our sickest surgical patients. Visceral hypoperfusion seen with cardiovascular instability, hypovolemia, or pressor therapy promotes decreased cystic arterial flow, gallbladder mucosal ischemia, and a low resistance to bacterial proliferation. Biliary stasis with bacterial proliferation is the end result of several clinical parameters seen in the critical illness. Prolonged ventilatory support with positive end-expiratory pressure (PEEP) has been shown to produce decreased portal blood flow and relative biliary stasis in animals [9]. Patients on parenteral nutrition or receiving nil per os demonstrate a lack of enterally mediated factors, via cholecystokinin, that promote gallbladder contraction. Hageman factor XII-dependent pathways, which can be triggered by multiple transfusion, endotoxemia, and injury, have been shown to be associated with gallbladder wall inflammation [10].

Secondary bacterial infection and gangrenous changes are seen in 40–100% of patients with AAC [8]. This is explained by the aforementioned factors of end-organ hypoperfusion and biliary stasis in a setting of critical illness. Difficulty in history taking and an unreliable physical examination, which is a common problem in these patients, may contribute to delays in diagnosis and an unappreciated progression of disease.

Prevention

A 5-year study of critically ill patients developing AAC was published in 1989 from a statewide trauma center. The 14 patients with AAC represented about 0.5% of all patients with at least a 7-day ICU stay [11]. Despite increased awareness over the ensuing decades, AAC remains an uncommon disease that affects less than 1% of critically ill patients. It is not at all unexpected that most surgeons may go many years without treating this disease.

While there are no large prospective clinical trials to scientifically evaluate the prophylactic efficiency of measures proposed to prevent AAC, emphasis on early enteral feeding, lower levels of PEEP, and a more restrictive policy on blood transfusions have all taken place since the 1989 publication.

Diagnosis

It is more practical to prevent the fatal consequences of AAC than to prevent its occurrence. Herein lies the critical importance of early diagnosis and intervention. The use of early ultrasound and computed tomography (CT) in patients with sepsis of undetermined cause has been documented to help decrease the rates of gangrene and perforation in patients with AAC [12]. Radiographic diagnostic criteria include the following [11].

1. Gallbladder wall thickness of ≥4 mm
2. Pericholecystic fluid or subserosal edema in the absence of ascites
3. Intramural gas
4. Sloughed mucosal membrane

Although HIDA scanning is nonspecific and less helpful in this population of patients who are frequently parenterally fed, a decrease in the rate of false positives by the intravenous administration of morphine sulfate during cholescintigraphy is possible [13].

Improvements in the management of critically ill and injured patients increases the number of candidates at risk for the development of AAC. Adherence to the fundamentals of critical care (i.e., maintenance of adequate volume and oxygen delivery and early initiation of enteral feedings) may have counteracted the tendency for this entity to increase. Early CT scanning or ultrasound examination in the critically ill patients with sepsis of undetermined cause will facilitate early diagnosis and improved outcome in those occasional patients who do have AAC.

Management

The treatment for AAC is with emergency cholecystectomy. The incidence of gangrene and/or perforation approaches 50% [8]. Tube cholecystostomy, generally reserved as a procedure of last resort when cholecystectomy is intolerable or technically impossible, has received mention as a therapeutic procedure but is probably more appropriate for obstructive calculus disease. Percutaneous cholecystostomy has also been mentioned, but this approach has the limitations of the greater likelihood of leaving foci of gangrene in place and the lack of surgical exploration to absolutely confirm the diagnosis. Cholecystostomy tube decompression when used in patients too sick to tolerate general anesthesia must be followed by a definitive procedure, i.e., laparoscopic cholecystectomy, once the patient is more stable.

References

1. Perez-Hernandez JL, et al. Acute abdominal pain in elderly patients evaluated in the emergency department at a tertiary level. Rev Gastroenterol Mex. 2010;75(3):261–6.
2. Everhart JE, et al. Prevalence and ethnic differences in gallbladder disease in the United States. Gastroenterology. 1999;117(3):632–9.
3. Friedman GD, Raviola CA, Fireman B. Prognosis of gallstones with mild or no symptoms: 25 years of follow-up in a health maintenance organization. J Clin Epidemiol. 1989;42(2):127–36.
4. Glasgow RE, et al. The spectrum and cost of complicated gallstone disease in California. Arch Surg. 2000;135(9):1021–5. discussion 1025–7.
5. Worthen NJ, Uszler JM, Funamura JL. Cholecystitis: prospective evaluation of sonography and 99mTc-HIDA cholescintigraphy. AJR Am J Roentgenol. 1981;137(5):973–8.
6. Zafar SN, et al. Optimal time for early laparoscopic cholecystectomy for acute cholecystitis. JAMA Surg. 2015;150(2):129–36.
7. Key A, Dawkins A, DiSantis D. Rigler's triad. Abdom Imaging. 2015;40(1):229–30.
8. Huffman JL, Schenker S. Acute acalculous cholecystitis: a review. Clin Gastroenterol Hepatol. 2010;8(1):15–22.
9. Johnson EE, Hedley-Whyte J. Continuous positive-pressure ventilation and portal flow in dogs with pulmonary edema. J Appl Physiol. 1972;33(3):385–9.
10. Becker CG, Dubin T, Glenn F. Induction of acute cholecystitis by activation of factor XII. J Exp Med. 1980;151(1):81–90.
11. Cornwell EE III, et al. Acute acalculous cholecystitis in critically injured patients. Preoperative diagnostic imaging. Ann Surg. 1989;210(1):52–5.
12. Shapiro MJ, et al. Acute acalculous cholecystitis in the critically ill. Am Surg. 1994;60(5):335–9.
13. Flancbaum L, et al. Morphine cholescintigraphy in the evaluation of hospitalized patients with suspected acute cholecystitis. Ann Surg. 1994;220(1):25–31.

33 Gastrointestinal Bleeding in the Elderly Patient

Russell J. Nauta

As with management of gastrointestinal bleeding in younger adults, successful therapy of gastrointestinal hemorrhage in the elderly depends on source identification and source control through directed intervention. Frailty, defined as age-associated declines in physiologic reserve and function across multiorgan systems, may influence the impact of the bleed and limit the options for treatment [1]. Not only dose, but also duration of exposure to self-administered toxins may have a cumulative effect, as with the long-term effect of cigarette smoking on duodenal ulcers and the effect of chronic alcohol use on the development of bleeding esophageal varices.

Elderly patients have often been subjected to more pharmacologic intervention than their youthful counterparts, and complete evaluation requires not only an identification and assessment of drugs contributory or causal to the bleed, but also a judgment as to which can be safely stopped while the source of GI hemorrhage is sought, identified, and controlled.

Aspirin, coumadin, and heparin no longer stand alone as the sole drugs affecting coagulation. Antiplatelet agent and nonsteroidal anti-inflammatory drug (NSAID) use is widespread. As more patients are treated with thrombin inhibitors and other novel oral anticoagulants (NOACs), the clinician must be familiar with which drugs can be safely stopped, which are readily reversed, and which have no identified antidote [2].

Many cancers and many cardiovascular disorders have peak incidences in the sixth through ninth decades and the drugs used to treat them may contribute to the tendency to bleed [3]. Additionally, surgical intervention for aortic disease may be associated with well-described acute and delayed hemorrhagic complications.

Lastly, urgency and choice of diagnostic modalities and treatment are intuitively inferred by the observation that crucial organ systems perform less efficiently over time and that individual organ performance, in general, is less robust in old age than in youth. As an example, glomerular filtration rate at age 90 is half that found at age 20 [4].

Initial Approach to the Patient

The approach to the geriatric patient must be individualized. As complete a history must be taken as the bleeding rate will allow. It should be determined whether the bleeding is rapid or slow, chronic or acute, and whether it has fostered hemodynamic compromise. As with blood loss incurred through trauma, initial resuscitation with isotonic fluid should be informed by trends

R.J. Nauta, M.D., F.A.C.S.
Harvard Medical School, Boston, MA, USA

Mount Auburn Hospital, 330 Mount Auburn Street, Cambridge, MA 02138, USA
e-mail: rnauta@mah.harvard.edu

A. Rodriguez et al. (eds.), *Geriatric Trauma and Acute Care Surgery*,
https://doi.org/10.1007/978-3-319-57403-5_33

in vital signs and should verify the presence of an adequate airway, adequate ventilation, adequate cerebral perfusion, and adequate urine output. Beta-blockers and calcium channel blockers may produce artificially low heart rates for the volume loss incurred, and the presence of a pacemaker may produce discordance between the rate of electrical discharges and actual hemodynamically significant systoles. Habitual use of alcohol, tobacco, antiplatelet agents, NSAIDs, heparin, coumadin, or NOACs should be identified.

Discontinuing an anticoagulant should occur with the advice and consent of the prescriber. Antiplatelet agents require 5 days without drug administration to fall to a subtherapeutic level. Combinations of fresh frozen plasma and vitamin K, or prothrombin complex concentrates, in increasing order of potency, can reverse heparin and warfarin, depending on clinical urgency. Of the NOACs, only one (dabigatran) has a Federal Drug Administration-approval antidote (idarucizumab) [2, 5].

Blood should be typed and crossed at the same time as a broad metabolic and hematologic screen is obtained, and blood resuscitation should supplement crystalloid resuscitation when more than 30% of the blood volume has been lost to hemorrhage. Initial vascular access should be obtained with short, large caliber intravenous catheters; placement of a central venous catheter and bladder catheterization may guide the resuscitation once volume repletion has been initiated. An impression should be formed as to whether the bleeding is an upper GI bleed (i.e., with a presumed source anywhere from the lips to the ligament of Treitz) or a lower GI bleed (originating somewhere between the ligament of Treitz and the anus). As in younger populations, upper gastrointestinal bleeding is more common, accounting for two-thirds of all gastrointestinal hemorrhage.

Nasogastric suction should be established early in the evaluation of upper gastrointestinal bleeds. Passage of a nasogastric tube in lower gastrointestinal bleeds has been said to be of low discriminatory yield, on the grounds that a competent pylorus may not yield a red aspirate even from a briskly bleeding duodenal source. However, a bilious effluent from a tube placed in the stomach remains a valuable tool to exclude bleeding from the stomach and duodenum; it is unlikely that green bile without blood would be recovered if either of those two organs were actively bleeding at the time of nasogastric intubation. Upper gastrointestinal bleeding produces tarry stools or coffee ground stools because of the effect of oxidation on hemoglobin, but the cathartic effect of a rapid upper GI bleed may produce bright red blood per rectum from a proximal source because of rapid transit. Thus, as with any diagnostic test, nasogastric suction is useful if one knows the limitations of the test and can interpret it appropriately.

Careful abdominal examination may disclose important peritoneal findings, the presence of organomegaly or a palpable tumor. Scars from previous gastrointestinal or vascular operations may contribute to a robust differential diagnosis, and Cope's dictum that it is more useful to place a gloved digit in the lower end of the GI tract than a thermometer in the upper end usually applies [6]. Thus, the digital rectal examination and analysis of the stool for blood should not be omitted.

As noted above, nonsteroidal anti-inflammatory drugs are taken for rheumatologic illness and antiplatelet agents are taken for cardiac prophylaxis, cardiac therapy (for example, to maintain stent patency), neurologic treatment, or prophylaxis of TIAs. They may be contributory to the bleed, and their use is therefore essential to uncover in the history taking.

Upper GI Hemorrhage

Hematemesis or melena suggests an upper gastrointestinal source. If a bleeding episode is thought to be from the upper gastrointestinal tract, all efforts should be directed toward the early performance of an emergent upper endoscopy and the preparation of the patient for this procedure. Such preparation begins with airway control and establishment of adequate vascular access and volume replacement. Medical management of prolonged clotting times, to include reversal of anticoagulants where appropriate, should begin.

The three leading causes of upper gastrointestinal bleeding are gastric and duodenal ulcer disease, varices, and arterial venous malformations. Mallory Weiss tears (from protracted vomiting), erosions (from NSAID use or ingested alcohol), tumors, and solitary protruding vessels such as the Dieulafoy abnormality, are less common. The mainstay of endoscopic control of peptic ulcer bleeding or arteriovenous malformation is injection of sclerosing agents in the submucosa adjacent to the offending vessel. An actively bleeding vessel, a vessel visible at endoscopy, or an ulcer with clot at its base makes subsequent bleeding more likely. Even if surgery is not immediately mandated in such patients by visible resumption of bleeding, identification of a high-risk source at the earliest possible opportunity is extraordinarily helpful should re-bleeding occur. Gastric ulcers are typically wedged or biopsied to exclude cancer, whereas duodenal ulcers are oversewn with three sutures placed in the bed of the ulcer where the bifurcating gastroduodenal ulcer is exposed. Mallory Weiss tears refractory to endoscopic management are oversewn through a gastrostomy, and Dieulafoy lesions are oversewn if endoscopic management fails.

Since nearly all sources of upper gastrointestinal bleeding by definition have eroded mucosa, it could be compellingly argued that all patients would profit by the administration of proton pump inhibitors, with the possible exception of variceal bleeds and Dieulafoy lesions. Proton pump inhibitors are more effective reducers of intraluminal acid than their historic H2 antagonist antecedents [7]. Also, an increasing appreciation has developed that all upper gastrointestinal hemorrhage is not, as was previously believed, simply a mismatch between the host's ability to produce acid and his or her ability to defend himself or herself against it. Gastric erosions, or so-called stress gastritis, more commonly seen two or three decades ago, illustrated the value of normalizing gastric pH in all seriously ill patients, but likely have as co-derivative origin a vasoconstriction at the mesenteric level. Whether presenting as stress ulcers in the ICU, Curling's ulcers in the burn unit, or Cushing's ulcers in the neurosurgical ICU, the unifying mechanism of illness appears to be shunting of blood away from the mucosa and resultant ischemia of the proximal gastrointestinal tract. Moreover, the bleeding of stress gastritis is diffuse, to be distinguished from the more focal bleeding seen in peptic ulcer disease. Many true ulcers of the gastric or duodenal mucosa are now attributed to *H. pylori*, an infectious organism, and are successfully treated with bismuth-based quadruple pharmacologic antimicrobial therapy rather than therapies exclusively directed at acid overproduction [8]. While the oversecretion of gastrin still plays a role in hypersecretion syndromes such as those occasioned by rare Zollinger–Ellison syndrome, acid probably plays less of a role in upper gastrointestinal hemorrhage than originally postulated.

Acutely, the treatment for bleeding ulceration is endoscopic intervention with injection or clips, intravenous proton pump inhibition, and appropriate volume resuscitation. Though some surgical textbooks still advocate early surgical intervention for visible vessels, visible bleeding, or ulcer with an adherent clot, most endoscopists would try a second round of endoscopy before embolization or surgical intervention.

Esophageal Varices

Esophageal varices represent an acute manifestation of an increase in portal venous pressure usually occasioned or abetted by the ingestion of alcohol. Derangement and scarring within the sinusoid cause venous pressure to rise in the portal vein and its valveless venous tributaries as the liver scars and obstructs blood flow through the sinusoids. Veins draining the foregut and midgut in particular dilate and collateralize with low-pressure systemic veins, producing varices. When traumatized by food ingestion, alcohol ingestion, or forceful vomiting, bleeding from these collateralized varices may result. The bleeding may be torrential because venous pressure in the torn varix is no longer relieved into the systemic veins, but into the atmosphere.

Bleeding gastroesophageal varices are predominantly treated endoscopically, with sclerosing or banding being utilized as the endoscopist prefers. Should endoscopy fail or the offending varix not be visualized, urgent transjugular intrahepatic portosystemic shunt (TIPS), a radiologic decompression of the portal vein into the systemic circulation, may be required. This intervention is effective only for esophageal varices, and only when the systemic and portal vessels are not obstructed with clot on preoperative imaging.

Surgical portosystemic shunts, where anastomoses are created between the main tributaries of the portal and systemic circulation, produce fewer interventions for subsequent bleeding than endoscopic sclerotherapy, but have fallen out of favor because they do not extend life when compared to repetitive endoscopic approaches. Gastric varices are more often caused by thrombosis of the splenic vein following episodes of pancreatitis; they produce dilated blood vessels because of obstruction of flow to the portal system through the occluded splenic vein. While they may transiently respond to endoscopic sclerotherapy or banding, splenectomy is the treatment of choice.

Lower Gastrointestinal Bleeding

Significant lower gastrointestinal bleeding is usually manifest by bright red blood per rectum, as hemoglobin from blood lost more proximally is oxidized and the stool darkens. As with bleeding in the upper tracts, adequate management of lower gastrointestinal hemorrhage requires visualization of the source with a fiber-optic instrument.

Some colonoscopists are highly skilled (and highly motivated) to perform the lavage necessary to reliably see the entire colon at presentation. Not infrequently, however, colonic bleeding is intermittent, and the patient is better served by resuscitation, normalization of hemodynamic parameters, bowel preparation, and colonoscopy on an urgent, rather than emergent, basis [9].

Anoscopy usually precedes colonoscopy and is successful in excluding bleeding from the last several centimeters of the GI tract. If no such active source is found, the observation that brisk bleeding is coming from the rectum has identified only the orifice of egress; efforts to identify the anatomic source should continue.

Lower gastrointestinal hemorrhage may occur from polyps (benign or malignant), diverticular hemorrhage, or arteriovenous malformations. Again, the colonoscope is exceptionally useful for diagnosis and therapy. Diverticula are preferentially concentrated in the sigmoid in non-Asians and Asians alike; however, arteriovenous malformations and diverticular bleeding from a right colon source are more common in Asian populations. Arteriovenous malformations in all ethnic groups are more commonly seen in the right colon.

If chronic bleeding originates from small or pedunculated polyps, it may be controlled by snare polypectomy. Larger, more sessile polyps, or overt cancers can be identified and marked for surgical removal with segmental resection. Bleeding from arteriovenous malformations can usually be controlled urgently with the electrocautery. Wherever possible, the entire colon should be seen before surgical management of an acute lower GI bleed is undertaken, unless the rate of bleeding dictates emergent segmental resection as treatment of a visualized bleeding lesion. In these instances, visualization of the entire colon may be postponed until the patient is more hemodynamically stable, but a mental note should be made to evaluate the entire colon at some point in the convalescence.

On occasion, the surgeon may encounter a referring physician strongly advocating for surgical intervention before a source of bleeding has been specifically identified. Within reason, the surgeon must resist performing such a procedure; in this situation, laparotomy produces an elegant view of the outside of the colon, while gastrointestinal bleeding continues unlocalized from the inside of the colon. The goal of source identification and source control must be reiterated and strongly defended. Four alternatives to colonoscopy may be useful in this circumstance. One involves the technetium labeling of an aliquot of red blood cells withdrawn from the patient, which are labeled with the radionuclide, and then reinfused [10, 11]. The abdomen is then imaged and clinically important blood loss is visualized as intraluminal appearance of the radionclide-tagged red cells as hemorrhage into the visceral lumen occurs. A second approach involves selective cannulation of the superior mesenteric artery and inferior mesenteric artery separately, in hopes of injecting an iodinated dye and identifying a "blush" as that dye leaves the bleeding vessel. As can be reasonably inferred, bleeding must be reasonably brisk to allow such a blush to be recognized at arteriography—typically in the range of 0.4 to 1.0 cm^3 per min. The technetium scan is slightly more sensitive, identifying bleeds in the range of 0.1 cm^3 per min, but such sensitivity comes at the expense of anatomic detail, as a mesenteric vessel is not selectively cannulated or recognizable by the nuclear camera.

A combined and sequential third approach first uses the less specific nuclear medicine study as a "yes/no" determination as to whether the patient is bleeding, with the radiologist standing by to perform a selective angiogram if the nuclear medicine shows technetium-labeled red cells leaving the intravascular space. Although conferring a risk of colonic infarction if too large a vessel is occluded in elderly patients, embolization of an angiographically identified bleed with metal coils or clot may stop a bleed completely. Great care needs to be taken not to infarct the injected segment of bowel and to limit the quantity of iodinated dye used, as the dye is nephrotoxic. Success in stopping hemorrhage with this technique still requires the subsequent investigation of the morphology of the bleed and characterization of the bleeding site as tumor, AVM, or diverticulosis.

Some centers utilize a fourth approach involving a carefully timed injection of dye during a CT scan to attempt anatomic localization. A second procedure for hemorrhage control is necessary if such an extravasation is demonstrated, but impressive sensitivity (85%) and specificity (92%) have been reported with CT angiography [12].

Barium is not used in the acute localization of gastrointestinal hemorrhage, as it obscures vascular imaging, thereby making subsequent diagnostic or therapeutic angiography difficult.

Slow Gastrointestinal Bleeding

Slow gastrointestinal bleeding is detected by stool guaiac or, more recently, by detection of DNA shed into the stool by neoplasms. Patients with hypoperfusion of the intestine due to severe atherosclerotic cardiovascular disease may also present with trace blood in the stool; the etiology in this instance is mucosal sloughing. Typically, of the three mesenteric vessels (celiac, SMA, and inferior mesenteric), two must be compromised to produce either detectable blood loss or ischemic gastrointestinal pain.

Slow bleeds may be identified by "push" endoscopy, where the abdomen is opened and the intestine is fed over a long scope introduced orally; telangiectasias or other arteriovenous malformations are often identified through this technique. Capsule endoscopy, where the patient ingests a camera which tumbles intraluminally from mouth to anus as it records, has become a useful diagnostic adjunct to endoscopic studies in hard-to-access areas of the small intestine.

Remote and Immediate History of Vascular Disease

Vascular reconstruction, particularly abdominal aortic reconstruction, may compromise blood flow to the colon acutely. In this instance, the wall of the graft occludes the orifice of the inferior mesenteric artery and collaterals from the middle colic or sigmoidal arteries prove insufficient to sustain colonic mural perfusion. Successful identification and therapy for this ischemic bleeding, are suggested by a septic or febrile presentation shortly after graft placement. Fiber-optic sigmoidoscopy shows the mucosa to be friable and easily enticed to bleed. Occasionally, in particularly in patients with severe ischemic colitis, a similar presentation may occur without aortic prior reconstruction.

In another graft-related catastrophe, the proximal end of an aortic vascular graft may erode into the lumen of the fourth portion of the duodenum many years after placement, producing upper gastrointestinal hemorrhage. This lethal presentation of aortic graft-related gastrointestinal bleeding is often heralded by a "sentinel" or herald bleed as the aortic graft placed decades earlier erodes the fourth portion of the duodenum. The initial bleed is followed by exsanguination. The diagnosis is only made when graft erosion is suspected in a bleeding patient with a remote history of aortic reconstruction. Graft removal, duodenal repair, and extra-anatomic bypass are the operations of choice.

Conclusions

The therapeutic approach should be methodical and logical, but not slow. Elderly patients with a gastrointestinal bleed require an initial resuscitation and a directed workup based on likely diagnoses for the patient's clinical context and his or her comorbid illnesses. The resuscitating surgeon must insist that his or her radiologic and gastroenterologic colleagues offer their expertise on a timely basis. Seldom is it required to blindly remove a segment of the gastrointestinal tract without having previously identified that it has a high likelihood of being the bleeding source; in particular, the historical practice of removing the entire colon blindly for gastrointestinal bleeding is to be discouraged except in extraordinarily rare circumstances.

Resection or control of the bleeding side is the therapeutic goal. In large bowel resection, reestablishment of intestinal continuity is dependent on the degree of soilage and the patient's comorbid illness. It is particularly true of the elderly that even though drugs taken for rheumatologic, neurologic, or cardiovascular illnesses may aid and abet bleeding, when patients with or without major coagulopathies bleed, they bleed from an anatomic source. The deliberate and knowledgeable clinician should be able to identify that source in the overwhelming majority of patients and deliver a satisfactory result.

References

1. Chen X, Mao G, Leng SX. Frailty syndrome: an overview. Clin Interv Aging. 2014;9:433–41.
2. Hu T, Vaidya V, Asirvatham S. Reversing anticoagulation effects of novel oral anticoagulants: role of ciraparantag, andexanet alfa, and idarucizumab. Vasc Health Risk Manag. 2016;12:35–44.
3. American Cancer Society Cancer Facts in Figures 2016. http://www.cancer.org.
4. Brown WW, David BB, Spry LA, et al. Aging and the kidney. Arch Intern Med. 1986;146:1790–6.
5. Babilonia K, Trujillo T. The role of prothrombin complex concentrates in reversal of target specific anticoagulants. Thromb J. 2014;12:8.
6. Cope Z, Silen W. Cope's early diagnosis of the acute abdomen. 22nd ed. New York: Oxford University Press; 2010.
7. Sachs G, Shin JM, Howden CW. Review article: the clinical pharmacology of proton pump inhibitors. Aliment Pharmacol Ther. 2006;23(2):2–8.
8. Papastergiou V, Georgopoulos S, Karatapanis S. Treatment of helicobacter pylori infection: past, present and future. World J Gastrointest Pathophysiol. 2014;5(4):392–9.
9. Hunter R, Kochman M. Lower gastrointestinal bleeding and colitis. In: Lanken P, Hanson III CW, Manaker S, editors. The intensive care unit manual. Philadelphia: WB Saunders; 2001. p. 683–91.
10. Tabibian J, Song LM, Enders F, et al. Technetium-labeled erythrocyte scintigraphy in acute gastrointestinal bleeding. Int J Color Dis. 2013;28:1099–105.
11. Suzman MS, Talmor M, Jennis R, et al. Accurate localization and surgical management of active lower gastrointestinal hemorrhage with technetium-labeled erythrocyte scintigraphy. Ann Surg. 1996;224(1):29–36.
12. Garcia-Blazquez V, Vicente-Bartulos A, Olavarria-Delgado A, et al. Accuracy of CT angiography in the diagnosis of acute gastrointestinal bleeding: systematic review of meta-analysis. Eur Radiol. 2013;23(5):1181–90.

34 Intestinal Obstruction in Geriatric Population

Paula Ferrada, Ashanthi Ratnasekera, and Ricardo Ferrada

Introduction

Intestinal obstruction is an interruption of the normal enteric flow in either small or large bowel. An obstruction before the ileocecal valve is considered a proximal bowel obstruction and after the valve is called a distal bowel obstruction. Both can have a mechanical or functional etiology. The management may differ depending on the cause of the bowel obstruction.

In the geriatric population, the presentation of bowel obstruction may be late. Comorbidities are frequently seen and as a result morbidity and mortality can be higher.

Types of Intestinal Obstruction by Location

- Small-bowel obstruction (proximal)
- Large-bowel obstruction (distal)
- Partial obstruction with gas flowing past the point of obstruction
- Volvulus and closed-loop obstruction

P. Ferrada, M.D.
Virginia Commonwealth University, USA

A. Ratnasekera, D.O.
Crozer Keystone Health System, Chester, PA, USA

R. Ferrada, M.D. (✉)
Centro Medico Imbanaco and Clinica Amiga, USA
e-mail: ricardoferrada@yahoo.com

Physiology of the Intestinal Tract

- *Intestinal secretions*

The GI tract produces 8–10 L of secretions daily. The contents contain water, electrolytes, glucose, and urea and the concentration is mostly isotonic. The amount of fluid excreted in a 24-h time frame in every level of the GI tract varies:

Saliva	1000 mL
Gastric secretions	2500 mL
Pancreatic secretions	800 mL
Biliary tract	1000 mL
Intestine	4000 mL

The small intestine plays a major role in digestion and absorption of carbohydrates, proteins, minerals, vitamins, and fats.

An adult normally consumes approximately 300 g of carbohydrates per day. Majority of dietary starch is long-chain polysaccharides which are broken down into simple saccharides such as amylose, maltotriose, and maltose by salivary and pancreatic amylases. When simple saccharides are passed into the duodenum and jejunum the remainder of the digestion occurs with the brush border enzymes. The brush border enzymes contain lactase, maltase, and trehalase which break down disaccharides into monosaccharides. Monosaccharides are absorbed via sodium transport channels via active transport. The main membrane transport channels are

A. Rodriguez et al. (eds.), *Geriatric Trauma and Acute Care Surgery*,
https://doi.org/10.1007/978-3-319-57403-5_34

sodium-glucose transporter 1 (SGLT-1), glucose transporter 5 (GLUT-5), and glucose transporter 2 (GLUT-2). Fructose is absorbed by facilitated diffusion via the GLUT-5 carrier.

Protein digestion is initiated in the stomach where the gastric secretions denature protein. Once denatured protein enters the duodenum inactive trypsinogen is activated to trypsin by brush border enzymes which activates other proteolytic enzymes. The proteolytic enzymes trypsin, chymotrypsin, and elastase act on peptide bonds and remove a single amino acid from the carboxyl end of the peptide. This splits complex peptides into dipeptides and tripeptides, which are absorbed from the intestinal lumen by a sodium-mediated active transport mechanism and digested further by enzymes in the brush border. 80–90% of protein digestion occurs in the jejunum.

Fat digestion occurs in the small intestine. An adult consumes about 60–100 g of fats per day. The process of emulsification occurs when the fat molecules are broken down to smaller sizes by water-soluble enzymes and lecithin and bile salts in bile. Fat digestion is furthered by forming micelles which are small spherical globules composed of 20–40 molecules of bile salts with a sterol nucleus that is highly fat soluble and a hydrophilic outer polar group. The monoglycerides and free fatty acids are formed by lipolysis and is absorbed through the brush border by simple diffusion due to its lipophilic nature.

Feces contains less than 200 cm^3 of fluids, which indicates that approximately 96% of fluid content is absorbed from food. The absorption in the large intestine and feces formation includes the succus coming from the small bowel. Each day approximately 1.5 L of chyme passes through the ileocecal valve into the colon. Most of the water and electrolytes are absorbed. Absorption occurs mainly in the proximal half of the colon, with a maximum of 6–8 L every day. The distal colon acts as storage area.

- *Intestinal gas*

Usually gas is scarce in stomach and colon. Small bowel has no gas. The total amount of gas in the GI is around 100 cm^3, but can be higher in older people due to lack of normal tone. The amount of gas expelled daily by the rectum is 200–2000 cm^3, and on average 600 cm^3.

Main source of intestinal gas is swallowed air. Other sources are CO_2 secondary to fermentation of hydrochloric acid by duodenal bicarbonate, and colonic methanol. These gases mixed with oxygen have the potential to be volatile when using electrocautery during colonoscopy.

Gastrointestinal function enteric nervous system.

The GI nervous system is composed of two plexus: Auerbach's plexus which is located between the outer muscle layers, and the Meissner's plexus which is located in the inner submucosa. The Auerbach's or myenteric outer plexus controls the GI movements, and the inner Meissner's plexus controls the secretions and blood flow.

A number of neurotransmitters are released by the nerve endings. The commonly known are effects of norepinephrine and acetylcholine. These are excitatory neurotransmitters. The receptors undergo change which allows ions across the cell membrane.

Etiology

There are three main types of intestinal obstructions: mechanical obstruction, pseudo-obstruction, and adynamic ileus.

- *Mechanical obstruction*

The most common cause of bowel obstruction. The causes of mechanical obstruction are:

- Extrinsic causes such as hernias, adhesions, volvulus, and extrinsic compression by tumor
- Intrinsic causes such as polyps, intestinal atresia, intussusception, intramural hematomas, cancer, inflammation, or edema
- Intraluminal causes such as foreign bodies (gallstones, fecal impaction, bezoars)

According to the level of the intestinal tract, the different causes of obstruction can be as follows:

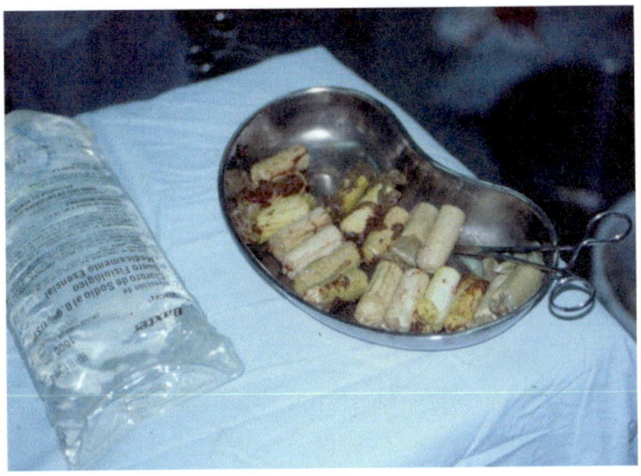

Fig. 34.1 Bowel obstruction caused by cocaine bags

Stomach. The most common are cancer, peptic ulcer disease, and bezoars (Fig. 34.1). Cancer and peptic ulcers can produce obstruction in the pyloric area, and as a consequence gastric emptying is impaired. Initially the obstruction improves by nasogastric tube. However, chronic fibrosis or mass effect produced by an ulcer warrants surgical intervention. Symptoms from bezoars are insidious: they appear and disappear with no explanation. Gastric cancer requires resection with oncologic principles of resection. The color of the emesis can give a clue of obstruction proximal to pylorus if absent of bile.

Duodenum. The most common causes are duodenal wall hematoma due to trauma. Wilkie syndrome or SMA syndrome is an obstruction produced by the superior mesenteric artery on the third part of duodenum compressing the duodenum against the aorta. This is infrequently found. The patient presents with weight loss and nausea vomiting.

Small bowel. Commonly, intestinal obstructions are located in the small bowel and majority are due to adhesions. Other causes of small-bowel obstruction include hernias, volvulus, gallstone ileus, and intussusception. Therefore it is imperative that all patients with abdominal pain receive a complete examination including the groin and a rectal exam.

Colon. The most frequent cause of colon obstruction is carcinoma, located in sigmoid or rectum. Volvulus, diverticulitis, fecal impaction, abdominal carcinomatosis, regional enteritis, foreign bodies, and endometriosis are frequent. Constipation is an emergency in the elderly patient since fecal impaction can cause ischemia by pressure and perforation of the large intestine.

Pseudo-Obstruction

Pseudo-obstruction of the large bowel, also known as Ogilvie's syndrome, is the lack of movement of colonic contents and succus forward. It is caused by the inhibition of the neuromuscular system. The most frequent causes are infections, both systemic and intra-abdominal; electrolyte disorders; and abdominal surgery. Small bowel recovers itself in 24 h, stomach in 48 h, and colon in 3–5 days. In the elderly population, pseudo-obstruction can present frequently due to infection and illness. The reduction of peristaltic waves results in impaired propulsive effect and accumulation of intestine fluids and gas. However the loss of electrolytes and fluids is less than that seen in mechanical obstruction.

Abdominal X-rays or computed tomography of the abdomen and pelvis will demonstrate dilated colon with no point of change in caliber. The treatment is supportive initially. These patients may require NG tube decompression if they also have small-bowel dilation from incompetent ileocecal valve. Patients will require rectal tube decompression for decompression of the colon. Underlying electrolyte abnormalities and infection may need to be reversed. Neostigmine injection has been shown to temporarily relieve the pseudo-obstruction. Neostigmine should be administered under cardiac monitoring and should be monitored for any bradyarrhythmias. If this condition is refractory to supportive management and patient re-presents with the same scenario, the benefits of a subtotal colectomy with end ileostomy should be considered. In elderly population with multiple comorbidities, the decision for a subtotal colectomy may be difficult. However, the incidences of multiple hospital admissions and chronic electrolyte abnormalities may aid in the decision to perform a subtotal colectomy.

Adynamic Ileus

Similar to Ogilvie's syndrome, an ileus is defined as the slowing or absence of propulsion of enteric contents. It is most commonly seen in elderly patients after major abdominal or cardiac surgery. Electrolyte imbalances, intra-abdominal infection, and pancreatitis are also other commonly seen states contributing to adynamic ileus. Anticholinergic medications, Haldol, and narcotics are also known to cause adynamic ileus. Patients will present similarly to bowel obstruction with symptoms of nausea, vomiting, and abdominal distention with no passage of gas or stool. Abdominal X-rays will demonstrate dilated small bowel throughout; air fluid levels may also be apparent. Treatment of an ileus is supportive with nasogastric tube decompression, IV fluids, and correction of underlying cause. Medications to increase motility have not shown to decrease length or resolution of ileus.

Incidence

Among the patients with intestinal obstruction 75–80%, the obstruction is located in the small bowel and the rest in the large bowel. As previously mentioned the more frequent cause of small-bowel obstruction (SBO) is adhesions, followed by hernias [1].

The most common cause of colon obstruction is malignancy with the majority located in sigmoid and rectum. Malignant tumors of the anal canal account for 10% of these patients. Both types are found in older patients. The most common nonmalignant cause of bowel obstruction is volvulus [2].

Pathophysiology

Most common cause of adhesions is previous surgery; however intra-abdominal infectious processes can produce adhesions as well. Surgical trauma, inflammation blood, or pus starts the process by fibrin deposits which are later colonized by fibroblasts. Finally a strong cord appears and serves as an obstruction, or in the worst case a twist with ischemia of the bowel.

Hernias are the second most common cause of bowel obstruction. The more dangerous hernia is a femoral hernia. However, the more frequently found is umbilical hernias. An indirect inguinal hernia becomes obstructed more easily than direct, because of a potential smaller ring. A direct inguinal hernia is usually due to a debilitated and weak abdominal wall. Ventral hernias can produce obstruction as well, particularly if the defect is smaller [3–5].

Gallstone ileus is a rare cause of obstruction. Most common presentation is in the elderly population in the distal ileum. It is produced by a gallstone which passes through a cholecystoduodenal fistula. The gallstone is lodged in the distal ileocecal valve causing a mechanical obstruction. Therefore "gallstone ileus" is a misnomer for this disease process [6].

Intussusception is commonly seen in the pediatric population. Enlargement of the Peyer's patches due to a viral cause will cause an intussusception of the ileum into the ascending colon. Most commonly it is palpated as a mass in the right upper quadrant. In the pediatric population air-contrast enema will reduce the intussusception majority of the time. On the contrary, in the adult population the most common cause of intussusception is small-bowel polyps which may be the lead point. Transient peristalsis can be seen as "intussusception" on CT of abdomen, with no proximal obstruction or symptoms. However, true intussusception will present as a mechanical obstruction. These patients should undergo surgical intervention and resection of bowel. The bowel should be examined for pathology for any malignancy [7].

Volvulus is a state where the bowel can be twisted in the mesenteric axis. In the pediatric population it is commonly seen in patients with Ladd bands causing midgut volvulus and can present with bilious emesis. In the elderly population, right colon and sigmoid volvulus are common. The ascending colon, cecum, and terminal ileum may twist and cause volvulus. The fixed points are the ileocecal valve and the ascending colon may be mobile. The cecum alone can be involved in volvulus and this is named cecal bascule. A radiographic diagnosis can be made by plain X ray and by computed tomography. A sigmoid volvulus may present as acute abdominal pain, obstipation, and abdominal distention (Fig. 34.2). On plain film the appearance of bent inner tube can present. On CT there may be a swirl in the mesentery. If the patient has no signs of peritonitis and perforation, the patient may undergo decompression with rigid proctoscope or flexible sigmoidoscopy with rectal tube placement. Decompression for 24–48 h may be necessary with interval sigmoid resection with primary anastomosis. If the patient presents with concerns of peritonitis and nonviable bowel, emergent operative intervention with sigmoid resection and colostomy may be required [8, 9]. Other causes such as Meckel's diverticulum causing small-bowel volvulus and bowel ischemia can present (Fig. 34.3).

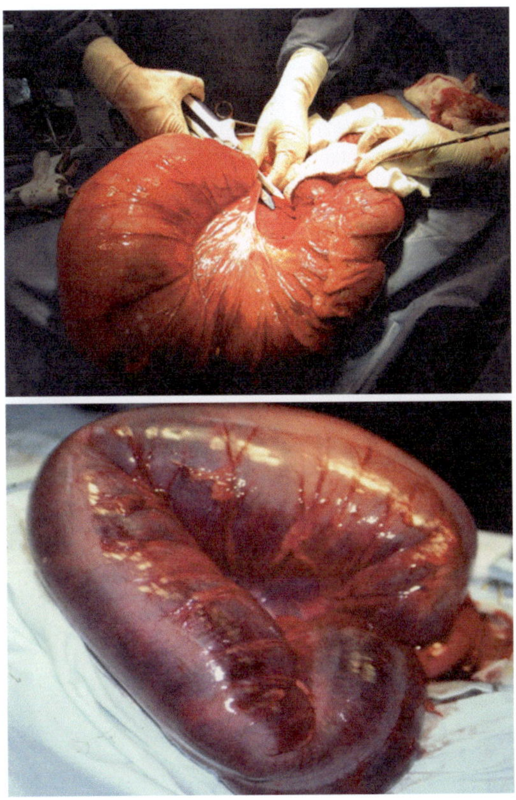

Fig. 34.2 Sigmoid volvulus causing obstruction with proximal sigmoid dilation

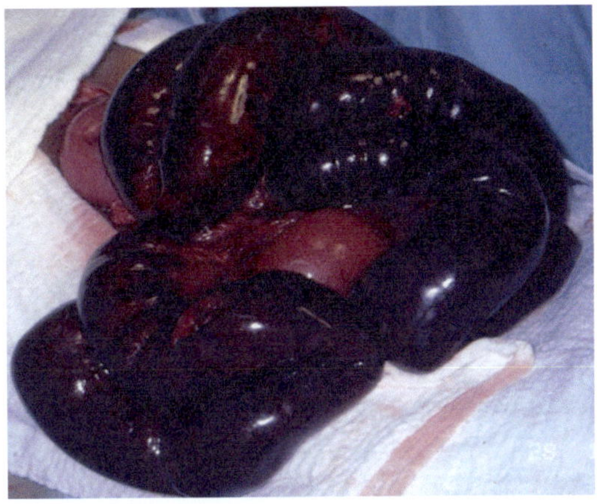

Fig. 34.3 Volvulus caused by Meckel's diverticulum

Bowel irregularity in the elderly population is prevalent due to multiple ailments, comorbidities, immobility, and infection. Geriatric patients may experience severe constipation for these reasons. The etiology must be attempted to be reversed or symptomatic management with an aggressive bowel regimen must be pursued. In the event, patients present with severe obstipation, and plans for evacuation of stool with mechanical and chemical bowel regimen must be considered. Geriatric patients with severe obstipation may also present with rectal thickening and stercoral ulcers. Perforation of stercoral ulcers may present with feculent peritonitis leading to sepsis requiring laparotomy and resection.

Management

Vomiting in the geriatric population carries increased morbidity due to impairment of reflexes which increases the possibility of bronchoaspiration. Hypovolemia due to the sequestration of the intestine can be masked, because a number of older patients suffer from hypertension. On the other hand older patients are also less compliant and are not able to communicate well regarding pain, and a complicated obstruction can occur with minimal or absent signs.

Initial management should include a thorough history and physical exam of the patient, including a rectal exam. Laboratory studies should be pursued for leukocytosis, lactic academia, and any electrolyte abnormalities. Radiographic studies can be initiated with abdominal X-rays followed by oral contrasted abdominal and pelvic CT scans. NG tube decompression and fluid resuscitation to euvolemia should be ensued. Resuscitation in the elderly population with multiple comorbidities should be judicious. If the patient presents with signs of peritonitis, sepsis and bowel nonviability emergent laparotomy should be considered.

Peritonitis on a patient with bowel obstruction is due to perforation or bowel necrosis and should be avoided at all cost. Small-bowel obstruction when partial can be observed in the absence of leukocytosis or tachycardia. A water-soluble study through the nasogastric tube can be diagnostic of a complete obstruction and in some cases therapeutic when the obstruction is partial or the patient has a dynamic ileus.

Colonic obstruction is always a surgical emergency. In the case of partial colonic obstruction the use of endoscopic stents has been of value to temporize surgery in colorectal carcinoma. This allows for neoadjuvant therapy before surgery and possibly better outcomes. However, the use of stents in benign disease has yet to be validated.

References

1. Springer JE, Bailey JG, Davis PJ, Johnson PM. Management and outcomes of small bowel obstruction in older adult patients: a prospective cohort study. Can J Surg. 2014;57:379–84.
2. Markogiannakis H, Messaris E, Dardamanis D, et al. Acute mechanical bowel obstruction: clinical presentation, etiology, management and outcome. World J Gastroenterol. 2007;13:432–7.
3. Alhambra-Rodriguez de Guzman C, Picazo-Yeste J, Tenias-Burillo JM, Moreno-Sanz C. Improved outcomes of incarcerated femoral hernia: a multivariate analysis of predictive factors of bowel ischemia and potential impact on postoperative complications. Am J Surg. 2013;205:188–93.
4. Kurt N, Oncel M, Ozkan Z, Bingul S. Risk and outcome of bowel resection in patients with incarcerated groin hernias: retrospective study. World J Surg. 2003;27:741–3.
5. Neutra R, Velez A, Ferrada R, Galan R. The risk of incarceration of inguinal hernia in Cali. Col J Chron Dis. 1981;34:561–4.
6. Alvarez LF, Bejarano W, Rojas OL. Biliary fistula and Bouveret's syndrome. The same but different. Rev Col Gastroenterol. 2010;25:86–93.
7. Gupta RK, Agrawal CS, Yadav R, Bajracharya A, Sah PL. Intussusception in adults: institutional review. Int J Surg. 2011;9(1):91–5.
8. Martin V, Shaw-Smith C. Review of genetic factors in intestinal malrotation. Pediatr Surg Int. 2010;26:769–81.
9. Nehra D, Goldstein AM. Intestinal malrotation: varied clinical presentation from infancy through adulthood. Surgery. 2010;149:386–93.

35 Acute Appendicitis

Tiffany N. Anderson, Frederick Moore, and Janeen Jordan

Introduction

Appendicitis is one of the most commonly treated diseases in the world. Reginald Fitz provided the first description in 1886 when he incidentally noted that in the pre-appendectomy era one-third of postmortem patients had evidence of prior appendiceal inflammation, thus identifying it as a cause for right lower quadrant pain [1]. Over the years many others have worked to further define its characteristics. McBurney famously stated, "The seat of greatest pain, determined by the pressure of one finger, has been very exactly between an inch and a half and 2 inches from the anterior spinous process of the ilium on the straight line drawn from that process to the umbilicus" [2]. In recent decades the understanding of appendicitis and its natural course has been challenged with evidence pointing to two different disease processes, one self-resolving and the other more complicated, necessitating surgery.

T.N. Anderson, M.D. • F. Moore, M.D. (✉)
J. Jordan, M.D.
University of Florida Academic Health Center, Gainesville, FL 32611, USA
e-mail: Frederick.Moore@surgery.ufl.edu; Jordanja29@gmail.com

Anatomy and Physiology

The appendix is an anti-mesenteric luminal appendage of the cecum extending from the coalescence of the tenia coli. On average, it is 9 cm in length and lies just over the right side of the pelvic brim. This location may be altered in pregnancy or those with visceral malrotation. Within the lamina propria are lymphoid aggregates, similar to Peyer's patches, containing B and T cells [3]. Although the appendix is no longer thought to be simply a vestigial organ, its overall role remains unclear. Some epidemiology studies suggest that the removal of the appendix, whether incidental, due to infection, inflammation, or malignancy, may be protective for developing ulcerative colitis, yet with a slight increased risk of Crohn's and severe *Clostridium difficile* [4].

Epidemiology

Acute appendicitis has been shown to affect 90–100/100,000 inhabitants in developed countries with an overall lifetime risk of 7–8% [4]. There appears to be a slight male predominance, more common in higher socioeconomic groups and less prevalent in non-white groups. There also appears to be geographic differences with higher incidence reported in South Korea (16%)

A. Rodriguez et al. (eds.), *Geriatric Trauma and Acute Care Surgery*, https://doi.org/10.1007/978-3-319-57403-5_35

compared to the USA and Africa (9% and 1.8%, respectively) [4]. Although this is a commonly treated pediatric disease, the peak incidence is found within the second and third decades of life, with the geriatric population making up about 5–10% of these cases [5].

Etiology and Pathogenesis

Despite its overall frequency the pathogenesis of acute appendicitis remains unclear. It has been associated with direct luminal obstruction, infectious etiology, summer months, and possibly genetic factors with a threefold increase in families with a positive history of appendicitis. In addition there appears to be reduced occurrences during pregnancy and in non-whites. For some patients with negative appendectomy, pain may be attributed to neurogenic factors related to excess proliferation of nerve fibers and neuropeptides (Table 35.1) [5–7].

Traditionally, acute appendicitis has been thought to have a linear progression from simple inflammation to frank perforation. However, there is growing evidence that simple and complex appendicitis are distinctly different disease processes with different fates. An inflamed appendix without gangrene or necrosis that *does not proceed to perforation* (reversible) can present as phlegmatous or advanced inflammation. A separate, more complex process involves a severe inflammatory response that will rapidly proceed to gangrene, perforation, or both [4, 6, 7].

Table 35.1 Potential etiologies

• Fecolith	• Ethnicity
• Lymphoid hyperplasia	• Positive family history
• Impacted stool	• Neurogenic
• Malignancy	• Environmental
• Infection (*E. coli*, Bacteroides, Fusobacterium, Chlamydia, Campylobacter)	• Less common in pregnancy

Clinical Characteristics

As with other visceral organs, there are no somatic fibers innervating the appendix making localization of early inflammation challenging. Pain is often described as starting in the periumbilical region and migrating to the right lower quadrant (RLQ) as a result of focal irritation of the peritoneum which does contain somatic pain innervations. Other associated symptoms in addition to pain are anorexia, nausea and/or vomiting, fevers, and leukocytosis. Other accessory physical exam findings include Dunphy's sign, Rovsing's sign, obturator sign, or iliopsoas sign (Table 35.2) [3]. For the elderly population, RLQ pain has been the most consistent finding; however due to socioeconomic factors, dementia, etc., these patients may have a delay in diagnosis. Often, infection in the elderly is associated with delirium or confusion preventing the patient from effectively communicating their symptoms. Therefore, the infectious process may be advanced at the time of diagnosis [5, 8, 9].

In an effort to improve clinical predictability the Alvarado score was developed in 1986. Its utility continues to be evaluated, and there is evidence for its ability to rule out appendicitis [10]. A more recently developed predictive scoring system, the appendicitis inflammation response (AIR) score, is suggested to have improved sensitivity and specificity than the Alvarado system (Table 35.3) [4, 11].

Table 35.2 Physical exam findings

Sign	Description	Significance
Dunphy's	Pain with coughing or movement	Diffuse peritonitis
Iliopsoas	Pain with extension of the right hip	Posterior displacement of appendix to the cecum
Obturator	Pain with internal rotation of the right hip	Inferior displacement of the appendix into the pelvis
Rovsing's	RLQ pain with LLQ palpation	Focal inflammation of the RLQ

Table 35.3 Comparison of Alvarado and AIR score

	Alvarado	AIR
Symptoms		
Nausea and vomiting	1	
Vomiting		1
Anorexia	1	
Migration of pain to the RLQ[a]	1	
Signs	1	
Rebound tenderness		
Light		1
Medium		2
Strong		3
RLQ tenderness	2	1
Temperature >37.5 °C	1	
Temperature >38.5 °C		1
Laboratory test		
Leukocytosis shift	1	
Polymorphonuclear leukocytes		
70–84%		1
≥85%		2
White blood cell count		
>10.0 × 109/L	2	
10.0–14.9 × 109/L		1
≥15.0 × 109/L		2
CRP[b] concentration		
10–49 g/L		1
≥50 g/L		2
Total score	10	12
Low probability	Intermediate probability	High probability
Alvarado score 1–4	Alvarado score 5–6	Alvarado score 7–10
AIR score 0–4	AIR score 5–8	AIR score 9–12

[a]*RLQ* Right lower quadrant
[b]*CRP* C-reactive protein

Diagnosis/Diagnostic Tests

With the advent of more advance imaging modalities, the rate of detection and accuracy of diagnosis have greatly increased.

Transabdominal ultrasound has become less frequently used due to its dependence on amenable body habitus and operator experience. In the optimum setting in adults there is 86% sensitivity and 81% specificity for diagnosing appendicitis assuming that the appendix is visualized [4, 6].

Computed tomography is the imaging modality of choice for evaluating the appendix. There is an approximately 93% sensitivity when detecting inflammatory changes in the appendix. For older populations at increased risk of malignancy, CT may be particularly useful for discovering occult malignancy possibly contributing to the clinical presentation [4].

Magnetic resonance imaging offers a lower radiation risk for patients with better accuracy than US. This can be particularly useful in pregnant patients where risk of radiation exposure can lead to teratogenesis of the fetus [4, 12]. The use of ultrasound in this patient population is also complicated by the displacement of the appendix due to the gravid uterus. The sensitivity and specificity of MRI have been found to be equivalent to CT, but may incur an increased cost [12].

For women, the differential diagnosis of right lower quadrant pain expands significantly and may confuse the diagnosis of appendicitis. It is often necessary to evaluate for a gynecological pathology concurrently. Transvaginal US may be useful for evaluating the adnexa for painful cystic disease or pelvic inflammatory disease, which may cause pathologic and radiographic changes in the vicinity of the appendix [4].

As useful as imagery may be, neither CT nor MRI can reliably predict whether the inflammation of the appendix (early) will develop into a complex or perforated disease process or remain simple or phlegmatous. Laboratory findings that suggest a low probability of appendicitis include creatinine-reactive protein (CRP) <60, white blood cell count (WBC) <12, and age <60. The presence of an appendicolith noted by imaging may influence the decision for removal due to the increased propensity for luminal obstruction [4–6].

Treatment

Traditionally, surgical removal is the cornerstone of treatment of appendicitis. The open approach remains the standard procedure. However with the advent and increasing utilization of laparoscopy, this method for many institutions is the procedure of choice. This approach is particularly useful in children and the obese population; however some studies have suggested a slightly higher risk of fetal loss compared to the open procedure in the pregnant population. Other techniques described including the single-incision approach and natural orifice (transvaginal and transgastric) have yet to demonstrate significant improvement over laparoscopic or open approach [3, 4, 13, 14].

Accurate data regarding spontaneous resolution of appendicitis is unclear, although it is estimated that 1 in 13 patients will resolve without antibiotics or resection [15, 16].

There has been growing interest in nonoperative management for uncomplicated appendicitis. In a recent study evaluating the treatment of acute appendicitis with antibiotics for patients deemed poor surgical candidates showed a 5.9% had treatment failure, 4.4% recurrence rate, and 3% complication rate [17]. This data suggests that appendicitis may resolve in 85% of patients without requiring surgical resection with an acceptably low recurrence and complication rate. Additional studies have likewise been conducted randomizing patients to resection vs. medical management and have found similar results [4, 6, 7, 14, 16]. The duration of intravenous antibiotics, overall course of antibiotics, and specific antibiotic regimen have yet to be defined. However, our institution is currently investigating the regimen of a 3-day course of IV gram negative and anaerobic coverage and PO antibiotics for a total therapy duration of 7 days. An additional noted benefit of this modality of treatment has been a reduction in hospital cost averaging $1800 less than surgical intervention, at the expense of slightly increased hospital length of stay [14].

Perforation with abscess occurs in 3–8% of patients on presentation. Percutaneous drainage is the preferred initial treatment. Immediate surgery is associated with a threefold increased risk of morbidity, by way of injury to adjacent organs [4]. Following drainage of the abscess, the recurrence rate of appendicitis is 4–7%. Interval appendectomy approximately 6 weeks following treatment has been utilized. However, the absolute necessity for interval appendectomy has also been challenged given this low rate of recurrent inflammation [4]. Additionally, recurrence with subsequent perforation is also significantly low. Some data suggest that interval appendectomy is not an absolute requirement and may be determined by the presence of recurrent symptoms [17].

Prognosis

Overall prognosis with treatment of acute appendicitis is excellent. Even with perforated appendicitis with sepsis, the expected mortality is 0.09–0.24% in developed health systems. This increases roughly to 1–4% in low- and middle-income countries. In 1–2% of patients presenting with appendicitis, malignancy has been found within the appendix including neuroendocrine (carcinoid), adenocarcinoma, and mucinous cystadenoma [4]. Appropriate follow-up may entail colonoscopy and/or repeat imaging.

Conclusion

Appendicitis is one of the most common pathologies of the abdomen. Surgery continues to be the mainstay of treatment. However there is growing enthusiasm for nonoperative management. The likelihood of presenting with a subsequent episode of perforated appendicitis following initial nonsurgical management may be sufficiently low to question the perceived risks associated with nonoperative management of uncomplicated appendicitis. There is apparent financial incentive for nonoperative management. In the context of the elderly it is important to recognize that this patient population often present atypically related to socioeconomic factors (i.e., transportation and communication difficulties) or age-related physiologic changes such as dementia or delirium. A high index of suspicion and early utilization of computed tomography have been found to be most effective at reducing morbidity and mortality. And for the particularly medically complex patient, poorly suited for surgery, antibiotics should be considered when treating acute appendicitis.

References

1. Fitz RH. Perforating inflammation of the vermiform appendix with special reference to its early diagnosis and treatment. Trans Assoc Am Phys. 1886;1:107–44.
2. McBurney C. Experience with early operative interference in cases of disease of the vermiform appendix. N Y Med J. 1889;50:676–84.
3. Mathews JB, Hodin RA. Acute abdomen and appendicitis. In: Mulholland MW, et al., editors. Greenfield's surgery: scientific principles and practice, vol. 1. 5th ed. Philadelphia: Lippincott Williams & Wilkins; 2011. p. 1199–211.
4. Bhangu A, Soreide K, Di Saverio S, Assarsson J, Drake F. Acute appendicitis: modern understanding of pathogenesis, diagnosis, and management. Lancet. 2015;386:1278–87.
5. Omari A, Khammash M, Qasaimeh G, Shammari A, Yaseen M, Hammori S. Acute appendicitis in the elderly: risk factors for perforation. World J Emerg Surg. 2014;9:6.
6. Livingston EH, Woodward WA, Sarosi GA, Haley RW. Disconnect between incidence of nonperforated and perforated appendicitis: implications for pathophysiology and management. Ann Surg. 2007;245:886–92.
7. Livingston E, Fomby T, Woodward W, Haley R. Epidemiological similarities between appendicitis and diverticulitis suggesting a common underlying pathogenesis. Arch Surg. 2011;146(3):308–14.
8. Lunca S, Bouras G, Romedea NS. Acute appendicitis in the elderly patient: diagnostic problems, prognostic factors and out-comes. Rom J Gastroenterol. 2004;13:299–303.
9. Nasa P, Juneja D, Singh O. Severe sepsis and septic shock in the elderly: an overview. World J Crit Care Med. 2012;1(1):23–30.
10. Ohle R, O'Reilly F, O'Brien KK, Fahey T, Dimitrov BD. The Alvarado score for predicting acute appendicitis: a systematic review. BMC Med. 2011;9:139.
11. de Castro SMM, Ünlü Ç, Steller E, van Wagensveld BA, Vrouenraets BC. Evaluation of the appendicitis inflammatory response score for patients with acute appendicitis. World J Surg. 2012;36(7):1540–5.
12. Repplinger MD, Levy JF, Peethumnoongsin E, Gussick ME, Svenson JE, Golden SK, Ehlenbach WJ, Westergaard RP, Reeder SB, Vanness DJ. Systemic review and meta-analysis of the accuracy of MRI to diagnose appendicitis in the general population. J Magn Reson Imaging. 2016;43(6):1346–54.
13. Madore J, Collins C, Ayturk MD, Santry H. The impact of acute care surgery on appendicitis outcomes: results from a national sample of university-affiliated hospitals. J Trauma Acute Care Surg. 2015;79:282–8.
14. Wu J, Dawes A, Sacks G, Brunicardi FC, Keeler E. Cost effectiveness of nonoperative management versus laparoscopic appenedectomy for acute uncomplicated appendicitis. Surgery. 2015;158:712–21.
15. Cobben LP, de Van Otterloo AM, Puylaert JB. Spontaneously resolving appendicitis: frequency and natural history in 60 patients. Radiology. 2000;215(2):349–52.
16. Salminen P, Paajanen H, Rautio T, et al. Antibiotic therapy vs appendectomy for treatment of uncomplicated acute appendicitis: the APPAC randomized clinical trial. JAMA. 2015;313:2340–8.
17. McCutcheon BA, Chang DC, Marcus LP, Inui T, Noorbakhsh A, Schallhorn C, et al. Long-term outcomes of patients with nonsurgically managed uncomplicated appendicitis. J Am Coll Surg. 2014;218:905–13.

Part XV

Critical Care

36 Critical Care: Pulmonary

Nicole L. Werner and Lena M. Napolitano

Pulmonary Function in the Geriatric Patient

Geriatric patients have age-related decreased pulmonary function that predisposes them to a higher risk of pulmonary complications post-injury and after emergent surgery [1]. These changes include decreased pulmonary compliance, "senile emphysema," mucociliary dysfunction, sarcopenia-induced reduction in intercostal and diaphragmatic function, and increased pulmonary vascular resistance. Specific changes that make weaning from mechanical ventilation difficult in the geriatric patient include decreased diffusion capacity, increased dead space ventilation, reduced respiratory drive (significant reduced response to hypoxemia and hypercapnia), and a higher prevalence of central sleep apnea among elderly patients.

N.L. Werner, M.D., M.S.
L.M. Napolitano, M.D. (✉)
Division of Acute Care Surgery (Trauma, Burns, Surgical Critical Care, Emergency Surgery), Department of Surgery, University of Michigan, Ann Arbor, MI 48109-0033, USA
e-mail: lenan@umich.edu

Pulmonary Issues in Geriatric Trauma and Acute Care Surgery

Pulmonary complications [atelectasis, pneumonia, pulmonary edema, COPD exacerbation, acute respiratory failure, acute respiratory distress syndrome (ARDS)] in the post-injury and postoperative period are a significant cause of morbidity and mortality. Risk factors for postoperative pulmonary complications include (1) *patient-related* and (2) *procedure-related* risk factors (Table 36.1). Among patient-related risk factors, advanced age is the leading risk factor. Smoking and sleep apnea are also significant predictors of postoperative pulmonary complications [2, 3]. The major procedure-related risk

Table 36.1 Patient-related risk factors for pulmonary complications

Pulmonary	Nonpulmonary
Smoking	Age
Chronic obstructive pulmonary disease	General health status
Asthma	Obesity
Interstitial lung disease	Obstructive sleep apnea
Upper respiratory infection	Pulmonary hypertension
	Heart failure
	Nutritional status
	Dependent functional status
	Neurologic impairment

A. Rodriguez et al. (eds.), *Geriatric Trauma and Acute Care Surgery*,
https://doi.org/10.1007/978-3-319-57403-5_36

factors (emergent surgery, major abdominal/vascular or thoracic surgery) confer higher risk for pulmonary complications than that of patient-related risk factors. Emergency surgery was associated with a greater than twofold increased risk of pulmonary complications.

A number of risk indices can be used to provide a numerical estimate of risk of pulmonary complications, including the Arozullah Respiratory Failure Index [4] (Table 36.2), the ARISCAT (Canet) Risk Index [5] (Table 36.3), and the Gupta Calculator for Postoperative Respiratory Failure [6] or Postoperative Pneumonia [7]. All of these risk indices include advanced age as a significant risk factor for pulmonary complications.

Table 36.2 Arozullah Respiratory Failure Index

Preoperative predictor	Point value
Type of surgery	
Abdominal aortic aneurysm	27
Thoracic	21
Neurosurgery, upper abdominal, peripheral vascular	14
Neck	11
Emergency surgery	11
Albumin <3.0 g/dL	9
BUN >30 mg/dL	8
Partially or fully dependent functional status	7
History of chronic obstructive pulmonary disease	6
Age (years)	
>70	6
60–69	4

Performance of the Arozullah Respiratory Failure Index

Class	*Point total*	*Percent respiratory failure*
1	≤10	0.5
2	11–19	1.8
3	20–27	4.2
4	28–40	10.1
5	>40	26.6

Adapted from Arozullah AM, Daley J, Henderson WG, et al. Multifactorial risk index for predicting postoperative respiratory failure in men after major noncardiac surgery. Ann Surg 2000;232(2):250

Table 36.3 The ARISCAT risk index includes seven independent risk factors of any severity that predict postoperative pulmonary complication rates

Factor	Adjusted odds ratio (95% CI)	Risk score
Age (years)		
≤50	1	–
51–80	1.4 (0.6–3.3)	3
>80	5.1 (1.9–13.3)	16
Preoperative oxygen saturation (%)		
≥96	1	–
91–95	2.2 (1.2–4.2)	8
≤90	10.7 (4.1–28.1)	24
Respiratory infection in the last month	5.5 (2.6–11.5)	17
Preoperative anemia (hemoglobin ≤10 g/dL)	3.0 (1.4–6.5)	11
Surgical incision		
Upper abdominal	4.4 (2.3–8.5)	15
Intrathoracic	11.4 (1.9–26.0)	24
Duration of surgery (h)		
≤2	1	
2–3	4.9 (2.4–10.1)	16
>3	9.7 (2.4–19.9)	23
Emergency surgery	2.2 (1.0–4.5)	8
Performance of the ARISCAT pulmonary risk index		
Risk class	*Number of points in risk score*	*Postoperative pulmonary complication rate (%)*
Low	<26	1.6
Intermediate	26–44	13.3
High	≥45	42.1

Each factor is assigned a weighted score and patients are stratified as low, intermediate, and high risk for developing pulmonary complications

Adapted from Canet J, Gallart L, Gomar C, et al. Prediction of postoperative pulmonary complications in a population-based surgical cohort. Anesthesiology 2010;113:1338

Prevention of Pulmonary Complications

Given the increased morbidity and mortality associated with pulmonary complications, all efforts to prevent these complications should be

Table 36.4 Strength of the evidence for specific interventions to reduce the risk for postoperative pulmonary complications

Risk reduction strategy	Strength of evidence[a]	Type of complication studied
Postoperative lung expansion modalities	A	Atelectasis, pneumonia, bronchitis, severe hypoxemia
Selective postoperative nasogastric decompression	B	Atelectasis, pneumonia, aspiration
Short-acting neuromuscular blockade	B	Atelectasis, pneumonia
Laparoscopic (vs. open) operation	C	Spirometry, atelectasis, pneumonia, overall respiratory complications
Smoking cessation	I	Postoperative ventilator support
Intraoperative neuraxial blockade	I	Pneumonia, postoperative hypoxia, respiratory failure
Postoperative epidural analgesia	I	Atelectasis, pneumonia, respiratory failure
Immunonutrition	I	Overall infectious complications, pneumonia, respiratory failure
Routine total parenteral or enteral nutrition[b]	D	Atelectasis, pneumonia, empyema, respiratory failure
Right-heart catheterization	D	Pneumonia

From Lawrence VA, Cornell JE, Smetana GW. Strategies to reduce postoperative pulmonary complications after noncardiothoracic surgery: Systematic review for the American College of Physicians. Ann Intern Med 2006;144:596–608

[a]Definitions for categories of strength of evidence, modified from the U.S. Preventive Services Task Force categories (II). A = good evidence that the strategy reduces postoperative pulmonary complications and benefit outweighs harm; B = at least fair evidence that the strategy reduces postoperative pulmonary complications and benefit outweighs harm; C = at least fair evidence that the strategy may reduce postoperative pulmonary complications, but the balance between benefit and harm is too close to justify a general recommendation; D = at least fair evidence that the strategy does not reduce postoperative pulmonary complications or harm outweighs benefit; I = evidence of effectiveness of the strategy to reduce postoperative pulmonary complications is conflicting, of poor quality, lacking, or insufficient or the balance between benefit and harm cannot be determined

[b]Evidence remains uncertain (strength of evidence I) on total parenteral or enteral nutrition for severely malnourished patients or when a protracted time of inadequate nutritional intake is anticipated

implemented. A systematic review of strategies to reduce postoperative pulmonary complications after noncardiothoracic surgery identified that few interventions have been shown to definitively reduce postoperative pulmonary complications (Table 36.4) [8, 9]. Postoperative strategies to prevent pneumonia focus on increasing lung volume, pulmonary toilet, pain control, and preventing aspiration. Lung expansion interventions via incentive spirometry (although widely used) have not shown definitive benefit in reducing postoperative pulmonary complications [10]. The use of nasal continuous positive airway pressure (nCPAP) may be of benefit [11]. For CPAP, the danger of gastric distention in patients with abdominal surgery is one prohibitive factor to take into consideration. Selective, rather than routine, use of nasogastric tubes is recommended to reduce postoperative pulmonary complications [12].

Pneumonia

Postoperative pneumonia incidence varies dependent on risk factors, ranging from an incidence of 1.5% to as high as 15.3% in high-risk groups [13, 14]. Postoperative pneumonia was significantly more common in patients undergoing emergent vs. elective surgery (11.1% vs. 2.9%) [15]. In 2005, the ATS/IDSA provided guidelines to further categorize pneumonia into hospital-acquired pneumonia (HAP), ventilator-associated pneumonia (VAP), and healthcare-associated pneumonia (HCAP) [16].

Pathophysiology

Under normal circumstances, the lower respiratory tract is sterile. Both HAP and VAP are generally associated with introduction of bacteria to the sterile lower respiratory tract. This can be exacerbated by impaired host defenses. The introduction of bacteria to the lower airways occurs by two important mechanisms: bacterial colonization of the aero-digestive tract and aspiration of contaminated secretions into the lower airway (Fig. 36.1). A variety of factors promote these mechanisms including presence of invasive devices, medications altering gastric emptying and pH, contaminated water, medications, and respiratory therapy equipment.

Diagnosis and Definitions

Pneumonia is an acute infection of the pulmonary parenchyma. It is important to distinguish between community- and hospital-acquired pneumonia, since the causative pathogens are different. In the post-injury and postoperative period, hospital-acquired pneumonia (HAP) is defined as pneumonia occurring >48 h after hospital admission. Ventilator-associated pneumonia (VAP) is a type of HAP that develops more than 48 h after endotracheal intubation. Healthcare-associated pneumonia (HCAP) is pneumonia that occurs in a patient with healthcare contact (Table 36.5) [3].

The diagnosis of pneumonia is difficult because the clinical findings are nonspecific,

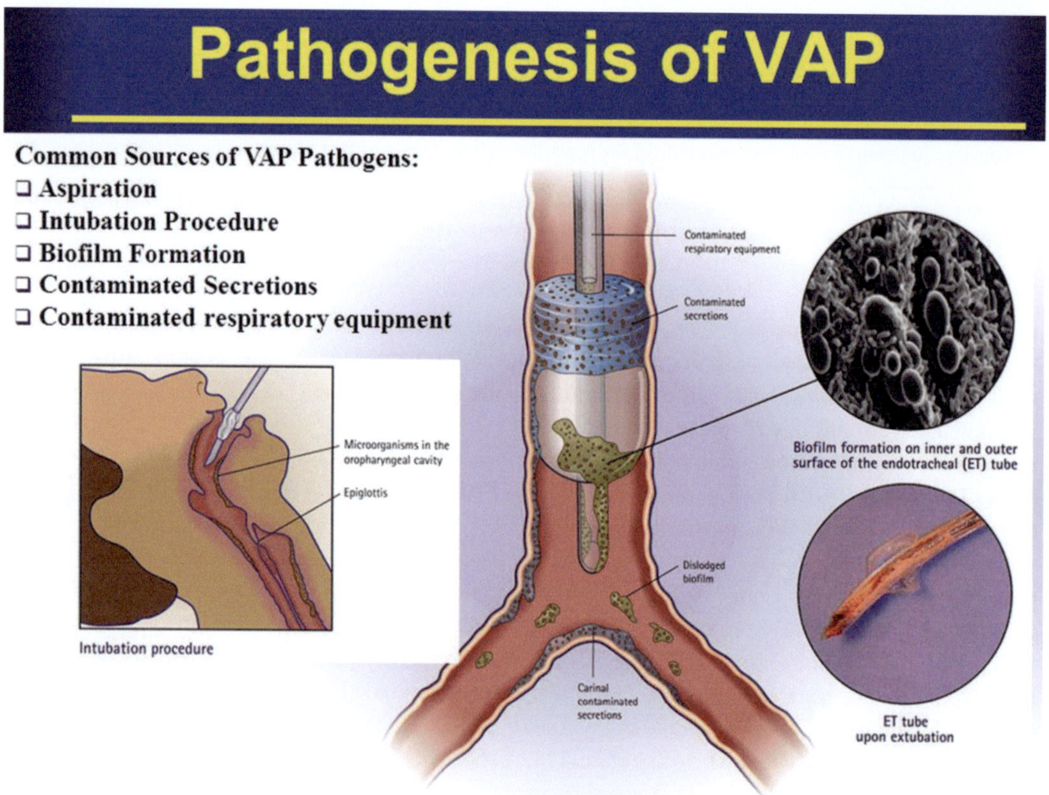

Fig. 36.1 Pathogenesis of ventilator-associated penumonia (VAP). Adapted from American Thoracic Society. Guidelines for the management of adults with hospital-acquired, ventilator-associated, and healthcare-associated pneumonia. Am J Respir Crit Care Med 2005; 171 (4): 388–416

Table 36.5 Risk factors for multidrug-resistant pathogens causing HAP, HCAP, and VAP

• Antimicrobial therapy in preceding 90 d
• Current hospitalization of 5d or more
• High frequency of antibiotic resistance in the community or in the specific hospital unit
• Presence of risk factors for HCAP
– Hospitalization for 2d or more in the preceding 90d
– Residence in a nursing home or extended-care facility
– Home infusion therapy (including antibiotics)
– Chronic dialysis within 30d
– Home wound care
– Family member with multidrug-resistant pathogen
• Immunosuppressive disease and/or therapy

Adapted from American Thoracic Society. Guidelines for the management of adults with hospital-acquired, ventilator-associated, and healthcare-associated pneumonia. Am J Respir Crit Care Med 2005; 171 (4): 388–416

including new or progressive infiltrate on chest radiograph and clinical characteristics (fever, purulent sputum, leukocytosis and hypoxia) [3]. When findings at autopsy are used as a reference, the combination of radiographic infiltrate plus two out of three clinical features (fever >38 °C, leukocytosis/leukopenia, purulent secretions) resulted in 69% sensitivity and 75% specificity for pneumonia [17].

The diagnosis of VAP is suspected when a patient on mechanical ventilation develops new pulmonary infiltrate with fever, leukocytosis, and purulent secretions. Further signs of increased ventilator support or oxygen requirements also raise this suspicion. However, the differential diagnosis for these findings can be broad (atelectasis, ARDS, chemical pneumonitis, contusion, pulmonary embolism, drug reaction, infiltrative tumor) [18]. Frequently radiographic and clinical abnormalities occur in patients without a true diagnosis of VAP. Only 43% of patients with radiographic evidence were found to have VAP by postmortem examination [19].

Currently, the CDC defines VAP using a combination of radiological, clinical, and laboratory criteria, in patients who are ventilated for greater than 48 h. Pneumonia is characterized into three types including clinically defined (PNEU-1); common bacterial, fungal, or atypical pneumonia (PNEU-2); and pneumonia in immunocompromised patients (PNEU-3) [20].

It has been documented that VAP rates in trauma patients are markedly different dependent on the specific definition used, since CDC and NHSN definitions are different than VAP criteria for the National Trauma Data Bank (NTDB) [21]. It has been identified that trauma factors play a critical role in VAP etiology, as rib fractures, pulmonary contusion, and failed prehospital intubation were significant predictors of VAP in a multivariate model [22].

Diagnostic testing is helpful when VAP is suspected because radiologic and clinical findings are nonspecific. Thus it is recommended that all patients with possible VAP undergo lower respiratory tract sampling with microscopic evaluation and culture. This can be done using bronchoscopic sampling of the lower respiratory tract (bronchoalveolar lavage, BAL) or without the use of a bronchoscope (mini-BAL) with similar safety and diagnostic accuracy [23]. In patients with left lower lobe infiltrates and possible VAP, bronchoscopic BAL is preferred in order to obtain a sample from the left lung, since mini-BAL sampling catheters most commonly advance into the right lower lobe bronchus. Bronchoscopic sampling is not associated with improved mortality, or reduced duration of ventilation, ICU, or hospital length of stay. However, it does influence antibiotic selection and de-escalation of antibiotics [24]. Given the severity of VAP and the frequency of serious conditions that can mimic VAP, additional tests that provide further evidence for VAP are clearly warranted [25]. At present, no sensitive and specific biomarker is currently available to confirm a diagnosis of VAP [26–32].

Ventilator-Associated Event (VAE) Surveillance Definitions

In 2011, the CDC convened a working group to address the limitations of the NHSN PNEU definitions and propose a new approach to surveillance for VAEs. The VAE surveillance definition algorithm (Fig. 36.2) was implemented by NHSN in 1/2013 and is based on objective, streamlined, and potentially automatable criteria that identify a broad

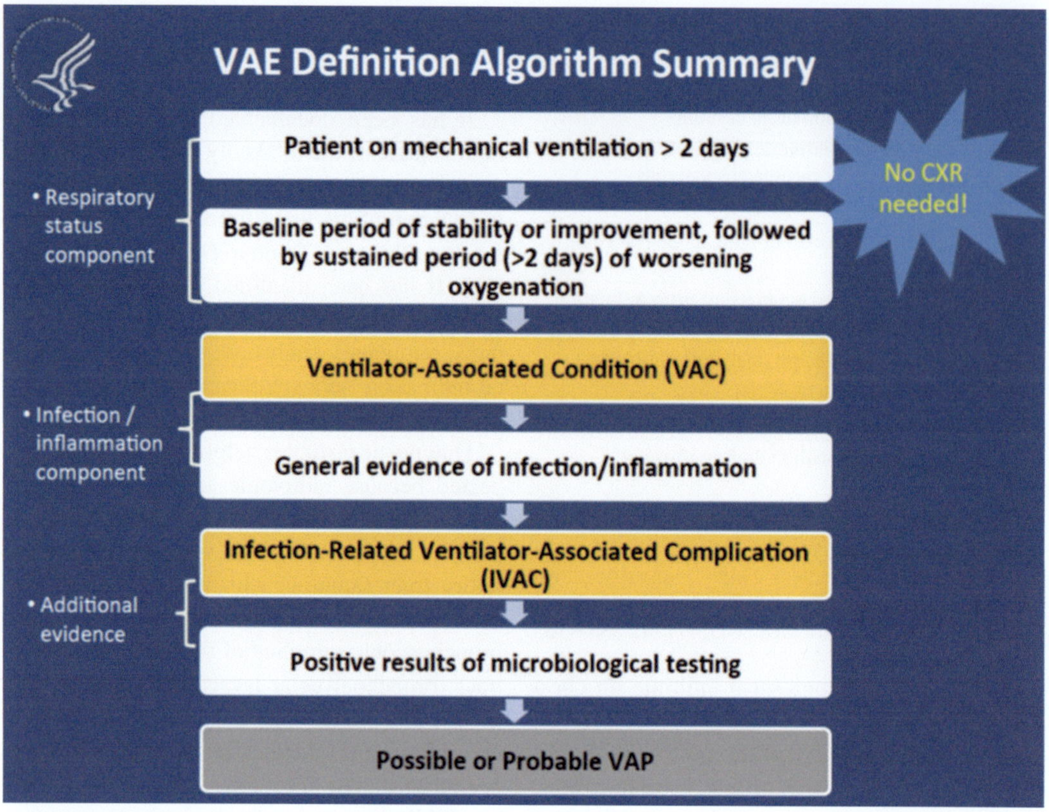

Fig. 36.2 Ventilator-associated event (VAE) CDC Definition Algorithm Summary-2016. *Adapted from* http://www.cdc.gov/nhsn/PDFs/pscManual/10-VAE_FINAL.pdf

range of conditions and complications which occur in mechanically ventilated adult patients. The VAE definition algorithm is for use in surveillance, and is not a clinical definition and is not intended for use in the clinical management of patients [33].

Treatment

When VAP is suspected based on clinical and radiographic findings, it is important first to obtain lower respiratory tract samples for cultures. Early empiric antimicrobial therapy for VAP is then initiated. Following this, in the next 48 h, an assessment of clinical response and cultures should be performed. If there is clinical improvement and culture results are negative, consider stopping antibiotics. If culture results are positive, consider de-escalating or narrowing the antibiotics. If there is no clinical response, consider searching for other causes.

The initiation of early, appropriate empiric broad-spectrum antibiotics to treat HAP, VAP, or HCAP significantly improves patient survival [3, 34, 35]. The three leading VAP pathogens are *S. aureus* (24.4% of all isolates, 54.4% as MRSA), *Pseudomonas aeruginosa*, and *Acinetobacter baumannii*. Inadequate antibiotic therapy is a strong predictor of death in VAP patients, irrespective of underlying disease state and severity of illness [36–40]. The choice of empiric antibiotics should be based on local antibiograms (particularly in surgical ICUs) [3] and on patient risk factors for MDR bacteria (Table 36.5).

Duration of Antibiotics for Pneumonia

A landmark multicenter RCT compared 8 vs. 15 days of antibiotic treatment in 401 patients in 51 ICUs [41]. No difference in 30-day mortality was identified (18.8% vs. 17.2%) and no differences in ventilator-free days, organ failure-free days, length of ICU stay, and 60-day mortality were identified. However there was a higher recurrence of infection rate for nonfermenting gram-negative bacilli, including *Pseudomonas aeruginosa*, and more MDR pathogens appeared in the 15-day treatment group (42% vs. 62%, $p = 0.038$). Based on the results of this study, optimal duration of therapy for VAP should be 8 days, except in those isolates that are nonfermenting gram-negative bacilli, including *Pseudomonas aeruginosa* and *acinetobacter* species where longer duration of antimicrobial therapy is recommended.

HAP/VAP Prevention

Aggressive HAP prevention efforts in surgical patients are successful in reducing postoperative pneumonia [42]. Reports from the U.S. National Healthcare Safety Network (NHSN) have documented a recent decline in VAP rates related to the implementation of prevention strategies. However, the highest rates of VAP remain in surgical ICUs, particularly in burn and trauma ICUs [43]. HAP/VAP preventive strategies are therefore very important to implement in all post-injury and postsurgical patients, and should particularly be used in geriatric patients.

The development of VAP is related to (1) bacterial colonization of the aero-digestive tract or (2) aspiration of contaminated secretions into the lower airway. The strategies to prevent infection are therefore aimed at (1) reducing bacterial colonization and (2) decreasing aspiration incidence. Decreasing aspiration incidence can be achieved through improved positioning, increased HOB elevation, and use of specialty endotracheal tubes that aspirate subglottic secretions. Bacterial colonization can be reduced by minimizing the days on mechanical ventilation through weaning protocols, use of chlorhexidine in the posterior pharynx, and silver-coated endotracheal tubes. Clinical guidelines for VAP prevention review all evidence-based strategies for VAP prevention [44]. Ventilator bundles are used as an effective method to reduce VAP rates in the intensive care unit (Table 36.6) [45, 46].

Table 36.6 Measures to include in VAP prevention bundle

Process measures	Structural measures
1. Head of bed elevation: use of a semirecumbent position (≥30°)	1. Use a closed endotracheal tube suctioning system
2. SATs and SBTs: make a daily assessment of readiness to wean with the use of the SAT and SBT	2. Change close suctioning catheters only as needed
3. Oral care: at least 6 times per day	3. Change ventilator circuits only if damaged or soiled
4. Oral care with chlorhexidine: 2 times per day	4. Change heat and moisture exchanger every 5–7 days and as clinically indicated
5. Subglottic suctioning: use subglottic suctioning in patients expected to be MV for >72 h	5. Provide easy access to noninvasive ventilation equipment and institute protocols to promote use
	6. Periodically remove the condensate from circuits, keeping the circuit closed during the removal, taking precautions not to allow condensate to drain toward patient
	7. Use an early mobility protocol
	8. Perform hand hygiene
	9. Avoid supine position
	10. Use standard precautions while suctioning respiratory tract secretions
	11. Use orotracheal intubation instead of nasotracheal
	12. Avoid use of prophylactic systemic antimicrobials
	13. Avoid nonessential tracheal suctioning
	14. Avoid gastric overdistention

MV mechanical ventilation, *SAT* spontaneous awakening trial, *SBT* spontaneous breathing trial
From Speck K, Rawat N, Weiner NC, Tujuba HG, Farley D, Berenholtz S. A systematic approach for developing a ventilator-associated pneumonia prevention bundle. Am J Infect Control. 2016 Jun 1;44(6):652–6

Noninvasive Ventilation

The foremost strategy for VAP prevention is to avoid intubation or reduce time of duration of mechanical ventilation. Noninvasive ventilation should therefore be considered where evidence exists to support its use, in COPD and pulmonary edema exacerbations, for acute respiratory failure following upper abdominal surgery, and as a weaning strategy for intubated adults with respiratory failure [47–51].

Spontaneous Awakening and Breathing Trials (SAT/SBT)

Prolonged mechanical ventilation is a risk factor for VAP (1–3% increased VAP risk with each day of mechanical ventilation) [52]. The use of a weaning protocol, a sedation protocol, or both has been shown to reduce the duration of mechanical ventilation [53] and is associated with lower ventilator-associated events (VAE) [54]. Routine use of SAT and SBT is now standard in all ventilated patients.

Semirecumbent Position

The semirecumbent (≥30°) position in mechanically ventilated patients has been associated with a reduced incidence of VAP [55]. Supine position and mechanical ventilation >7 days were independent VAP risk factors. Other studies have not confirmed this finding, but compliance with the target semirecumbent position was not reached in these studies [56–58].

Specialized Endotracheal Tubes

CASS Tubes

A number of randomized trials have shown a decreased rate of VAP in patients with CASS (continuous aspiration of subglottic secretions) tubes. A meta-analysis of ten RCTs with 2213 patients showed significantly reduced incidence of VAP (RR 0.56, 95% CI 0.45–0.69, $p < 0.00001$) and early-onset VAP (RR = 0.23, 95% CI: 0.13–0.43, $p < 0.00001$), shortened ventilation duration by 1.55 days (95% CI: −2.40 to −0.71 days, $p = 0.0003$), and prolonged time to VAP by 3.90 days (95% CI: 2.56–5.24 days). No significant differences were observed regarding incidence of late-onset VAP, overall mortality, or length of intensive care unit or hospital stay [59].

Silver-Coated Tube

Silver-coated endotracheal tubes aim to prevent biofilm formation, delay airway colonization, and reduce bacterial burden due to bactericidal activity. The NASCENT RCT (2003 patients) reported that use of the silver-coated endotracheal tube was associated with a significant VAP (defined as BAL >10^4 CFU/mL) reduction (4.8% vs. 7.5%; 36% relative risk reduction) and was associated with a significant delay in time to VAP [60]. Other trials have confirmed this benefit [61].

Chlorhexidine Gluconate

One strategy to reduce bacterial colonization is to use oral chlorhexidine gluconate (0.12%). One trial in cardiac surgical patients documented a significant decrease in the incidence of nosocomial pneumonia and mortality [62]. A meta-analysis of similar trials concluded that oral chlorhexidine in mechanically ventilated ICU patients was associated with a 40% reduction in VAP [63].

Selective Decontamination (SDD/SOD)

Selective decontamination of the digestive tract (SDD) and oropharynx (SOD) is a strategy aimed at preventing airway colonization. Several studies have shown modest benefit in pneumonia rate and mortality [64–66]. However, this has not been used widely in the United States due to significant concern regarding potential emergence of MDR bacteria [67].

Tracheostomy

A number of large RCTs have found no difference in mortality, VAP, or other outcome measures comparing early (4–8 days) vs. late (10–15 days) tracheostomy [68, 69]. Thus, early tracheostomy should not be performed for VAP prevention or survival benefit, but may be considered for other reasons, such as patient comfort and airway protection, as in patients with severe traumatic brain injury.

Acute Respiratory Failure

Acute respiratory failure can be due to loss of airway protection, failure to oxygenate (hypoxemic respiratory failure, type I), or failure to ventilate (hypercapnia respiratory failure, type 2) (Fig. 36.3). Initial assessment of the airway is first priority. Several risk factors common in geriatric patients contribute to loss of airway including neurological impairment, absent cough/gag reflex, aspiration events, or laryngeal edema. For these reasons, close attention must be paid to elderly patients, those with head trauma, and patients that have had airway procedures. A single event of aspiration in this setting can be disastrous and often is fatal.

Hypoxic respiratory failure (type 1) is defined by a $PaO_2 < 60$ mmHg. Hypocapnia can often accompany hypoxia because of increased ventilatory drive. Hypoxic respiratory failure is more common, with the underlying problem at the pulmonary capillary-alveolar interface (either fluid filling or collapse of alveolar units) resulting in diffusion defects or ventilation perfusion mismatch. Diffusion defects can be caused by fluid accumulation in the extracellular space leading to pulmonary edema which leads to impaired oxygenation. There are two spectrums in ventilation/perfusion mismatch: (1) dead-space ventilation (alveoli get ventilation but no perfusion, i.e., pulmonary embolism) and (2) shunt (alveoli get perfusion, but no ventilation). Hypoxic respiratory failure can also be caused by inability to extract oxygen at a cellular level (carbon monoxide or cyanide poisoning and sepsis).

Hypercapneic respiratory failure (type 2) is defined by a $PaCO_2 > 50$ mmHg. Hypoxemia can be common in these patients, because elevated alveolar CO_2 can displace alveolar O_2. Determination of the causative etiology of type 2 respiratory failure requires a careful systematic assessment from the brain to the lung. A central loss of ventilation can be due to sedation, narcotic overdose, stroke, or medication. Spinal cord procedures or traumatic injuries can result in loss of diaphragm or accessory chest wall muscle use. Thoracic trauma (rib fractures, flail chest, pneumothorax, hemothorax, pleural effusions) can impair ventilation. The airway should be evaluated for distal obstruction (right main-stem intubation, foreign object, mucous plug). Issues with gas exchange or V/Q mismatch at the alveolar level can also cause hyperventilation (atelectasis, pneumonia, contusion, ARDS).

Faced with a patient in acute hypoxemic respiratory failure, a brief period of noninvasive ventilation [70] or high-flow oxygen via nasal cannula should be considered if there is a promptly reversible cause of the acute respiratory failure. A recent study documented that treatment with high-flow oxygen via nasal cannula was associated with reduced 90-day mortality but no difference in intubation rates (38% for high-flow nasal) compared with standard face mask oxygen (47%) or noninvasive positive-pressure ventilation (50%) [71]. Many patients with severe acute respiratory failure (hypoxemic or hypercapneic) require early intubation and initiation of mechanical ventilation. All patients with signs and symptoms of acute respiratory failure must be monitored and treated in an intensive care unit.

One-year mortality of critically ill patients treated with prolonged mechanical ventilation (>14 days) was 62% and only 50% were successfully liberated from mechanical ventilation [72]. Additional studies document that elderly patients treated with mechanical ventilation did not have worse outcomes than younger patients, suggesting that mechanical ventilation should not be restricted in elderly patients with respiratory failure on the basis of chronologic age [73, 74].

Mode of Mechanical Ventilation

There is currently no evidence to support one mode (volume vs. pressure, Table 36.7) of mechanical ventilation for patients with acute respiratory failure [75]. All efforts to reduce ventilator-induced lung injury should be implemented in all ventilator modes used. Early transition to spontaneous ventilation (pressure support, proportional assist, adaptive support) should be encouraged to avoid diaphragm and intercostal muscle weakness and prevent ventilator dyssynchrony, especially in geriatric

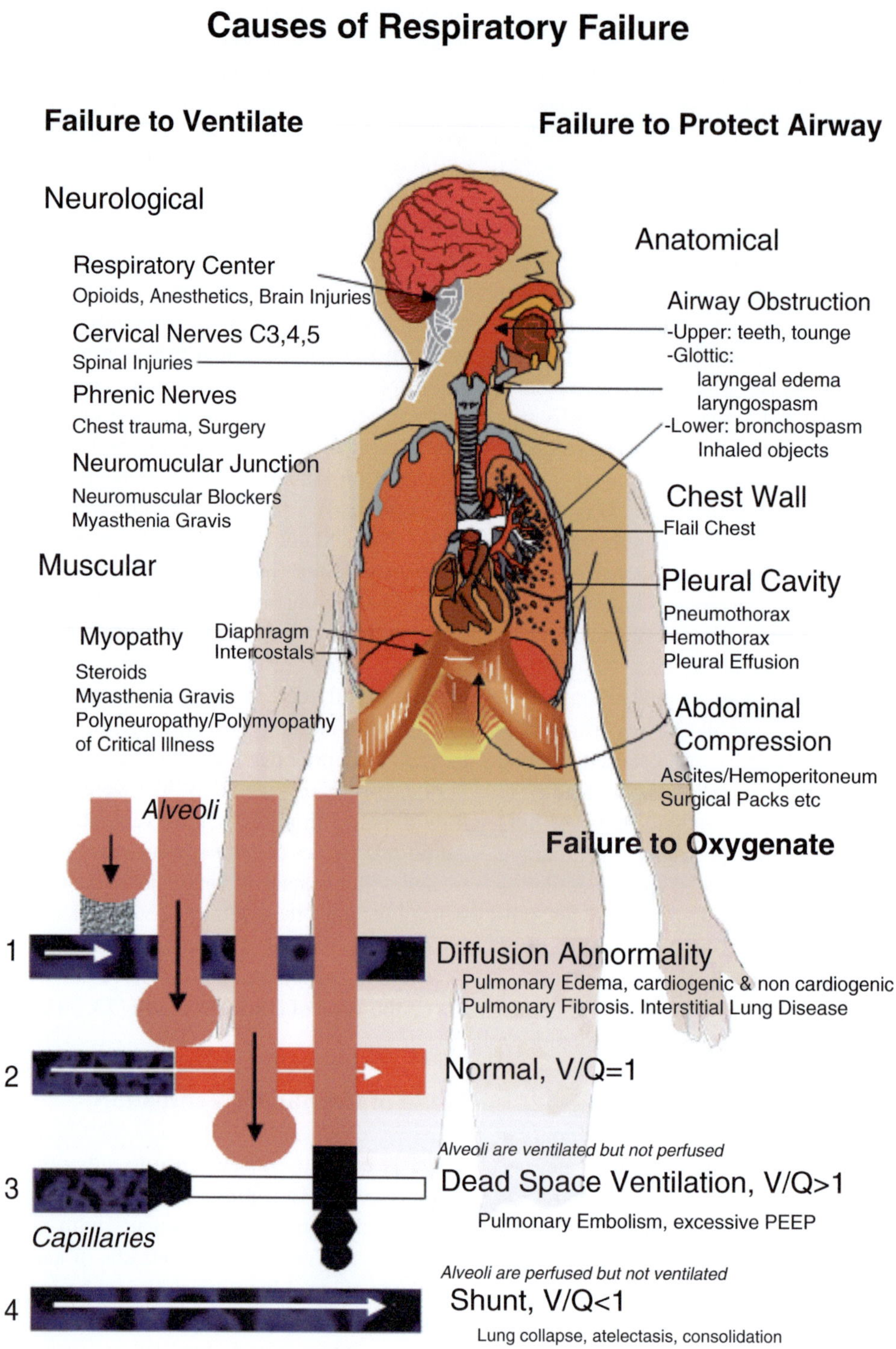

Fig. 36.3 Causes of acute respiratory failure

Table 36.7 Ventilator settings and changes in modes of mechanical ventilation (volume vs. pressure)

	Volume (assist control)	Pressure (pressure control)
Minute ventilation	VT × RR	VT delivered by set pressure × RR
Flow	Constant	Variable with changes in compliance and resistance
Inspiratory time	Constant	Constant
Decreased compliance	Volume constant, PIP increases	Pressure constant, VT decreases
Increased resistance	Volume constant, PIP increases	Pressure constant, VT decreases
Favorable characteristics of ventilator mode	Known tidal volume, minute ventilation	Control of plateau pressures, decelerating inspiratory flow pattern
Weakness of ventilator mode	Uncontrolled peak airway pressure may increase the risk for VILI	No guarantee of tidal volume
Control of pH and pCO_2	Adjust minute ventilation by either VT or RR	Adjust minute ventilation by either inspiratory pressure or RR
Control of PaO_2	Adjust FiO_2 and PEEP	Adjust FiO_2 and PEEP or increase mean airway pressure by changing inspiratory time and I:E ratio

patients. Automated weaning is associated with reduced duration of ventilation and ICU length of stay [76, 77].

Acute Respiratory Distress Syndrome (ARDS)

The Berlin ARDS definition (mild, moderate, severe ARDS based on severity of hypoxemia defined by PaO_2/FiO_2 ratio) was established in 2012 (Fig. 36.4) to address the limitations of the previous American-European Consensus Conference definition of 1994 [78]. Using the Berlin Definition, stages of mild, moderate, and severe ARDS were associated with increased mortality (27%, 32%, and 45%, respectively) and increased median duration of mechanical ventilation in survivors (5 days; IQR 2–11; 7 days; IQR 4–14; and 9 days; IQR 5–17).

The recent Large Observational Study to Understand the Global Impact of Severe Acute Respiratory Failure (LUNG SAFE) examined patients undergoing invasive or noninvasive ventilation in 459 ICUs. ARDS represented 10.4% of ICU admission and 23.4% of patients requiring mechanical ventilation. Hospital mortality was 34.9% for mild ARDS patients, 40.3% for moderate ARDS patients, and 46.1% for those with severe ARDS, confirming overall high mortality rates for ARDS [79].

A number of evidence-based ARDS treatment strategies should be considered [low tidal volume (6 mL/kg predicted body weight) ventilation, optimal PEEP dependent on lung recruitability, neuromuscular blockade, early (≤48 h after ARDS onset) and prolonged (repletion of 16-h session) prone position, recruitment maneuvers, inhaled nitric oxide, monitoring transpulmonary pressures to identify adequate PEEP, high-frequency oscillatory ventilation, and extracorporeal membrane oxygenation, ECMO) in addition to standard infection management if pneumonia is present and conservative fluid management. Higher risk and higher cost therapies should be matched with increased severity of ARDS (Fig. 36.4) [80]. Targeting oxygenation of 88–92% and tolerating a moderate level of hypercapnia are safe in ARDS treatment [81, 82]. For patients with severe ARDS and severe hypoxemia, transfer to an ARDS referral center with ECMO capability is recommended.

Summary

Pulmonary issues in geriatric trauma and acute care surgery patients are common, particularly pneumonia and acute respiratory failure, which are significant causes of morbidity and mortality. National rates of VAP remain highest in surgical, trauma, and burn ICUs. Prevention of VAP can

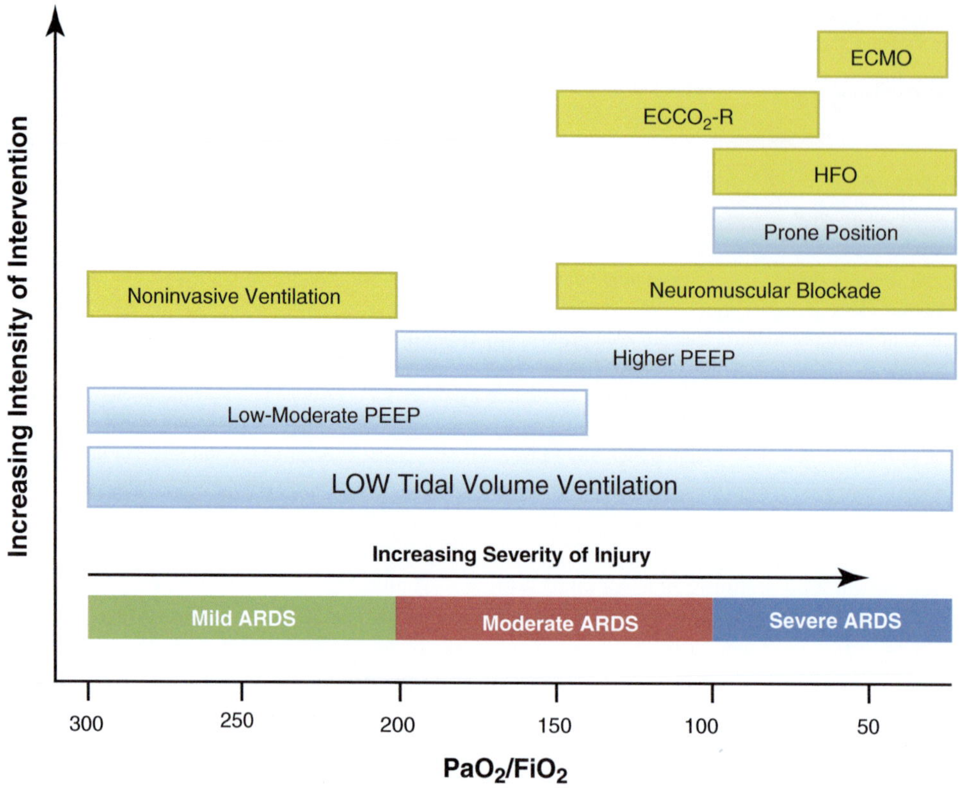

Fig. 36.4 The Berlin definition of ARDS and therapies for ARDS treatment. Mild ARDS: $PaO_2/FiO_2 > 200$ to ≤ 300 mm Hg. Moderate ARDS: $PaO_2/FiO_2 > 100$ to ≤ 200 mm Hg. Severe ARDS: $PaO_2/FiO_2 \leq 100$ mm Hg. Adapted from The ARDS Definition Task Force. Acute Respiratory Distress Syndrome: The Berlin Definition. JAMA 2012;307(23):2526–2533

be optimized by reducing the risk of aspiration and bacterial colonization of the airway through evidence-based preventive strategies (chlorhexidine, semirecumbent position, specialized endotracheal tubes, spontaneous awakening and breathing trials, and ventilator weaning protocols). New CDC surveillance definitions for ventilator-associated events are used to track pulmonary complications in the ICU. The new Berlin definition of ARDS has confirmed the high rates of mortality associated with ARDS, and allows us to match treatment strategies to hypoxemia-related severity of ARDS.

References

1. Ramly E, Kaafarani HM, Velmahos GC. The effect of aging on pulmonary function: implications for monitoring and support of the surgical and trauma patient. Surg Clin North Am. 2015;95(1):53–69.
2. Chun KY, Annabelle T, David YL, et al. Pulmonary complications after major abdominal surgery: National Surgical Quality Improvement Program analysis. J Surg Res. 2015;198:441–9.
3. Memtsoudis S, Liu SS, Ma Y, Chiu YL, Walz JM, Gaber-Baylis LK, Mazumdar M. Perioperative pulmonary outcomes in patients with sleep apnea after noncardiac surgery. Anesth Analg. 2011;112(1):113–21.
4. Arozullah AM, Daley J, Henderson WG, et al. Multifactorial risk index for predicting postoperative respiratory failure in men after major non cardiac surgery. The National Veterans Administration Surgical Quality Improvement Program. Ann Surg. 2000;232:242.
5. Canet J, Gallart L, Gomar C, et al. Prediction of postoperative pulmonary complications in a population based cohort. Anesthesiology. 2010;113:1338.
6. Gupta H, Gupta PK, Fang X, et al. Development and validation of a risk calculator predicting respiratory failure. Chest. 2011;140:1207.
7. Gupta H, Gupta PK, Schuller D, et al. Development and validation of a risk calculator for predicting postoperative pneumonia. Mayo Clin Proc. 2013;88:1241.
8. Lawrence VA, Cornell JE, Smetana GW, American College of Physicians. Strategies to reduce postoperative pulmonary complications after noncardiothoracic

surgery: systematic review for the American College of Physicians. Ann Intern Med. 2006;144(8):596–608. Review
9. Qaseem A, Snow V, Fitterman N, Hornbake ER, Lawrence VA, Smetana GW, Weiss K, Owens DK, Aronson M, Barry P, Casey DE Jr, Cross JT Jr, Fitterman N, Sherif KD, Weiss KB. Clinical efficacy assessment Subcommittee of the American College of Physicians. Risk assessment for and strategies to reduce perioperative pulmonary complications for patients undergoing noncardiothoracic surgery: a guideline from the American College of Physicians. Ann Intern Med. 2006;144(8):575–80.
10. do Nascimento Junior P, Módolo NS, Andrade S, et al. Incentive spirometry for prevention of postoperative pulmonary complications in upper abdominal surgery. Cochrane Database Syst Rev. 2014;2:CD006058.
11. Zarbock A, Mueller E, Netzer S, et al. Prophylactic nasal continuous positive airway pressure following cardiac surgery protects from postoperative pulmonary complications: a prospective, randomized, controlled trial in 500 patients. Chest. 2009; 135:1252.
12. Nelson R, Edwards S, Tse B. Prophylactic nasogastric decompression after abdominal surgery. Cochrane Database Syst Rev. 2007;3:CD004929.
13. Arozullah AM, Khuri SF, Henderson WG, et al. Development and validation of a multifactorial risk index for predicting postoperative pneumonia after major noncardiac surgery. Ann Intern Med. 2001;135(10):847–57.
14. Napolitano LM. Use of severity scoring and stratification factors in clinical trials of hospital-acquired and ventilator-associated pneumonia. Clin Infect Dis. 2010;51(Suppl 1):S67–80.
15. Ozhathil DK, Li Y, Smith JK, Witkowski E, Coyne ER, Alavi K, Tseng JF, Shah SA. Colectomy Performance improvement within NSQIP 2005-2008. J Surg Res. 2011;171(1):e9–e13.
16. American Thoracic Society; Infectious Diseases Society of America. Guidelines for the management of adults with hospital-acquired, ventilator-associated, and healthcare-associated pneumonia. Am J Respir Crit Care Med. 2005;171(4):388–416.
17. Fàbregas N, Ewig S, Torres A, et al. Clinical diagnosis of ventilator associated pneumonia revisited: comparative validation using immediate post-mortem lung biopsies. Thorax. 1999;54:867.
18. Meduri GU. Diagnosis and differential diagnosis of ventilator-associated pneumonia. Clin Chest Med. 1995;16:61.
19. Wunderink RG, Woldenberg LS, Zeiss J, et al. The radiologic diagnosis of autopsy-proven ventilator-associated pneumonia. Chest. 1992;101:458.
20. http://www.cdc.gov/nhsn/PDFs/pscManual/6pscVAPcurrent.pdf
21. Leonard KL, Borst GM, Davies SW, et al. Ventilator-associated pneumonia in trauma patients: different criteria, different rates. Surg Infect. 2016;17(3):363–8.
22. Mangram AJ, Sohn J, Zhou N, et al. Trauma-associated pneumonia: time to redefine ventilator-associated pneumonia in trauma patients. Am J Surg. 2015;210(6):1056–61. discussion 1061-2
23. Kollef MH, Bock KR, Richards RD, Hearns ML. The safety and diagnostic accuracy of minibronchoalveolar lavage in patients with suspected ventilator-associated pneumonia. Ann Intern Med. 1995;122:743.
24. Shorr AF, Sherner JH, Jackson WL, Kollef MH. Invasive approaches to the diagnosis of ventilator-associated pneumonia: a meta-analysis. Crit Care Med. 2005;33:46.
25. Klompas M. Does this patient have ventilator-associated pneumonia? JAMA. 2007;297(14):1583–93.
26. Luyt CE, Combes A, Reynaud C, et al. Usefulness of procalcitonin for the diagnosis of ventilator-associated pneumonia. Intensive Care Med. 2008;34(8):1434–40.
27. Ramirez P, Garcia MA, Ferrer M, et al. Sequential measurements of procalcitonin levels in diagnosing ventilator-associated pneumonia. Eur Respir J. 2008;31(2):356–62.
28. Linssen CF, Bekers O, Drent M, Jacobs JA. C-reactive protein and procalcitonin concentrations in BAL fluid as a predicctor of ventilator-associated pneumonia. Ann Clin Biochem. 2008;45:293–8.
29. Gibot S, Cravoisy A, Levy B, et al. Soluble triggering receptor expressed on myeloid cells and the diagnosis of pneumonia. N Engl J Med. 2004;350(5):451–8.
30. Determann RM, Millo JL, Gibot S, et al. Serial changes in soluble triggering receptor expressed on myeloid cells in the lung during development of ventilator-associated-pneumonia. Intensive Care Med. 2005;31(11):1495–500.
31. Anand NJ, Zuick S, Klesney-Tait J, Kollef MH. Diagnostic implications of soluble triggering receptor expressed on myeloid cells-1 in BAL fluid of patients with pulmonary infiltrates in the ICU. Chest. 2009;135(3):641–7.
32. Oudhuis GJ, Beuving J, Bergmans D, et al. Soluble triggering receptor expressed on myeloid cells-1 in bronchoalveolar lavage fluid is not predictive for ventilator-associated pneumonia. Intensive Care Med. 2009;35(7):1265–70.
33. http://www.cdc.gov/nhsn/PDFs/pscManual/10-VAE_FINAL.pdf
34. Meduri GU, Johanson WG Jr. International consensus conference: clinical investigation of ventilator-associated pneumonia. Chest. 1992;102:551S.
35. Hidron AI, Edwards JR, Patel J, et al. NHSN annual update: antimicrobial-resistant pathogens associated with healthcare-associated infections: annual summary of data reported to the National Healthcare Safety Network at the Centers for Disease Control and Prevention 2006–2007. Infect Control Hosp Epidemiol. 2008;29:996–1011.
36. Iregui M, Ward S, Sherman G, et al. Clinical importance of delays in the initiation of appropriate antibiotic treatment for ventilator-associated pneumonia. Chest. 2002;122:262.
37. Habarth S, Garbino J, Pugin, et al. Inappropriate initial antimicrobial therapy and its effect on survival in a clinical trial of immunomodulating therapy for severe sepsis. Am J Med. 2003;115(7):529–35.

38. Luna CM, Vujacich P, Niederman MS, et al. Impact of BAL data on the therapy and outcome of ventilator-associated pneumonia. Chest. 1997;111:676.
39. Kollef MH, Sherman G, Ward S, et al. Inadequate antimicrobial treatment of infections: a risk factor for hospital mortality among critically ill patients. Chest. 1999;115(2):462–74.
40. Teixeira PJ, Seligman R, Hertz FT, et al. Inadequate treatment of ventilator-associated pneumonia: risk factors and impact on outcomes. J Hosp Infect. 2007;65(4):361–7.
41. Chastre J, Wolff M, Fagon JY, et al. Comparison of 8 vs 15 days of antibiotic therapy for ventilator-associated pneumonia in adults: a randomized trial. JAMA. 2003;290:2588.
42. Wren SM, Martin M, Yoon JK, Bech F. Postoperative pneumonia-prevention program for the inpatient surgical ward. J Am Coll Surg. 2010;210:491–5.
43. Napolitano LM. Perspectives in surgical infections: what does the future hold? Surg Infect. 2010;11(2):111–23. Review
44. Muscedere J, Dodek P, Keenan S, Fowler R, Cook D, Heyland D. VAP guidelines committee and the Canadian critical care trials group. Comprehensive evidence-based clinical practice guidelines for ventilator-associated pneumonia: prevention. J Crit Care. 2008;23(1):126–37.
45. Wip C, Napolitano L. Bundles to prevent ventilator-associated pneumonia: how valuable are they? Curr Opin Infect Dis. 2009;22(2):159–66.
46. Speck K, Rawat N, Weiner NC, Tujuba HG, Farley D, Berenholtz S. A systematic approach for developing a ventilator-associated pneumonia prevention bundle. Am J Infect Control. 2016;44(6):652–6.
47. Cabrini L, Landoni G, Oriani A, Plumari VP, Nobile L, Greco M, Pasin L, Beretta L, Zangrillo A. Noninvasive ventilation and survival in acute care settings: a comprehensive systematic review and metaanalysis of randomized controlled trials. Crit Care Med. 2015;43(4):880–8.
48. Bajaj A, Rathor P, Sehgal V, Shetty A. Efficacy of noninvasive ventilation after planned extubation: a systematic review and meta-analysis of randomized controlled trials. Heart Lung. 2015;44(2):150–7.
49. Vital FM, Ladeira MT, Atallah AN. Non-invasive positive pressure ventilation (CPAP or bilevel NPPV) for cardiogenic pulmonary oedema. Cochrane Database Syst Rev. 2013;5:CD005351.
50. Faria DA, da Silva EM, Atallah ÁN, Vital FM. Noninvasive positive pressure ventilation for acute respiratory failure following upper abdominal surgery. Cochrane Database Syst Rev. 2015;10:CD009134.
51. Burns KE, Meade MO, Premji A, Adhikari NK. Noninvasive positive-pressure ventilation as a weaning strategy for intubated adults with respiratory failure. Cochrane Database Syst Rev. 2013;12:CD004127.
52. Garrard CS, A'Court CD. The diagnosis of pneumonia in the critically ill. Chest. 1995;108(2 Suppl):17S–25S.
53. Girard TD, Kress JP, Fuchs BD, et al. Efficacy and safety of a paired sedation and ventilator weaning protocol for mechanically ventilated patients in intensive care (awakening and breathing controlled trial): a randomised controlled trial. Lancet. 2008;371(9607):126–34.
54. Klompas M, Anderson D, Trick W, et al. The preventability of ventilator-associated events. The CDC prevention epicenters wake up and breathe collaborative. Am J Respir Crit Care Med. 2015;191(3):292–301.
55. Drakulovic MB, Torres A, Bauer TT, et al. Supine body position as a risk factor for nosocomial pneumonia in mechanically ventilated patients: a randomised trial. Ann Intern Med. 1999;354:1851.
56. van Nieuwenhoven CA, Vandenbroucke-Grauls C, van Tiel FH, Joore HC, van Schijndel RJ, van der Tweel I, Ramsay G, Bonten MJ. Feasibility and effects of the semirecumbent position to prevent ventilator-associated pneumonia: a randomized study. Crit Care Med. 2006;34(2):396–402.
57. Alexiou VG, Ierodiakonou V, Dimopoulos G, Falagas ME. Impact of patient position on the incidence of ventilator-associated pneumonia: a meta-analysis of randomized controlled trials. J Crit Care. 2009;24(4):515–22.
58. Wang L, Li X, Yang Z, Tang X, Yuan Q, Deng L, Sun X. Semi-recumbent position versus supine position for the prevention of ventilator-associated pneumonia in adults requiring mechanical ventilation. Cochrane Database Syst Rev. 2016;1:CD009946.
59. Wang F, Bo L, Tang L, Lou J, Wu Y, Chen F, Li J, Deng X. Subglottic secretion drainage for preventing ventilator-associated pneumonia: an updated meta-analysis of randomized controlled trials. J Trauma Acute Care Surg. 2012;72(5):1276–85. https://doi.org/10.1097/TA.0b013e318247cd33.
60. Kollef MH, Afessa B, Anzueto A, et al. Silver-coated endotracheal tubes and incidence of ventilator-associated pneumonia: the NASCENT randomized trial. JAMA. 2008;300(7):805–13.
61. Tokmaji G, Vermeulen H, Müller MC, Kwakman PH, Schultz MJ, Zaat SA. Silver-coated endotracheal tubes for prevention of ventilator-associated pneumonia in critically ill patients. Cochrane Database Syst Rev. 2015;8:CD009201.
62. DeRiso AJ, Ladowski JS, Dillon TA, et al. Chlorhexidine gluconate 0.12% oral rinse reduces the incidence of total nosocomial respiratory infection and nonprophylactic systemic antibiotic use in patients undergoing heart surgery. Chest. 1996;109:1556.
63. Shi Z, Xie H, Wang P, et al. Oral hygiene care for critically ill patients to prevent ventilator-associated pneumonia. Cochrane Database Syst Rev. 2013;13(8):CD008367.
64. de Smet AM, Kluytmans JA, Cooper BS, et al. Decontamination of the digestive tract and oropharynx in ICU patients. N Engl J Med. 2009;360:20.
65. D'Amico R, Pifferi S, Leonetti C, et al. Effectiveness of antibiotic prophylaxis in critically ill adult patients: systematic review of randomised controlled trials. BMJ. 1998;316:1275.

66. Silvestri L, van Saene HK, Casarin A, et al. Impact of selective decontamination of the digestive tract on carriage and infection due to gram-negative and gram-positive bacteria: a systematic review of randomised controlled trials. Anaesth Intensive Care. 2008;36:324.
67. Wunderink RG. Welkommen to our world. Emergence of antibiotic resistance with selective decontamination of the digestive tract. Am J Respir Crit Care Med. 2010;181:426.
68. Siempos II, Ntaidou TK, Filippidis FT, Choi AM. Effect of early versus late or no tracheostomy on mortality and pneumonia of critically ill patients receiving mechanical ventilation: a systematic review and meta-analysis. Lancet Respir Med. 2015;3(2):150–8.
69. Hosokawa K, Nishimura M, Egi M, Vincent JL. Timing of tracheotomy in ICU patients: a systematic review of randomized controlled trials. Crit Care. 2015;19:424.
70. Piroddi IM, Barlascini C, Esquinas A, Braido F, Banfi P, Nicolini A. Non-invasive mechanical ventilation in elderly patients: a narrative review. Geriatr Gerontol Int. 2017;17(5):689–96. https://doi.org/10.1111/ggi.12810.
71. Frat JP, Thille AW, Mercat A, et al. High-flow oxygen through nasal cannula in acute hypoxemic respiratory failure. N Engl J Med. 2015;372(23):2185–96.
72. Damuth E, Mitchell JA, Bartock JL, et al. Long-term survival of critically ill patients treated with prolonged mechanical ventilation: a systematic review and meta-analysis. Lancet Respir Med. 2015;3(7):544–53.
73. Ely EW, Evans GW, Haponik EF. Mechanical ventilation in a cohort of elderly patients admitted to an intensive care unit. Ann Intern Med. 1999;131(2):96–104.
74. Lai CC, Ko SC, Chen CM, Weng SF, Tseng KL, Cheng KC. The outcomes and prognostic factors of the very elderly requiring prolonged mechanical ventilation in a single respiratory care center. Medicine (Baltimore). 2016;95(2):e2479.
75. Chacko B, Peter JV, Tharyan P, John G, Jeyaseelan L. Pressure-controlled versus volume-controlled ventilation for acute respiratory failure due to acute lung injury (ALI) or acute respiratory distress syndrome (ARDS). Cochrane Database Syst Rev. 2015;1:CD008807.
76. Rose L, Schultz MJ, Cardwell CR, Jouvet P, McAuley DF, Blackwood B. Automated versus non-automated weaning for reducing the duration of mechanical ventilation for critically ill adults and children. Cochrane Database Syst Rev. 2014;6:CD009235.
77. McConville JF, Kress JP. Weaning patients from the ventilator. N Engl J Med. 2012;367(23):2233–9.
78. ARDS Definition Task Force, Ranieri VM, Rubenfeld GD, Thompson BT, Ferguson ND, Caldwell E, Fan E, Camporota L, Slutsky AS. Acute respiratory distress syndrome: the Berlin definition. JAMA. 2012;307(23):2526–33.
79. Bellani G, Laffey JG, Pham T, et al. Epidemiology, patterns of care, and mortality for patients with acute respiratory distress syndrome in intensive care units in 50 countries. JAMA. 2016;315(8):788–800.
80. Pipeling MR, Fan E. Therapies for refractory hypoxemia in acute respiratory distress syndrome. JAMA. 2010;304(22):2521–7.
81. Chiumello D, Brioni M. Severe hypoxemia: which strategy to choose. Crit Care. 2016;20(1):132.
82. Bein T, Grasso S, Moerer O, et al. The standard of care of patients with ARDS: ventilatory settings and rescue therapies for refractory hypoxemia. Intensive Care Med. 2016;42(5):699–711.

37 Cardiac/Hemodynamic Monitoring

Jay Menaker and Thomas M. Scalea

Introduction

Patients over the age of 65 [1–4] represent one of the fastest growing sections of the US census. This increase in the number of elderly is multifactorial, but is due in large part to longer life expectancy due to advances in health care as well as the aging baby boomers. In 2012, there were 43.1 million people aged 65 and older, 12 times the number in 1900 [5, 6]. It is estimated that by the year 2050, the population of elderly will be approximately 84 million people and account for almost 21% of the US population [5, 6]. Additionally, it is predicted that by the year 2030, those over the age of 85, the oldest-old, will number more than 9 million and by year 2050 almost 20 million [5, 7].

Physiologic Changes

As people age their physiologic reserve decreases. This loss of physiologic decline varies from organ to organ and individual to individual [8]. Under normal conditions, most elderly people can overcome this decrease in reserve and meet their physiologic needs. However, when stress occurs, including acute trauma or illness, the demand is overwhelming and the elderly are unable to compensate and achieve the physiologic demand to ensure adequate perfusion.

Age is a major risk factor for the development of cardiovascular disease (CVD). Over 40% of deaths in patients older than 65 years have been attributed to CVD [9]. Myocardial changes as one ages affect anatomical, physiologic, and electro-physiologic activity of the heart [10]. Older patients can often have decreased myocardial contractility and ventricular compliance for a given preload [11]. Additionally, changes in the make-up of the myocardium result in conduction abnormalities. These alterations in the conduction system increase the likelihood of arrhythmias, including sick sinus syndrome, bundle branch blocks, and atrial arrhythmias and subsequent syncope in the elderly [12–14].

As people age, their systolic blood pressure increases. This is due to a decrease in compliance of the outflow tract, resulting from an increased afterload. During times of acute illness or injury, this results in decreases in ejection fraction and cardiac output [11, 15–17]. Unfortunately, the elderly's maximum heart rate can decrease by as much as 30%, making it impossible to compensate for the decreased cardiac function [18]. Furthermore, aged myocardium does not respond as well to increased levels of endogenous and

J. Menaker, M.D. • T.M. Scalea, M.D. (✉)
Division of Surgical/Critical Care, Department of Surgery, Program in Trauma, R Adams Cowley Shock Trauma Center, University of Maryland School of Medicine, 22 South Greene Street, T1R60, Baltimore, MD 21201, USA
e-mail: jmenaker@umm.edu; tscalea@umm.edu

A. Rodriguez et al. (eds.), *Geriatric Trauma and Acute Care Surgery*,
https://doi.org/10.1007/978-3-319-57403-5_37

exogenous catecholamine [19]. This requires the elderly patient to be volume resuscitated to maintain adequate stroke volume and cardiac output [11, 20]. However, clinicians must be very careful with aggressive volume resuscitation in the elderly patient and balance the need for adequate cardiac output with the potential for pulmonary edema.

Atrial Fibrillation

Atrial fibrillation (AF) is the most common arrhythmia and increases in incidence as one ages [21–25]. Although its reported incident varies, the true rate is unknown due to a lack of continuous monitoring outside an intensive care unit [25]. AF has been shown to be associated with significantly longer intensive care unit (ICU) and hospital length of stay (LOS). Additionally, it is associated with the need for vaso-active and inotropic support, higher daily fluid requirements, and rate of severe infections [23–25].

When considering treatment options for the elderly patient in AF, clinicians need to focus on two things. One is the symptomatic treatment of AF; the second is the underlying cause. Treatable causes including thyroid dysfunction, electrolyte abnormalities, or acute cardiac ischemia need to be investigated and corrected if possible. Therapy goals should focus on rate control, rhythm control, and the prevention of thromboembolism [25]. Patients with compromised hemodynamics warrant immediate cardioversion. For those who remain hemodynamically stable and without symptoms, medical therapy should be initiated.

The benefits of rate control versus rhythm control have been debated. Two large studies demonstrated no benefit from rhythm control over rate control [26, 27]. Thus many clinicians focus their pharmacological interventions on controlling the ventricular rate using atrioventricular nodal blockers [25]. Treatment options include amiodarone, which for many has become the initial drug of choice for atrial fibrillation. It is a class III antiarrhythmic agent that depresses atrioventricular conduction and controls the ventricular rate. Many clinicians like amiodarone because it is safe to use in patients with reduced ejection fraction. Side effects include bradycardia, thyroid dysfunction acutely, and the development of pulmonary fibrosis with long-term use. Additionally, amiodarone has many drug-drug interactions, specifically warfarin. Intravenous (IV) amiodarone has been associated with acute elevation in liver enzymes; however levels normalize with its discontinuation [28]. Dronedarone, similar to amiodarone, has been studied for rate and rhythm control in AF. It reduces morbidity and mortality in patients with high-risk AF; however it is contraindicated in patients with acute severe heart failure [29].

β-blockers and calcium channel blockers (CCB) are other pharmacological options. β-blockers may be more suitable for postoperative hyper-adrenergic states, while CCB, specifically diltiazem, may be more ideal in patients with severe pulmonary disease. Side effects of both include hypotension and bradycardia. Typically CCB are avoided in patients with underlying heart failure. Digoxin, despite being one of the oldest antiarrhythmic agents for AF, is still used by many clinicians. It works by slowing down conduction at the atrioventricular node by parasympathetic activation. Many consider it the ideal choice for patients with evidence of heart failure. Digoxin can be synergistic with β-blockers or CCB; however, it is less effective in postoperative patients with high sympathetic tone [25]. Similar to amiodarone, digoxin has many drug-drug interactions which often limit its use in critically ill patients. Additionally, as digoxin is renally metabolized, levels must be closely monitored and adjusted.

Some patients do not respond to any of medications discussed above and remain in AF. Those in AF for more than 48 h have an increased risk of atrial thrombus formation and anticoagulation therapy should be considered [25]. The CHADS2 score and now the newer CHA2DS2—Vasc score have been used to stratify who should be anticoagulated based on risk factors [30]. However, the risks of systemic anticoagulation in the elderly who are prone to falls, as well as have the potential for many drug-drug interactions, need to be taken into account. The HAS-BLED score has been used to calculate the 1-year bleeding risk in patients with AF [31]. It has shown to be a better predictor of bleeding than other scores [32–34]. The HAS-BLED score should not be used to exclude patients from anticoagulation therapy, but rather as a tool to correct any modifiable risk factors [34]. Additionally because it uses readily available clinical data it is easier to use than other scores [34].

Myocardial Ischemia/Infarction

Cardiac complications occur from 12 to 16.7% in the elderly [35–37]. They are one of the highest causes of mortality in the elderly surgical patient. Myocardial infarction (MI) has been shown to be the leading cause of postoperative death in patients over the age of 80 [38]. The prevalence of postoperative MI in patients over 65 years of age ranges from 0.1 to 4% and usually occurs within 72 h following surgery [39–41].

β-blockers have historically been considered a standard treatment to help prevent perioperative cardiac events in the elderly. They help minimize flow across plaques decreasing the incidence of rupture. This plaque rupture can cause as many as 50% of perioperative MI [42]. β-blockers minimize ventricular dysrhythmias, improve myocardial oxygen balance, and decrease sympathetic tone. A number of publications supported the use of β-blockade to prevent postoperative complications [43–47]. Based on these studies the use of perioperative blockade was quickly adopted due to the potential benefit with few adverse side effects [43, 48]. Subsequent studies, however, have demonstrated no differences in cardiac complications or mortality with the use of β-blockers [49, 50]. Furthermore, in some literature, it has been shown that the use of β-blockers actually increases surgical mortality [43, 51, 52]. In 2008 the POISE study group evaluated the use perioperative β-blockade and concluded that although the treatment group has significantly lower rates of MI, there was a significantly higher death rate and stroke rate in patients receiving β-blockers [53]. As a result, there is little consensus on the use of perioperative β-blockers. Some believe patients having one or two risk factors (high-risk surgery, known ischemic heart disease, history of congestive heart failure or cerebrovascular disease, baseline creatinine >2 mg/dL) would benefit, while others believe patients with more than three risk factors are more appropriate [42, 52, 54]. The 2014 ACC/AHA guidelines state that those taking β-blockers at the time of surgery should continue therapy [43]. Additionally, they suggest starting a β-blocker in high-risk patients [43]. Despite these guidelines, it is clear that larger randomized trials are needed.

Hemodynamic Monitoring

Elderly patients are often unable to increase their native cardiac output in times of stress. Instead, they increase their systemic vascular resistance which produces a normal blood pressure [55]. Unfortunately, despite a normal blood pressure, elderly patients a have severely depressed and compromised cardiac function, causing poor systemic perfusion. In 1990, Scalea et al. published a landmark study of geriatric trauma patients demonstrating that as many as 50% geriatric trauma patients who appeared clinically stable with "normal" blood pressure had unrecognized cardiogenic shock and a poor outcome [56]. In this study, a pulmonary artery catheter was used to guide and optimize resuscitation with volume, inotropes, and afterload reduction. The authors demonstrated a survival increase from 7 to 53%. The study concluded that clinicians could improve outcome by identifying occult shock early in the geriatric population with the use of invasive monitoring.

For years clinicians have struggled with identifying the ideal method to measure a critically ill patient's volume status [57]. Physical exam has not been shown to be helpful in accurately determining intravascular volume. Additionally, traditional measurements of preload including CVP and PCWP have been unreliable in predicting cardiac preload and the need for volume to optimize cardiac function [58]. Changes produced by passive leg raises (PLR) have been shown to predict the need for fluid administration in mechanically ventilated patients [59]. The pulmonary artery catheter (PAC), first described and used in 1970 by Swan and Ganz, had traditionally been considered the gold standard of hemodynamic monitoring [60]. Unfortunately the literature supporting its use in critically ill patients is highly variable. Some studies have demonstrated no effect on patient outcome [61, 62], others have showed decreased mortality [56, 63, 64], and still others have shown an increase in mortality as well as utilization of resources [65, 66]. Some suggested that the studies demonstrating a negative outcome were due to misinterpretation of PAC data and subsequent clinical decision making rather than the use of PAC itself [67–69]. Despite the ongoing arguments of the value and utility of the PAC, newer and less invasive hemodynamics monitoring methods have been developed.

Continuous Central Venous Oximetry

Continuous central venous oximetry (ScvO2) has been used as an alternative to the PAC (SvO2). It allows clinicians to continuously monitor venous oxygenation in the superior vena cava. ScvO2 is generally higher than SvO2 in the critically ill; however the correlation between the two is variable [70–72]. ScvO2 can help identify global tissue hypoxia, which allows earlier intervention in the clinical course and affect outcome [73, 74].

Pulse Contour Analysis

Other alternatives to the PAC include pulse contour analysis. The idea is based on the Windkessel model where stroke volume can be continuously estimated using arterial waveform [75]. Using the area under the curve of the systolic arterial pressure waveform, stroke volume can then be calculated [76]. Unfortunately pulse contour technology has a number of limitations including its accuracy in patients with irregular heart rhythms, evidence of right heart failure, and low tidal volume mechanical ventilation [77].

Examples of pulse contour technology include the FloTrac™ (Edwards Lifesciences, Irvine, CA). It provides continuous cardiac output, stroke volumes, and stroke volume variation using only an arterial catheter. Cardiac output is calculated using arterial wave form analysis and the principle that the pulse pressure and stroke volume are proportional [59]. Some studies demonstrated clinically acceptable agreements between the PAC and FloTrac™ [78, 79], while others have not [57, 80, 81].

Another pulse contour analysis devise is the PiCCO™ (Pulsion Medical Systems; Munich, Germany). It requires both an arterial line, placed either in the femoral or in the axillary artery, and a central venous catheter. In addition to measuring cardiac output, stroke volumes, and stroke volume variation, it has the ability to calculate intra-thoracic blood volume (ITBV), global end diastolic volume (GEDV), and extravascular lung water (EVLW). These volumes measure cardiac preload better than central venous pressure (CVP) and pulmonary capillary wedge pressure (PCWP) [82, 83]. Additionally, they are not affected by mechanical ventilation. The PiCCO™ system requires calibration on a regular basis, depending on the hemodynamics of the patient. As with other hemodynamic monitoring modalities, the literature of their effectiveness is variable [84, 85].

Stroke volume variation (SVV) is a simple and accurate measurement of fluid responsiveness [86]. A low SVV represents a patient who does not require ongoing resuscitation while a high SVV implies a volume responsive patient. The exact threshold for SVV remains unknown [87]. Values between 9.5 and 10.5% have been suggested as cut-offs to predict fluid responsiveness [88, 89]. Both the FlorTrac™ and the PiCCO™ have been shown to equally predict fluid responsiveness; however the FloTrac™ had a lower threshold [87].

Noninvasive Methods

A number of noninvasive techniques have been used to measure hemodynamic parameters. These techniques include partial gas rebreathing (NICO system), thoracic bioimpedance, impedance plethysmography, and portable Doppler devices. Currently these techniques are not widely available and have not been validated versus other more invasive techniques [90].

Echocardiography

The role of bedside echocardiography has become a mainstay in the management of the critically ill patient. Fluid status and inferior vena cava diameter and collapsibility can rapidly be attained at the bedside providing reliable monitoring of intravascular volume in the mechanically ventilated patient [91]. Although it cannot provide continuous monitoring, it can easily be repeated to quickly evaluate the response to an intervention [92].

The first focused echocardiography ultrasound protocol for noncardiologists was the "Focused Assessment with Transthoracic Echocardiography" (FATE) [93]. It allowed clinicians to measure hemodynamics and optimize care. Since then a number of similar protocols have been created. The "Bedside Echocardiographic Assessment in Trauma" (BEAT) was described in 2008 and compared function and volume status with a PAC in critically ill patients [94]. In 2011, Ferrada et al. first described the "Focused Rapid Echocardiographic Examination" (FREE) [95]. It was designed to be performed by both surgeons and intensivists. It is a "transthoracic examination, incorporating hemodynamic information from the echocardiogram with the patient's clinical scenario to generate broad treatment recommendations about fluid, inotropic agents and vasopressors" [95]. The FREE demonstrated similar results when compared to a PAC: however, there was less agreement with the FloTrac™ especially in patients with low (<40%) ejection fractions [96].

Conclusion

The elderly population continues to increase. As people age, their physiologic reserve decreases, and when stressed, they are often unable to effectively compensate and meet the physiologic demand to ensure adequate perfusion. Underlying cardiac dysfunction becomes more pronounced, and complications including cardiac dysrhythmia, myocardial ischemia, and infarction occur. Early aggressive hemodynamic monitoring has been shown to improve survival in the elderly patient population; however, the optimal method by which to do this has yet to be definitively determined.

References

1. Osler T, Baker SP, Long W. A modification of the injury severity score that both improves accuracy and simplifies scoring. J Trauma. 1997;43:922–6.
2. Champion HR, Copes WS, Buyer D. Major trauma in geriatric patients. Am J Public Health. 1989;79:1278–82.
3. Grossman MD, Miller D, Scaff DW. When is elder old? Effect of preexisting conditions on mortality in geriatric trauma. J Trauma. 2002;52:242–6.
4. Taylor MD, Tracy JK, Meyer W. Trauma in the elderly: intensive care unit resource use and outcome. J Trauma. 2002;53:407–14.
5. Ortman JM, Velkoff VA. An aging nation: the older population in the United States. Population estimates and projections. Current Population Reports 2014; P25–1140.
6. US Census Bureau 65 + in the United States. 2010. https://www.census.gov/content/dam/Census/library/publications/2014/demo/p23-212.pdf. Accessed 10 Nov 2015.
7. United States Census Bureau. U.S. population projections. National population projections. 2014. https://www.census.gov/population/projections/data/national/2014.html. Accessed 10 Nov 2015.
8. Boss GR, Seegmiller JE. Age related physiologic changes and their clinical significance. West J Med. 1981;135:434–40.
9. Lakatta EG. Age-associated cardiovascular changes in health. Impact on cardiovascular disease in older persons. Heart Fail Rev. 2002;7:29–49.
10. Harris R. Cardiovascular diseases in the elderly. Med Clin North Am. 1983;67:379–94.
11. Morley JE, Reese SS. Clinical implications of the aging heart. Am J Med. 1989;86:77–86.
12. Marik PE. Management of the critically ill geriatric patient. Crit Care Med. 2006;34:S176–82.

13. Rosenthal RA, Kavic SM. Assessment and management of the geriatric patient. Crit Care Med. 2004;4:S92–S105.
14. Watters JM, McClaran JC. The elderly surgical patient. In: the American College of Surgeons: care of the surgical patient, vol. 1. New York: Scientific American; 1991.
15. Pisani MA. Consideration in the caring for the critically ill older patient. J Intensive Care Med. 2009;24:83–95.
16. Sollott SJ, Lakatta EG. Normal aging changes in the cardiovascular system. Cardiol Elderly. 1993;1:349–58.
17. Stratton JR, Levy WC, Cerqueira MD, et al. Cardiovascular response to exercise. Effects of aging and exercise training in healthy men. Circulation. 1994;59:1648–55.
18. Lakatta EG, Levy D. Arterial and cardiac aging: major shareholders in cardiovascular disease enterprises: part II: the aging heart in health: links to heart disease. Circulation. 2003;107:346–54.
19. Lakatta EG. Age-related alterations in the cardiovascular response to adrenergic mediated stress. Fed Proc. 1980;39:3173–7.
20. Green JS, Crouse SF. Endurance training, cardiovascular function and the aged. Sports Med. 1993;16:331–41.
21. Ryu JK. Postoperative atrial fibrillation after noncardiothoracic surgery: is it different from after cardiothoracic surgery? Korean Circ J. 2009;39:93–4.
22. Brathwaite D, Weissman C. The new onset of atrial arrhythmias following major noncardiothoracic surgery is associated with increased mortality. Chest. 1998;114:462–8.
23. Polanczyk CA, Goldman L, Marcantonio ER. Supraventricular arrhythmia in patients having noncardiac surgery: clinical correlates and effect on length of stay. Ann Intern Med. 1998;129:279–85.
24. Seguin P, Signouret T, Laviolle B. Incidence and risk factors of atrial fibrillation in a surgical intensive care unit. Crit Care Med. 2004;32:722–6.
25. Joshi KK, Tiru M, Chin T, Fox MT, Stefan MS. Postoperative atrial fibrillation in patients undergoing non-cardiac non-thoracic surgery: a practical approach for the hospitalist. Hosp Pract (1995). 2015;43(4):235–44.
26. Van Gelder IC, Hagens VE, Bosker HA, et al. A comparison of rate control and rhythm control in patients with recurrent persistent atrial fibrillation. N Engl J Med. 2002;347:1834–40. Abstract
27. Wyse DG, Waldo AL, Di Marco JP, the Atrial Fibrillation Follow-up Investigation of Rhythm Management (AFFIRM) Investigators. A comparison of rate control and rhythm control in patients with atrial fibrillation. N Engl J Med. 2002;347:1825–33.
28. Grecian R, Ainslie M. Acute hepatic failure following intravenous amiodarone. BMJ Case Rep. 2012. doi: 10.1136/bcr-2012-007080.
29. Patel C, Yan GX, Kowey PR. Dronedarone. Circulation. 2009;120:636–44.
30. Mason PK, Lake DE, DiMarco JP, Ferguson JD, Mangrum JM, Bilchick K, et al. Impact of the CHA2DS2-VASc score on anticoagulation recommendations for atrial fibrillation. Am J Med. 2012;125(6):603.e1.
31. Pisters R, Lane DA, Nieuwlaat R, de Vos CB, Crijns HJ, Lip GY. A novel user-friendly score (HAS-BLED) to assess 1-year risk of major bleeding in patients with atrial fibrillation: the euro heart survey. Chest. 2010;138:1093–100.
32. Roldán V, Marín F, Fernández H, Manzano-Fernandez S, Gallego P, Valdés M, Vincente V, Lip GY. Predictive value of the HAS-BLED and ATRIA bleeding scores for the risk of serious bleeding in a 'real world' population with atrial fibrillation receiving anticoagulant therapy. Chest. 2013;143:179–84.
33. Apostolakis S, Lane DA, Guo Y, Buller H, Lip GY. Performance of the HEMORR(2)HAGES, ATRIA, and HAS-BLED bleeding risk-prediction scores in patients with atrial fibrillation undergoing anticoagulation: the AMADEUS (evaluating the use of SR34006 compared to warfarin or acenocoumarol in patients with atrial fibrillation) study. J Am Coll Cardiol. 2012;60:861–7.
34. Lane DA, Lip GYH. Use of the CHA2DS1-Vasc and HAS-BLED scores to aid decision making for thromboprophylaxis in nonvalvular atrial fibrillation. Circulation. 2012;126:860–5.
35. Seymour DG, Pringle R. Post-operative complications in the elderly surgical patient. Gerontology. 1983;29:262–70.
36. Pedersen T, Eliasen K, Henriksen E. A prospective study of risk factors and cardiopulmonary complications associated with anaesthesia and surgery: risk indicators of cardiopulmonary morbidity. Acta Anaesthiol Scand. 1990;34:144–55.
37. Liu LL, Leung JM. Predicting adverse postoperative outcomes in patients aged 80 years or older. J Am Geriatr Soc. 2000;48:405–12.
38. Djokovic JL, Hedley-Whyte J. Prediction of outcome of surgery and synesthesia in patients over 80. JAMA. 1979;242:2301–6.
39. Plumlee JE, Boettner RB. Myocardial infarction during and following anesthesia and operation. South Med J. 1972;65:886–9.
40. Pedersen T, Eliasen K Henriksen E. A prospective study of mortality associated with anaesthesia and surgery: risk indicators of mortality in hospital. Acta Anaesthesiol Scand. 1990;34:176–82.
41. Seymour DG. Medical assessment of the elderly surgical patient. London: Croom Helm; 1986. p. 80.
42. Kertai MD, Bax JJ, Klein J. Is there any reason to withhold beta blockers from high risk patients with coronary artery disease during surgery? Anesthesiology. 2004;100:4–7.
43. Fleisher LA, Fleischmann KE, Auerbach AD, Barnason SA, Beckman JA, Bozkurt B, Davila-Roman VG, Gerhard-Herman MD, Holly TA, Kane GC, Marine JE, Nelson MT, Spencer CC, Thompson A, Ting HH, Uretsky BF, Wijeysundera DN, American

College of Cardiology; American Heart Association. 2014 ACC/AHA guideline on perioperative cardiovascular evaluation and management of patients undergoing noncardiac surgery: a report of the American College of Cardiology/American Heart Association task force on practice guidelines. J Am Coll Cardiol. 2014;64(22):e77–e137.
44. Boersma E, Poldermans D, Bax JJ, et al. Predictors of cardiac events after major vascular surgery: role of clinical characteristics, dobutamine echocardiography, and beta-blocker therapy. JAMA. 2001;285:1865–73.
45. Poldermans D, Boersma E, Bax JJ, Thomson IR, van de Ven LL, Blankensteijn JD, Baars HF, Yo TI, Trocino G, Vigna C, Roelandt JR, van Urk H. The effect of bisoprolol on perioperative mortality and myocardial infarction in high-risk patients undergoing vascular surgery. Dutch echocardiographic cardiac risk evaluation applying stress echocardiography study group. N Engl J Med. 1999;341(24):1789–94.
46. Mangano DT, Layug EL, Wallace A, Tateo I. Effect of atenolol on mortality and cardiovascular morbidity after noncardiac surgery. Multicenter study of perioperative ischemia research group. N Engl J Med. 1996;335(23):1713–20.
47. Auerbach AD, Goldman L. β-blockers and reduction of cardiac events in noncardiac surgery. JAMA. 2002;287:1435–44.
48. Lindenauer PK, Fitzgerald J, Hoople N, Benjamin EM. The potential preventability of postoperative myocardial infarction: underuse of perioperative beta-adrenergic blockade. Arch Intern Med. 2004;164(7):762–6.
49. Brady AR, Gibbs JS, Greenhalgh RM, Powell JT, Sydes MR, POBBLE trial investigators. Perioperative beta-blockade (POBBLE) for patients undergoing infrarenal vascular surgery: results of a randomized double-blind controlled trial. J Vasc Surg. 2005;41(4):602–9.
50. Yang H, Raymer K, Butler R, Parlow J, Roberts R. The effects of perioperative beta-blockade: results of the Metoprolol after vascular surgery (MaVS) study, a randomized controlled trial. Am Heart J. 2006;152(5):983–90.
51. Devereaux PJ, Beattie WS, Choi PT, Badner NH, Guyatt GH, Villar JC, Cinà CS, Leslie K, Jacka MJ, Montori VM, Bhandari M, Avezum A, Cavalcanti AB, Giles JW, Schricker T, Yang H, Jakobsen CJ, Yusuf S. How strong is the evidence for the use of perioperative beta blockers in non-cardiac surgery? Systematic review and meta-analysis of randomised controlled trials. BMJ. 2005;331(7512):313–21.
52. Lindenauer PK, Pekow P, Wang K. Perioperative beta-blocker therapy and mortality after major noncardiac surgery. N Engl J Med. 2005;353:349–61.
53. Devereaux PJ, Yang H, Yusuf S, Guyatt G, Leslie K, Villar JC, et al. Effects of extended-release metoprolol succinate in patients undergoing non-cardiac surgery: a randomised controlled trial. Lancet. 2008;371:1839–47.
54. Priebe HJ. Perioperative myocardial infarction – aetilogy and prevention. Br J Anaesth. 2005;95:3–19.
55. Oleske DM, Wilson RS, Bernard BA. Epidemiology of injury in people with Alzheimer's disease. J Am Geriatr Soc. 1995;43:741–6.
56. Scalea TM, Simon HM, Duncan AO, et al. Geriatric blunt multiple trauma: improved survival with early invasive monitoring. J Trauma. 1990;30:129–34.
57. Eiferman DS, Davido HT, Howard JM, Gerckens J, Evans DC, Cook CH, Stawicki SP. Two methods of hemodynamic and volume status assessment in critically ill patients: a study of disagreement. J Intensive Care Med. 2016;31:113–7.
58. Kumar A, Anel R, Bunnell E, Habet K, Zanotti S, Marshall S, et al. Pulmonary artery occlusion pressure and central venous pressure fail to predict ventricular filling volume, cardiac performance or the response to volume infusion in normal subjects. Crit Care Med. 2004;3:691–9.
59. Boulain T, Achard JM, Teboul JL. Changes in BP induced by passive leg raising predict response to fluid loading in critically ill patients. Chest. 2002;121:1245–52.
60. Swan HJC, Ganz W, Forrester J. Catheterization of the heart in man with the use of a flow directed balloon-tipped catheter. N Engl J Med. 1970;283:447–51.
61. Harvey S, Harrison DA, Singer M, Ashcroft J, Jones CM, Elbourne D, Brampton W, Williams D, Young D, Rowan K, PAC-Man study collaboration. Assessment of the clinical effectiveness of pulmonary artery catheters in management of patients in intensive care (PAC-man): a randomised controlled trial. Lancet. 2005;366:472–7.
62. Wu AW, Rubin HR, Rosen MJ. Are elderly people less responsive to intensive care? J Am Geriatr Soc. 1990;38:621–7.
63. Sandham JD, Hull RD, Brant RF, Knox L, Pinero GF, Doig CJ, et al. A randomized, controlled trial of the use of pulmonary artery catheters in high risk surgical patients. NEJM. 2003;348:5–14.
64. Boyd O, Grounds RM, Bennett ED. A randomized clinical trial of the effect of deliberate perioperative increase of oxygen delivery on mortality in high-risk surgical patients. JAMA. 1993;270:2699–707.
65. Savino JA, Del Guercio LR. Preoperative assessment of high-risk surgical patients. Surg Clin North Am. 1985;65:763–91.
66. Connors AF Jr, Speroff T, Dawson NV, Thomas C, Harrell FE Jr, Wagner D, Desbiens N, Goldman L, Wu AW, Califf RM, Fulkerson WJ Jr, Vidaillet H, Broste S, Bellamy P, Lynn J, Knaus WA. The effectiveness of right heart catheterization in the initial care of critically ill patients. SUPPORT investigators. JAMA. 1996;276(11):889–97.
67. Polanczyk CA, Rohde LE, Goldman L, Cook EF, Thomas EJ, Marcantonio ER, et al. Right heart catheterization and cardiac complications in patients undergoing noncardiac surgery: an observational study. JAMA. 2001;286:309–14.
68. Shoemaker WC, Appel PL, Kram HB. Prospective trial of supranormal values of survivors as thera-

peutic goals in high risk surgical patients. Chest. 1988;94:1176–86.
69. Iberti TJ, Fischer EP, Leibowitz AB. A multicenter study of physicians' knowledge of the pulmonary artery catheter. Pulmonary artery catheter study group. JAMA. 1990;264:2928–32.
70. Reinhart K, Kuhn HJ, Hartog C. Continuous central venous and pulmonary artery oxygen saturation monitoring in the critically ill. Intensive Care Med. 2004;30:1572–8.
71. Goodrich C. Continuous central venous oximetry monitoring. Crit Care Nurs Clin North Am. 2006;18:203–9.
72. Martin C, Auffray JP, Badetti C, Perrin G, Papazian L, Gouin F. Monitoring of central venous oxygen saturation versus mixed venous oxygen saturation in critically ill patients. Intensive Care Med. 1992;18(2):101–4.
73. Rady MY, Rivers EP, Martin GB. Continuous central venous oximetry and shock index in the emergency department: use in the evaluation of clinical shock. Am J Emerg Med. 1992;10:538–41.
74. Scalea TM, Hartnett RW, Duncan AO, Atweh NA, Phillips TF, Sclafani SJ, et al. Central venous oxygen saturation: a useful clinical tool in trauma patients. J Trauma. 1990;30:1539–43.
75. Otto F. Die Grundform des arteriellen Pulses. Zeitung für Biologie. 1899;37:483–586.
76. Wesseling KH, Smith NT, Nichols WW. Beat-to-beat cardiac output from the arterial pressure pulse contour. In: Feldman SA, Leigh JM, Spierdijk J, editors. Measurement in anaesthesia. Leiden: Leiden University Press; 1974. p. 148–64.
77. Porhomayon J, El-Solh A, Papadakos P. Cardiac output monitoring devices: an analytic review. Intern Emerg Med. 2012;7:163–71.
78. Cannesson M, Attof Y, Rosamel P. Comparison of FloTrac cardiac output monitoring system in patients undergoing coronary artery bypass grafting with pulmonary artery cardiac output measurements. Eur J Anaesthesiol. 2007;24:832–9.
79. Button D, Weibel L, Reuthebuch O. Clinical evaluation of the FloTrac/Vigileo system and two established continuous cardiac output monitoring devices in patients undergoing cardiac surgery. Br J Anaesth. 2007;99:329–36.
80. Saraceni E, Rossi S, Persona P, Dan M, Rizzi S, Meroni M, et al. Comparison of two methods for cardiac output measurement in critically ill patients. Br J Anaesth. 2011;106:690–4.
81. Mayer J, Boldt J, Schöllhorn T, Röhm KD, Mengistu AM, Suttner S. Semi-invasive monitoring of cardiac output by a new device using arterial pressure waveform analysis: a comparison with intermittent pulmonary artery thermodilution in patients undergoing cardiac surgery. Br J Anaesth. 2007;98(2):176–82.
82. Boussat S, Jacques T, Levy B, Laurent E, Gache A, Capellier G, et al. Intravascular volume monitoring and extravascular lung water in septic patients with pulmonary edema. Intensive Care Med. 2002;28:712–8.
83. Bindels AJ, van der Hoeven JG, Graafland AD. Relationships between volume and pressure measurements and stroke volume in critically ill patients. Crit Care. 2000;4:193–9.
84. Della Rocca G, Costa MG, Coccia C, Pompei L, Di Marco P, Vilardi V, et al. Cardiac output monitoring: aortic transpulmonary thermodilution and pulse contour analysis agree with standard thermodilution methods in patients undergoing lung transplantation. Can J Anaesth. 2003;50:707–11.
85. Uchino S, Bellomo R, Morimatsu H, Sugihara M, French C, Stephens D, et al. PAC/PiCCO use and likelihood of success evaluation [PULSE] study group pulmonary artery catheter versus pulse contour analysis: a prospective epidemiological study. Crit Care. 2006;10:R174.
86. Michard F. Changes in arterial pressure during mechanical ventilation. Anesthesiology. 2005;103:419–28.
87. Hofer CK, Senn A, Weibel L. Assessment of stroke volume variation for prediction of fluid responsiveness using the modified FloTrac™ and PiCCOplus™ system. Crit Care. 2008;12:R82.
88. Berkenstadt H, Margalit N, Hadani M, Friedman Z, Segal E, Villa Y, et al. Stroke volume variation as a predictor of fluid responsiveness in patients undergoing brain surgery. Anesth Analg. 2001;92:984–9.
89. Suehiro K, Okutani R. Stroke volume variation as a predictor of fluid responsiveness in patients undergoing one-lung ventilation. J Cardiothorac Vasc Anesth. 2010;24:772–5.
90. Mehta Y, Arora D. Newer methods of cardiac output monitoring. World J Cardiol. 2014;6(9):1022–9.
91. Feissel M, Michard F, Faller JP. The respiratory variation in inferior vena cava diameter as a guide to fluid therapy. Intensive Care Med. 2004;30:1834–7.
92. Cecconi M, De Backer D, Antonelli M, Beale R, Bakker J, Hofer C, Jaeschke R, Mebazaa A, Pinsky MR, Teboul JL, Vincent JL, Rhodes A. Consensus on circulatory shock and hemodynamic monitoring. Task force of the European Society of Intensive Care Medicine. Intensive Care Med. 2014;40(12):1795–815.
93. Jensen MB, Sloth E, Larsen KM. Transthoracic echocardiography for cardiopulmonary monitoring in intensive care. Eur J Anaesthesiol. 2004;21:700–7.
94. Gunst M, Ghaemmaghami V, Sperry J, Robinson M, O'Keeffe T, Friese R, et al. Accuracy of cardiac function and volume status estimates using bedside echocardiographic assessment in trauma/critical care. J Trauma. 2008;65:509–16.
95. Ferrada P, Murthi S, Anand RJ. Transthoracic focused rapid echocardiographic examination: real-time evaluation of fluid status in critically ill trauma patients. J Trauma. 2011;70:56–62.
96. Murthi SB, Hess JR, Hess A. Focused rapid echocardiographic evaluation versus vascular catheter-based assessment of cardiac output and function in critically ill trauma patients. J Trauma. 2012;72:1158–64.

38 Nutrition Assessment and Therapy

Kimberly Joseph

Introduction

Elderly patients are at particularly high risk for malnutrition. The French National Authority for Health (HAS) in its 2007 guidelines for nutrition support in the elderly estimated that protein-energy malnutrition occurs in 4–10% of persons over 70 who live at home, 15–38% of those in institutional care, and 30–70% of those who are hospitalized [1]. Similar estimates have been made for the elderly population in America [2, 3]. Elderly patients may present with pre-existing functional limitations, including the capacity for volitional feeding. The elderly patient is also known to have reduced appetite, longer periods of illness/duration of hospital stay, higher infection rates, and delayed wound healing [4]. The addition of a traumatic injury and/or critical illness and subsequent catabolic stress in such patients only exacerbates what may be an already precarious situation. Literature specific to nutrition assessment and therapy in elderly trauma victims is limited; however, malnourished elderly patients with hip fractures have been noted to have increased morbidity [5]. A retrospective analysis that compared trauma and nontrauma patients as well as older vs. younger trauma patients [6] documented lower prescribed nutrition support and greater caloric deficits.

In 2016, the American Society for Parenteral and Enteral Nutrition (ASPEN) and the Society of Critical Care Medicine (SCCM) published updated guidelines for the assessment and provision of nutrition support therapy in adult critically ill patients [7]. The guidelines included updated and expanded recommendations for a variety of patient populations, including for trauma patient subsets such as general trauma, traumatic brain injury, burns, and patients with "open abdomens." The guidelines did not include grouped recommendations for geriatric populations specifically. Although aspects of the guideline recommendations can certainly be extrapolated for use in geriatric trauma patients, more work is needed to better define protocols for this population.

Physiologic and Metabolic Changes in the Elderly

Basal Metabolic Rate may decrease as much as 16% in elderly persons, accompanied by a redistribution of body content with higher fat and decreased lean body mass [8, 9]. Data from Weijs and colleagues [10] suggests that low skeletal muscle area is a risk factor for mortality in

K. Joseph, M.D., F.A.C.S., F.C.C.M
Department of Trauma and Burns, John H. Stroger Hospital of Cook County, 1900 W Polk St., Rm. 1300, Chicago, IL 60612, USA
e-mail: kjoseph@cookcountytrauma.org; kjtrauma@gmail.com

A. Rodriguez et al. (eds.), *Geriatric Trauma and Acute Care Surgery*,
https://doi.org/10.1007/978-3-319-57403-5_38

mechanically ventilated patients. Certain disease states, such as congestive heart failure, may incur on an elderly person persistent catabolic stress, impairing optimal nutritional status. Renal, pulmonary, and cardiac functions decline in elderly persons [11–15], all of which may influence metabolic, fluid, electrolyte, and nutritional status. Further complicating the picture is the likelihood of baseline dehydration, considered to be the most common fluid problem in older people [16–18]. The gastrointestinal tract is also affected: aging can result in the loss of cells in the myenteric plexus, decreased gastric emptying, increased gastrointestinal reflux, dysphagia, constipation, and inappropriately prolonged satiety [19–21]. Chronic gastritis and prolonged use of proton pump inhibitors may result in small bowel bacterial overgrowth and reduced absorption of micronutrients [22]. In animal studies, data suggests that aging may result in reduced gastric lipase and bile acid secretion along with decreased lipid solubility, and can result in decreased lipid absorption; the data in humans is less clear [23, 24]. Subclinical hypothyroidism is also seen in the elderly, although the indications for treatment remain controversial [25].

The risk for vitamin and nutrient deficiencies increases with aging. There has been much interest recently in vitamin D deficiency in many population subsets; in the elderly this deficiency is multifactorial and can be due to decreased appetite, the inability to masticate certain foods, and limited direct sunlight exposure. It is associated with muscle weakness, particularly in the proximal muscle groups, and has been associated with increased fall risk [26]. To prevent deficiency, vitamin D 600 IU daily should be added to the diet of elderly persons along with efforts to provide adequate exposure to sunlight. Vitamin B12 is another common deficiency seen in the elderly. Signs of B12 deficiency include anemia, neuropathy, and dementia [27]. The recommended daily allowance of B12 is 2.4 micrograms; elderly persons should try to obtain their B12 from either supplements or fortified foods. Vitamin K deficiency is less common, but may be associated with osteoporosis, osteoarthritis, and atherosclerosis [28]. Vitamin K supplementation is not recommended in patients receiving warfarin therapy, as it will counteract the anticoagulant effect of the drug. However, consideration should be given to its administration in the acutely ill trauma patient with evidence of coagulopathy. Supplementation with vitamin C, vitamin A, and zinc should be considered if would healing is of concern.

Estimating Energy Requirements

Indirect calorimetry is still considered the "gold standard" for estimating resting energy expenditure and caloric needs in ICU patients. This methodology is relatively expensive and not widely available; its use in trauma patients may be problematic as well if the patient has a chest tube or any other source of air leak. The ASPEN/SCCM guidelines recommend the use of Indirect Calorimetry when available; in its absence, the guidelines recommend the use of a weight-based equation (25–30 kcal/kg/day). Other predictive equations and protein markers are not believed to be as effective at estimating energy requirements [7, 29]. In addition to caloric needs, practitioners should consider evaluation for and replacement of vitamin and micronutrient deficiencies. Caloric and protein requirements must also be adjusted in the presence of obesity and potentially for the mechanism and severity of injury in a trauma or burn patient. Table 38.1 summarizes nutritional requirements that should be considered.

Table 38.1 Calorie, protein, and nutrient requirements

Variable	Baseline ICU patient	Trauma ICU patient with wound	Burn patient	Obese trauma ICU patient with wound
Energy requirements, calories	IC or 25–30 kcal/kg/day	IC or 25–30 kcal/kg/day	IC or Toronto equation	BMI 30–50: 11–14 kcal/kg/day, ABW
				BMI ≥50: 22–25 kcal/kg/day, IBW
Protein	1.2–2.0 g/kg/day	1.5–2.0 g/kg/day	1.5–2.0 g/kg/day	BMI 30–40: 2 g/kg/day
				BMI ≥50: up to 2.5 g/kg/day
IVF	25–30 mL/kg/day	Variable: increased with open abdomen, acute resuscitation	Based on TBSA	Variable: increased with open abdomen, acute resuscitation
Vitamin D	600 IU/day	600 IU/day	600 IU/day	600 IU/day
Vitamin B12	2.4 mcg/day	2.4 mcg/day	2.4 mcg/day	2.4 mcg/day
Vitamin C	200–400 mg/day	500 mg/day	500 mg/day	500 mg/day
Vitamin A	2300–3000 IU/day	2300–3000 IU/day	2300–3000 IU/day	2300–3000 IU/day
Zinc	2.5–5 mg/day	2.5–5 mg/day	2.5–5 mg/day	2.5–5 mg/day

IC indirect calorimetry, *ABW* actual body weight, *IBW* ideal body weight, *IVF* intravenous fluid, *IU* international units, *mcg* micrograms, *mg* milligrams

Nutrition Risk Assessment: Screening Tools

In 2012, ASPEN and the Academy of Nutrition and Dietetics released a consensus statement on characteristics recommended for use in the identification of malnutrition [30], expanding the concept to factor in sequelae of inflammation. Nutrition risk assessment should include consideration of disease states that result in chronic inflammation (e.g., obesity, rheumatoid arthritis) as well as those that lead to significant acute inflammation (e.g., trauma, burns, closed head injury, sepsis). In elderly patients, consideration should also be given to the existence of comorbidities.

A variety of screening tools exist to assess nutritional status, some of which are validated in elderly populations. None of these are trauma-specific; however, some have been validated in critically ill patient populations. Examples of widely used screening tools include:

Mini Nutritional Assessment (*MNA*): initially an 18-item questionnaire [31] that was condensed into a shorter version (MNA-SF) that includes assessment of appetite, intake, weight loss, history of psychological stress or acute disease, and BMI (or calf circumference if BMI not available). This tool was specifically developed to assess elderly patients.

Nutrition Risk Screening (*NRS 2002*): consists of a two-part assessment process, the first part assessing BMI, weight loss/decreased intake, or the presence of severe illness. Any positive finding in the initial screen is followed by an assessment of the degree of malnutrition; a mildly malnourished patient might be one with a hip fracture not requiring ICU care or who has mildly decreased food intake. A moderate score would be obtained in a patient with severe pneumonia or

Table 38.2 Comparison of nutrition risk assessment tools

Factors→	Weight loss	Food intake	BMI	Illness acuity, severity	Age	Validated in elderly	Validated in critical illness	Can use without history information
Tool↓	–	–	–	–	–	–	–	–
MNA	√	√	√	√	√	√		
MUST	√		√	√		√	√	
GNRI			√	√	√	√	√	√
NRS2002	√	√	√	√			√	√
NUTRIC				√	√		√	√

MNA Mini Nutritional Assessment, *MUST* Malnutrition Universal Screening tool, *GNRI* Geriatric Nutrition Risk Index, *NRS 2002* Nutrition Risk Score 2002, *NUTRIC* Nutrition Risk in Critically Ill, *BMI* Body Mass Index

who has had major abdominal surgery. A patient with rapid weight loss, significant decrease in recent food intake, or requiring ICU care would be classified as severely malnourished [32].

Malnutrition Universal Screening Tool (*MUST*): takes into account BMI, weight loss, and acute disease effect (patient is acutely ill and is unlikely to have volitional nutritional intake for >5 days) and has been used to predict hospital length of stay and mortality in acutely ill elderly patients [33].

Geriatric Nutrition Risk Index (*GNRI*): risk assessment formula incorporating ideal body weight (IBW), weight loss, and albumin [34], used as a proxy for chronic illness severity.

Nutrition Risk in Critically Ill (*NUTRIC*) *score* [35]: developed specifically for ICU patients, it factors in age, Acute Physiologic and Chronic Health Evaluation (APACHE II) and Sequential Organ Failure Assessment (SOFA) scores, comorbidities, days from hospital to ICU admission, and Interleukin-6 (IL-6) levels; a modification exists which leaves out the IL-6 measurement.

Table 38.2 compares the attributes of the above screening tools.

The current ASPEN/SCCM guidelines suggest the use of a validated screening tool such as the NRS-2002 or NUTRIC score to evaluate any patient admitted to the ICU in whom volitional intake is anticipated to be insufficient [7]. Tripathy and Mishra studied 111 elderly ICU patients and compared the utility of the MUST vs. the GNRI [36]; they determined that either scoring system was valid for use in that population, although the MUST appeared easier to use.

Another assessment concept that is gaining in popularity is the measurement of muscle mass by computed tomography (CT) scan [37]. A study of elderly ICU patients who had admission abdominal CT scans [38] demonstrated correlation between muscle mass at the L3 level and ventilator-free days and mortality. The advantage of such a technique is that it could be repeated to evaluate progress of nutritional therapy; however, it also requires repeated patient radiographic exposure.

Nutrition Therapy Monitoring

Multiple validated tools exist to assess nutrition risk as noted above. The techniques to monitor adequacy of delivery of nutrition therapy, other than indirect calorimetry, are more controversial. Literature regarding monitoring of adequate delivery of nutrition support has tended to focus on whether or not the delivered therapy met the original prescription. However, this presumes that the original estimates of overall caloric and protein requirements are correct and adequate. McClave et al. noted that volume-based enteral feeding protocols resulted in a higher percentage of delivery of goal calories [39]. However, no data was collected on morbidity, length of stay, etc. Improved nutrient delivery has also been reported with the PEP uP protocol by Heyland [40]. CT scanning, used to evaluate sarcopenia on admission, may be useful as a monitoring tool for adequacy of therapy; issues regarding recurrent radiation exposure and confounders such as degree of mobility will need to be considered as protocols are developed.

Timing and Route of Nutrition Therapy

Several studies were published in the 1980s and 1990s making the case for early enteral nutrition in trauma patients. The patients studied tended to be younger patients who sustained penetrating trauma. Results suggested that enteral nutrition was preferable to parenteral nutrition and that early enteral nutrition resulted in decreased septic morbidity [41–43]. Provision of nutrients directly into the small intestine has been demonstrated to maintain mucosal integrity and to support the cells that make up the gut-associated lymphoid tissue (GALT), decreasing overall gut permeability [44, 45]. The current ASPEN/SCCM guidelines recommend the initiation of enteral nutrition within 24–48 h in high-risk critically ill and trauma patients as long as the patient is hemodynamically stable [7]. The guidelines further recommend that high-risk patients (e.g., a high NRS 2002 or NUTRIC score) in the ICU should have enteral feedings increased to the prescribed goal as soon as feasible. Until recently, the literature seemed weighted towards delaying initiation of parenteral nutrition for 5–7 days in ICU patients [46]; however, data from recent trials suggests that provision of parenteral nutrition within 24–36 h of ICU admission may not result in adverse consequences [47, 48], and perhaps should be considered in high-risk patients if enteral nutrition is not expected to be possible/tolerated.

Nutrition Therapy Components

Like their younger counterparts, geriatric trauma and critically ill patients require adequate macronutrient and micronutrient provision. Based on a variety of studies, the ASPEN/SCCM guidelines place particular emphasis on provision of adequate protein [7]. For medical ICU patients, doses in the range of 1.2–2.0 g/kg/day are recommended, with higher doses suggested for trauma and burn patients [7]. More controversial is the provision of what is often termed "immunonutrition" or "immune-modulating" nutrition. Early studies done in trauma patients suggested that enteral nutrition modulated with antioxidants, nucleotides, and glutamine resulted in improved outcomes [49]. The more recent REDOXS trial called into question the safety of glutamine in patients admitted to the ICU with organ failure [50]; however, the majority of the study patients were medical patients, and the study used doses of glutamine that had not been routinely employed in trauma patients. The implications for trauma patients, particularly those with penetrating trauma and bowel injuries, remain unclear. A randomized trial in burn patients demonstrated reduction in gram-negative bacteremia in severely burned patients receiving enteral glutamine [51]. The ASPEN/SCCM guidelines recommend that immune-modulating formulas, with an emphasis on arginine and fish oils, be considered in traumatic brain injury patients, perioperative surgical ICU patients, and severely injured trauma patients [7].

Special Considerations

Sepsis: The definitions for sepsis are being updated currently, but it is not anticipated that recommendations regarding nutrition therapy will change. The ASPEN/SCCM guidelines recommend that enteral nutrition be initiated as soon as possible after the patient is hemodynamically stable. Parenteral nutrition should be avoided in the acute septic phase regardless of nutrition risk, as should immune-modulating formulas [7].

Obesity: The ASPEN/SCCM guidelines recommend that "hypocaloric" nutrition therapy be considered in critically ill/injured obese patients, with preservation of protein administration. In the absence of indirect calorimetry, 11–14 kcal/kg/d based on *actual body weight* is recommended for patients with BMI 30–50; for patients with BMI > 50, the recommendation is for 22–25 kcal/kg/day based on *ideal body weight.* 2 g/kg ideal body weight/day of protein should be provided to patients with BMI 30–40 and as much as 2.5 g/kg/day ideal body weight for patients with BMI ≥50 [7].

Early Mobility and Nutrition Therapy: early mobilization protocols in the ICU are thought to decrease delirium and prevent ICU-acquired weakness, among other complications [52]. Protocols are being developed to pair intensive nutrition and physical therapy to evaluate possible synergies. For the "Chronically Critically Ill" (expected to stay in the ICU for more than 21 days), the ASPEN/SCCM guidelines recommend aggressive enteral nutrition therapy in combination with a resistance exercise program [7].

Burn patients: there is controversy regarding how to assess energy requirements in burn patients when indirect calorimetry is not available. The ASPEN/SCCM guidelines recommend the standard weight-based equation; however, the European Society for Parenteral and Enteral Nutrition recommends that use of the Toronto equation be considered in adult severely burned patients [53].

End of Life Considerations: specific therapies are secondary to determining the wishes of the patient and the family involved. Artificial Nutrition and Hydration (ANH) are not obligatory in futile cases; effective communication, including provision of accurate information and mindful listening, are crucial in order to avoid confusion and discomfort.

Summary

Geriatric trauma patients present both an assessment and management challenge to the practitioner. Assessment tools that take age into account are not trauma-specific, and much of the literature regarding provision of therapy in critically ill patients is not directed specifically at the elderly. It is important to be cognizant of characteristics that are more likely to be seen in elderly patients—declining organ function, baseline nutrient and fluid abnormalities, and, perhaps most relevant to nutrition therapy, loss of lean body mass. Patients who are assessed to be high risk should have early enteral nutrition if possible; consideration may be given to starting parenteral nutrition earlier if it is anticipated the patient will not be able to tolerate enteral nutrition. Frequent re-evaluation of the patient's status is necessary to ensure that adequate nutrient delivery is maintained. By culling pertinent recommendations from the existing literature, it should be possible to tailor an appropriate nutrition therapy plan for the elderly trauma patient (Fig. 38.1).

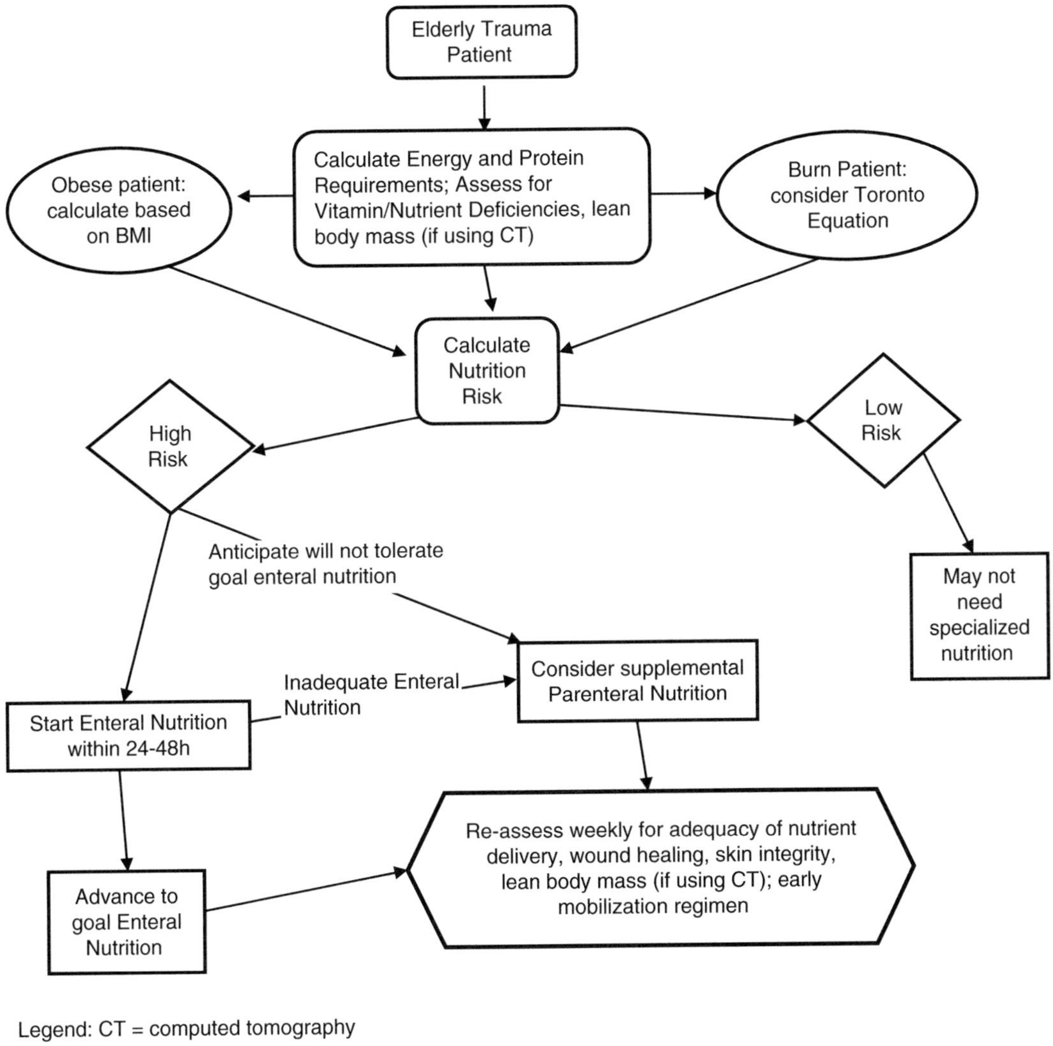

Fig. 38.1 An approach to nutrition therapy in elderly trauma patient. *Legend*: *CT* computed tomography

References

1. Raynaud-Simon A, Revel-Delhom C, Hébuterne X, French Nutrition and Health Program, French Health High Authority. Clinical practice guidelines from the French Health high authority: nutritional support strategy in protein-energy malnutrition in the elderly. Clin Nutr. 2011;30(3):312–9.
2. Guigoz Y, Lauque S, Vellas BJ. Identifying the elderly at risk for malnutrition. The Mini nutritional assessment. Clin Geriatr Med. 2002;18(4):737–57.
3. Saka B, Kaya O, Ozturk GB, Erten N, Karan MA. Malnutrition in the elderly and its relationship with other geriatric syndromes. Clin Nutr. 2010;29(6):745–8.
4. Feldblum I, German L, Castel H, HarmanBoehm I, Bilenko N, Eisinger M, et al. Characteristics of undernourished older medical patients and the identification of predictors for undernutrition status. Nutr J. 2007;6:37.
5. Symeonidis PD, Clark D. Assessment of malnutrition in hip fracture patients: effects on surgical delay, hospital stay and mortality. Acta Orthop Belg. 2006;72(4):420–7.
6. Wade CE, Kozar RA, Dyer CB, Bulger EM, Mourtzakis M, Heyland DK. Evaluation of nutrition deficits in adult and elderly trauma patients. JPEN J Parenter Enteral Nutr. 2015;39(4):449–55.
7. McClave SA, Taylor BE, Martindale RG, Warren MM, Johnson DR, Braunschweig C, McCarthy MS, Davanos E, Rice TW, Cresci GA, Gervasio JM, Sacks GS, Roberts PR, Compher C, Society of Critical Care Medicine; American Society for Parenteral and Enteral Nutrition. Guidelines for the Provision and Assessment of Nutrition Support Therapy in the Adult Critically Ill patient: Society of Critical Care Medicine (SCCM) and American Society for Parenteral and Enteral Nutrition (A.S.P.E.N.). JPEN J Parenter Enteral Nutr. 2016;40(2):159–211.
8. Busse EW. How mind, body, and environment influence nutrition in the elderly. Postgrad Med. 1978;63(3):118–22. 125
9. Thompson M. Geriatric nutrition. J Natl Med Assoc. 1980;72(8):795–7. 801-803
10. Weijs PJ, Looijaard WG, Dekker IM, Stapel SN, Girbes AR, Oudemans-van Straaten HM, Beishuizen A. Low skeletal muscle area is a risk factor for mortality in mechanically ventilated critically ill patients. Crit Care. 2014;18(2):R12.
11. Ramly E, Kaafarani HMA, Vlehamos GC. The effect of aging on pulmonary function implications for monitoring and support of the surgical and trauma patient. Surg Clin N Am. 2015;95(1):53–69.
12. Gulshan S, Goodwin J. Effect of aging on respiratory system physiology and immunology. Clin Interv Aging. 2006;1(3):253–60.
13. Baldea AJ. Effect of aging on renal function plus monitoring and support. Surg Clin N Am. 2015;95(1):71–83.
14. Weinstein JR, Anderson M. The aging kidney: physiologic changes. Adv Chronic Kidney Dis. 2010;17(4):302–7.
15. Martin RS, Farrah JP, Chang MC. The effect of aging on cardiac function plus monitoring and support. Surg Clin N Am. 2015;95(1):23–35.
16. Bossingham MJ, Carnell NS, Campbell WW. Water balance, hydration status, and fat-free mass hydration in younger and older adults. Am J Clin Nutr. 2005;81:1342–50.
17. Bennett JA, Thomas V, Riegel B. Unrecognized chronic dehydration in older adults: examining prevalence rate and risk factors. J Geront Nurs. 2004;30(11):22–8.
18. Mentes J. Oral hydration in older adults. Am J Nurs. 2006;106(6):40–9.
19. Nohra E, Bochicchio GV. Management of the gastrointestinal tract and nutrition in the geriatric surgical patient. Surg Clin N Am. 2015;95:85–101.
20. Morley JE. Pathophysiology of the anorexia of aging. Curr Opin Clin Nutr Metab Care. 2013;16(1):27–32.
21. Chapman IM. The anorexia of aging. Clin Geriatr Med. 2007;23(4):735–56.
22. Elphick HL, Elphick DA, Sanders DS. Small bowel bacterial overgrowth. An under-recognized cause of malnutrition in older adults. Geriatrics. 2006;61(9):21–6.
23. Holt PR, Balint JA. Effects of aging on intestinal lipid absorption. Am J Phys. 1993;264(1):G1–6.
24. Peachey SE, Dawson JM, Harper EJ. The effect of ageing on nutrient digestibility by cats fed beef tallow-, sunflower oil- or olive oil-enriched diets. Growth Dev Aging. 1999;63(1):61–70.
25. Gesing A. The thyroid gland and the process of aging. Thyroid Res. 2015;8(Suppl 1):A8.
26. Janssen HCJP, Samson MM, Verhaar HJJ. Vitamin D deficiency, muscle function, and falls in elderly people. Am J Clin Nutr. 2002;75(4):611–5.
27. Baik HW, Russell RM. Vitamin B12 deficiency in the elderly. Annu Rev Nutr. 1999;19:357–77.
28. Booth SL, Vitamin K. Status in the elderly. Curr Opin Clin Nutr Metab Care. 2007;29(5):21–8.
29. Ferrie S, Allman-Farinelli M. Commonly used "nutrition" indicators do not predict outcome in the critically ill: a systematic review. Nutr Clin Pract. 2013;28(4):463–84.
30. White JV, Guenter P, Jensen G, Malone A, Schofield M, Academy of Nutrition and Dietetics

Malnutrition Work Group; A.S.P.E.N. Malnutrition Task Force; A.S.P.E.N. Board of Directors. Consensus statement of the Academy of Nutrition and Dietetics/American Society for Parenteral and Enteral Nutrition: characteristics recommended for the identification and documentation of adult malnutrition (undernutrition). J Acad Nutr Diet. 2012;112(5):730–8.
31. Guigoz Y, Vellas B, Garry PJ. Mini- nutritional assessment: a practical assessment tool for grading the nutritional state of elderly patients. Facts Res Gerontol. 1994;4(suppl 2):15–59.
32. Kondrup J, Rasmussen HH, Hamberg O, Stanga Z, Ad Hoc ESPEN Working Group. Nutritional risk screening (NRS 2002): a new method based on an analysis of controlled clinical trials. Clin Nutr. 2003;22(3):321–36.
33. Stratton RJ, King CL, Stroud MA, Jackson AA, Elia M. Malnutrition Universal screening tool predicts mortality and length of hospital stay in acutely ill elderly. Br J Nutr. 2006;95(2):325–30.
34. Bouillane O, Morineau G, Dupont C, Coulombel I, Vincent J-P, Nicolis I, Benazeth S, Cynober L, Aussel C. Geriatric nutritional risk index: a new index for evaluating at-risk elderly medical patients. Am J Clin Nutr. 2005;82(4):777–83.
35. Heyland DK, Dhaliwal R, Jiang X, Day AG. Identifying critically ill patients who benefit the most from nutrition therapy: the development and initial validation of a novel risk assessment tool. Crit Care. 2011;15(6):R268.
36. Tripathy S, Mishra JC. Assessing nutrition in the critically ill elder patient: a comparison of two screening tools. Indian J Crit Care Med. 2015;19(9):518–22.
37. Prado CM, Heymsfield SB. Lean tissue imaging: a new era for nutritional assessment and intervention. JPEN J Parenter Enteral Nutr. 2014;38(8):940–53.
38. Moisey LL, Mourtzakis M, Cotton BA, Premji T, Heyland DK, Wade CE, Bulger E, Kozar RA, Nutrition and Rehabilitation Investigators Consortium (NUTRIC). Skeletal muscle predicts ventilator-free days, ICU-free days, and mortality in elderly ICU patients. Crit Care. 2013;17(5):R206.
39. McClave SA, Saad MA, Esterle M, Jotautas AE, Glen A, Franklin GA, Heyland DK, Hurt RT. Volume-based feeding in the critically ill patient. JPEN J Parenter Enteral Nutr. 2015;39(6):707–12.
40. Heyland DK, Dhaliwal R, Lemieux M, Wang M, Day AG. Implementing the PEP uP protocol in critical care units in Canada: results of a multicenter, quality improvement study. JPEN J Parenter Enteral Nutr. 2015;39(6):698–706.
41. Moore EE, Jones TN. Benefits of immediate Jejunostomy feeding after major abdominal trauma- a prospective, randomized study. J Trauma. 1986;26(10):874–81.
42. Kudsk KA, Croce MA, Fabian TC, Minard G, et al. Enteral vs parenteral feeding: effects of septic morbidity after blunt and penetrating abdominal trauma. Ann Surg. 1992;215(5):503–11.
43. Moore FA, Feliciano DV, Andrassy RJ, McArdle AH, et al. Enteral feeding, compared with parenteral, reduces postoperative septic complications: results of a meta-analysis. Ann Surg. 1992;216(2):172–83.
44. Kudsk KA. Current aspects of mucosal immunology and its influence by nutrition. Am J Surg. 2002;183(4):390–8.
45. Jabbar A, Chang WK, Dryden GW, McClave SA. Gut immunology and the differential response to feeding and starvation. Nutr Clin Pract. 2003;18(6):461–82.
46. Casaer MP, Mesotten D, Hermans G, Wouters PJ, et al. Early versus late parenteral nutrition in critically ill adults. N Engl J Med. 2011;356(6):506–17.
47. Doig GS, Simpson F, Sweetman EA, Finfer S, et al. Early parenteral nutrition in critically ill patients with short-term relative contraindications to early enteral nutrition. JAMA. 2013;309(20):2130–8.
48. Harvey SE, Parrott F, Harrison DA, Bear DE, Segaran E, Beale R, Bellingan G, Leonard R, Mythen MG, Rowan KM, CALORIES Trial Investigators. Trial of the route of early nutritional support in critically ill adults. N Engl J Med. 2014;71(18):1673–84.
49. Moore FA, Moore EE, Kudsk KA, Brown RO, et al. Clinical benefits of an immune enhancing diet for early post-injury enteral feeding. J Trauma. 1994;37(4):607–15.
50. Heyland D, Muscedere J, Wischmeyer PE, Cook D, Jones G, Albert M, Elke G, Berger MM, Day AG, Canadian Critical Care Trials Group. A randomized trial of glutamine and antioxidants in critically ill patients. N Engl J Med. 2013;368(16):1489–97.
51. Wischmeyer PE, Lynch J, Liede J, Wolfson R, Riehm J, Gottlieb L, Kahana M. Glutamine administration reduces gram-negative bacteremia in severely burned patients: a prospective, randomized, double-blind trial versus isonitrogenous control. Crit Care Med. 2001;29:2075–2080a.
52. Hodgson CL, Berney S, Harrold M, Saxena M, Bellomo R. Clinical review: early patient mobilization in the ICU. Crit Care. 2013;17(1):207.
53. Rousseau A-F, Losser M-R, Ichai C, Berger MM. ESPEN endorsed recommendations: nutrition therapy in major burns. Clin Nutr. 2013;32(4):497–502.

Acute Kidney Injury (AKI)

39

Ajai Malhotra

Introduction

Kidneys perform a multitude of essential functions within the human body. Of these the most important are (1) maintaining pH through regulation of acid/base levels and (2) excreting end products of metabolism. These functions are especially important for healing following trauma and/or surgery. The essential functions of the kidney take place in two distinct yet connected microscopic entities within the renal parenchyma—glomerulus and the tubules. The process of removing the end products of metabolism starts with the glomerular capillaries filtering the blood and passing the filtrate onto the renal tubules. One of the measures of renal function is the glomerular filtration rate (GFR)—volume of fluid passing from the glomerulus onto the renal tubules per minute. Within the renal tubules two processes control what is excreted in the urine: (1) selective reabsorption by which almost 99% of the filtrate volume is reabsorbed back into the circulation and (2) active secretion from the blood into the tubules of substances that are to be excreted, creatinine being one of them. Through glomerular filtration and tubular active secretion, nearly all the creatinine in the renal artery blood is removed with hardly any present in the renal veins. Thus creatinine clearance rate (CCR) defined as the volume of blood cleared of creatinine per minute closely approximates the GFR and is commonly used as a measure of GFR, which is more difficult to directly measure. Normal values of CCR are given in Table 39.1. There are gender differences in CCR, being lower in females likely due to their lower average muscle mass, which is the principal source of creatinine.

There are major morphologic changes that occur in the kidney with increasing age (Table 39.2). These morphologic changes directly affect renal function. The renal blood flow declines to half by age 80 from its peak at age 20 with a progressive decline in GFR. This decline in GFR is manifested by decrease in CCR that is maximum at age 20 and, on average, declines by about 6.5 mL/min per decade post age 20 [1].

Table 39.1 Normal values for renal function measurements by age and gender

Parameter	Value
Serum creatinine	Adult males: 0.6–1.2 mg/dL
	Adult females: 0.5–1.1 mg/dL
	Teen: 0.5–1.0 mg/dL
	Child: 0.3–0.7 mg/dL
Creatinine Clearance Rate (CCR)	Adult male (<40 years): 107–139 mL/min
	Adult female (<40 years): 87–107 mL/min

A. Malhotra, M.D.
Acute Care Surgery,
University of Vermont College of Medicine,
Burlington, VT, USA
e-mail: ajai.malhotra@uvmhealth.org

A. Rodriguez et al. (eds.), *Geriatric Trauma and Acute Care Surgery*,
https://doi.org/10.1007/978-3-319-57403-5_39

Table 39.2 Morphologic changes in the kidney with age

Morphologic change	Quantification
Loss of renal mass	20–25% loss by age 80
Loss of functioning glomeruli and glomerulosclerosis	30–50% loss by age 70
Decreased tubular number and size and increased fibrosis	
Thickened basement membranes of capillaries and tubules	
Increased arteriosclerosis and decreased afferent arteriolar lumen	

Table 39.3 RIFLE criteria for renal dysfunction

Category	Serum Cr/GFR criteria	Urine output criteria
Risk	Cr increase ×1.5 above baseline	<0.5 mL/kg/h for 6 h
	GFR decline by >25%	
Injury	Cr increase ×2 above baseline	<0.3 mL/kg/h for 24 h
	GFR decline by >50%	
Failure	Cr increase ×3 above baseline	<0.3 mL/kg/h for 24 h or anuria
	GFR decline by 75%	
Loss	Persistent AKI for >4 weeks	
End stage	AKI for >3 months	

Sensitivity for AKI is highest for "risk" category and specificity highest for "end stage" category

The overall impact of these changes is loss of renal concentrating and diluting ability, decreased ability to conserve sodium, lower levels of renin and aldosterone with decreased prostaglandin production and an enhanced vasoconstrictive response leading to increased susceptibility to ischemia and nephrotoxic medications [2]. One of the important reasons of poorer tolerance to injury and surgery among elderly is the decline in renal function and reserve.

Acute renal failure is the term that was utilized in the past to describe injury to the kidney resulting in the kidney unable to perform its essential functions. Usually renal failure is associated with oliguria (urine output <20 mL/h—oliguric renal failure), though it can be observed with more normal or even excessive urine output (non-oliguric renal failure). Multiple studies demonstrated that the development of acute renal failure was associated with a 50% increase in the relative risk of inhospital mortality. More recently it has been realized that even smaller insults to the kidneys that do not result in overt acute renal failure can adversely affect outcomes [3, 4]. Hence the concept and term acute renal failure has been replaced by RIFLE criteria, which encompasses a spectrum of renal dysfunction from "risk" of damage to overt "end stage" renal failure with AKI in the middle of that spectrum. RIFLE includes both urinary output criteria and metabolic criteria (Serum creatinine or GFR) (Table 39.3) [5]. At the "risk" category, the sensitivity for injury is high though the specificity relatively poor. Hence patients diagnosed at risk *may* have suffered renal injury, but if not meeting the risk criteria, the probability of renal injury is very low. These criteria have been shown to correlate with outcomes [6, 7].

While the outcome of any patient who develops AKI is worse, multiple studies and meta-analysis have demonstrated that the incidence of AKI is higher and the degree to which AKI adversely impacts outcomes is more pronounced in the elderly [8, 9].

Causes of AKI

Causes of AKI are multitude and are classified into prerenal, renal, and post-renal (Table 39.4). Prerenal denotes a reduction in renal perfusion either total perfusion in terms of volume and/or reduction in perfusion pressure. This leads to the kidney being unable to perform its function even though there is no inherent renal pathology. Renal causes are those where the kidney does not perform its function due to inherent renal disease either acute or chronic. Post-renal includes any disease or condition causing an obstruction to the free flow of urine from the renal collecting system down to the external urethral meatus. Large majority (>75%) of patients with AKI encountered in the surgical intensive care unit (ICU) are either hypovolemia causing prerenal AKI, or acute tubular necrosis (ATN) causing renal AKI.

Table 39.4 Cases of various forms of AKI—prerenal, renal and post-renal

Prerenal	Hypovolemia from blood/fluid losses
	Hemorrhage
	Gastro-intestinal: Vomiting, diarrhea, GI fistula, etc.
	Urinary: Diuretics, salt wasting states, adrenal insufficiency, etc.
	Cutaneous: Burns, excessive sweating, etc.
	Third spacing: Sepsis, pancreatitis, postoperative, etc.
	Reduced "effective" circulating volume
	Hypoalbuminemia
	Cirrhosis
	Cardiac failure
	Failure of "auto-regulation"
	Use of NSAIDS or ACE inhibitors
Renal	Vascular
	Large vessel: occlusion of bilateral renal artery/vein
	Small vessel: intrarenal micro-angiopathic occlusions
	Thrombotic-thrombocytopenic purpura, hemolytic uremic syndrome, etc.
	Glomerular dysfunction: glomerulonephritis
	Acute tubular necrosis (ATN)
	All prerenal causes when prolonged
	Nephrotoxic agents
	Acute interstitial nephritis (AIN)
	Allergic reactions to medications
	Certain infections: Brucellosis, Epstein–Barr virus, etc.
Post-renal	Genitourinary malignancy: prostate, urinary bladder
	Urinary stone disease
	Acute papillary necrosis, e.g., due to NSAID use

Prerenal AKI

In surgical patients with prerenal AKI, the cause is most often related to reduction in effective circulating volume either due to blood loss or redistribution. The later occurs in ill patients from systemic inflammation and loss of intravascular volume into the interstitial space. It can also occur in patients with heart failure where, while there is overall fluid retention, the intravascular volume is depleted. Auto-regulatory mechanisms present within the kidneys allow them to function despite reduced perfusion, but these mechanisms too are less effective with age, can be overwhelmed by extreme reduction in perfusion, and can be interfered with. These auto-regulatory pathways are dependent upon chemical signaling involving prostaglandins and renin–angiotensin II pathway. Thus use of nonsteroidal anti-inflammatory medications affecting the production of prostaglandins and ACE inhibitors interfering with the renin pathway adversely affect auto-regulation and can cause severe AKI in an at-risk patient [10, 11].

Reduced renal perfusion directly leads to a reduction in GFR. Less filtrate reaching the tubules results in increased reabsorption of urea causing an increase in blood urea nitrogen (BUN). Since creatinine is principally secreted into the tubular lumen and is less dependent upon glomerular filtration, creatinine rise is limited in prerenal AKI. This leads to a higher BUN/creatinine ratio (>20) in prerenal AKI. Although this elevated ratio is a strong pointer to prerenal AKI, by itself it is not diagnostic since it could be elevated in hyper-catabolic states as well. The sine qua non of prerenal AKI is the intense conservation of Na and water by the kidneys. This is demonstrated by oliguria, highly concentrated urine (urine osmolality >500 mOsm/kg) with very low Na concentration (usually <10 mEq/L) and low fractional excretion of Na ($FE_{Na} < 1\%$—see below).

Renal AKI

Renal AKI results from reduced renal function as a result of renal parenchymal disease. These states may be classified as vascular, glomerular, and tubulointerstitial. Vascular causes include bilateral occlusions of the major renal vessels (renal artery and/or vein) or widespread microscopic thrombosis of intrarenal vasculature occurring in a variety of syndromes (thrombotic thrombocytopenic purpura, hemolytic uremic syndrome, etc.). Glomerular dysfunction is seen in the multiple types of acute glomerulonephritis that lead to renal dysfunction. Glomerular and vascular causes of renal AKI are quite rare in the surgical ICU and beyond the scope of this text. The large majority of renal AKI observed in this setting are caused by tubulointerstitial disease—acute tubular necrosis (ATN) and acute interstitial nephritis (AIN).

ATN is by far the most common form of renal AKI. Pathologically ATN is associated with (1) necrosis and sloughing of the epithelial cells lining the lumen of the tubules causing obstruction; (2) back leak of the filtrate into the circulation through the disrupted tubular epithelium; and (3) reduced glomerular blood flow likely due to afferent arterial vasoconstriction. These three together result in severe renal dysfunction associated with significant rise in the serum BUN and creatinine with a BUN/Cr ratio of <20. Additionally, the sloughed off epithelial cells from the tubular lumen make their way down the urinary passage and can appear on urinalysis as cellular casts. Since renal function is directly affected, the urine is usually not concentrated and has osmolality that is similar to plasma. For the same reason, the kidneys fail to conserve Na and hence FE_{Na} is elevated to >3%. As noted above, reduction in renal perfusion leads to prerenal AKI that is often rapidly reversible by improving renal perfusion. When the reduced perfusion is severe it leads to ATN where recovery is slower since the epithelial lining of the tubules has to be regenerated [12]. A rare but very severe form of AKI is caused by bilateral acute cortical necrosis (ACN). Unlike ATN, where the tubules are primarily affected and glomeruli spared, in ACN both the tubules and glomeruli are affected by the necrotic process. The inciting event is usually very severe shock from any cause though majority of cases are seen in association with obstetric emergencies—placental abruption, amniotic fluid embolism, toxemia of pregnancy, etc. Pathologically there are fibrin thrombi within the capillary beds of the kidney with necrosis. Severe oliguria is the norm with CAN and unlike ATN recovery is uncommon.

AIN can be caused by multiple disorders and is characterized by acute inflammation of the renal interstitium and tubules. The nature of the interstitial infiltrate is dependent upon the primary condition. Since AIN is often seen as an allergic reaction to medications, it is associated with eosinophilic infiltrate within the renal parenchyma and cutaneous manifestations. It can also be caused by some rare infections such as brucellosis and Epstein–Barr viral infection.

Post-renal AKI

Post-renal AKI is also known as "obstructive uropathy." It is caused by complete obstruction to urinary outflow. For a patient to develop post-renal AKI, the obstruction needs to be complete or near complete and affect both kidneys. Long-standing partial obstruction can lead to inability of the kidneys to concentrate urine and an acquired form of nephrogenic diabetes insipidus [13]. The common causes of complete bilateral obstruction leading to post-renal form of AKI include genitourinary malignancy, enlarged prostate, and urinary stone disease. A sometime missed cause is papillary necrosis caused by NSAID use where the renal papilla undergo necrosis, slough off and causes obstruction. Such patients can present with painless hematuria. A complete or near complete cessation of urinary flow should prompt consideration of post-renal AKI, since with prerenal and renal causes, the decrease in urinary output is rarely complete. While renal and prerenal AKI is diagnosed in the appropriate settings by laboratory tests of blood and urine, post-renal AKI requires imaging to arrive at the correct diagnosis.

Approach to AKI in the Surgical ICU (Fig. 39.1)

Prevention

Even relatively mild degrees of renal dysfunction are associated with worse outcomes; hence, preventing AKI from occurring in the first place must be an important goal of all critical care in the ICU. Since in most instances AKI is, or at

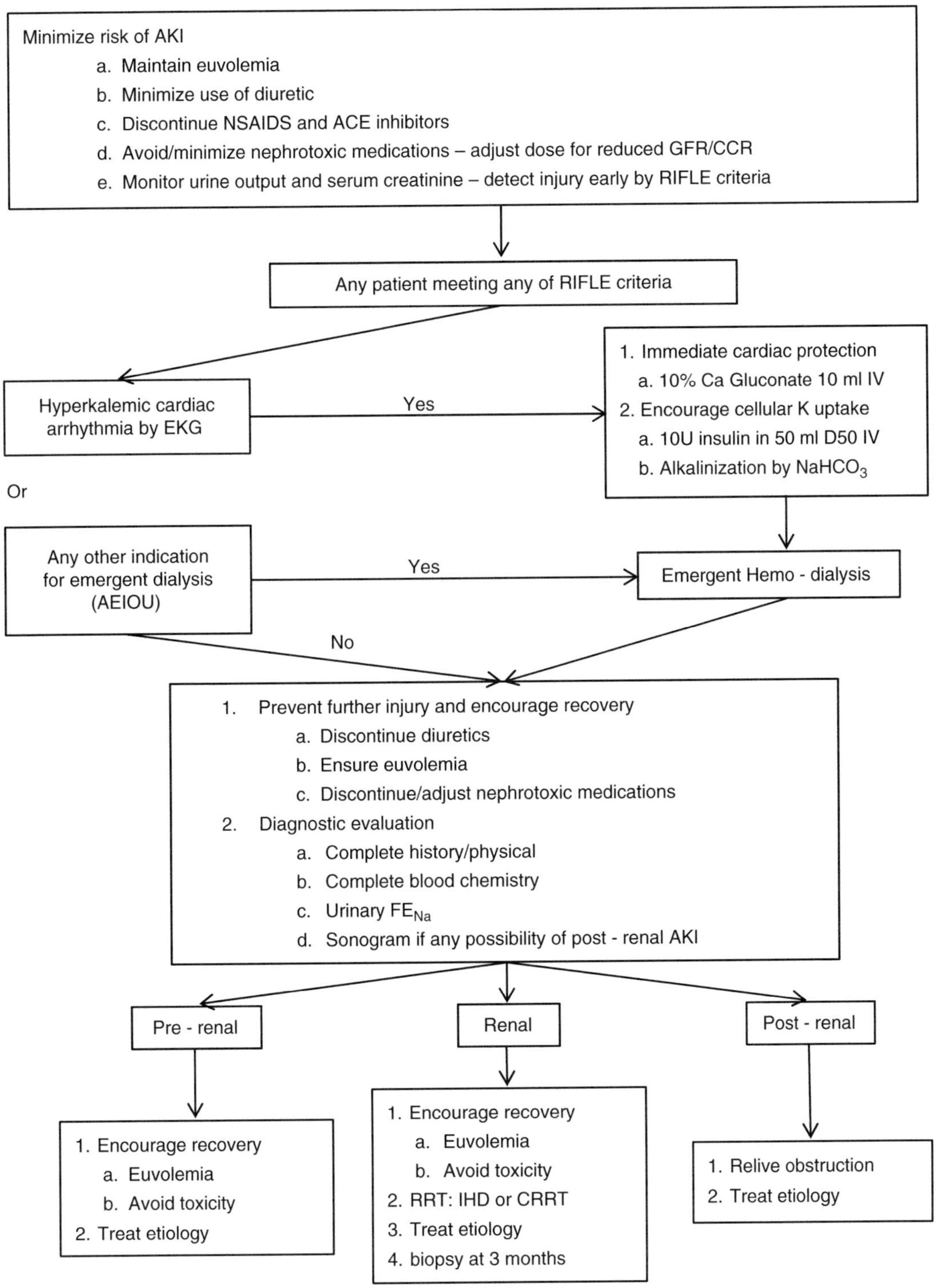

Fig. 39.1 Stepwise algorithm for any ICU patient at risk of AKI

least starts as, prerenal from loss of effective circulating volume, keeping a patient euvolemic is extremely important. In the past in the surgical ICUs, in an attempt to prevent the development of AKI, patients were often given too much volume especially in the form of crystalloids. This was directly related to development of multiple complications related to too much volume, namely ARDS, abdominal compartment syndrome, etc. The current understanding is that while hypoperfusion due to hypovolemia should be avoided to prevent organ dysfunction such as AKI, hypervolemia is to be avoided as well and the goal should be euvolemia. Instead of relying completely on provider judgment in assessing the intravascular volume status of a patient, more objective criteria—stroke volume/systolic pressure variation; intensivist performed point of care Echocardiogram and passive leg raise tests, etc.—should be utilized. Secondly when using nephrotoxic medications a careful risk/benefit analysis should be performed to ensure that the benefit of the medication clearly outweighs the risk of nephrotoxicity. If such nephrotoxic medications are utilized, the dose should be carefully adjusted for the individual patient to account for age or other factors related to poorer clearance.

While general principles of prevention outlined above apply to almost all patients admitted to the ICU, they are especially important in patients that have conditions placing them at greater risk of developing AKI. Surgical patients at particular risk of developing AKI are (1) patients suffering hemorrhagic shock due to trauma or any other surgical condition, e.g., ruptured aneurysm and severe necrotizing pancreatitis; (2) postoperative patients following major abdominal, vascular, or open heart surgery; (3) traumatized patients with massive crush injury releasing myoglobin and causing pigment induced nephropathy (see below); (4) major burn patients; (5) patients with preexisting renal disease; (6) patients suffering from systemic sepsis; and (7) geriatric patients. There have been attempts to quantify risk in specific populations but these remain imprecise and of moderate sensitivity at best [14]. There have also been attempts at developing interventions that could prevent the development of AKI in these at-risk patients. These include use of low dose Dopamine, diuretics, renal protective agents such as Mannitol, and alkalinizing agents such as sodium bicarbonate. To date no such strategy has proven effective in preventing AKI [15, 16]. The best strategy for prevention as mentioned above is maintenance of euvolemia, and strict attention to the use of nephrotoxic agents.

Diagnostic Approach to AKI in the ICU

Despite all preventative measures, some critically ill patients will develop AKI. All patients at risk should be carefully monitored with hourly urine output and at least once daily checking of BUN and serum creatinine. If there is an abrupt decrease in urinary output, the catheter should be checked for blockage. If no blockage is found patients meeting "at risk" RIFLE criteria should have another careful evaluation of (1) intravascular volume; (2) mean arterial pressures; (3) use of diuretics and nephrotoxic agents. In addition, patients should be evaluated by checking FE_{Na} to differentiate prerenal from renal AKI and microscopic urine analysis to detect presence and type of casts. The presence and type of casts seen on microscopic examination can help determine the cause of the AKI. A 24-hour urine collection is necessary to accurately determine FE_{Na} by the following formula:

$$FE_{Na} = [\text{Urinary Na} \times \text{Plasma Creatinine}/\text{Plasma Na} \times \text{Urinary Creatinine}] \times 100.$$

In a patient in prerenal AKI, all diuretics should be suspended and intravascular volume replenished to euvolemic levels. After adequate volume resuscitation, pressors should be utilized to increase the renal perfusion pressure. In most cases of prerenal AKI, these measures should suffice in reversing the process. In specific patients where post-renal AKI is suspected, a sonogram should be performed to evaluate any dilatation of the urinary passage suggesting obstruction. If such an obstruction is found, it will need to be relieved to reverse the AKI. In patients where the prerenal AKI does not reverse, obstruction has been ruled out, or renal AKI is diagnosed, the treatment of AKI should be as outlined below.

AKI Therapy

Treatment for AKI should be done in the following stepwise fashion (Fig. 39.1):

1. Evaluation for immediate threats to life: The most immediate threat to life from AKI is from acute increase in serum K. Patients should have a serum K measured immediately and frequently. Patients with AKI due to pigment nephropathy are especially prone to hyperkalemia. Patients demonstrating hyperkalemia should have an immediate EKG performed to check for cardiac effects of hyperkalemia. If such effects are detected, immediate therapy consists of calcium gluconate that is cardioprotective from hyperkalemia. Along with cardioprotection, measures to reduce serum K by driving the K from the extracellular compartment intracellularly should be undertaken—alkalization with sodium bicarbonate, and infusion of dextrose with insulin. While these immediate measures are carried out, preparations should be made for urgent dialysis (see renal replacement therapy below).
2. Evaluation for other indications for urgent dialysis: Even in the absence of immediate threat to life from hyperkalemia, patients may have other indications for urgent dialysis (see below). If any of these exist, preparations should be made for urgent dialysis.
3. In the absence of immediate threat to life, and any indication for urgent dialysis, supportive expectant therapy is appropriate:
   (a) Intravascular volume: Maintaining euvolemia
   (b) Drugs: Avoiding nephrotoxic drugs as much as possible and modifying the dose of all renally excreted drugs
   (c) Diet: In the past protein restriction to <40 g daily was the norm. However in this day and age of easy availability of renal replacement therapy restricting proteins and placing patients at risk of protein calorie malnutrition is not considered appropriate. Patients should be provided with adequate calories and proteins as per their needs preferably via the enteral route.
   (d) Fluids: As with diet, in the past patients were strictly restricted to 1–1.5 L of fluid per day. This created problems with essential therapeutic drugs and also led to severe thirst. Now with relative ease of renal replacement therapy, fluid restriction is not necessary and patients should get adequate fluids to maintain euvolemia, get appropriate medications, and be supplied with adequate calories and proteins.

Common Syndromes Associated with AKI

Pigment Induced Nephropathy

Increased plasma levels of oxygen transporting pigments—myoglobin and hemoglobin—can lead to AKI. Myoglobinemia, seen with injuries involving muscle crush and sometimes after heavy use of street drugs [17, 18], is the more common form since its low molecular weight of ~17,000 Daltons allows it to be filtered by the glomerulus and form proteinaceous casts within the tubular lumen. The pigment is directly toxic to the tubular cells via free oxygen radicals. Serum levels of creatine kinase are elevated to >5000 U/L though often run much higher. Free hemoglobin is a less common cause of AKI since the molecule is much larger and is usually not filtered through the glomerulus. Additionally, free hemoglobin binds to haptoglobin forming a large complex that cannot be filtered. Only when there is massive hemolysis that exhausts the supply of haptaglobin does free hemoglobin appear in the circulation and cause hemoglobinuric AKI. The pathophysiology is the same for both the pigments.

Therapy for pigment nephropathy follows the same general principles outlined. The major difference is the addition of forced diuresis with volume expansion and use of furosemide. Mannitol can also be used though judiciously since it can acutely increase the circulating volume and if diuresis does not occur, lead to volume overload [19]. Both pigments tend to be more soluble in alkaline urine, hence using sodium bicarbonate to alkalinize the urine to pH > 6.5 is also recommended, especially to prevent the development of AKI in at-risk patients.

Contrast Induced Nephropathy (CIN)

Intravenous radiocontrast agents can lead to AKI that has been termed CIN. With rapid expansion of diagnostic and therapeutic radiologic interventions coupled with an aging population with significant comorbidities, the incidence of CIN is rising. Risk factors for CIN are presented in Table 39.5. The actual incidence even in prospective studies varies from a low of <5% to a high of 50%. This is likely due to different study populations and differing definitions of CIN. The most commonly accepted definition is an absolute increase in serum creatinine of 0.5 mg/dL or increase of 25% above baseline. The increase commonly occurs 48–72 h post contrast exposure [20]. The proposed mechanism CIN likely involves vasoconstriction within the renal parenchyma leading to AKI with prerenal type of presentation though there is some evidence of direct toxicity mediated by free radicals [21]. A number of interventions have been studied to reduce the incidence of CIN. Interventions that have shown benefit at least in some, though not all, studies are: volume expansion, alkalanization, use of *N*-acetylcystein, limiting volume of contrast agent, using lower osmolarity agents, and discontinuing other nephrotoxic medications [22–27]. Hemodialysis either before or after radiocontrast administration to dialyze out the agent has not been shown to be beneficial [28].

Table 39.5 Risk factors for contrast induced nephropathy (CIN)

Age > 60 years
Hypovolemia
Use of diuretics
Preexisting renal insufficiency
Diabetic nephropathy
Congestive heart failure
Hepatic failure
Large volume of contrast (>2 mL/kg)

HepatoRenal Syndrome (HRS)

HRS is a unique form of AKI that is seen in patients with advanced hepatic disease. The onset can vary from fairly acute to quite insidious. The typical clinical presentation is very similar to prerenal forms of AKI likely due to severe intrarenal vasoconstriction rather than inherent renal parenchymal disease. This is supported by the observation that HRS rapidly resolves if the hepatic disease is reversed or a functioning liver is transplanted. The pathophysiology likely involves vasodilatation in the splanchnic circulation caused by portal hypertension. This vasodilatation results in pooling of the blood volume within the splanchnic circulation especially in the large dilated mesenteric veins. This in turn leads to poor venous return to the heart and reduced perfusion to the rest of the body including the kidney. The kidneys respond to this relative hypo perfusion by afferent arteriolar vasoconstriction that leads to reduced GFR. Patients with HRS are prone to developing hepatic encephalopathy. Electrolyte disturbances—hypokalemia and hyponatremia—and acid-base disorders are more often seen in HRS as compared to other causes of AKI. While the principles of care are similar in this form of AKI, fluid balance becomes much more challenging since for the AKI a relatively full intravascular compartment and avoidance of diuretics is preferred, while to prevent ascites and peripheral edema from hepatic insufficiency, a mild degree of hypovolemia with diuretic use is preferred. Drainage of ascites especially if causing abdominal compartment syndrome (see below), either externally or internally via a peritoneovenous shunts may offer partial relief. Portal-systemic shunts too may ameliorate the AKI, but AKI in and of itself is not an indication to perform such shunts [29–32].

Abdominal Compartment Syndrome (ACS) Associated AKI

Over the past two decades ACS has been accepted as a distinct nosologic entity where an increase in intra-abdominal pressure leads to organ system dysfunction [33]. Kidneys, along with the lungs, are the most sensitive organs to elevated intra-abdominal pressures. Initially renal function is affected by the elevated intra-abdominal pressure compressing the renal veins. In later stages as the ACS progresses and cardiac output falls due to diminished venous return, this further contributes to AKI. Initially the presentation is that of oliguric with a prerenal picture, but if the ACS progress, ATN sets in. The only effective therapy is rapid relief of the intra-abdominal hypertension usually by surgical decompression [34].

Prognosis and Outcome

The majority (~80%) of the patients that develop AKI and survive will have return of renal function and be dialysis free [35]. While that maybe so, the prognosis for renal function is dependent upon the severity of the initial insult that caused the AKI. Patients with brief vascular insults will likely recover near baseline function within 72 h, while those with more severe and prolonged insults requiring dialysis for the AKI will likely have some long term effect where the serum creatinine remains 1–2 mg/dL above the pre-insult baseline value [36, 37]. During the recovery phase it is extremely important to avoid a second insult in the form of hypovolemia and nephrotoxic medications, etc. Recovery from AKI is heralded by increasing urine output and lack of rise or decrease in serum creatinine despite not getting dialysis. Differing functions of the kidney may recover at different time intervals. Urine output may increase first followed by reduction in serum creatinine and finally the ability to regenerate bicarbonate and maintain body pH. During the recovery phase electrolyte imbalances are common, hence careful monitoring is essential to avoid life-threatening abnormalities from developing.

It has long been known that the development of AKI is associated with a higher mortality. The reasons for this remain a bit unclear and maybe related to the adverse impact of AKI on the immune function [38]. Reported mortality rates range from 25 to 64% [39, 40]. The variation likely represents differing study populations. Overall mortality rates are lower for non-oliguric forms of AKI and AKI due to CIN, while very high rates are reported for HRS. The exact contribution of AKI as an independent risk factor for mortality among critically ill patients is debated. In a prospective study by Hoa et al. on post-cardiac surgery patients, 145 of 843 (17%) developed AKI and AKI was found to be an independent risk factor for mortality with a hazard ratio of 7.8. The overall numbers in terms of outcome for patients developing AKI in the ICU have not changed significantly for the past five decades [41].

As mentioned in the early part of the chapter, multiple studies and meta-analysis have demonstrated that the overall outcomes in general and the return of renal function after AKI in particular are adversely affected by age [8, 9].

Renal Replacement Therapy (RRT)

In critically ill patients with rapidly deteriorating renal function coupled with a hyper-catabolic state from the primary illness, unless renal replacement therapy is provided, the patient will likely die. In broad terms RRT can be provided in two forms—hemodialysis (HD) and peritoneal dialysis (PD). In both types of dialysis the principle of solute and fluid removal is the same. In both blood and dialysate fluid are separated by a semipermeable membrane. Solutes and fluid moves across this membrane following concentration and osmotic gradients. The two main processes are convection, where hydrostatic pressure serves as the driving force and diffusion where concentration gradients and osmotic pressure serve as the driving forces. By manipulating flow rates of blood and dialysate, and the composition of the dialysate, it is possible to control what gets removed—fluid or solute—and, in the case of solute, what types of solute—high molecular weight or low/medium molecular weight. In the case of HD the semipermeable membrane is in a cartridge called the hemofilter or hemodialyzer, while in case of PD, the peritoneal surface serves as the semipermeable membrane. For the most part, in the ICU setting PD is not used, and the focus of RRT in this chapter will be HD.

There are two forms of HD—intermittent (IHD) and continuous (CRRT). IHD is the main form of RRT utilized for the large majority of patients with end stage renal disease and is also utilized in the ICU for more stable patients. CRRT is less taxing to the hemodynamics of the patient and hence is often utilized for critically ill more unstable patients that need fluid and or solute removal due to AKI. RRT is associated with a host of complications. The complete discussion of all the complications and their management is beyond the scope of this chapter and discussed elsewhere in the text. The common complications are—thrombosis of the access or dialysis circuit, infection, hypotension, and electrolyte imbalances. The decision to initiate RRT should be taken with a careful evaluation of risks and benefits, and if initiated, meticulous attention to detail is paramount to minimize complications.

Indications

Indications for dialysis maybe divided into emergent and non-emergent. Emergent indications are those where without dialysis the patient may die probably within a very short period of time. These can be summarized by the mnemonic AEIOU: A—acidosis; E—electrolytes principally hyperkalemia; I—ingestions or overdose of medications/drugs; O—overload of fluid causing heart failure; U—uremia leading to encephalitis/pericarditis. The principal non-emergent indication for dialysis is ESRD where the renal function has deteriorated to the point that without dialysis, the patient cannot survive long term. In between these two extremes is the use of dialysis for AKI where there is an expectation of return of renal function sufficient for the patient to live without dialysis. Despite AKI being a very common disorder encountered in the ICU, surprisingly there is little consensus on the indications for dialysis. Some units start dialysis quite early with the expectation that by doing so, the ultimate outcome is improved. Other units tend to delay dialysis till the uremia leads to encephalopathy or an emergent indication emerges. The results of studies to determine the ideal indication and timing of initiating dialysis for AKI are mixed. Combining the results of multiple studies by meta-analysis is hampered by differing studies using differing definitions of early and late dialysis, and also that the older studies were performed with IHD, while the more recent ones have been done with CRRT [42, 43]. In an attempt to provide some objective guidance, the AKI Network has published guidelines [44]. The guidelines emphasize: (1) the indications maybe taken as absolute and relative. Absolute indications are such that by itself each absolute indication would merit dialysis. On the other hand, relative indications are such that while by itself the individual indication may not merit dialysis, however when taken with the entire clinical scenario, the patient merits dialysis. The latter occurs most often in the face of MSOF. The indications are summarized in Table 39.6; (2) fluid overload in critically ill patients is associated with worse outcomes, hence in critically ill patients with fluid overload early CRRT may help with fluid management and possibly improve outcomes [45]; and (3) in line with #2, there is a tendency towards initiating dialysis early in patients with oliguric AKI as opposed to non-oliguric AKI. The above discussion notwithstanding, all agree that dialysis should be administered to treat severe uremia even in the absence of any of the emergent indications. Severe uremia is usually defined as BUN of >100 mg/dL. Lastly the panel did not critically evaluate some emerging evidence of the early use of CRRT in patients with sepsis where the investigators claim that by dialyzing early and vigorously, inflammatory cytokines are removed and outcomes improved. The hypothesis while intriguing remains unproven [46, 47].

Table 39.6 Indications for renal replacement therapy in patients with acute kidney injury as per Acute Renal Failure Trial Network

Indication	Parameter	Absolute/Relative
Metabolic abnormality	BUN >76 mg/dL	Relative
	BUN >100 mg/dL	Absolute
	Hyperkalemia >6 mEq/L	Relative
	Hyperkalemia >6 mEq/L with EKG changes	Absolute
	Dysnatremia	Relative
Acidosis	pH > 7.15	Relative
	pH < 7.15	Absolute
	Lactic acidosis related to Metformin use	Absolute
Anuria/oliguria	Urine output <0.5 mL/kg/h × 6 h	Relative
	Urine output <0.5 mL/kg/h × 12 h	Relative
	Urine output <0.3 mL/kg/h × 24 h	Relative
	Anuria × 12 hours	Relative
Fluid overload	Diuretic sensitive	Relative
	Diuretic resistant	Absolute

Access

In patients with ESRD, dialysis is often anticipated and planned for by creation of an arteriovenous fistula or graft even before the patient actually needs dialysis. In patients with AKI encountered in the ICU, dialysis is usually performed via large (12-15Fr) dual lumen catheters inserted percutaneously into a large vein or directly into the right atrium. These catheters are of two types—cuffed, tunneled and uncuffed, non-tunneled. Un-cuffed non-tunneled catheters are placed in the unit just as central venous lines. The commonly used ones are made of polyurethane and usually placed acutely for urgent dialysis in the internal jugular or femoral veins. Insertion into the subclavian vein is avoided to prevent stricture of vein that may hamper future placement of fistula or graft in the ipsilateral upper extremity. When placed with appropriate antiseptic precautions, they are safe to use for 2–3 weeks duration. If it is anticipated that dialysis maybe required for a longer duration, a cuffed tunneled catheter is preferred. These are made of silicone usually inserted with fluoroscopic guidance and have a cuff that sits in a subcutaneous tunnel. The tunnel and cuff tend to prevent catheter infection and hence these can be used for longer periods of time.

Dose

As is the case with exact indications and timing, there is also no consensus regarding the ideal dose or intensity of dialysis. While a number of smaller and usually retrospective studies suggest that higher intensity dialysis is associated with improved outcomes [48–50], larger prospective studies failed to demonstrate that [51, 52]. Guidelines as to how much dialysis should be administered to patients with AKI are published by the Acute Renal Failure Trial Network (ATN Trial) [52]. Most centers tend to keep the BUN at about 70 mg/dL. Besides solute reduction, the other component of dialysis is intravascular volume management. In patients that are septic and in the state of systemic inflammation, the capillaries remain hyper-permeable and any removal of fluid from the intravascular compartment leads to hemodynamic instability even though the total body water is increased. On the other hand, in patients that are recovering and the state of inflammation is subsiding, the capillaries regain their selective permeability and removing fluid from the intravascular compartment does not lead to hemodynamic compromise, rather there is resorption of the "third" space fluid from the interstitial compartment. Objective measures of intravascular volume should be utilized in determining how much volume should be removed.

Modality

As in other issues related to AKI, there is ongoing debate as which modality—IHD or CRRT—is superior. It is generally accepted that CRRT is better tolerated specially by critically ill patients that may have some degree of hemodynamic compromise. The results of studies are mixed in terms of overall mortality and return of renal function [53–57]. The modalities can be difficult to directly compare since it is difficult to dialyze the same amount of solute and volume with IHD when it is performed a few hours usually on alternate days, as with CRRT that can be performed round the clock. In the largest randomized prospective study to date, the outcomes were similar for the two forms of dialysis [58]. One surprising result of that study, unlike many others, was that even critically ill patients could tolerate IHD if the dialysate had a very high concentration of Na. In the US most ICUs will opt for CRRT in critically ill patients especially those with unstable or tenuous hemodynamic status, and utilize IHD for the stable patients. In UK and Australia, CRRT is the modality of choice for AKI in the ICU.

Summary

The large majority of patients admitted to the surgical ICU are at risk of AKI as defined by the RIFLE. Due to a host of anatomic and physiologic changes within the kidney that occur with age, the risk of AKI is significantly higher. The occurrence of even mild AKI adversely affects overall outcomes with the elderly often having the worst outcomes of all. Meticulous attention to fluid management and minimizing the use of nephrotoxic medications can help reduce the incidence. All at-risk patients that do develop AKI should have a reexamination of intravascular volume and discontinuation or adjustment of dosage of nephrotoxic medications. RRT therapy is often required for managing patients that do develop AKI.

References

1. Skorecki K, Chertow GM, Marsden PA, Taal MW, Yu ALS. Brenner & Rector's the kidney. 10th ed. Philadelphia: Saunders Elsevier; 2015.
2. Lindeman RD, Goldman R. Anatomic and physiologic age changes in the kidney. Exp Gerontol. 1986;21:379.
3. Lassnigg A, Schmidlin D, Mouhieddine M, et al. Minimal changes of serum creatinine predict prognosis in patients with cardiothoracic surgery: a prospective cohort study. J Am Soc Nephrol. 2004;15:1597.
4. Levy MM, Marcias WL, Vincent JL, et al. Early changes in organ function predict eventual survival in severe sepsis. Crit Care Med. 2005;33:2194.
5. Bellomo R, Ronco C, Kellum JA, et al. Acute dialysis quality initiative workgroup: acute renal failure – definition, outcome measures, animal models, fluid therapy and information technology needs: the second international consensus conference of the acute dialysis quality initiative (ADQI) group. Crit Care. 2004;8:R204.
6. Hoste EA, Clermont G, Kersten A, et al. RIFLE criteria for acute kidney injury are associated with hospital mortality in critically ill patients: a cohort analysis. Crit Care. 2006;10:R73.
7. Uchino S, Bellomo R, Goldsmith D, et al. An assessment of RIFLE criteria for acute renal failure in hospitalized patients. Crit Care Med. 2006;34:1913.
8. Pascual J, Orofino L, Liano F, et al. Incidence and prognosis of acute renal failure in older patients. J Am Geriatr Soc. 1990;38:25.
9. Schmitt R, Coca S, Kanbay M, et al. Recovery of kidney function after acute kidney injury in the elderly: a systematic review and meta-analysis. Am J Kidney Dis. 2008;52:262.
10. Clive DM, Stoff JS. Renal syndromes associated with nonsteroidal anti-inflammatory drugs. N Engl J Med. 1984;310:563.
11. Hricik DE, Browning PJ, Kopelman R, et al. Captopril-induced functional renal insufficiency in patients with bilateral renal-artery stenosis or renal-artery stenosis in a solitary kidney. N Engl J Med. 1983;308:373.
12. Hou S, Bushinsky DA, Wish JB, et al. Hospital acquired renal insufficiency: a prospective study. Am J Med. 1993;44:27.
13. Early LE. Extreme polyuria in obstructive uropathy. N Engl J Med. 1956;255:600.
14. Thakar CV, Arrigain S, Worley S, et al. A clinical score to predict renal failure after cardiac surgery. J Am Soc Nephrol. 2005;6:162.
15. Zacharias M, Conlon NP, Herbison GP, et al. Interventions for protecting renal function in the perioperative period. Cochrane Database Syst Rev. 2008;4:CD003590.
16. Lassnigg A, Donner E, Grubhofer G, et al. Lack of renoprotective effects of dopamine and furose-

mide during cardiac surgery. J Am Soc Nephrol. 2000;11:97.
17. Honda N, Kurokawa K. Acute renal failure and rhabdomyolysis. Kidney Int. 1983;23:888.
18. Roth D, Alacron FJ, Fernandez JA, et al. Acute rhabdomyolysis associated with cocaine intoxication. N Engl J Med. 1990;319:673.
19. Better OS, Stein JH. Early management of shock and prophylaxis of acute renal failure in traumatic rhabdomyolysis. N Engl J Med. 1990;322:825.
20. Berns AS. Nephrotoxicity of contrast media [clinical conference]. Kidney Int. 1989;36:730.
21. Detrenis S, Meschi M, Musini S, et al. Lights and shadows on the pathogenesis of contrast-induced nephropathy: state of the art. Nephrol Dial Transplant. 2005;20:1542.
22. Heymen SN, Brezis M, Greenfield Z, et al. Protective role of furosemide and saline in radiocontrast-induced acute renal failure in rat. Am J Kidney Dis. 1989;14:377.
23. Solomon R, Werner C, Mann D, et al. Effects of saline, mannitol and furosemide to prevent acute decreases in renal function induced by radio-contrast agents. N Engl J Med. 1994;331:1416.
24. Tepel M, van der Giet M, Schwarzfeld C, et al. Prevention of radiographic-contrast agent-inducedreductions in renal function by acetylcysteine. N Engl J Med. 2000;343:210.
25. Gonzalez DA, Norsworthy KJ, Kern SJ. A meta-analysis of N-acetylcysteine in contrast-induced nephrotoxicity: unsupervised clustering to resolve heterogeneity. BMC Med. 2007;5:32.
26. Merten GJ, Burgess WP, Gray LV, et al. Prevention of contrast-induced nephropathy with sodium bicarbonate: a randomized controlled trial. JAMA. 2004;291:2328.
27. Kuhn MJ, Chen N, Sahani DV, et al. The PREDICT study: a randomized double-blind comparison of contrast-induced nephropathy after low- or isoosmolar contrast agent exposure. AJR Am J Roentgenol. 2008;191:151.
28. Cruz DN, Perazella MA, Bellomo R, et al. Extracorporeal blood purification therapies for prevention of radiocontrast-induced nephropathy: a systematic review. Am J Kid Dis. 2006;48:361.
29. Ariyan S, Sweeney T, Kerstein MD. The hepatorenal syndrome: recovery after portacaval shunt. Ann Surg. 1975;181:847.
30. Fisher JE, Foster GS. Survival from acute hepatorenal syndrome following splenorenal shunt. Ann Surg. 1976;814:22.
31. Epstein M. Peritoneovenous shunt in the management of ascites and hepatorenal syndrome. Gastroenterology. 1982;82:790.
32. Epstein M. The LeVeen shunt for ascites and hepatorenal syndrome. N Engl J Med. 1980;302:628.
33. Malbrain ML, Cheatham ML, Kirkpatrick A, et al. Results from the international conference of experts on intra-abdominal hypertension and abdominal compartment syndrome: I. Definitions. Intensive Care Med. 2006;32:1722.
34. Shibagaki Y, Tai C, Nayak A, et al. Intra-abdominal hypertension is an under-appreciated cause of acute renal failure. Nephrol Dial Transplant. 2006;21:567.
35. Liano F, Felipe C, Tenorio MT, et al. Long term outcome of acute tubular necrosis: a contribution to its natural history. Kidney Int. 2007;71:676.
36. Myers BD, Miller C, Mehigan JT, et al. Nature of renal injury following total renal ischemia in man. J Clin Invest. 1984;73:329.
37. Spurney RF, Fulkerson WJ, Schwab SJ, et al. Acute renal failure in critically ill patients: prognosis of recovery of kidney function after prolonged dialysis support. Crit Care Med. 1991;19:8.
38. Kleinknecht D, Jungers P, Chanard J, et al. Uremic and non-uremic complications of acute renal failure: evaluation of early and frequent dialysis on prognosis. Kidney Int. 1972;1:190.
39. Hou S, Bushinsky DA, Wish JB, et al. Hospital-acquired renal insufficiency: a prospective study. Am J Med. 1983;74:243.
40. Spiegel DM, Ullian ME, Zerbe GO, et al. Determinants of survival and recovery in acute renal failure patients dialyzed in intensive-care units. Am J Nephrol. 1991;11:44.
41. Ympa YP, Sakr Y, Reinhart K, et al. Has mortality from acute renal failure decreased? A systematic review of the literature. Am J Med. 2005;118:827.
42. Seabra VF, Balk EM, Liangos O, et al. Timing of renal replacement therapy in acute renal failure: a meta-analysis. Am J Kidney Dis. 2008;52:272.
43. Palevsky PM. Indications and timing of renal replacement therapy in acute kidney injury. Crit Care Med. 2008;36(S4):S224.
44. Gibney N, Hoste E, Burdmann EA, et al. Timing of initiation and discontinuation of renal replacement therapy in AKI: unanswered key questions. Clin J Am Soc Nephrol. 2008;3:876.
45. Foland JA, Fortenberry JD, Warshaw BL, et al. Fluid overload before continuous hemofiltration and survival in critically ill children: a retrospective analysis. Pediatrics. 2004;32:1771.
46. Piccinni P, Dan M, Barbacini S, et al. Early isovolemic hemofiltration in oliguric patients with septic shock. Intensive Care Med. 2006;32:80.
47. Cole L, Bellomo R, Hart G, et al. A phase II randomized, controlled trial of continuous hemofiltration in sepsis. Crit Care Med. 2002;30:100.
48. Schiffl H, Lang SM, Fischer R. Daily hemodialysis and the outcome of acute renal failure. N Engl J Med. 2002;346:305.
49. Ronco C, Bellomo R, Homel P, et al. Effects of different dose in continuous veno-venous hemofiltration on outcomes of acute renal failure: a prospective randomized trial. Lancet. 2000;356:26.
50. Saudan P, Niederberger M, De Seigneux S, et al. Adding a dialysis dose to continuous hemofiltration

increases survival in patients with acute renal failure. Kidney Int. 2006;70:1312.
51. Bellomo R, Cass A, Cole L, et al. Intensity of continuous renal-replacement therapy in critically ill patients. N Engl J Med. 2009;361:1627.
52. Palevsky PM, Zhang JH, O'Connor TZ, et al. Intensity of renal support in critically ill patients with acute kidney injury. N Engl J Med. 2008;359:7.
53. Uchino S, Bellomo R, Kellum JA, et al. Patient and kidney survival by dialysis modality in critically ill patients with acute kidney injury. Int J Artif Organs. 2007;30:281.
54. Bell M, Granath F, Schon S, et al. Continuous renal replacement therapy is associated with less chronic renal failure than intermittent hemodialysis after acute renal failure. Intensive Care Med. 2007;33:773.
55. Rabindranath K, Adams J, Macleod AM, et al. Intermittent versus continuous renal replacement therapy for acute renal failure in adults. Cochrane Database Syst Rev. 2007;3:CD003773.
56. Pannu N, Klarenbach S, Wiebe N, et al. Renal replacement therapy in patients with acute renal failure: a systematic review. JAMA. 2008;299:793.
57. Bagshaw SM, Berthiaume LR, Delaney A, et al. Continuous versus intermittent renal replacement therapy for critically ill patients with acute kidney injury: a meta-analysis. Crit Care Med. 2008;36:610.
58. Vinsonneau C, Camus C, Combes A, et al. Continuous venovenous hemodiafiltration versus intermittent hemodialysis for acute renal failure in patients with multiple-organ dysfunction syndrome: a multicentre randomized trial. Lancet. 2006;368:379.

40 Infections in the Geriatric Person Following Trauma

Wayne Campbell[†] and Alexander Chen

Introduction

Compared to younger adults, geriatric trauma patients have higher mortality rates, longer length of hospital stay, and higher rates of infectious complications [1, 2]. The population of elderly persons continues to increase with improvements in public health and nutrition. In 2010, 8% of the world population, or an estimated 524 million people, were above the age of 65. This number is expected to increase to 1.5 billion people by 2050, which will be 16% of the projected world population [3]. As such, we will need to be prepared for an increasing number of elderly trauma patients.

The older patient who suffers an injury is more susceptible to infection for reasons including immune senescence as well as comorbidities such as diabetes, obesity, peripheral arterial disease, vascular disease, and pulmonary disease [4–6]. The presence of infection leads to increased length of stay (LOS), intensive care length of stay (ICU LOS), and mortality. Furthermore, other comorbidities, including obesity, renal dysfunction, and liver disease, can complicate antibiotic dosing [7].

Alterations in the Immune System with Aging

Immunosenescence, the term given to the gradual decline in immune function with advancing age, is characterized by an attenuated ability to respond to infection. During normal aging, there are numerous changes to the immune system. Neutrophils chemotaxis and phagocytosis are reduced. Phagocytosis by monocytes is also impaired, as is the respiratory burst required to generate microbicidal reactive oxygen species. TNF-α production is decreased, along with IL-6, while other cytokines such as IL-8 are increased. There is impaired maturation and proliferation of natural killer (NK) cells, as well as decreased expression of cytotoxicity activating receptors, diminished responsiveness to cytokines, and decreased cytotoxicity via impairment of perforin release. Response to immunizations is also diminished as we age [8, 9].

Some authors have attributed excess infection and mortality in older human and animal models to a chronic inflammatory state of aging (inflammaging) [1]. Inflammaging includes chronic elevations in cytokines including C-reactive protein and IL-6, and although these alterations are

[†]Deceased

W. Campbell, M.D.
Department of Medicine-Infection Deseases, Union Memorial Hospital, 201 East University Parkway, Baltimore, MD, USA
e-mail: Wayne.Campbell@medstar.net

A. Chen
Medstar Union Memorial Hospital, 201 E University Parkway, Baltimore, MD 212014, USA
e-mail: alexander.chen@medstar.net

A. Rodriguez et al. (eds.), *Geriatric Trauma and Acute Care Surgery*, https://doi.org/10.1007/978-3-319-57403-5_40

considered important, their exact role remains unclear [10]. CMV seropositivity, which increases with age, is hypothesized to drive chronic T-cell proliferation, leading to shortened telomeres and the above changes in T-cell populations, which then results in proliferative exhaustion and inability to respond to infection and immunization [11].

Following trauma, there is a complex immune response involving both pro- and anti-inflammatory cytokines which is still not well understood. The initial insult triggers the systemic inflammatory response syndrome (SIRS), causing the release of proinflammatory mediators including IL-6 and IL8, as well as platelet activating factors. Within hours, the body moves to an immunosuppressive phase with increased IL-10 and interferon gamma, while production of proinflammatory cytokines decreases [8]. Unchecked, these alterations are thought to have deleterious effects for the host. Unfortunately, the attempts to modulate these host responses have yet to yield improvement in clinical outcomes in humans [12].

This biphasic response of the immune system to trauma is also effected by increasing age. After trauma, the usual inflammatory response is attenuated in older patients, then fails to return to baseline for weeks afterward, suggesting the prolonged occurrence of long-term inflammation and immune suppression [1]. Numerous studies have shown multiple alterations to neutrophil function, including decreased phagocytosis and CD16 expression [13] as well as decreased production of reactive oxygen compounds [14]. Much of the impairment in neutrophil function can be linked to alterations in gene transcription that lead to an incomplete immune response in the older subject, with simultaneous difficulty resolving the initial inflammatory response [2, 15].

Presentation and Diagnosis of Infection

The diagnosis of infection requires a high index of suspicion in the elderly. Fever can be diminished or absent, and tachycardia is less common, and confusion may be the only sign of illness [16]. Leukocytosis is generally a reliable sign of significant infection even in the elderly [17], although the systemic inflammation caused by injury may make evaluation more difficult. Unsuccessful attempts have been made to diagnose infection by the use of specific inflammatory markers such as C-reactive protein (CRP). In contrast, procalcitonin (PCT) is emerging as a specific test for bacterial infections, allowing avoidance of antibiotics in low-risk subjects. When studied in cohorts of elderly trauma patients, CRP tends to rise slowly over several days following major injury, and remain elevated even at 1 week, while PCT rises within a few hours of injury, peaks within 1–2 days, then returns to normal over the next few days due to its half-life of approximately 1 day [18]. The magnitude of the initial peak is correlated with Injury Severity Score (ISS), increased blood loss, abdominal trauma, and mortality, indicating that the level within the first 1–2 days is more useful as a prognostic indicator rather than a diagnostic test for infection; serial measurements are likely necessary to gain the full benefit of testing [19, 20].

All older patients should be screened on admission for pneumonia and urinary tract infection [21]. Elderly patients often present with existing infections on arrival to the trauma service; in one series, up to 18% of the elderly had a community-acquired infection, which was nearly twice as frequent as the non-elderly. In addition, more than half of those with existing infections would later acquire nosocomial infections, with resulting increase in ICU stay, total length of stay, and mortality [22–24].

Nosocomial Infections

Among trauma patients, hospital-acquired infections are associated with greater than double the cost and length of stay, with substantial increases in mortality [25]. Hospital-acquired infections can affect up to 40% of elderly trauma patients. Pneumonia and urinary tract infections combine to form the majority of nosocomial-acquired infections in this age group, with lower rates of bloodstream, skin and wound, and CNS infections than younger patients [22, 24, 26]. This is likely due to the fact that most patients are admitted due to falls or motor vehicle collisions with non-penetrating trauma. Comorbidities including COPD and urinary incontinence play a significant risk factor.

Prevention of nosocomial infection in the trauma patient is an area for ongoing exploration. Routine use of antibiotics for prophylaxis against VAP and meningitis is not supported by the literature. Antibiotic courses for penetrating wounds should be limited to no more than 48 hours due to risk of selection for resistant organisms [27]. The use of daily chlorhexidine baths has shown promise for the reduction of HAI in the general ICU setting [28]. Use of bundles may improve care and reduce infectious complications as well as mortality, although care needs to be taken to make sure the bundle is properly implemented and enforced [29]. The Institute for Healthcare Improvement has published a number of guides for the use of care bundles to prevent many infections, including VAP, CLABSI, and CA-UTI (http://www.ihi.org/Topics/Bundles/Pages/default.aspx). It should be noted that the bundles are an evolving process and differ among geographic regions. There is recent interest in the use of probiotics in the critically ill, but data is preliminary and safety is unclear [30–32].

Ventilator associated pneumonia (VAP) is a major cause of prolonged hospital stay. The estimated prevalence of VAP varies from 8 to 17.8% due to differing diagnostic criteria [33–36]. Risk factors for pneumonia in the aged include comorbidities such as swallowing disorders, congestive heart failure, renal disease, immunosuppressive therapy, alcohol abuse, malnourishment, and diaphragmatic weakness [37]. In patients with closed head injury and subdural hematomas, prolonged mechanical ventilation is not surprisingly associated with increased complications, including pneumonia [38, 39]. The presence of four or more rib fractures also portends worse outcome; a multidisciplinary approach may reduce the risk of pneumonia as well as mortality and LOS [40]. Guidelines for the management of VAP from the Infectious Disease Society of America are currently being revised and will be available in late 2016 at http://www.idsociety.org/Organ_System/#HospitalAcquiredVentilatorAssociatedPneumoniaHAPVAP.

CDC criteria for diagnosis of ventilator-associated pneumonia in adults
At least one of the following:
• Fever (>38.0 °C or >100.4 °F)
• Leukopenia (≤4000 WBC/mm^3) or leukocytosis (>12,000 WBC/mm^3)
• For adults >70 years old, altered mental status with no other recognized cause
AND at least two of the following:
• New onset of purulent sputum or change in character of sputum, or increased respiratory secretions, or increased suctioning requirements
• New onset or worsening cough, or dyspnea, or tachypnea
• Rales or bronchial breath sounds
• Worsening gas exchange (e.g., O_2 desaturations (e.g., P $PaO_2/FiO_2 < 240$), increased oxygen requirements, or increased ventilator demand)

The "Ventilator Associated Pneumonia Prevention Bundle" includes five components, including elevation of the head of the bed to a minimum of 30°, daily sedative interruption with assessment of readiness for extubation, prophylaxis against peptic ulcers and deep venous thrombosis, and daily use of chlorhexidine as an oral rinse [41, 42]. Again, the method appears to be effective in small studies. However, when each intervention is assessed separately, the benefit is unclear. Individual methods which have been shown to have benefit are numerous, but of varied quality of evidence; the strongest evidence exists for minimizing or avoiding sedation, daily sedation interruption, daily assessment of readiness for extubation, and avoidance of unnecessary ventilator circuit changes (Klompas et al. 2014). Selective oral decontamination alone has shown decreases in the rate of VAP, but not in mortality [43]. Likewise, patient positioning may reduce risk of pneumonia but the effect on mortality is unclear [43, 44].

Selective digestive decontamination (SDD) and selective oral decontamination (SOD) are strategies to reduce VAP by using nonabsorbable antimicrobials and antifungals, often with systemic antibiotics. SOD and SDD have been shown to be effective at reducing VAP and also reducing mortality, but remain controversial due to the risk of selection of resistant organisms and *Clostridium difficile*-associated diarrhea [45]. A recent systematic review of oral decontamination alone or digestive decontamination alone did find a mortality benefit for either strategy, although there is great heterogeneity among studies [46]. In addition, many of the studies have been performed in areas of low prevalence of antibiotic resistance. Studies performed in other areas have yielded conflicting results regarding risk of future harm from antibiotic resistance [47].

Several authors have reported an increased risk of pneumonia in trauma patients associated with increasing amounts of red cell transfusion [35, 48, 49]. These data are difficult to interpret due to lack of randomization, but a review of controlled trials for transfusion in the setting of hip fracture repair did find a troubling trend toward pneumonia and wound infection in the "liberal" threshold arm [50]. Therefore, in less severe trauma such as uncomplicated hip fracture, a goal hemoglobin of 7–8 g/dL may be desirable as long as the patient is otherwise stable.

Urinary tract infections account for up to 40% of nosocomial infection in trauma patients and affect over 4% of elderly trauma patients; the vast majority are due to indwelling catheters. Trauma patients are particularly prone to UTI because the patient in a state of physiologic stress may enter a catabolic state with urinary spillage of glucose, amino acids, and catecholamines, which can all enhance bacterial growth. Age, female gender, and higher injury severity score are all predictive for UTI. Patients with UTI were significantly more likely to be older, female, and have higher injury severity score. Mortality also increased with age [51, 52]. The use of a care bundle to prevent CA-UTI has also been shown to be effective in observational studies. Key features are the avoidance of unnecessary urinary catheters, attention to aseptic technique during insertion, proper maintenance of the urinary drainage system, and daily assessment of necessity of catheters ([41, 42, 53]).

The older patient may is at increased risk of MRSA colonization due to a higher level of prior contact with the healthcare system; female gender and diabetes are also risk factors [54]. Trauma patients colonized with MRSA have been found to have significantly higher risk of MRSA infection and mortality [55]. Decolonization of patients has been effective in certain non-trauma settings, and the topic is currently being investigated in trauma patients.

C. difficile infection (CDI) is another area of concern, particularly since the emergence of hypervirulent strains in North America and Europe. Up to 10% of elderly patients may be colonized at the time of hospital admission, with risk of increased colonization during hospitalization [56]. Mortality of affected trauma patients is nearly double that of unaffected patients [25]. Prevention of infection is primarily via hand hygiene with soap and water and appropriate isolation of the patient, as well as antibiotic stewardship. Decolonization and prophylactic antibiotics have not been shown to be effective [57].

The use of care bundles to prevent CLABSI has been shown to be effective in multiple studies [41, 42, 58–60]. Key measures include strict adherence to hand hygiene, full barrier precautions during line insertion, and skin antisepsis, with avoidance of the femoral vein and prompt removal of unnecessary catheters. Antiseptic (chlorhexidine) impregnated foam rings placed against the skin at the insertion site have found broad acceptance.

Diabetes mellitus is an important risk factor for infections and mortality in trauma; studies have shown that hyperglycemia is correlated with increased mortality, as well as LOS and ICU LOS. As of 2012, more than one-quarter of US adults over the age of 65 were estimated to have diabetes, with most new diagnoses occurring in those over age 45 [61]. Similar trends are expected worldwide due to aging population and changes in lifestyle and diet [62]. However, tight control has not been shown to improve patient outcomes, and recommendations remain to keep blood sugars between 140 and 180 mg/dL [63]. Computerized algorithms to maintain euglycemia via insulin infusions are early in development and show promise in reducing infection but have yet to show improvement in mortality in the setting of trauma [64].

Criteria for Catheter-associated Urinary Tract Infection (CAUTI):

A UTI where an indwelling urinary catheter was in place for >2 calendar days on the date of event, with day of device placement being Day 1,

AND

An indwelling urinary catheter was in place on the date of event or the day before. If an indwelling urinary catheter was in place for >2 calendar days and then removed, the date of event for the UTI must be the day of discontinuation or the next day for the UTI to be catheter-associated.

CAUTI Criteria 1a:
Patient must meet 1, 2, **and** 3 below:

1. Patient has an indwelling urinary catheter in place for the entire day on the date of event and such catheter had been in place for >2 calendar days, on that date (day of device placement = Day 1)
2. Patient has at least **one** of the following signs or symptoms:
   - Fever >38.°C
   - Suprapubic tenderness with no other recognized cause
   - Costovertebral angle pain or tenderness with no other recognized cause
3. Patient has a urine culture with no more than two species of organisms, at least one of which is a bacteria >10^5 CFU/ml

OR

CAUTI Criteria 1b
Patient must meet 1, 2, **and** 3 below:

1. Patient had an indwelling urinary catheter in place for >2 calendar days which was removed on the day of, or day before the date of event.
2. Patient has at least one of the following signs or symptoms
   - Fever >38.°C
   - suprapubic tenderness with no other recognized cause
   - costovertebral angle pain or tenderness with no other recognized cause
   - urinary urgency with no other recognized cause
   - dysuria with no other recognized cause
3. Patient has a urine culture with no more than two species of organisms, at least one of which is a bacteria >10^5 CFU/ml

Adapted from FACS 2016 definitions

Source: Trauma Quality Improvement Program (http://mtqip.org/sites/default/files/downloads/MICHIGAN%20TQIP%20VARIABLE%20AN%20DEFINITIONS%203.1.pdf)

Antibiotic Dosing in the Elderly Trauma Patient

The clinician should expect challenges to antimicrobial dosing in the severely ill trauma patient. The effects of sepsis and fluid shifts lead to an increase in the volume of distribution of hydrophilic antibiotics, including beta-lactams, aminoglycosides, and glycopeptides. In addition, hypoalbuminemia, which is found in over 50% of elderly trauma patients, can also necessitate increased doses for highly protein bound antibiotics including ceftriaxone, ertapenem, and daptomycin [65, 66]. The elderly patient is also likely to have a lower lean body weight, so volume of distribution of lipophilic antibiotics will be relatively higher. Augmented renal clearance, defined as creatinine clearance exceeding 130 mL/min and generally seen in younger patients, can speed the elimination of many medications [7]. Many older patients have reduced renal function, and serum creatinine is a poor substitute for GFR due to low body mass and nutrition. MDRD, CKD-EPI, and Cockroft-Gault equations are all reasonable estimates in stable elderly patients, but direct measurement of renal function may be necessary in the most ill patients [67, 68].

Since the effects of fluid shifts and sepsis are more pronounced in the most severely ill, these patients are likely to receive underdosing of antibiotics. Notably, cefazolin, a commonly used antibiotic for perioperative prophylaxis, is likely underdosed in trauma patients, who may need doses of up to 2 g every 6 h [69]. Vancomycin likewise requires increased dosing or continuous infusion to maintain adequate trough levels [70, 71]. Guidance from an experienced pharmacist is recommended. Care should also be taken to minimize polypharmacy and to monitor QTc prolongation, particularly in patients who require macrolides, fluoroquinolones, and azoles [72, 73].

Tissue penetration of antibiotics can be compromised by vascular injury and sepsis. Plasma levels may also not reflect alveolar drug penetration; lipophilic compounds such as fluoroquinolones and linezolid are best used in this compartment [7]. Specific recommendations for the selection of antimicrobials can be obtained from an antibiotic guide such as the Sanford Guide (http://www.sanfordguide.com/) or the Johns Hopkins ABX Guide (http://www.hopkinsguides.com/hopkins).

VENTILATOR-ASSOCIATED PNEUMONIA

A pneumonia where the patient is on mechanical ventilation >2 calendar days on the date of the event, with day of ventilator placement being Day 1

AND

The ventilator was in place on the date of the vent or the day before. If the patient is admitted or transferred into a facility on a ventilator, the day of admission is considered Day 1

VAP Algorithm for Bacterial or Filamentous Fungal Pathogens:

RADIOLOGY	SIGNS/SYMPTOMS	LABORATORY
Two or more serial radiographs with at least **one** of the following • New or progressive **and** persistent infiltrate • Consolidation • Cavitation NOTE: In patients **without** underlying pulmonary or cardiac disease (e.g., respiratory distress syndrome, bronchopulmonary dysplasia, pulmonary edema, or chronic obstructive pulmonary disease), **one definitive** chest radiograph is acceptable.	At least **one** of the following: • Fever (>38°C) • Leukopenia (<4000 WBC/mm^3 or leukocytosis (≥ 12,000 WBC/mm^3 • For adults ≥ 70 years old, altered mental status with no other recognized cause AND at least 2 of the following: • New onset of purulent sputum, or change in character of sputum, or increased respiratory secretions, or increased suctioning requirements • New onset or worsening cough, or dyspnea, or tachypnea • Rales or bronchial breath sounds • Worsening gas exchange (e.g., O2 desaturations (e.g., $PaO_2/FiO_2 \leq 240$), increased oxygen requirements, or increased ventilator demand)	At least **one** of the following: • Positive growth in blood culture not related to another source of infection • Positive growth in culture of pleural fluid • Positive quantitative culture from minimally-contaminated LRT specimen (e.g, BAL or protected specimen brushing) • ≥ 5% BAL-obtained cells contain intracellular bacteria on direct microscopic exam (e.g., Gram's stain) • Positive quantitative culture of lung tissue • Histopathologic exam shows at least **one** of the following evidences of pneumonia o Abscess formation or foci of consolidation with intense PMN accumulation in bronchioles and alveoli o Evidence of lung parenchyma invasion by fungal hyphae or pseudohyphae

VAP Algorithm for Viral, Legionella, and other Bacterial Pneumonias:

RADIOLOGY	SIGNS/SYMPTOMS	LABORATORY
Two or more serial radiographs with at least **one** of the following • New or progressive **and** persistent infiltrate • Consolidation • Cavitation NOTE: In patients **without** underlying pulmonary or cardiac disease (e.g., respiratory distress syndrome, bronchopulmonary dysplasia, pulmonary edema, or chronic obstructive pulmonary disease), **one definitive** chest radiograph is acceptable.	At least **one** of the following: • Fever (>38°C) • Leukopenia (<4000 WBC/mm^3 or leukocytosis (≥12,000 WBC/mm^3 • For adults ≥70 years old, altered mental status with no other recognized cause AND at least 2 of the following: • New onset of purulent sputum, or change in character of sputum, or increased respiratory secretions, or increased suctioning requirements • New onset or worsening cough, or dyspnea, or tachypnea • Rales or bronchial breath sounds • Worsening gas exchange (e.g., O2 desaturations (e.g., $PaO_2/FiO_2 \leq 240$), increased oxygen requirements, or increased ventilator demand)	At least **one** of the following: • Positive culture of virus, Legionella or Chlamydia from respiratory secretions • Positive non-culture diagnostic laboratory test of respiratory secretions of tissue for virus, Bordetella, Chlamydia, Mycoplasma, Legionella (e.g., EIA<FAMA<shell vial assay, PCR, micro-IF) • Fourfold rise in paired sera (IgG) for pathogen (e.g., influenza virus, Chlamydia) • Fourfold rise in L. pneumophila serogroup antibody titer to ≥1:128 in paired acute and convalescent sera by indirect IFA • Detection of L. pneumophila serogroup 1 antigens in urine by RIA or EIA

Adapted from FACS definitions 2016. Abbreviations: EIA: enzyme immunoassay. FAMA: fluorescence-activated microsphere assay. PCR: polymerase chain reaction. Micro-IF: micro immunofluorescence assay

UTI: Defined as an infection anywhere along the urinary tract with clinical evidence of infection, which includes at least one of the following symptoms with no other recognized cause:

1. Fever of 38°C or greater
2. White blood cell (WBC) count greater than 100,000/μL or less than 3,000/μL
3. Urgency
4. Frequency
5. Dysuria
6. Suprapubic tenderness

AND positive urine culture (≥100,000 microorganisms per microliter of urine with no more than two species of microorganisms)

OR at least two of the following signs or symptoms with no other recognized cause:

1. Fever of 38°C or greater
2. WBC count greater than 100,000/μL or less than 3,000/μL
3. Urgency
4. Frequency
5. Dysuria
6. Suprapubic tenderness

AND at least one of the following:

1. Positive dipstick for leukocyte esterase and/or nitrate
2. Pyuria (urine specimen with >10 WBC/μL or >3 WBC/high-power field of unspun urine)
3. Organisms seen on Gram stain of unspun urine
4. At least two urine cultures with repeated isolation of the same uropathogen (gram-negative bacteria or *Staphylococcus saprophyticus*) with equal to or greater than 102 colonies per milliliter in nonvoided specimens
5. Equal to or less than 105 colonies per milliliter of a single uropathogen (gram-negative bacteria or *S. saprophyticus*) in a patient being treated with an effective antimicrobial agent for a UTI
6. Physician diagnosis of a UTI
7. Physician institutes appropriate therapy for a UTI

References

1. Hazeldine J, et al. Immunesenescence and inflammaging: a contributory factor in the poor outcome of the geriatric trauma patient. Ageing Res Rev. 2015;24:349–57.
2. Vanzant E, et al. Advanced age is associated with worsened outcomes and a unique genomic response in severely injured patients with hemorrhagic shock. Crit Care. 2015;19:77. https://doi.org/10.1186/s13054-015-0788-x.
3. National Institute on Aging. 2011. Global health and aging. https://www.nia.nih.gov/research/publication/global-health-and-aging
4. Elliott DC, Kufera JA, Myers RA. Necrotizing soft tissue infections. Risk factors for mortality and strategies for management. Ann Surg. 1996;224(5):672–83.
5. Kaye KS, et al. Risk factors for surgical site infections in older people. J Am Geriatr Soc. 2006;54(3):391–6.
6. Serrano PE, et al. Obesity as a risk factor for nosocomial infections in trauma patients. J Am Coll Surg. 2010;211:61–7.
7. Roberts JA, et al. Challenges and potential solutions-individualised antibiotic dosing at the bedside for critically ill patients: a structured review. Lancet Infect Dis. 2014;14(6):498–509.
8. Nomellini V, et al. Aging and animal models of systemic insult: trauma, burns and sepsis. Shock. 2009;31(1):11–20.
9. Pera A, et al. Immunosenescence: implications for response to infection and vaccination in older people. Maturitas. 2015;82:50–5.
10. Franceschi C, Campisi J. Chronic inflammation (inflammaging) and its potential contribution to age-associated diseases. J Geront. 2014;69(S1):S4–9.
11. Pawelec G, Derhovanessian E, Larbi A, Strindhall J, Wikby A. Cytomegalovirus and human immunosenescence. Rev Med Virol. 2009;19(1):47–56.
12. Groeneveld KM, et al. Immunotherapy after trauma: timing is essential. Curr Opin Anesthesiol. 2001;24:219–23.
13. Butcher SK, et al. Senescence in innate immune responses: reduced neutrophil phagocytic capacity and CD16 expression in elderly humans. J Leuk Biol. 2001;70:881–6.
14. Butcher SK, et al. Effect of age on susceptibility to post-traumatic infection in the elderly. Biochem Soc Trans. 2003;31(pt 2):449–51.
15. Nacionales D, et al. A detailed characterization of the dysfunctional immunity and abnormal myelopoiesis induced by severe shock and trauma in the aged. J Immun. 2015;195:2396–407.
16. Van Duin D. Diagnostic challenges and opportunities in older adults with infectious diseases. CID. 2012;54(7):973–8.
17. Lee CC, et al. Comparison of clinical manifestations and outcome of community acquired bloodstream infections among the oldest old, elderly, and adult patients. Medicine. 2007;86:138–44.
18. Meisner M, et al. Correlation of procalcitonin and CRP to inflammation, complications and outcome during ICU course of multitrauma patients. Crit Care. 2006;10:R1.
19. Castelli GP. Procalcitonin as a prognostic and diagnostic tool for septic complications afer major trauma. Crit Care Med. 2009;37:1845–9.
20. Sakran JV, et al. The utility of procalcitonin in critically ill trauma patients. J Trauma. 2012;73:413–8.
21. American College of Surgeons. Trauma Quality Improvement Program. Geriatric Trauma Management Guidelines 2012. https://www.facs.org/quality-programs/trauma/tqip/best-practice
22. Bochicchio GV, et al. Impact of community-acquired infection on acquisition of nosocomial infection, length of stay, and mortality in adult blunt trauma patients. Surg Infect. 2002a;3(1):21–8.
23. Bochicchio GV, et al. Community-acquired infections in the geriatric trauma population. Shock. 2000;14(3):338–42.
24. Bochicchio GV, et al. Nosocomial infections in elderly trauma patients: incidence and microbiology. Inf Med. 2002b;19(11):1–5.

25. Glance LG, et al. Increases in mortality, LOS, and cost associated with HAI in trauma patients. Arch Surg. 2011;146:794–801.
26. Bochicchio GV, et al. Impact of nosocomial infections in trauma: does age make a difference? J Trauma. 2001;50:612–9.
27. Poole D, et al. Systematic review of the literature and evidence based recommendations for antibiotic prophylaxis in trauma: results from an Italian consensus of experts. PLoS One. 2014;9(11):e113676.
28. Climo MW, et al. Effect of daily chlorhexidine bathing on hospital acquired infection. NEJM. 2013;368:533–42.
29. Reiff D, et al. Use of a bundle checklist combined with physician confirmation reduces risk of nosocomial complications and death in trauma patients compared to documented checklist use alone. Ann Surg. 2015;262:647–52.
30. Bo L, Li J, Tao T, Bai Y, Ye X, Hotchkiss RS, Kollef MH, Crooks NH, Deng X. Probiotics for preventing ventilator-associated pneumonia. Cochrane Database Syst Rev 2014, Issue 10. Art. No.: CD009066. DOI:https://doi.org/10.1002/14651858.CD009066.pub2.
31. Gu WJ, et al. The effects of probiotics in early enteral nutrition on the outcomes of trauma: a meta-analysis of randomized controlled trials. JPEN. 2013;37(3):310–7.
32. Urben LM, et al. Bugs or drugs: are probiotics safe for use in the critically ill? Curr Gastroenterol Rep. 2014;16(7):388.
33. Cook A. Ventilator associated pneumonia is more common and of less consequence in trauma patients compared with other critically ill patients. J Trauma. 2010;69:1083–91.
34. Leonard KL, et al. Ventilator-associated pneumonia in trauma patients: different criteria, different rates. Surg Infect. 2016;17(3):363–8.
35. Magnotti LJ, et al. Is ventilator-associated pneumonia in trauma patients an epiphenomenon or a cause of death? Surg Infect. 2004;5:237–42.
36. Mangram AJ, et al. Geriatric trauma service: a one-year experience. J Trauma. 2012;72:119–22.
37. Meyer KC. Lung infections and aging. Ageing Res Rev. 2004;3:55–67.
38. Busl KM, et al. Prolonged mechanical ventilation is associated with pulmonary complications, increased length of stay, and unfavorable discharge destination among patients with subdural hematoma. J Neurosurg Anesthesiol. 2015;27(1):31–6.
39. Hui X, et al. Increased risk of pneumonia among ventilated patients with traumatic brain injury: every day counts. J Surg Res. 2013;184:438–43.
40. Todd SA, et al. A multidisciplinary clinical pathway decreases rib fracture-associated infectious morbidity and mortality in high-risk trauma patients. Am J Surg. 2006;192(6):806–11.
41. How-to Guide. Prevent central-line associated bloodstream infections (CLABSI). Cambridge, MA: Institute for Healthcare Improvement; 2012a. www.ihi.org
42. How-to Guide. Prevent ventilator-associated pneumonia. Cambridge, MA: Institute for Healthcare Improvement; 2012b. www.ihi.org
43. Shi Z, Xie H, Wang P, Zhang Q, Wu Y, Chen E, Ng L, Worthington HV, Needleman I, Furness S. Oral hygiene care for critically ill patients to prevent ventilator-associated pneumonia. Cochrane Database Syst Rev 2013, Issue 8. Art. No.: CD008367.
44. Wang L, Li X, Yang Z, Tang X, Yuan Q, Deng L, Sun X. Semi-recumbent position versus supine position for the prevention of ventilator-associated pneumonia in adults requiring mechanical ventilation. Cochrane Database Syst Rev 2016, Issue 1. Art. No.: CD009946.
45. Chaari A. Does selective digestive decontamination prevent ventilator associated pneumonia in trauma patients? Am J Therap. 2014;21:470–6.
46. Price R, MacLennan G, Glen J. Selective digestive or oropharyngeal decontamination and topical oropharyngeal chlorhexidine for prevention of death in general intensive care: systematic review and network meta-analysis. Br Med J. 2014;348:g2197. https://doi.org/10.1136/bmj.g2197.
47. Plantinga NL, Bonten MJ. Selective decontamination and antibiotic resistance in ICUs. Crit Care. 2015;19(1):259. https://doi.org/10.1186/s13054-015-0967-9.
48. El Solh AA, et al. Nosocomial pneumonia in elderly patients following cardiac surgery. Respir Med. 2006;100:729–36.
49. Torrance HDT, Pearse RM, O'Dwyer MJ. Does major surgery induce immune suppression and increase the risk of postoperative infection? Curr Opin Anaesth. 2016;29:376–83.
50. Brunskill SJ, Millette SL, Shokoohi A, Pulford EC, Doree C, Murphy MF, Stanworth S. Red blood cell transfusion for people undergoing hip fracture surgery. Cochrane Database Syst Rev 2015, Issue 4. CD009699.
51. Monaghan SF. The development of a urinary tract infection is associated with increased mortality in trauma patients. J Trauma. 2011;71(6):1569–74.
52. Polites SF, et al. Urinary tract infection in elderly trauma patients: review of the trauma quality improvement program identifies the population at risk. J Trauma Acute Care Surg. 2014;77(6):952–9.
53. Lo E, et al. Strategies to prevent catheter-associated urinary tract infections in acute care hospitals: 2014 update. Inf Cont Hosp Epidem. 2014;35:S32–47.
54. Graham PL, et al. A U.S. population-based survey of *Staphylococcus aureus* colonization. Ann Intern Med. 2006;144:318–25.
55. Croft CA, et al. MRSA in a trauma population. Am Surg. 2009;75:458–62.
56. Ghose C. Clostridium Difficile infection in the twenty-first century. Emerg Microb Infect. 2013;2:e62. https://doi.org/10.1038/emi.2013.62.

57. Dubberke E, Carling P, Carrico R, Donskey C, Loo V, McDonald L, et al. Strategies to prevent Clostridium Difficile infections in acute care hospitals: 2014 update. Infect Control Hosp Epidemiol. 2014;35(6):628–45. https://doi.org/10.1086/676023. http://www.jstor.org/stable/10.1086/676023
58. Berenholtz SM. Eliminating catheter related bloodstream infections in the ICU. Crit Care Med. 2004;32:2014–20.
59. Blot K, et al. Prevention of central line-associated bloodstream infections through quality improvement interventions: a systematic review and meta-analysis. Clin Infect Dis. 2014;59(1):96–105.
60. Marschall J, Mermel L, Fakih M, Hadaway L, Kallen A, O'Grady N, et al. Strategies to prevent central line–associated bloodstream infections in acute care hospitals: 2014 update. Infect Control Hosp Epidemiol. 2014;35(7):753–71. https://doi.org/10.1086/676533. http://www.jstor.org/stable/10.1086/676533
61. CDC National Diabetes Statistics Report 2014. http://www.cdc.gov/diabetes/pubs/statsreport14/national-diabetes-report-web.pdf
62. Wild S, et al. Global prevalence of diabetes. Estimates for the year 2000 and projections for the year 2030. Diabet Care. 2004;27:1047–53.
63. American Diabetes Association. Standards of medical care in diabetes-2013. Diabetes Care. 2013;36(Suppl 1):S11–66. http://dx.doi.org/10.2337/dc13-S011
64. Toschlog EA, et al. Morbidity reduction in critically ill trauma patients through use of a computerized insulin infusion protocol: a preliminary study. J Trauma. 2007;62:1370–6.
65. Garwe T, et al. Hypoalbuminemia at admission is associated with increased incidence of in-hospital complications in geriatric trauma patients. Am J Surg. 2016;212(1):109–15.
66. Ulldemolins M. The effects of Hypoalbuminemia on optimizing antibacterial dosing in critically ill patients. Clin Pharmacokinet. 2011;2011(50):99–110.
67. Michels WM, et al. Performance of the Cockcroft-Gault, MDRD, and new CKD-EPI formulas in relation to GFR, age, and body size. Clin J Am Soc Nephrol. 2010;5(6):1003–9.
68. Stevens LA, et al. Comparison of drug dosing recommendations based on measured GFR and kidney function estimating equations. Am J Kidney Dis. 2009;54(1):33–42.
69. Roberts JA, et al. Plasma and target-site subcutaneous tissue population pharmacokinetics and dosing simulations of cefazolin in post-trauma critically ill patients. J Antimicrob Chemother. 2015;70:1495–502.
70. Medellın-Garibay SE, et al. Pharmacokinetics of vancomycin and dosing recommendations for trauma patients. J Antimicrob Chemother. 2016;71:471–9.
71. Schmelzer TM, et al. Vancomycin intermittent dosing versus continuous infusion for treatment of ventilator associated pneumonia in trauma patients. Amer Surg. 2013;79:1185–90.
72. Corbett SM, Rebuck JA. Medication-related complications in the trauma patient. J Int Care Med. 2008;23:91–108.
73. Owens RC, Nolin TD. Antimicrobial-associated QT interval prolongation: pointes of interest. Clin Infect Dis. 2006;43:1603–11.

Part XVI

Post-Acute Care: Considerations in Disposition

41 Perioperative Management of the Geriatric Patient

Bellal Joseph and Peter Rhee

The Impact of Aging Physiology in Critical Care

It is obvious and well known that the geriatric population is growing in number and complexity in modern surgical practice. Advances in surgical and anesthetic techniques, combined with sophisticated perioperative monitoring are some of the reasons for the complexity. Therefore, a more comprehensive and multidisciplinary approach is necessary to adequately address the significant differences in physiology and outcomes presented by this challenging group. The optimal goal of surgical critical care for geriatric patients is not only to reduce mortality rates, but for them to maintain and preserve a good quality of life and increase their ability to return to their pre-injury level of function and independence. Ideally, following discharge, patients should be able to live independently, healthfully, and be reintegrated into their previous social life. The mortality of intensive care patients increases gradually with age and reaches around 20% in patients between 60 and 75 years of age. Obviously the mortality rate of older patients is much greater than for the younger cohorts [1].

Likewise, the burden of comorbid disease and dependency rises with age and predicts the need for hospitalization. Not surprisingly, the demand for critical care services and admissions to intensive care units is projected to dramatically increase through the next decade [2, 3]. Presently, in the US, patients aged ≥65 years occupy approximately 55% of all ICU bed-days and an estimated 14% of those patients aged ≥85 years die in the ICU [3]. This irrefutable reality means that the growing population of elderly intensive care patients with multiple medical problems and functional impairment can only be best served by surgeons with a good working knowledge of the changes associated with aging, including the physiological transformations that directly impact the efficacy of surgery and anesthesia. With the aging population there is a definite need for more geriatric services to aid the surgeons but this is currently a limited resource and surgeons need to be able to become our own geriatric service.

Clinical Presentation of Elderly Patients

Primary evaluation of the elderly patient with a suspected surgical emergency is challenging. Presentation of the elderly patient is often atypical, delayed, and vague. Preexisting mental

B. Joseph, M.D. (✉) • P. Rhee, M.D.
Division of Trauma, Department of Surgery, University of Arizona, 1501 N. Campbell Ave, Room 5411, P.O. Box 245063, Tucson, AZ 85724, USA
e-mail: bjoseph@surgery.arizona.edu; prhee@GMH.EDU

A. Rodriguez et al. (eds.), *Geriatric Trauma and Acute Care Surgery*, https://doi.org/10.1007/978-3-319-57403-5_41

illness or neurologic deficits (e.g., dementia, delirium, prior stroke, and diabetic neuropathy) commonly contribute to atypical or delayed presentation by the patient. These widespread factors also make it difficult for primary care providers to detect issues [4]. Moreover, the history of present illness may be difficult to obtain as it is often complex, deficient, and imprecise. Similarly, the results of a physical examination may be misleadingly benign and, therefore, leave the well-intended care provider unaware of a serious underlying condition. Among patients hospitalized for intensive care, the following conditions contribute to delays and difficulties in consummate surgical evaluation and treatment: altered mental status, absence of peritoneal signs, analgesics, antibiotics, and mechanical ventilation. Consequently, such factors further contribute to increased rates of morbidity and mortality among the elderly with surgical conditions [5, 6].

Outcomes for Surgical Care in Geriatric

The quality of healthcare services has become increasingly important over the past couple of decades, and it is clear that a better understanding of the outcomes following traumatic injury or acute care surgery involving the elderly can be an excellent tool for advancing evidence-based healthcare as well as for guiding patients in making informed decisions.

Multiple factors help determine outcomes in geriatric trauma, including, for instance, general clinical condition, demographics, and the severity of the injury. The general clinical condition of the patient has a critical role in predicting outcomes of geriatric trauma. It is a cumulative effect of age, comorbidities, decline in physiologic reserve, cognition, and functional ability. In contrast to younger adults who suffer the same severity of injury, for example, geriatric patients are more likely to have higher mortality or to develop more long-term complications due to the fact that aging is associated with certain physiologic changes and multiple comorbidities that impede healing and recovery. Researchers have extensively studied the following outcomes in geriatric patients: inhospital mortality (IHM), post-hospitalization mortality (PMH), inhospital complications, functional status, and ICU and hospital length of stay. Multiple studies have shown a significant association between mortality, inhospital complications, and increasing age. Post-injury functional status of the elderly patient is a sensitive indicator of the patient's health and quality of life after traumatic injury and acute care surgery. Elderly patients admitted to the hospital for an acute illness or a traumatic injury are more prone than younger patients to develop functional disability and to be discharged to skilled nursing facilities for long-term care. Notably, more than 90% of geriatric trauma patients require skilled nursing care facilities at least for 1 year after the injury [7]. Complications resulting from a functional decline after such an injury include loss of independence, falls, incontinence, depression, malnutrition, and the lack of socialization.

Fortunately, an early evaluation via a team assessment of the general clinical condition, injury severity, and functional and cognitive impairments of the elderly patient can enable rapid and appropriate management by utilizing geriatric principles to minimize the risk of adverse outcomes.

Challenges in Pre- and Postoperative Care for the Elderly

In recent years, there has been a growing interest in the impact of surgery on the elderly. As life spans increase and more elderly patients undergo surgery, it is crucial that healthcare systems and providers gain enough knowledge to understand how elderly patients are different and how to modify their care to improve their outcomes. Pre and postoperative care is critical in the elderly because they have higher rates of morbidity and mortality. Of course, these characteristics can seriously undercut the benefits of surgery for this population.

Preoperative Care

The aim of the preoperative assessment is to identify perioperative risks and factors that increase patient risk for postoperative complications or death. Surgical disease itself and the type of surgical procedure could be a part of those factors. However, the two most important factors in the determination of postoperative morbidity and mortality relate to the general health and physiological reserve of the patient. Diminished physiologic reserves have a direct impact on the patient's ability to have an optimal response to the additional stress of surgery and possible postoperative complications. A preoperative assessment includes a complete history with a full medication list, a physical examination, and laboratory examinations. Additionally, an assessment of surgical risks should be included in a preoperative evaluation of an elective surgery. Regarding informed consent, the patient and consenting family member(s) or legal guardian(s) should be told about the procedure and any potential complications or disabilities. It is also worth highlighting that the prevalence of undernutrition and malnutrition in older patients is considerable. From 9 to 15% of persons over the age of 65 years are found to be malnourished in outpatient clinics, 12 to 50% in acute inpatient hospitals, and 25 to 60% or more in chronic institutional setting. The laboratory assessment of malnutrition generally includes a complete blood cell count, albumin and transferrin levels. An albumin level of less than 3.2 g/dl in a frail elderly person is a risk factor for increased mortality. A body mass index of less than 20 kg/m^2 also suggests a high risk. A complete and careful physical examination is necessary. It is important to note hydration, nutritional status, the neck (lymph nodes, thyroid masses, carotid pulsations, and bruits), blood pressure, and an abdominal examination for lesions such as hernia, aortic aneurysm, and masses. A rectal examination is also a necessity, as is a pelvic examination in women. Any evidence of peripheral vascular disease should be identified. While age as an isolated factor has a minimal effect on postoperative morbidity or mortality, current data shows that comorbid status has the greatest effect on the surgical outcome.

Postoperative Care

Infection

Postoperative infections are an important cause of morbidity and mortality in elderly patients. Although the mechanism of how the aging process decreases the immunologic response is still not clear, the relevant literature demonstrates that elderly patients have diminished immune function that makes them more liable to infection [8]. The most common sites of postoperative infection are the urinary tract, the lungs, and the surgical site [8].

Surgical site infection (SSI) is a major postoperative complication, and it is the most common nosocomial infection in surgical patients, accounting for 38% of nosocomial infections in such patients [9]. A SSI is an infection related to an operative procedure that occurs at or near the surgical incision within 30 days of the procedure or within 1 year if prosthetic material is implanted during surgery. It has a considerable impact on morbidity, and it can create a substantial economic burden for both patients and the healthcare system [10]. Most significantly, elderly patients with a SSI have a three times higher mortality rate than that elderly patients without infections [10, 11]. It is associated with the operative procedure/technique as well as patient-specific factors. Advanced age is a host-derived risk factor for SSI [12]. This infection is caused by organisms introduced into the surgical wound at the time of the operative procedure [10]. Most of these organisms originate from the patient's own flora; however, exogenous sources of bacteria can also lead to infection. Fortunately, the application of preventive practices can prevent a SSI. These include appropriate antibiotic selection and administration, intraoperative maintenance of normothermia, not shaving the surgical site until just prior to incising the skin, and ensuring perioperative euglycemia [12, 13]. Close monitoring of surgical wounds postoperatively is necessary to ensure the early detection and treatment of wound infections. Treatment of SSI involves opening the incision and allowing adequate drainage. The results of culture and sensitivity tests should guide the use of antibiotics [10]. The fear of not detecting SSI early is necrotizing fasciitis, which can be very rapid and deadly.

A urinary tract infection (UTI) is typically due to prolonged bladder catheterization. Approximately 25% of hospitalized patients undergo urinary bladder catheterization. Of these, 10–27% develop UTIs [14]. Around 80% of patients with nosocomial UTIs undergo urinary bladder catheterization. There is a greater need for urinary bladder catheterization in elderly patients, especially due to the need for careful monitoring of urine output, medication side effects, preexisting incontinence, prostatism, and decreased mobility. Elderly patients usually present with the classic symptoms of dysuria, fever, and frequency. These are also common in younger people, but the elderly may have more vague presentations, such as an acute confusional state, decreased mobility, or newly developed urinary incontinence. It is noteworthy that UTI examination findings can reflect many possible causes. Consequently, it is necessary to examine the patient completely for other possible diagnoses, send a urine sample to confirm the diagnosis, and to perform an antibiotic sensitivity test.

Postoperative confusion may be the first and only sign of a UTI. One of the most efficacious preventive strategies for elderly patients is to minimize the use of urinary catheters as well as the early removal of the catheters [8]. Other strategies used to minimize bacterial colonization and subsequent infection include disinfecting the skin regularly and using disinfectants in the collecting system. Although every effort should be made to discontinue the catheter as soon as possible, the worse scenario is acute kidney injury as the urine output was not known.

ICU patients are at risk of dying not only from their primary disease, but also from secondary processes such as nosocomial infections. Nosocomial pneumonia (NP) is the second most common nosocomial infection. It is the leading cause of postoperative mortality in elderly patients [15]. NP occurs primarily in patients undergoing general surgery. Ventilator-associated pneumonia (VAP) is pneumonia that occurs more than 48 h after patients have been intubated and received mechanical ventilation. Diagnosing VAP requires a high clinical suspicion combined with a bedside examination, a radiographic examination, and a microbiologic analysis of respiratory secretions. Although NP has the same presentation and management for all age groups, certain risk factors including age and depleted physiological reserve make the elderly more vulnerable to NP. Additionally, nasogastric tubes, tracheal intubation, dementia, aspiration, recent chest or abdominal surgery, and immobility can increase the risk for developing NP [15]. Underlying comorbid conditions, malnutrition, and impaired immune function also increase the mortality associated with postoperative pneumonia in the elderly [8].

Neuropsychiatric Disorders

Neuropsychiatric problems are common among older patients. Delirium, dementia, and depression are pernicious conditions that have to be taken into account. 15% of all patients admitted for repair of hip fractures, for instance, have dementia. An acute illness or hospitalization can also exacerbate depression among older patients. An abrupt change in cognition and consciousness is the major manifestation of delirium, defined as a temporary, altered mental status. New onset visual hallucinations in the elderly patients are more suggestive of delirium than of a new psychiatric disorder. Two types of delirium usually present in the postoperative phase: emergence delirium (ED) and postoperative delirium (POD). ED is a benign cognitive disorientation that can occur during the transition from anesthesia to wakefulness that resolves within minutes or hours, while POD is an acute organic brain syndrome that usually develops within the first few postoperative days [16, 17]. POD is an acute disorder, but it has been associated with a wide range of negative long-term outcomes for the elderly, even though patients may initially recover completely. Approximately 15% of all elderly patients experience POD after elective procedures, with a higher incidence (30–70%) among elderly who have undergone emergency operations [18]. Postoperative delirium (POD) can prolong the length of stay in the hospital as well as the postoperative dependence of elderly people. It is also associated with reduced function and independence, increased short- and long-term mortality, and prolonged cognitive impairment in survivors [19]. The definitive mechanism that underlies delirium is not clearly known; many hypotheses, however, concur that delirium is the final clinical consequence of complicated neurotransmitter abnormalities. Researchers have identified several factors, including infection, inflammation, metabolite disturbances, substance withdrawal, medications, discomfort, environmental disturbances (including sleep disruption), and severe pain due to inadequate analgesia. There are several criteria to diagnose delirium: disturbed consciousness, cognitive changes, rapid onset and fluctuating course, presence of a causal medical condition, or a change of substance usage [19, 20].

Cardiac Complications

Myocardial Ischemia and Infarction

Cardiac complications such as myocardial infarction and heart failure are common causes of postoperative morbidity and mortality that occur in 1–5% of patients undergoing noncardiac surgery [21, 22]. At least 10% of all perioperative deaths result from myocardial complications. The most common postoperative cardiac complications in elderly patients are myocardial ischemia and myocardial infarction. The elderly are also more liable to suffer from post-myocardial infarction heart failure [23]. The mortality associated with perioperative myocardial infarction is approximately 30% for older patients [19]. Comorbid conditions such as hypertension, diabetes mellitus, and a history of cardiac or renal failure are risk factors for a higher incidence of perioperative myocardial infarction (5.1%), cardiac death (5.7%), or ischemia (12–17.7%) in elderly patients [23].

The majority of perioperative myocardial infarctions occur within the first 3 days after surgery, and frequently on the first postoperative day [24]. Although chest pain is the most common presenting symptom of myocardial ischemia in young patients, elderly patients may present with minimal chest pain, which may be misleading. Myocardial ischemic events are silent in over 80% of elderly patients [25]. Incisional pain, residual anesthetic effects, postoperative analgesia, and the lack of typical angina pain in elderly patients during the postoperative period often leads to doctors to miss a diagnosis of a cardiac ischemic attack. Among the elderly, atypical presentations, such as tachycardia hypotension, dyspnea, respiratory failure, syncope, confusion, nausea, and excessive hyperglycemia in diabetics, are more common characteristics of myocardial ischemia.

Dysrhythmias

Postoperative arrhythmias are common and represent a major source of morbidity after both cardiac and noncardiac surgical procedures [26]. Postoperative atrial arrhythmias occur in 6.1% of elderly patients undergoing noncardiac surgery [27]. Postoperative electrolyte disturbances and increased sympathetic nervous system activity may lead to cardiac dysrhythmias, although myocardial ischemia or congestive heart failure should be taken in account [28].

The only proven preoperative risk factor for developing an atrial arrhythmias following surgery is an age of 60 years or older [28]. Patients aged more than 60 years and undergoing elective thoracic surgery are independently associated with a higher risk for developing atrial fibrillation [27]. Cardiac arrhythmias may also be stimulated by pulmonary disease, such as pneumonia or pulmonary embolism, volume overload, hyperthyroidism, or sympathomimetic drugs. Atrial arrhythmia-onset peaks 2–3 days following surgery. Perioperative atrial arrhythmias are usually well tolerated by younger patients. However, it can be associated with hemodynamic instability in elderly patients. The complications of atrial fibrillation include stroke and congestive heart failure. Atrial fibrillation is also associated with higher inpatient mortality when accompanied by myocardial infarction

(25 vs. 16%) [29]. Management of atrial fibrillation consists of heart rhythm and rate control as well as prophylaxis against of thromboembolism.

Pulmonary Complications

Postoperative pulmonary complications are common, especially in elderly patients with comorbidities. Nearly 5% of all patients undergoing noncardiac surgery experience significant pulmonary complications. These are a common cause of postoperative morbidity and mortality. They account for up to 40% of all postoperative complications and 20% of potentially preventable deaths [30]. The most common pulmonary complications are lung collapse, hypoxemia, hypoventilation, acute respiratory distress syndrome, and pneumonia. Development of these complications can extend the ICU unit stay and increase mortality. Compared to younger patients, patients 70 years of age and older have a higher risk of respiratory complications, including bacterial pneumonia, non-cardiogenic pulmonary edema, and respiratory failure requiring intubation [31]. Age-related alterations in pulmonary function combined with postoperative pulmonary pathophysiologic changes place the elderly patient at greater risk for complications. Clinical predictors of adverse pulmonary outcomes include site of surgery (chest, abdomen), duration and type of anesthesia, chronic obstructive pulmonary disease (COPD), asthma, preoperative hyper-secretion of mucus, chest deformation, and perioperative nasogastric tube placement [32].

Aspiration

Aspiration is the inhalation of oropharyngeal or gastric contents into the larynx and lower respiratory tract. Normal deglutition is a smooth, coordinated process that involves a complex series of voluntary and involuntary neuromuscular contractions. Age-related changes affect each phase of the swallowing process, increasing the risk of aspiration in the elderly [33]. The presence of other risk factors in the elderly that make them particularly vulnerable to oropharyngeal aspiration include dysphagia, poor oral hygiene, altered level of consciousness, and gastroesophageal reflux disease [33]. Dysphagia and recurrent pneumonia in elderly patients are alarming factors for physicians. Patients found to be aspirating should undergo swallow therapy, modification of dietary consistency, training in specific swallowing techniques, and upright positioning while feeding. Surgery is rarely indicated.

Pain Management

Effective pain management is more complex in the elderly than it is for younger patients. Nonetheless, it is essential for a smooth recovery and early rehabilitation. This complexity is due to certain factors that include impaired cognition, medical comorbidities, drug interactions, and problems with appropriate dosing. Age-related suboptimal renal function often limits the ability to adopt a standardized protocol for pain management after surgery. Obviously, pain may have a substantial impact on recovery and may also exacerbate underlying pulmonary or cardiac comorbidities. Fear of pain results in less postoperative mobility, thereby increasing the risk of thromboembolism, urinary retention, fecal impaction, and atelectasis [34]. The treatment plan should anticipate the need for pain control. Also, it should be individualized and assessed/modified frequently based on the patient's response. Medical and non-pharmacologic approaches should also be used. These include physical agents and cognitive behavioral approaches [35]. Opioids are the ideal agents for treating acute postoperative pain because they have no ceiling to the analgesic effect. However, ways to diminish the need for opioids are being explored due to the possible adverse effects on respiratory, gastrointestinal, and cognitive function in older patients. Managing pain is very difficult in the elderly as it can easily alter mental status and this derangement can be confused with delirium. The geriatric mantra is "start low, go slow, but go" when dealing with titrating pain medication. Combination of benzodiazepines and opiates are a dangerous combination. Elderly patients with injuries from fractures and the desire to treat the pain must be weighed against iatrogenic complications. The use of regional and local anesthesia is highly recommended when applicable. One approach is to decrease the analgesic requirements with minimally invasive surgery. Because minimally invasive procedures result in shorter hospitalization, earlier ambulation, decreased postoperative pain, and more rapid return to routine activities, laparoscopic surgery would appear to be the ideal surgical choice for elderly patients [36].

Geriatrics and GCS

A low Glasgow coma scores (GCS) in patients >65 years upon arrival to the hospital is an accurate predictor of poor functional outcomes and high mortality rates. The mortality rate in patients >60 years with an admission GCS < 8 is 87%. It is 100% in patients with ≥80 years with a GCS of <11 [37].

A low energy mechanism of trauma can lead to serious injury and complications in geriatric trauma patients, especially in patients with traumatic brain injury (TBI), due to the effect of anticoagulant drugs commonly prescribed to older patients [38].

Elderly patients with a brain injury sustained higher mortality and poorer functional outcomes due to physiological changes that occur during the aging process. As the brain decreases in size with age, the clinical symptoms of brain tissue compression may present late [39]. Therefore, close observation of elderly patients with a GCS score is necessary for 24 h after the injury to avoid devastating complications of TBI [39, 40].

Geriatrics and Injury Scores

In younger populations, the accuracy of the injury severity score (ISS) has been validated. Among the elderly, however, there is a lack of consistency in the ISS application [41]. Patients >60 years of age with an average ISS of 19.7 have an 18% mortality rate [41]. The mortality rate in geriatric patients is twice that in younger patients with the same ISS [41]. Current studies have demonstrated that a combination of the ISS with the APACHE II scores is a more accurate predictor of mortality in the elderly than using the ISS or the APACHE II alone [42].

Ethical and End-of-Life Decisions

As people approach the end of their lives, they and their families face tasks and decisions ranging from the simple to the extremely complex. They may be practical, psychosocial, spiritual, legal, existential, or medical in nature. The central component of the physician–patient relationship is the patient's best interest. The patient has the right to determine the level of care or type of therapy. The goal of end-of-life care is to provide comfort throughout the dying process. Experts suggest that open patient–doctor communication and decisions about care should occur early in the illness. This helps to prepare the individual for the progression and treatment of the illness. It also guides patients and their families toward realistic expectations about the entire process. Advance directives may aid decision-making by physicians and family members when an elderly patient cannot participate in the decision-making process. Advance directives are only activated when the treating physician has determined that the patient is incapacitated. Unfortunately, many patients presenting with acute surgical processes have no advance directive. In the absence of such a document, healthcare providers may give more aggressive care than the patient desired. For the elderly patient who presents with a life-threatening acute surgical process, therefore, the physician should use clearly understandable terms to explain to the patient or surrogate the diagnoses, management options, and expected outcomes. Management of unrealistic expectations is often difficult to manage with the family members who do not want the guilt of ending a loved one's life. Ideally, this will allow for a more scrupulous determination of the level of aggressiveness of treatment/intervention desired by the patient or surrogate. Without this thorough effort, the patient or his/her surrogate may complain about the patient suffering as a result of either a deficiency or an excess of care.

Frailty

The physiological changes associated with aging are unique in each individual. Patients with same chronological age may have different physiological age. Frailty is defined as a syndrome of decreased physiological reserve and a diminished resistance to stressors resulting in increased vulnerability to poor health outcomes. Studies have demonstrated that frailty index is superior to age in predicting the outcomes in geriatric trauma patients and the use of age alone for clinical decision may be misleading [43, 44]. However, the impact of frailty on outcomes in trauma patients decreases at the extremes of age. There are numerous functional tests, questionnaires, and indexes for measuring frailty and there is no consensus on which is best to use across all clinical settings. According to recent studies, a frailty measuring instrument should include nutritional status, physical activity, mobility, strength, energy (physical domain), cognition, mood (psychological domain), and social relations (social domain) as essential factors [45].

Several models exist for the calculation of the frailty index. The most comprehensive frailty questionnaire is the Rockwood frailty model based on 70 variables that assess the cognitive, physiological, physical, and social well-being of the individual. This index has been validated in patients undergoing elective surgery. The frailty index is so much more than just a predictor of outcome. It can be used to manage and advise as well as to predict the need for resources. In general, this is a more expanded form of learning how old a patient is physiologically compared to their mere chronological age. The physiology is exceedingly varied for a given age. A person 70 years of age may have little to no reserves with abundant comorbidities whereas someone in the 90s may be fully independently functional. Thus using a standardized set of questions, the frailty score and index is much more meaningful than just the chronological age. More recently, a modified 50-variable Rockwood frailty index has been shown to reliably predict morbidity in patients undergoing emergency general surgery [46]. Interestingly, using the 15 strongest predictors out of the 50 variables, a similar predictability can be achieved. The use of this 15-variable Emergency General Surgery (EGS) specific frailty index allows for a more rapid yet accurate assessment of the frailty status of patients undergoing emergency general surgery. For each question in the frailty index, a patient receives a score varying from 0 to 1. The sum of final score is then divided by 15 to calculate the frailty index of the patient. Patients with a frailty index of >0.325 are considered frail and are at a high risk for morbidity following emergency general surgery.

Another important healthcare quality matrix is failure to rescue, which is defined as death from a major complication. It indicates how well a hospital performs once a patient develops a complication. Existing literature suggests that reducing failure to rescue events might be the most important target for quality improvement in the geriatric population. A recent study by Joseph et al. has shown that presence of frailty in elderly trauma patients increases the odds of failure to rescue by threefold as compared to the non-frail patients [47]. Frailty index can be utilized as a tool to identify patients at increased risk of failure to rescue. Appropriate resource allocation to prevent complications and early initiation of aggressive management can significantly impact the failure to rescue rate and improve the quality of care provided to these patients.

Conclusion

Care of the elderly surgical patient is an important part of perioperative medicine. In this respect, awareness of specific pathophysiological and pharmacological aspects of this group of patients is required in order to preserve quality assurance. A combination of surgical, geriatric, and anesthesia risk factors seems to be responsible for a prolonged hospital stay and an increased morbidity and mortality. Recent developments focus on early recovery by multidisciplinary team for perioperative care, which includes minimal invasive surgery, postoperative anesthesiology rounds, and proactive geriatric consultation. Surgeons, anesthetists, and geriatricians should be aware of the responsibility and challenges for the development and successful implementation of such programs in perioperative practice.

Acknowledgement There are no identifiable conflicts of interests to report.

The authors have no financial or proprietary interest in the subject matter or materials discussed in the manuscript.

References

1. Horn J. Intensive care and the elderly. Arch Gerontol Geriatr. 1997;25(1):101–10.
2. Angus DC, Barnato AE, Linde-Zwirble WT, Weissfeld LA, Watson RS, Rickert T, Rubenfeld GD. Use of intensive care at the end of life in the United States: an epidemiologic study. Crit Care Med. 2004;32(3):638–43.
3. Bagshaw SM, Webb SA, Delaney A, George C, Pilcher D, Hart GK, Bellomo R. Very old patients admitted to intensive care in Australia and New Zealand: a multicentre cohort analysis. Crit Care. 2009;13(2):R45.
4. Kim PK, Kauder DR, Schwab CW. Acute care surgery and the elderly, Acute Care Surgery. New York: Springer; 2007. p. 187–93.
5. Levkoff SE, Cleary PD, Wetle T, Besdine RW. Illness behavior in the aged. J Am Geriatr Soc. 1988;36(7):622–9.
6. Watters JM, Blakslee JM, March RJ, Redmond ML. The influence of age on the severity of peritonitis. Can J Surg. 1996;39(2):142.
7. Joseph B, Hassan A. Geriatric trauma patients: what is the difference? Current Surgery Reports. 2016;4(1):1–6.
8. Beliveau MM, Multach M. Perioperative care for the elderly patient. Med Clin N Am. 2003;87(1):273–89.
9. Neumayer L, Hosokawa P, Itani K, El-Tamer M, Henderson WG, Khuri SF. Multivariable predictors of postoperative surgical site infection after general and vascular surgery: results from the patient safety in surgery study. J Am Coll Surg. 2007;204(6):1178–87.
10. Kirby JP, Mazuski JE. Prevention of surgical site infection. Surg Clin N Am. 2009;89(2):365–89.
11. Kaye KS, Anderson DJ, Sloane R, Chen LF, Choi Y, Link K, Sexton DJ, Schmader KE. The effect of surgical site infection on older operative patients. J Am Geriatr Soc. 2009;57(1):46–54.
12. Barie PS. Surgical site infections: epidemiology and prevention. Surg Infect. 2002;3(S1):s9–s21.
13. Dellinger EP, Hausmann SM, Bratzler DW, Johnson RM, Daniel DM, Bunt KM, Baumgardner GA, Sugarman JR. Hospitals collaborate to decrease surgical site infections. Am J Surg. 2005;190(1):9–15.
14. Cunha BA. Urinary tract infections in males. In: Bope E, Rakel R, editors. Conn's current therapy, 2003. Philadelphia: Elsevier Science; 2003. p. 733–5. ISBN 0–7216-8745–8.
15. Feldman C. Pneumonia in the elderly. Med Clin N Am. 2001;85(6):1441–59.
16. Radtke F, Franck M, Hagemann L, Seeling M, Wernecke K, Spies C. Risk factors for inadequate emergence after anesthesia: emergence delirium and hypoactive emergence. Minerva Anestesiol. 2010;76(6):394–403.
17. Young J, Inouye SK. Delirium in older people. BMJ: British Medical Journal. 2007;334(7598):842.
18. Ansaloni L, Catena F, Chattat R, Fortuna D, Franceschi C, Mascitti P, Melotti R. Risk factors and incidence of postoperative delirium in elderly patients after elective and emergency surgery. Br J Surg. 2010;97(2):273–80.
19. Lagoo-Deenadayalan SA, Newell MA, Pofahl WE. Common perioperative complications in older patients. In: Principles and practice of geriatric surgery. New York: Springer; 2011. p. 361–76.
20. Strøm C, Rasmussen L. Challenges in anaesthesia for elderly. Singap Dent J. 2014;35:23–9.
21. McGory ML, Maggard MA, Ko CY. A meta-analysis of perioperative beta blockade: what is the actual risk reduction? Surgery. 2005;138(2):171–9.
22. Auerbach AD, Goldman L. β-blockers and reduction of cardiac events in noncardiac surgery: scientific review. JAMA. 2002;287(11):1435–44.
23. Mehta RH, Rathore SS, Radford MJ, Wang Y, Wang Y, Krumholz HM. Acute myocardial infarction in the elderly: differences by age. J Am Coll Cardiol. 2001;38(3):736–41.
24. Ryder DL. The use of β-blockers to decrease adverse perioperative cardiac events. Dimens Crit Care Nurs. 2008;27(2):47–53.
25. Badner NH, Knill RL, Brown JE, Novick TV, Gelb A. Myocardial infarction after noncardiac surgery. Anesthesiology. 1998;88(3):572–8.
26. Loran DB, Hyde BR, Zwischenberger JB. Perioperative management of special populations: the geriatric patient. Surg Clin N Am. 2005;85(6):1259–66.
27. Amar D, Zhang H, Leung DH, Roistacher N, Kadish AH. Older age is the strongest predictor of postoperative atrial fibrillation. The Journal of the American Society of Anesthesiologists. 2002;96(2):352–6.
28. Ramsay JG. Cardiac management in the ICU. Chest J. 1999;115(suppl_2):138S–44S.
29. Amar D. Prevention and management of perioperative arrhythmias in the thoracic surgical population. Anesthesiol Clin. 2008;26(2):325–35.
30. Ergina PL, Gold SL, Meakins JL. Perioperative care of the elderly patient. World J Surg. 1993;17(2):192–8.
31. Polanczyk CA, Marcantonio E, Goldman L, Rohde LE, Orav J, Mangione CM, Lee TH. Impact of age on perioperative complications and length of stay in

patients undergoing noncardiac surgery. Ann Intern Med. 2001;134(8):637–43.
32. McAlister FA, Bertsch K, Man J, Bradley J, Jacka M. Incidence of and risk factors for pulmonary complications after nonthoracic surgery. Am J Respir Crit Care Med. 2005;171(5):514–7.
33. Feinberg MJ, Knebl J, Tully J, Segall L. Aspiration and the elderly. Dysphagia. 1990;5(2):61–71.
34. Wood DL. Failure of pain relief after surgery: attitudes of ward staff and patients toward postoperative analgesia. Plast Reconstr Surg. 1996;97(7):1523.
35. Katz PR. Geriatrics syllabus for specialists: the American Geriatrics Society; 2002.
36. Brunt L, Quasebarth M, Dunnegan D, Soper N. Outcomes analysis of laparoscopic cholecystectomy in the extremely elderly. Surg Endosc. 2001;15(7):700–5.
37. Cagetti B, Cossu M, Pau A, Rivano C, Viale G. The outcome from acute subdural and epidural intracranial haematomas in very elderly patients. Br J Neurosurg. 1992;6(3):227–31.
38. Joseph B, Pandit V, Aziz H, Kulvatunyou N, Hashmi A, Tang A, O'Keeffe T, Wynne J, Vercruysse G, Friese RS, et al. Clinical outcomes in traumatic brain injury patients on preinjury clopidogrel: a prospective analysis. The journal of trauma and acute care surgery. 2014;76(3):817–20.
39. Pennings JL, Bachulis BL, Simons CT, Slazinski T. SUrvival after severe brain injury in the aged. Arch Surg. 1993;128(7):787–94.
40. Chang W-H, Tsai S-H, Su Y-J, Huang C-H, Chang K-S, Tsai C-H. Trauma mortality factors in the elderly population. International Journal of Gerontology. 2008;2(1):11–7.
41. Watts HF, Kerem Y, Kulstad EB. Evaluation of the revised trauma and injury severity scores in elderly trauma patients. Journal of emergencies, trauma, and shock. 2012;5(2):131.
42. Carillo E, Richardson J, Malias M, Cryer H, Miller F. Long term outcome of blunt trauma in the elderly. Surg Gynecol Obstet. 1993;176:559–64.
43. Jokar TO, Rhee PM, Zangbar B, Kulvatunyou N, Khalil M, O'Keeffe T, Tang AL, Friese RS, Gries LM, Joseph B. Redefining the association between old age and poor outcomes after trauma: the impact of the frailty syndrome. J Am Coll Surg. 2015;221(4):S83–S4.
44. Joseph B, Pandit V, Zangbar B, Kulvatunyou N, Hashmi A, Green DJ, O'Keeffe T, Tang A, Vercruysse G, Fain MJ. Superiority of frailty over age in predicting outcomes among geriatric trauma patients: a prospective analysis. JAMA Surg. 2014;149(8):766–72.
45. de Vries NM, Staal JB, van Ravensberg CD, Hobbelen JS, Olde Rikkert MG. Nijhuis-van der Sanden MW. Outcome instruments to measure frailty: a systematic review. Ageing Res Rev. 2011;10(1):104–14.
46. Joseph B, Pandit V, Zangbar B, Kulvatunyou N, Tang AL, O'Keeffe T, Green DJ, Fain MJ, Friese RS, Rhee PM. Emergency general surgery in the elderly: too old or too frail? J Am Coll Surg. 2014;219(3):S53–S4.
47. Joseph B, Phelan H, Hassan A, Jokar TO, O'Keeffe T, Azim A, Gries L, Kulvatunyou N, Latifi R, Rhee P. The impact of frailty on failure-to-rescue in geriatric trauma patients: a prospective study. J Trauma Acute Care Surg. 2016;81(6):1150–5.

Part XVII

Perioperative Management

Check for updates

42 Post-acute Considerations in Disposition

Laura Harmon, Leah Kohri, and Rosemary Kozar

Triaging Disposition

Older injured adults are at risk for poor outcomes [1]. Understanding the unique complexities specific to the geriatric trauma population is paramount. Injury severity score (ISS), age, and admitting Glasgow Coma Scale (GCS) are known predictive factors for mortality but older age is also predictive of complications and discharge to skilled nursing facilities [1, 2]. The importance of discharge destination after the index hospitalization is being increasingly recognized as a determinant of long-term survival in the injured elderly [3]. For a variety of reasons, the injured elderly are less likely to meet the criteria for discharge to home or inpatient rehabilitation. Rather, many are being discharged to skilled nursing facilities, one of the most important independent predictors of poor long-term outcomes [4]. In a retrospective analysis of 38,707 patients, Richmond et al. found that the presence of preexisting comorbid medical conditions increased the odds of experiencing complications during the acute hospitalization period. Increasing age, number and types of injuries, injuries due to falls, and lower functional level all predicted discharge to a skilled nursing facility [5]. In another study from the Queensland Trauma Registry, predictors of discharge to a nursing home for older trauma patients included older age, greater injury severity scores (ISS), longer hospital stay, and injury caused by a fall [1]. Beaulieu et al. identified early independent variables predictive of non-home discharges from a review of 2800 geriatric trauma patients. As expected, patients with lower burden of injury were more likely to be discharged home. Independent predictors of disposition to nursing home were female sex, age, intensive care stay, and hospital length of stay. Comorbidities most associated with non-home disposition were neurologic disorders, coagulopathy, and diabetes mellitus [6]. Delirium occurs in approximately 50% of patients while in the intensive care unit and more frequently in geriatric patients [7]. Implementation of bundled care protocols and early occupational and physical therapy

L. Harmon, M.D. • R. Kozar, M.D., Ph.D. (✉)
Department of Surgery, R Adams Cowley Shock Trauma Center, University of Maryland School of Medicine, 22 S Greene Street S4DO7, Baltimore, MD 21201, USA
e-mail: laura.harmon@yahoo.com; rkozar@umm.edu

L. Kohri, B.S.N., C.C.R.N.
Multitrauma Critical Care, R Adams Cowley Shock Trauma Center, 22 S Greene Street, Baltimore, MD 21201, USA
e-mail: lkohri@umm.edu

A. Rodriguez et al. (eds.), *Geriatric Trauma and Acute Care Surgery*,
https://doi.org/10.1007/978-3-319-57403-5_42

involvement have all proven effective measures at decreasing delirium [8, 9].

Of 1352 geriatric admissions after ground level falls, Ayoung-Chee et al. found 51% of elderly patients were discharged to a skilled nursing facility, 39% to home, and only 5% to inpatient rehabilitation facilities [9]. The overall one year mortality for those surviving to discharge was 24%. Patients discharged to a skilled nursing facility, however, had a threefold greater risk of mortality by one year compared with patients discharged to home, with 48% dead by two years. The majority of deaths occurred while patients were residents of the skilled nursing facility [9].

These data strongly suggest that efforts to minimize discharge to skilled nursing facilities are important to long-term outcomes. Potentially modifiable factors during the acute hospitalization include early mobilization, adequate nutrition, avoidance of delirium, prevention of falls, and early discharge planning [10]. In a systematic review and meta-analysis of nine trials involving 1736 patients, Fox et al. compared usual care to early discharge planning [11]. These investigators found that early discharge planning was associated with fewer hospital readmissions and lower readmission lengths of hospital stay. Though there were no differences in index length of hospital stay, mortality, or satisfaction with discharge planning, several of the trials indicated that early discharge planning was associated with greater overall quality of life.

Multidisciplinary Team Approach

Disposition of the geriatric trauma patient is complex and is best handled with a multidisciplinary team approach. Prior to discharge, geriatric patients often need to be evaluated by physical therapists, occupational therapists, speech pathologists, social services, nursing teams, and physicians. Though optimal for discharge planning, multiple teams and multiple disciplines can contribute to delays in discharge. There can be up to a 30% increase in length of hospitalization attributable to delays in communication between disciplines [12]. Early identification and treatment of underlying comorbidities and involvement of appropriate subspecialist is also necessary. At the R. Adams Cowley Shock Trauma Center, we have implemented daily multidisciplinary discharge rounds that are attended by nursing, respiratory care, physical therapy, social services and trauma and orthopedic physicians to discuss the disposition of the patient and attempt to reduce delays in discharge.

Preventing Readmissions

Unplanned rehospitalization in geriatric trauma patients is commonplace with a 25% occurrence within one year [13]. Older patients with severe head injury and those discharged to nursing facility have the highest risk of readmissions. This may reflect severity of injury, specifically in patients requiring higher level of care post hospitalization. Most common causes for readmission include Atrial fibrillation, anemia, and congestive heart failure [13]. During the index hospitalization, the team should clarify home medications, comorbidities, baseline functional and cognitive impairments, and degree of frailty to facilitate discharge planning and prevent readmissions. Geriatric consultation during the index hospitalization may assist with these but can also provide advanced care planning, management of medication changes, improvement in pain management, and reduction in discharges to long-term care [14–16]. Geriatric nursing, using an acute care elderly unit model, has also been reported to improve care by providing comprehensive discharge planning and management [17]. Accurate discharge instructions and early follow-up with not only the trauma physicians but also the patient's primary care physician or gerontologist can prevent readmissions.

Perhaps most important is being able to help the patient and families set realistic expectations. Soberg et al. studied the long-term multidimensional functional consequences of patients with multiple severe injuries two years after trauma. Soberg found a considerable gap in the functional status of post-traumatic patients when compared to the general population [18]. Helping the patient and family to understand the transition of care is paramount to the patient's long-term success [19]. Families should be encouraged to take an active role participating in inpatient care and focus should be centered on rehabilitation as an active process with goals to regaining independence [19, 20].

Keys to Successful Disposition

- Identification of predictors of disposition location.
- Early discharge planning.
- Multidisciplinary team approach.
- Good communication team members.
- Early follow-up to prevent readmission.

References

1. Aitken LM, Burmeister E, Lang J, Chaboyer W, Richmond TS. Characteristics and outcomes of injured older adults after hospital admission. J Am Geriatric Soc. 2010;58(3):442–9.
2. Botwinick I, Johnson J, Safadjou S, Cohen-Levy W, Reddy SH, McNelis J, Teperman SH, Stone ME. Geriatric nursing home falls: A single institution cross-sectional study. Arch Gerontol Geriatr. 2016;63:42–8.
3. Claridge JA, Leukhardt WH, Golob JF, McCoy AM, Malangoni MA. Moving beyond traditional measurement of mortality after injury: evaluation of risks for late death. J Am Coll Surg. 2010;210(5):788–94.
4. Davidson GH, Hamlat CA, Rivara FP, Koepsell TD, Jurkovich GJ, Arbabi S. Long-term survival of adult trauma patients. JAMA. 2011;305(10):1001–7.
5. Richmond TS, Kauder D, Strumpf N, Meredith T. Characteristics and outcomes of serious traumatic injury in older adults. J Am Geriatr Soc. 2002;50:215–22.
6. Beaulieu RA, McCarthy MC, Markert RJ, Parikh PJ, Ekeh AP, Parikh PP. Predictive factors and models for trauma patient disposition. J Surg Res. 2014;190(1):264–9.
7. Mori S, Takeda RJ, Carrara FS, Cohrs CR, Zanei SS, Whitaker IY. Incidence and factors related to delirium in an intensive care unit. Rev Esc Enferm USP. 2016;50(4):587–93.
8. Alvarez EA, Garrido MA, Tobar EA, Prieto SA, Vergara SO, Briceno CA, Gonzalez FJ. Occupational therapy for delirium management in elderly patients without mechanical ventilation in an intensive care unit: A pilot randomized clinical trial. J Crit Care. 2016;37:85–90.
9. Ayoung-Chee P, McIntyre L, Ebel BE, Mack CD, McCormick W, Maier RV. Long-term outcomes of ground-level falls in the elderly. J Trauma Acute Care Surg. 2014;76(2):498–503.
10. Yeh DD, Fuentes E, Quraishi SA, Cropano C, Kaafarani H, Lee J, King DR, DeMoya M, Fagenholz P, Butler K, Chang Y, Velmahos G. Adequate nutrition may get you home: Effect of caloric/protein deficits on the discharge destination of critically ill surgical patients. JPEN J Parenter Enteral Nutr. 2016;40(1):37–44.
11. Fox MT, Persaud M, Maimets I, Brooks D, O'Brien K, Tregunno D. Effectiveness of early discharge planning in acutely ill or injured hospitalized older adults: a systematic review and meta-analysis. BMJ Geriatric. 2013 Jul 6;13:70.
12. Agency for Healthcare Research and Quality. Heart disease, cancer and trauma-related disorders among the most costly conditions for men. Res Activities. 2011; 376.
13. Fawcett V, Flynn-O'brian KT, Shorter Z, Davidson GH, Bulger E, Rivara FP, Arbabi S. Risk factors for unplanned readmissions in older adult trauma patients in Washington State: a competing risk analysis. J Am Coll Surg. 2015;220(3):330–3.
14. Fallon WF, Rader E, Zyzanski S, et al. Geriatric outcomes are improved by a geriatric trauma consultation service. J Trauma. 2006;61(5):1040–6.
15. Mangram AJ, Mitchell CD, Shifflette VK, et al. Geriatric trauma service: a one-year experience. J Trauma Acute Care Surg. 2012;72(1):119–22.
16. Lenartowicz M, Parkovnick M, McFarlan A, et al. An evaluation of a proactive geriatric trauma consultation service. Ann Surg. 2012;256:1098–101.
17. www.jhartfound.org/images/upoads/resources/Business_Case_5-17_3.pdf.
18. Soberg HL, Bautz-Holter E, Roise O, Finset A. Long-term multidimensional duration consequences of severe multiple injuries two years after trauma: A prospective longitudinal cohort study. J Trauma. 2007;62(2):461–70.
19. Hardin SR. Engaging families to participate in care of older critical care patients. Critical Care Nurse. 2012;32(3):35–40.
20. McKevitt EC, Calvert E, Ng A, Simons RK, Kirkpatrick AW, Appleton L, Brown RG. Geriatric trauma: resource use and patient outcome. Can J Surg. 2003;46(3):211–5.

Part XVIII

Nursing Considerations in the Geriatric Patient

43 Nursing Considerations in General Evaluation, Risk Management, and Goals of Care

Cathy A. Maxwell

Introduction

In the context of a rapidly growing population of older adults, nursing care of geriatric trauma patients calls for the integration of knowledge and skills, as well as interdisciplinary approaches to optimize patient management in acute care settings. Older adults are hospitalized for injury in far greater numbers than younger adults despite lower injury severity [1]. In 2014, over 1.3 million adults were admitted to US hospitals with a primary injury diagnosis and 55% were age 65 or older [2]. Sixty-seven percent of adults age 18–64 were discharged to a home setting while only 17% of adults age 65 and older were discharged home [2]. These differences underscore the evolving complexity and needs of older adults and compel the importance of stellar nursing care during and after hospitalization.

The care of older adults entails a fundamental understanding of physiologic changes associated with aging, management of chronic conditions, polypharmacy, and models of frailty. Nurses equipped with this knowledge can provide proactive assessment of geriatric syndromes, including depression, delirium, dementia, pain, pressure ulcers, sarcopenia, and frailty. Among the geriatric trauma population, general assessment involves attention to both injury-specific and geriatric-specific considerations. Consistent with the directives presented in the Dr. Mangram's chapter, the following sections present approaches to general evaluation, risk management, and goals of care from a nursing perspective. Traumatic injury in older adults is a public health crisis and nurses are uniquely positioned to impact the continuum of care at the point of entry and beyond.

C.A. Maxwell, Ph.D., R.N.
Assistant Professor, Vanderbilt University School of Nursing, Nashville, TN, USA
e-mail: cathy.maxwell@vanderbilt.edu

Person-Centered Care

Holistic care is a foundational concept within theoretical models of nursing. Biomedical models of care are shifting to person-centered care approaches that recognize the role of nursing within interdisciplinary teams to address the complex needs of older adults [3]. Kogan et al. [3] identified five essential elements of person-centered care (Table 43.1). This person-centered care model supports an emerging

Table 43.1 Elements of person-centered care

Essential elements of person-centered care
• Care is coordinated across the health system, medical and supportive services
• Focus and targeted to defined populations
• Team-based and multidisciplinary
• Connections between medical care and supportive services
• Emphasis on the patient and family experience as a critical outcome

Kogan, AC, Wilber, K, Mosqueda, L (2016). Person-centered care for older adults with Chronic conditions and functional impairment: A systematic literature review. JAGS, 64:e1-e7

A. Rodriguez et al. (eds.), *Geriatric Trauma and Acute Care Surgery*,
https://doi.org/10.1007/978-3-319-57403-5_43

priority to focus on "geriatric trauma" as defined patient population and to coordinate care across trauma systems, interdisciplinary teams and transitional settings [4]. Within this framework, nurses are central to assessing and understanding the needs of patients with chronic conditions and functional impairments.

Geriatric trauma patients are admitted to hospitals with an array of chronic conditions. The Centers for Medicare and Medicaid Services (CMS) reported the prevalence of 19 chronic conditions within the US for 2014 (Fig. 43.1). The top ten chronic conditions include: hypertension (55%), hyperlipidemia (44.7%), ischemic heart disease (27%), arthritis (29.4%), diabetes (26.7%), chronic kidney disease (16.6%), depression (16.2%), heart failure (13.7%), chronic obstructive pulmonary disease (COPD) (11%), and Alzheimer's disease/dementia (10%) [5]. Eighty-seven percent of older adults have at least one chronic condition. Van Walraven et al. [6] developed a weighting algorithm based on the association of comorbidity and death to produce a comorbidity index. Among injured older adults admitted to US hospitals, over 44% of patients have a comorbidity index >3.0 with the highest percentage in level III/IV trauma centers (46.8%) and non-trauma centers (45.2%) [7] as compared to level I (40.2%) and level II (43.9%) trauma centers [7].

Nursing care of patients with injuries and chronic conditions requires early and accurate assessment. Nurses should be knowledgeable of specific chronic conditions and associated medical management. Chronic conditions and acute hospitalization for injury cannot be separated since conditions are intertwined and entail individualized assessment of needs, standardized approaches to care, and continuous process improvement efforts [8, 9]. Geriatric education is a first step that all trauma centers should employ to ensure that trauma nurses demonstrate competencies required to provide optimal care. Education initiatives should include: physiologic changes associated with age, effects of aging of safety of older adults, functional decline and cognitive impairment, frailty trajectories and end-of-life.

Continuity of care and care coordination are other essential nursing considerations. Yakusheva et al. [10] reported an association between discontinuity of nursing care and decline in clinical condition scores. Continuity enables greater familiarity with patient and family needs and increases patient satisfaction. Care coordination ensures that patient needs and preferences are met in terms of health services and the exchange of information across providers, functions and settings [11].

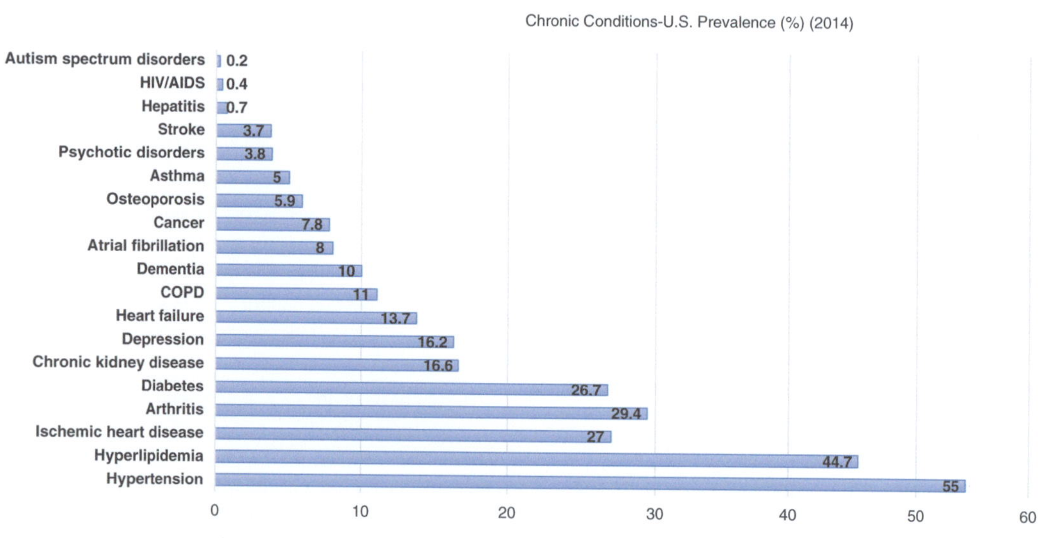

Fig. 43.1 Chronic conditions of older adults in the US (2014)

Polypharmacy is defined as the use of drugs in numbers exceeding medical necessity [12]. Nurses play a central role in reducing polypharmacy and associated risks. Patient care approaches should include accurate documentation of medication lists, patient/family education regarding the purpose and effect of medications, adverse effects, proper administration and use of a single pharmacy if possible. Counseling regarding avoidance of shared medications and disposal of expired medications are other issues often overlooked.

As adults age and develop functional impairments, they often underestimate the risk of falling, as well as the sequelae after a fall. Increased risk occurs as older adults experience muscle weakness, balance problems, orthostatic hypotension, decreased reflexes, sensory impairment, vision impairments, confusion, and effects of medication. Nurses on interdisciplinary teams should seek opportunities to educate patients and families regarding risk, including discussions about physical activity, strength and balance training and reducing risk within the home through environmental modifications. Hospitalization following injury provides an opportunity to discuss these issues with patients and family caregivers.

General Evaluation and Risk Assessment

The nurse's role with geriatric trauma patients on the trauma team requires complex decision-making skills in tandem with an understanding of physiologic systems impacted by injury. Nurses build on basic skills acquired through initial training (i.e., Trauma Nurse Core Course [TNCC]) and gain experience over time in rapid assessment and triage. As with the physician-based Advanced Trauma Life Support (ATLS), nurses also follow ABCDE language (i.e., Airway, Breathing, Circulation, Disability and Exposure) to conduct initial evaluation of the geriatric trauma patient. In agreement with Mangram et al. in the earlier section, the condition of "F" or "frailty" should be the next step in geriatric risk assessment.

Frailty

Frailty is syndrome of vulnerability that places patients at risk for poor outcomes following even a minor injury, highlighting the importance of early assessment. Physical frailty is defined as "a medical syndrome with multiple causes and contributors that is characterized by *diminished strength, endurance, and reduced physiologic function* that increases an individual's vulnerability for developing increased dependency and/or death (p. 393)" [13]. Consistent with physical frailty, Fried et al. [14] described the frailty phenotype as consisting of five characteristics: exhaustion, weakness, slowness, low physical activity, and weight loss. Rockwood et al. [15] described the broader concept of frailty that incorporates additional psychological and social factors that contribute to frailty. Enumeration of 20 to 70 factors allows for creation of a frailty index and risk stratification based on risk values. The distinction between the broader concept of frailty and physical frailty should be understood since frailty screening methods are based on one or both definitions. For example, the five-item FRAIL questionnaire [16] is based primarily on the Fried phenotype, while the Trauma Specific Frailty Index (TSFI) [17] is based on the Rockwood Frailty Index. Both approaches are statistically sensitive in identifying frailty, while the Rockwood model is better able to discriminate levels of frailty at the lower to middle end of the frailty continuum [18, 19]. Aging is associated with trajectories of frailty, and the occurrence of injury within these trajectories is an external stressor from which many older adults are unable to recover fully, and many experience functional decline and death (Fig. 43.2) [20].

Recent studies, specific to the geriatric trauma population demonstrate the vulnerability of frail injured older adults in striking ways for multiple patient outcomes. As already noted, frailty predicts discharge disposition to facilities other than

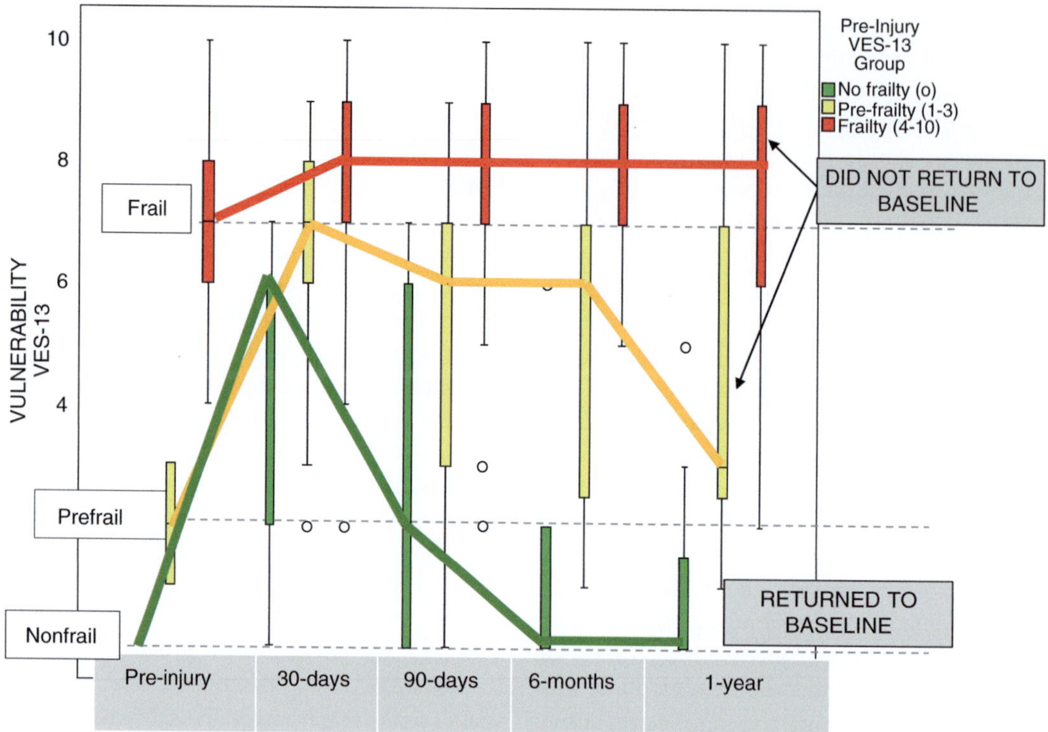

Fig. 43.2 Trajectories of frailty after injury

home, as well as development of complications or adverse events [17, 21–23]. Maxwell et al. [24–26] advanced this work in a prospective longitudinal cohort study at a level I trauma center. One hundred and eighty-eight older adults, aged 65 and older, were screened for pre-injury cognitive impairment and physical frailty and were followed for one-year, post-injury. Several important findings were reported from these studies. First, the prevalence of physical frailty among the geriatric trauma population (>50%) [24] is much higher than among community dwelling elders (~13%) [27]. Second, cognitive impairment among injured older adults is high (49.5%) and contributes to functional decline post-injury [26]. Thirdly, significant difficulties were identified in screening actual older patients after admission to the hospital secondary to cognitive impairment, delirium, sedation, and pain; however, studies have established the feasibility of screening via proxy respondents [24, 28], and have determined that proxy reports of older adults' pre-injury functional status are in an acceptable range of agreement with those of patients [25]. Finally, Maxwell et al. conducted multivariable logistic and linear regression models and determined pre-injury physical frailty to be the predominant predictor of 6-month and 1-year functional decline and mortality [26]. These studies emphasize the importance of frailty screening upon admission to acute care following injury.

A number of brief screening instruments for frailty and functional status are available for clinicians. Table 43.2 provides a list of commonly used screening instruments. Another option specific to trauma is the Trauma Specific Frailty Index (TSFI) which consists of 15 variables that can be identified upon admission to the hospital to derive a numerical index ranging from 0 to 1.0 [17]. Joseph et al. [17] identified a range between 0.12 and 0.38 among geriatric trauma patients and established an optimal cutoff of 0.27 (sensitivity 85%, specificity 75%) for identification of frailty.

Table 43.2 Screening instruments for risk identification

Screening instruments for identification of risk among older adults
• Vulnerable Elders Survey (VES-13) [29]
• Barthel Index [30]
• Life Space Assessment [31]
• Katz Activities of Daily Living [32]
• Frailty Index [15]
• Gerontopole Frailty Screening Tool [33]
• FRAIL Questionnaire [16]
• Cardiovascular Health Study Frailty Screening Scale [14]
• Identification of Seniors at Risk (ISAR) [34]
• Trauma Specific Frailty Index (TSFI) [17]

Goals of Care

Guidelines for Best Practice

Beyond the initial evaluation and risk assessment of geriatric trauma patients, nurses provide care throughout the hospital stay and prepare patients for transitions to other health care settings. Space precludes the ability to fully explore clinical practice guidelines in every area of geriatric care. Table 43.3 provides a list of quality elements for nursing care of the geriatric patient. Nurses are encouraged to explore areas identified in the list. Other online resources are available for individual study and development of geriatric trauma education programs.

The Hartford Institute for Geriatric Nursing provides a clinical website with online resources for nurses in clinical settings identified as "ConsultGeri" (https://consultgeri.org/our-team). This resource includes a curriculum guide for advanced certification in gerontology and information (textual, videos) on competencies to improve care of older adults. E-learning resources include webinars and an extensive list of other geriatric care organizations that offer important content on the care of older adults. Of particular interest is the "Try This," an inclusive set of assessment tools on topics relevant to the care of older adults. Each topic includes short video clips of demonstrations about particular assessment skills. These resources are free, downloadable, and ideal for customizing an education curriculum for trauma nurses.

Table 43.3 Elements for evidence-based nursing practice for geriatric patients

Elements for evidence-based nursing practice for geriatric patients [35]
• Assessment and maintenance of functional status
• Assessment and maintenance of cognitive status
• Screening for depression
• Screening for dementia
• Prevention, recognition and treatment of delirium
• Communication with family caregivers
• Preventing falls in acute care
• Pain management
• Preventing iatrogenic complications
• Reducing adverse drug events
• Addressing urinary incontinence
• Addressing mealtime difficulties
• Maintaining nutrition
• Oral care
• Preventing pressure ulcers and skin tears
• Age-related changes in health
• Excessive sleepiness or insomnia
• Elder abuse
• Addressing sensory impairments (vision, hearing
• Physical restraints and side rails: ethical, legal, and practical issues
• Health care decision-making
• Critical Care of older adults
• Advance directives and End-of-Life

Another important resource is *Nurses Improving Care for Healthsystem Elders* (NICHE) (http://www.nicheprogram.org/). NICHE focuses on protocols that are under the control of nursing practice or areas where nursing interventions have a substantive and positive impact on patient care. Guiding principles are based on: geriatric care at the bedside, patient/family-centered environments, healthy and productive practice environments, and multidimensional quality metrics.

Derived from leading experts in geriatric nursing, the following sections highlight overarching goals of care during hospitalization [35, 36], including maintaining physical and cognitive functioning, maximizing independence at discharge, assisting transitions of care to prevent unplanned readmissions, and early geriatric palliative care.

Maintaining Physical and Cognitive Function

Creditor [37] described *hazards of hospitalization in the elderly* over 20 years ago, and discussed physiologic factors associated with prolonged bedrest. These factors contribute to a cascade that leads to decline and dependency. Recent systematic reviews [38, 39] outline interventions to prevent functional and cognitive decline during hospitalization with an emphasis on multidisciplinary teams and multicomponent interventions. Nurses are in a unique position to advocate for aggressive attention to specific measures.

Functional decline is a primary complication following injury in older adults [26]. Early mobilization should be instituted upon admission with the goal of maximizing patients' physical abilities. Ambulation and/or structured exercises should occur three times a day (or more) as the patient is able to tolerate. Routine daily activities can be facilitated through transfers from bed to chair for meals, reading, and interactions with visitors. Care should be individualized to determine the most effective measure for enhancing functional status.

Delirium, or acute confusion, is a common problem for hospitalized older adults. Predisposing factors include: dementia, severe illness/injury, sensory impairment, surgery, ICU, psychoactive medications, and sleep deprivation [40]. Prevention strategies include frequent patient re-orientation to time, person, and place. Reorientation is assisted through white boards with names of care team members and daily schedules. Orienting communication by health care personnel, family and other visitors facilitates re-orientation and provides cognitive stimulation. Vision and hearing impairments contribute to the development of delirium during hospitalization. Personal glasses and hearing aids should be readily available to patients and other measures should be provided as needed, including magnifying lenses, materials for written communications, and use of fluorescent tape on floors and doorways. Portable amplifying devices are particularly helpful for patients with hearing impairments. Adequate sleep during hospitalization can be facilitated through reduced noise and less care interruptions, use of sleep aids (music, soft background sounds [e.g., rain]), and appropriate medications (e.g., melatonin). Daily nursing assessment of cognitive function is important for detecting subtle changes that can escalate and lead to complications, including urinary incontinence, pressure ulcers, falls, aspiration, and increased hospital length of stay.

Maximizing Independence at Discharge

Geriatric trauma highlights the relative influence of injury with aging. Hospitalized patients are often categorized according to their baseline frailty status (robust, prefrail, frail), yet all three categories are at risk for functional decline during hospitalization and beyond. Maximizing independence at discharge involves discussions with patients and family caregivers about the influence of frailty on patient outcomes and the importance of physical activity in mitigating decline. Prognostic indices are useful for clinical decision-making and promotion of interventions [41] (i.e., physical therapy, physical activity). However, no studies have assessed the influence of prognostic indicators on outcomes of geriatric trauma patients.

Decisions regarding inpatient rehabilitation, skilled nursing facility rehabilitation, and home health care should be individualized and based on comprehensive geriatric assessment, as well as assessment of physical capabilities. A recent systematic review found that older adults' acceptance and willingness to engage in exercise or physical activity was dependent on the perceived value of the activity, as well as the ability to find enjoyment in the activity [42]. Recommended guidelines for physical activity in older adults (age 65 and older) include at least 150 minutes of moderate activity or 75 minutes of vigorous activity per week, and muscle-strengthening activities on at least 2 days a week [43]. The discharge process is an opportunity to provide information on the importance of physical activity and fall prevention. The *National Council on Aging* (NCOA) (https://www.ncoa.org/) is an excellent resource offering fall prevention strategies, self-management resources, and information on programs available to seniors in communities throughout the US

Assisting Transitions of Care and Preventing Unplanned Readmissions

Transitions from acute care are recognized as a risk point for breakdowns in care coordination and continuity of care. Geriatric trauma patients and their families often find themselves at crossroads following hospitalization for injury. Injury is often a tipping point that identifies needs for a higher level of care from independent living, a change in driving status, psychosocial adaptation and acceptance of end points associated with aging. A heightened awareness by trauma nurses of these potential needs can facilitate appropriation of resources to assist transitions to other facilities (including home), as well as measures to help prevent unplanned readmissions.

A systematic review [44] of interventions to improve patient safety in transitional care identified three types of interventions employed primarily upon discharge from acute care: (1) profession-oriented interventions (patient education, physical therapy), (2) patient- or family-focused interventions (patient awareness, discharge support), and (3) organizational/culture interventions (transfer nurse, discharge protocols, medication reconciliation, standardized discharge forms). Studies [44–46] demonstrate the importance of key individuals (e.g., advanced practice nurse, case manager, social worker) who are knowledgeable of potential risks and who address diverse needs of patients and family caregivers in a systematic way before and after discharge.

Watkins et al. [45] reported a decrease in hospital readmissions and correlated cost savings through utilization of a *navigator transitional care model* that focused on social support and health education after discharge. Support included attention to services such as transportation (to appointments), housekeeping, and meal preparation, and education-reinforced medical management and measures to ensure safety in the home [45]. Naylor et al. [46] compared the effects of three interventions (standard care, resource nurse care, transitional care model) on rehospitalization and found that the *transitional care model* (TCM) demonstrated lower mean rehospitalization rates per patient. The TCM was administered by an advanced practice nurse, extended from the index hospitalization and 60 days beyond, and included home visits, a physician follow-up visit, telephone outreach, and 7 days–a–week phone support. These measures underscore the importance of focused attention on the discharge process.

Driving safety is a particularly important transition topic for geriatric trauma patients. Up to 25% [7, 24] of older adult injuries involve motor vehicle events and often highlight the need to address driving retirement. Betz et al. [47] conducted a metasynthesis to identify older adults' preferences for communication about driving with health care providers. Nurses and other providers are encouraged to be mindful of the following related themes.

- Driving discussions are emotionally charged and necessitate sensitivity and time to process.
- Discussions should be placed within the context of the event (illness, injury) to emphasize importance of safety.
- Providers are trusted resources to initiate sensitive conversations.
- Communication must occur over a period of time rather than suddenly.
- Older adults desire autonomy and agency in the decision to stop driving.

Models of care for transitions primarily focus on the medical and physical needs of patients.

However, among older adults, health changes that entail loss of independence call for interventions that address psychosocial needs as well. Nurses play a vital role at this juncture of care. Sullivan et al. [48] conducted a metasynthesis of qualitative studies and identified themes associated with older adults' transition experiences:

- Transitions to long-term care represent a painful loss that requires time for mourning;
- Patients seek stability through gaining autonomy to sustain a new sense of self; and
- Acceptance occurs when a unique inner balance is reached.

Being mindful of the time needed to process loss, and sensitivity to individual patients' needs are key components of nursing care. Interdisciplinary teams must also be sensitive to the psychological adjustments and adaptations that occur during transitions and offer support and opportunities for open dialogue and communication. Gilbert et al. [49] discussed the necessity for older adults to *recognize the need* for increased levels of care to facilitate transfers and/or relocations. The influence of family, friends and providers plays a key role in guiding patients through the process.

Geriatric Palliative Care and Advance Care Planning

Palliative care after injury may be an appropriate option for geriatric trauma patients with advanced frailty. Integrating palliative care for frail patients acknowledges the life-limiting nature of frailty and aims to improve quality of life through: (1) relief of physical and emotional suffering, (2) facilitation of patient-family-provider communication, and (3) coordination of care across settings.

The role of palliative care for geriatric trauma patients deserves special attention related to goals of care. Physical frailty is the primary clinical marker of biologic aging [50, 51] and the leading prognostic indicator for palliative care [52, 53]. The prevalence of frailty among this patient population calls for interventions to help patients and families understand changes associated with aging that lead to end-of-life. Admission to acute care following injury provides a window of opportunity in which patients and their families are often open to discussions about the implications of frailty, including the delivery of early geriatric palliative care (GPC). Early initiation and staging of GPC dialogue enhances receptivity to sensitive discussions. Discussion components of greatest importance to patients and family caregivers include prognosis [54, 55] and exploration of values and needs [54, 56]. A growing body of evidence supports the need for earlier models of palliative care aimed at meeting the needs of frail elders and addressing the inevitability or longitudinal nature of decline and death [57–59].

Advance care planning (ACP) is the process in which patients and families prepare for medical decision making. Uncertainty about end-of-life, difficulty acknowledging frailty, and reluctance to think about death in real terms are common narratives of frail elders [60, 61]. A recent systematic review of frail older adults with no over-riding diagnoses revealed that 61–91% of older adults want to engage in end-of-life discussions sooner than later, while family members are more reluctant to accept that their relatives are near the end of life [62]. Experts suggest that ACP is not a one-time event, but rather is a process that occurs over time. Shared decision-making (SDM) is a process in which health care decisions are made jointly by the patient, health professional(s), and family members or significant others. SDM is optimal under conditions of uncertainty and when decisions are preference sensitive [60, 63]. Hospitalization for injury provides an opportunity to begin these crucial conversations.

Summary

The preceding sections offer guiding principles, based on empirical evidence, from which nurses and other health care providers can approach the care of geriatric trauma patients. While the initial assessment of trauma is similar for the young and old, the emphasis on frailty assessment within the general evaluation for older adults is paramount. Regarding goals of care, vigilance to maximizing function, cognition and independence is crucial, and the significance of early geriatric palliative care within the context of care transitions warrants increased attention and future research. As trauma nurses have the opportunity to employ these approaches, they will impact the field of geriatric trauma care in greater capacity for years to come.

References

1. Agency for Healthcare Research and Quality (AHRQ). Healthcare Cost and Utlization Project (HCUPnet). 2012. http://hcupnet.ahrq.gov. Accessed 23 Oct 2014.
2. Agency for Healthcare Research and Quality (AHRQ). Healthcare Cost and Utilization Project. 2016. http://hcupnet.ahrq.gov. Accessed 2 Nov 2016.
3. Kogan AC, Wilber K, Mosqueda L. Person-centered care for older adults with chronic conditions and functional impairment: a systematic literature review. J Am Geriatr Soc. 2016;64(1):e1–7.
4. Cooper Z, Maxwell CA, Fakhry SM, et al. A position paper: the convergence of aging and injury and the need for a geriatric trauma coalition (GeriTraC). J Trauma Acute Care Surg. 2017;82(2):419–22.
5. CfMaMS. (CMS) Chronic Conditions- Dashboard. 2016. https://www.cms.gov/Research-Statistics-Data-and-Systems/Statistics-Trends-and-Reports/Dashboard/Chronic-Conditions-HRR/CC_HRR_Dashboard.html. Accessed 20 Nov 2016.
6. van Walraven C, Austin PC, Jennings A, Quan H, Forster AJ. A modification of the Elixhauser comorbidity measures into a point system for hospital death using administrative data. Med Care. 2009;47(6):626–33.
7. Maxwell CA. The aging of America: a comprehensive look at over 25,000 geriatric trauma admissions to United States hospitals. Crit Care Nurs Clin North Am. 2015;81(6):630–6.
8. Maxwell CA. Trauma in the geriatric population. Crit Care Nurs Clin North Am. 2015;27(2):183–97.
9. Bortz KL. Creating a geriatric-focused model of Care in Trauma with Geriatric Education. J Trauma Nurs. 2015;22(6):301–5.
10. Yakusheva O, Costa DK, Weiss M. Patients negatively impacted by discontinuity of nursing care during acute hospitalization. Med Care. 2016. (55):421–427.
11. Association AN. The value of nursing care coordination: a white paper of the american nurses association. Acedido em; 2012.
12. Maher RL, Hanlon J, Hajjar ER. Clinical consequences of polypharmacy in elderly. Expert Opin Drug Saf. 2014;13(1):57–65.
13. Morley JE, Vellas B, Abellan van Kan G, et al. Frailty consensus: a call to action. J Am Med Dir Assoc. 2013;14(6):392–7.
14. Fried LP, Tangen CM, Walston J, et al. Frailty in older adults: evidence for a phenotype. J Gerontol A Biol Sci Med Sci. 2001;56(3):M146–56.
15. Rockwood K, Song X, MacKnight C, et al. A global clinical measure of fitness and frailty in elderly people. Can Med Assoc J. 2005;173(5):489–95.
16. Morley JE, Malmstrom T, Miller D. A simple frailty questionnaire (FRAIL) predicts outcomes in middle aged African Americans. J Nutr Health Aging. 2012;16(7):601–8.
17. Joseph B, Pandit V, Zangbar B, et al. Validating trauma-specific frailty index for geriatric trauma patients: a prospective analysis. J Am Coll Surg. 2014;219(1):10–17. e11.
18. Blodgett J, Theou O, Kirkland S, Andreou P, Rockwood K. Frailty in NHANES: comparing the frailty index and phenotype. Arch Gerontol Geriatr. 2015;60(3):464–70.
19. Rockwood K, Andrew M, Mitnitski A. A comparison of two approaches to measuring frailty in elderly people. J Gerontol Ser A Biol Med Sci. 2007;62(7):738–43.
20. Maxwell CA, Mion LC, Mukherjee K, et al. Preinjury physical frailty and cognitive impairment among geriatric trauma patients determine postinjury functional recovery and survival. J Trauma Acute Care Surg. 2016;82(2):195–203.
21. Joseph B, Pandit V, Rhee P, et al. Predicting hospital discharge disposition in geriatric trauma patients: is frailty the answer? J Trauma Acute Care Surg. 2014;76(1):196–200.
22. Joseph B, Pandit V, Zangbar B, et al. Superiority of frailty over age in predicting outcomes among geriatric trauma patients: a prospective analysis. JAMA Surg. 2014:766–72.
23. Mangram AJ, Mitchell CD, Shifflette VK, et al. Geriatric trauma service: a one-year experience. J Trauma Acute Care Surg. 2012;72(1):119–22.
24. Maxwell CA, Mion LC, Mukherjee K, et al. Feasibility of screening for preinjury frailty in hospitalized injured older adults. J Trauma Acute Care Surg. 2015;78(4):844–51.
25. Maxwell CA. Preinjury physical function and frailty in injured older adults: self- versus proxy responses. 2015;63(7):1443–1447.
26. Maxwell CA, Mion LC, Mukherjee K, et al. Preinjury physical frailty and cognitive impairment among geriatric trauma patients determine postinjury functional recovery and survival. J Trauma Acute Care Surg. 2016;80(2):195–203.
27. Bandeen-Roche K, Seplaki CL, Huang J, et al. Frailty in older adults: a nationally representative profile in the United States. J Gerontol A Biol Sci Med Sci. 2015:1427–34.
28. Maxwell CA. Screening hospitalized injured older adults for cognitive impairment and pre-injury functional impairment. Appl Nurs Res. 2013;26(3):146–50.

29. Saliba D, Elliott M, Rubenstein LZ, et al. The vulnerable elders survey: a tool for identifying vulnerable older people in the community. J Am Geriatr Soc. 2001;49(12):1691–9.
30. Collin C, Wade DT, Davies S, Horne V. The Barthel ADL index: a reliability study. Int Disabil Stud. 1988;10(2):61–3.
31. Baker PS, Bodner EV, Allman RM. Measuring life-space mobility in community-dwelling older adults. J Am Geriatr Soc. 2003;51(11):1610–4.
32. Katz S. Assessing self-maintenance: activities of daily living, mobility, and instrumental activities of daily living. J Am Geriatr Soc. 1983;
33. Subra J, Gillette-Guyonnet S, Cesari M, Oustric S, Vellas B. The integration of frailty into clinical practice: preliminary results from the Gérontopôle. J Nutr Health Aging. 2012;16(8):714–20.
34. McCusker J, Bellavance F, Cardin S, Trepanier S, Verdon J, Ardman O. Detection of older people at increased risk of adverse health outcomes after an emergency visit: the ISAR screening tool. J Am Geriatr Soc. 1999;47(10):1229–37.
35. Kluger M, Capezuti E, Zwicker D, Mezey M, Fulmer TT, Gray-Miceli D. Evidence-based geriatric nursing protocols for best practice: Springer Publishing Company; 2007.
36. Reuben DB, Inouye SK, Bogardus ST, Baker DI, Leo-Summers L, Cooney LM. Models of geriatrics practice; the hospital elder life program: a model of care to prevent cognitive and functional decline in older hospitalized patients. J Am Geriatr Soc. 2000;48(12):1697–706.
37. Creditor MC. Hazards of hospitalization of the elderly. Ann Intern Med. 1993;118(3):219–23.
38. Martinez FT, Tobar C, Beddings CI, Vallejo G, Fuentes P. Preventing delirium in an acute hospital using a non-pharmacological intervention. Age Ageing. 2012;41(5):629–34.
39. Hickman LD, Phillips JL, Newton PJ, Halcomb E, Davidson PM. Multidisciplinary team interventions to optimise health outcomes for older people in acute care settings: a systematic review. Arch Gerontol Geriatr. 2015;
40. Inouye SK. Delirium in hospitalized older patients: recognition and risk factors. J Geriatr Psychiatry Neurol. 1998;11(3):118–25.
41. Yourman LC, Lee SJ, Schonberg MA, Widera EW, Smith AK. Prognostic indices for older adults: a systematic review. JAMA. 2012;307(2):182–92.
42. Devereux-Fitzgerald A, Powell R, Dewhurst A, French DP. The acceptability of physical activity interventions to older adults: a systematic review and meta-synthesis. Soc Sci Med. 2016;158:14–23.
43. Organization WH. Global strategy on diet, physical activity and health: a framework to monitor and evaluate implementation. 2006.
44. Laugaland K, Aase K, Barach P. Interventions to improve patient safety in transitional care–a review of the evidence. Work. 2012;41(Supplement 1):2915–24.
45. Watkins L, Hall C, Kring D. Hospital to home: a transition program for frail older adults. Prof Case Manag. 2012;17(3):117–23.
46. Naylor MD, Hirschman KB, Hanlon AL, et al. Comparison of evidence-based interventions on outcomes of hospitalized, cognitively impaired older adults. Journal of comparative effectiveness research. 2014;3(3):245–57.
47. Betz ME, Scott K, Jones J, DiGuiseppi C. "are you still driving?" Metasynthesis of patient preferences for communication with health care providers. Traffic Inj Prev. 2016;17(4):367–73.
48. Sullivan GJ, Williams C. Older adult transitions into long-term care: a meta-synthesis. J Gerontol Nurs. 2016;
49. Gilbert S, Amella E, Edlund B, Nemeth L. Making the move: a mixed research integrative review. Paper presented at: Healthcare2015.
50. Chang S-F, Lin P-L. Frail phenotype and mortality prediction: a systematic review and meta-analysis of prospective cohort studies. Int J Nurs Stud. 2015;52(8):1362–74.
51. Pialoux T, Goyard J, Hermet R. When frailty should mean palliative care. J Nurs Educ Pract. 2013;3(7):75–85.
52. Gott M, Ingleton C, Gardiner C, et al. Transitions to palliative care for older people in acute hospitals: a mixed-methods study. Health Serv Deliv Res. 2013;1(11)
53. O'Callaghan A, Laking G, Frey R, Robinson J, Gott M. Can we predict which hospitalised patients are in their last year of life? A prospective cross-sectional study of the gold standards framework prognostic indicator guidance as a screening tool in the acute hospital setting. Palliat Med 2014:0269216314536089.
54. You JJ, Dodek P, Lamontagne F, et al. What really matters in end-of-life discussions? Perspectives of patients in hospital with serious illness and their families. Can Med Assoc J. 2014;186(18):E679–87.
55. Wagner GJ, Riopelle D, Steckart J, Lorenz KA, Rosenfeld KE. Provider communication and patient understanding of life-limiting illness and their relationship to patient communication of treatment preferences. J Pain Symptom Manag. 2010;39(3):527–34.
56. Ko FC, Morrison RS. Hip fracture: a trigger for palliative care in vulnerable older adults. JAMA Intern Med. 2014;174(8):1281–2.
57. Goldstein NE, Morrison RS. The intersection between geriatrics and palliative care: a call for a new research agenda. J Am Geriatr Soc. 2005;53(9):1593–8.
58. Reyes-Ortiz CA, Williams C, Westphal C. Comparison of early versus late palliative care consultation in end-of-life care for the hospitalized frail elderly patients. Am J Hosp Palliat Care. 2015;32(5):516–20.

59. Buckinx F, Rolland Y, Reginster J-Y, Ricour C, Petermans J, Bruyère O. Burden of frailty in the elderly population: perspectives for a public health challenge. Archives of public health. 2015;73(1):19.
60. Légaré F, Witteman HO. Shared decision making: examining key elements and barriers to adoption into routine clinical practice. Health Aff (Millwood). 2013;32(2):276–84.
61. Kendall M, Carduff E, Lloyd A, et al. Different experiences and goals in different advanced diseases: comparing serial interviews with patients with cancer, organ failure, or frailty and their family and professional careers. J Pain Symptom Manag. 2015;50(2):216–24.
62. Sharp T, Moran E, Kuhn I, Barclay S. Do the elderly have a voice? Advance care planning discussions with frail and older individuals: a systematic literature review and narrative synthesis. Br J Gen Pract. 2013;63(615):e657–68.
63. Politi MC, Lewis CL, Frosch DL. Supporting shared decisions when clinical evidence is low. Med Care Res Rev. 2013;70(1 Suppl):113S–28S.

44 Geriatric Trauma: Emergency Nursing Considerations

Jessica Jurkovich

Introduction

Trauma is currently the fifth leading cause of death for the older adult and patients >65 years of age which accounts for nearly 25% of all trauma [1]. Age-related physiologic changes, comorbidities, polypharmacy, and lower physiologic reserve contribute to the complexity of care for the older adult. Worse outcomes in geriatric trauma patients occur with lower injury severity scores than their younger counterparts [2]. These patients are often under-triaged due to masked signs and symptoms of clinical decline. However, timely exams and appropriate interventions can lead to successful resuscitations and allow older adults to return to their prior baseline [3]. Thus, a prepared and investigative trauma team is necessary to recognize subtle changes and anticipate injuries unique to the elderly trauma patient.

The emergency nurse is one of the first hospital members to interact with the older adult patient and is linked to their care from admission to transfer or discharge. Acting as the voice for the patient and their family, the nurse provides insight to the medical team through goal-directed questioning and family-centered care. Within the trauma team the nurse optimizes critical communication and assists in the continuity of care with other providers such as laboratory and radiology staff, surgery personnel, acute and critical care nursing, and the receiving hospital staff [4]. An understanding of geriatric traumatic injuries, physiology, and comorbidities guides the nurse's interventions and understanding of the clinical provider's care. As an educated and dynamic team member, the nurse is able to assist in the successful resuscitation while respecting patient and family wishes. This chapter, using recommendations from the Emergency Nurses Association and American College of Surgeons, will discuss these geriatric considerations for the emergency nurse in both the primary and secondary survey incorporating common mechanisms of injury seen in the geriatric trauma patient.

Age-Related Changes

An understanding of the age-related changes in the older adult is crucial for the emergency nurse to accurately assess and anticipate traumatic injuries and complications. Physiologic alterations are present in each major system and comorbidities are present in >80% of older adults, predisposing this population to higher morbidity and mortality rates [5]. The impact of these changes in trauma is discussed throughout, and further chapters will address specific injury and system characteristics in more depth. However, a general overview of the common variations associated with aging is displayed in Fig. 44.1.

J. Jurkovich, AGACNP-BC, MSN, CCRN
Department of Trauma, Critical Care & Acute Care Surgery, Oregon Health Science University, Portland, OR, USA
e-mail: jurkovic@ohsu.edu

A. Rodriguez et al. (eds.), *Geriatric Trauma and Acute Care Surgery*,
https://doi.org/10.1007/978-3-319-57403-5_44

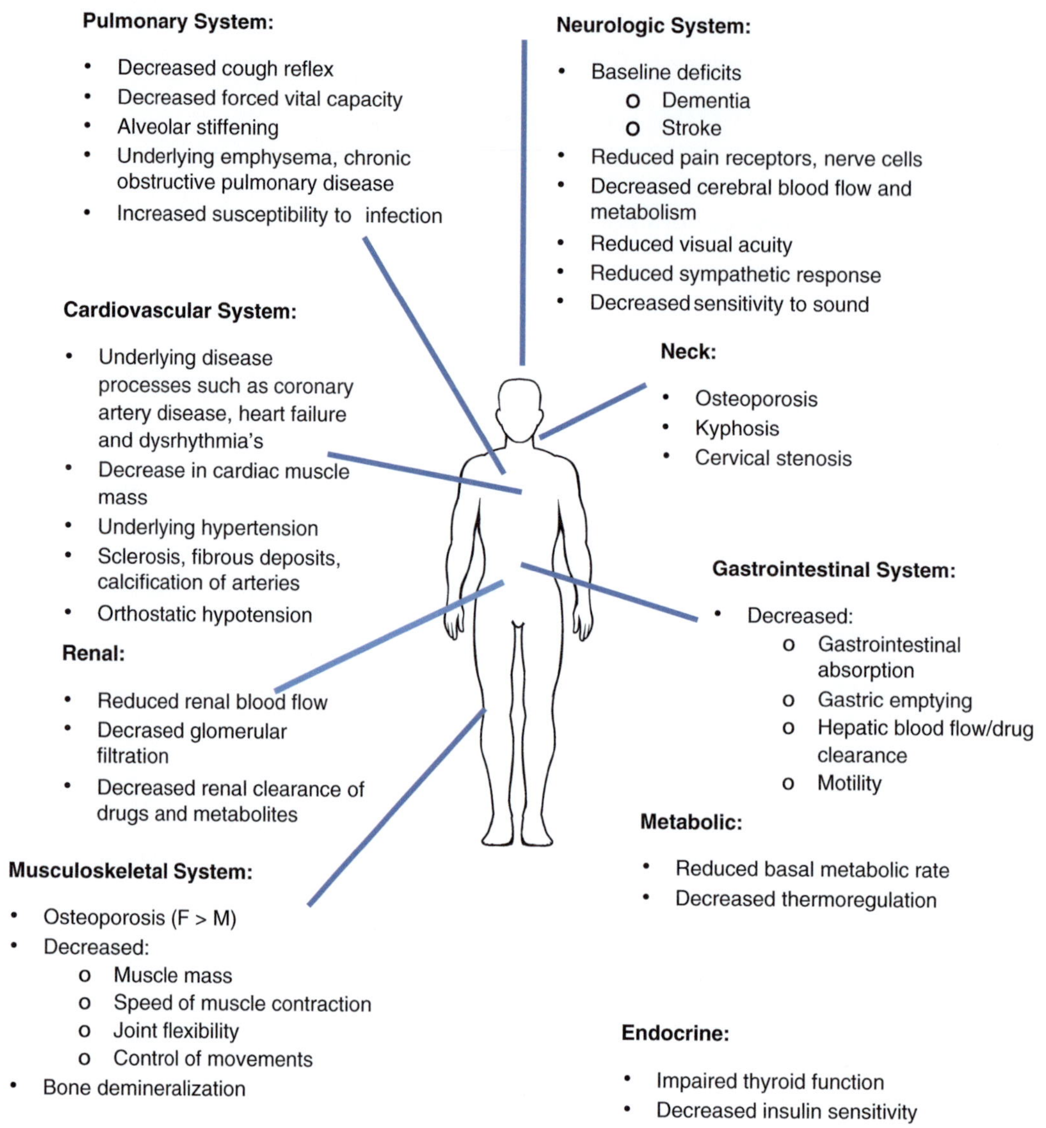

Fig. 44.1 Normal physiologic changes in the older adult

Mechanism of Injury

The geriatric patient is at risk for similar traumatic injuries seen across the lifespan, but less severe blunt force results in significant injuries as the osteoporotic changes in bone density reduce the body's ability to absorb energy [2]. The older adult is also at risk for burns and penetrating trauma. Yet the three most common mechanisms of injury are [6]:

- Falls
- Motor vehicle accidents (MVA)
- Pedestrian-related collisions

Epidemiology, risk factors, and common injuries are considered in Table 44.1. Additionally, all injured older adults should be screened for elder abuse or suicide-related origins [7].

Table 44.1 Geriatric trauma mechanisms of injury, risk factors, and associated injury

Mechanism of injury (MOI)	Epidemiology	Risk factors [8]	Common injuries [8]
Falls	• *Leading cause of geriatric trauma-related mortality* [18] • One in three adults ≥65 years of age fall annually [5] • Falls account for 25% of geriatric hospital admissions and 40% of nursing home admissions [1] • Less than 40% of patients return to independent living after a fall, and over 25% of patient's die within 1 year of injury [1] • *Leading cause of traumatic brain injury* in the geriatric population [2]	• Medication, cardiac, or volume induced orthostatic hypotension • Decreased reaction time • Poor balance and strength • Environmental factors such as wet surfaces, obstructed or cluttered pathways, rugs, poor footwear	• Lacerations or ecchymosis • Traumatic brain injuries • Subdural hematoma • Fractures, specifically pelvic fractures resulting in high rates of hemorrhage, transfusion and critical care admission. • Secondary complications from prolonged time down can lead to rhabdomyolysis. This may cause acute renal failure, hyperkalemia, fat embolisms, coagulopathies, or multi-system organ failure
Motor vehicle accidents (MVA)	• Second most common MOI in geriatric trauma [1] • Most frequently occurs when driver is making left turns [9]	• Decreased peripheral and night vision, cataracts, poor hearing, and delayed reflexes • Osteoporosis and bone demineralization increases risk of fractures upon impact	• Blunt chest trauma seen in 25% of older adults involved in MVC • Sternal, rib, clavicle, and pelvic fractures are common.
Pedestrian-related accidents	• Third most common MOI in geriatric trauma [1] • Older adults are victims of pedestrian-related collisions second only to pediatric patients [2] • Represent the largest percentage of fatalities [2]	• Kyphosis, decreased reaction time, slower pace, decreased visual and auditory acuity	• Similar blunt injury pattern as seen in MVA's

Geriatric Considerations of Emergency Room Care

As the emergency nurse, priorities of patient care are similar across the lifespan but special considerations in the primary and secondary survey are crucial for early recognition of geriatric trauma complications. Whether in a rural hospital or urban Level I Trauma Center, the nurse's role will focus on safety, efficiency, and closed-loop communication [3]. Traditional nursing roles of documentation of the primary and secondary assessment, recording and reporting vital signs, establishing peripheral intravenous (IV) access, oxygenation, and cataloging personal effects are key. Additionally, the emergency nurse has a vital role in providing patient and family support, and establishing the patient's care directive goals. Perhaps the most central role relative to this chapter's discussion is the ability of the emergency nurse to anticipate priorities of care, and to understand the physiologic differences in the elderly that may not be readily apparent to all team members. To facilitate this comprehensive role, both provider and nursing interventions are intertwined in the sections below.

Preparation and Triage

It is important to remain aware that the injury pattern and body's response to trauma is different in the elderly patient; their mechanism of injury and vital signs are not indicative of severity of injury [1]. For this reason the American College of Surgeons recommend triaging older adults to trauma centers for lower physiologic indicators than their younger counterpart [6]. Prior to the patient's arrival, the trauma team's roles and responsibilities should be assigned and the nurse should prepare resuscitation equipment by emergency department policy. As communication is critical for successful triage, models such as SBAR—situation, background, assessment, recommendation—are recommended [3].

Primary Survey

The initial survey begins the minute the patient crosses the emergency room threshold. Assess the patient from across the room; observe for obvious signs of hemorrhage, level of consciousness, and movement [3]. Attach patient to heart rate and pulse oximetry monitors, take blood pressure reading, and apply oxygen to maintain saturations of 94–98% [8]. It is critical to communicate readings and individual assessment throughout triage to the provider or team leader. Provide emotional support for the patient and consider normal geriatric physiologic changes, comorbidities, and mechanism of injury. Depending on the size of your team, the steps below may occur simultaneously with primary consideration for the greatest threat [9]. In general, the priority of airway and breathing is first, followed by hemorrhage control and circulatory resuscitation.

Airway and Alertness

Geriatric Considerations

Physiologic: Decreased cough and gag, thin mucous membranes, and reduced salivation place patients at increased risk for aspiration [8]. Kyphosis, cervical stenosis, and spinal misalignment may cause difficulty with airway patency [9].

Comorbidities: History of previous stroke with residual deficits such as dysphagia may impair swallowing and clearing of airway [8]. Patients may wear dentures, which often must be removed and saved.

Trauma*:* Assume for cervical trauma. Any report of bruising or facial laceration should increase suspicion for facial fractures [8]. Nasotracheal suction and nasal airway adjuncts are not commonly used in the elderly due to the concern for cribriform plate and nasal fractures [3].

Interventions

- Inspect airway carefully and consider partial and full denture dislodgement, if removed label and keep with patients clothing.
- Use the pneumonic AVPU to guide your adjunct airway needs [9]:
  - Alertness: Is the patient alert?
  - Verbal: Is the patient responding to verbal stimuli?
  - Pain: Does the patient respond only to pain?
  - Unresponsive: Is the patient unresponsive?

**If the patient is not fully alert and requires verbal or painful stimuli an airway adjunct is necessary. If the patient is unresponsive immediately check for a pulse and communicate the findings to the physician or team leader.*

- To open the airway, use the jaw thrust maneuver and maintain cervical spine stability.
- If dentures are present, consider leaving dentures in place to assist with bag-mask ventilation [3].
- Carefully insert airway adjuncts and suction catheters and assess for signs of traumatic insertion such as bleeding or edema [6].
- Anticipate the need for early intubation by ensuring adequate IV access, suction, pulse oximetry, bag-valve-mask ventilation, and easy access to the head of the bed.

Breathing

Geriatric Considerations:

Physiologic: Normal aging changes include alterations in gas exchange and decreased functional capacity, elastic recoil, and lung compliance [10].

Comorbidities*:* Obstructive disease such as chronic obstructive pulmonary disease (COPD) cause stiff parenchyma tissue, thereby increasing pulmonary vascular and airway resistance [11].

Trauma: Blunt chest trauma and rib fractures commonly lead to pneumothoraces, which paired with poor accessory muscle compliance results in early hypoxia [11].

Interventions

- Apply oxygen to patient, maintain oxygenation saturations at 94–98%
- Respiratory rates >24 breaths per minute are associated with looming respiratory decline [8]
- Perform your own pulmonary exam in conjunction with the provider; document and assess for peri-oral cyanosis; note patient's breathing quality, use of accessory muscles, and tracheal alignment
- Ensure adequate pain control and positioning to facilitate maximum ventilation, anticipating the patient may not be a candidate for pharmaceutical adjuncts

Circulation and Control of Hemorrhage

The common presence of comorbidities and the use of intentional anticoagulation place the geriatric trauma patient at an elevated risk for hemorrhage and hypovolemic shock. Coupled with this is the normal loss of physiologic reserve in the elderly, as they poorly tolerate sudden changes in their baseline perfusion pressures and tissue oxygenation [8]. Normal warning signs such as tachycardia and hypotension are often delayed, absent, or occur too late in the course of care to allow adequate time for restoration of circulation [12]. Subtle changes in vital sign trends and mentation can guide the provider's care, thus the nurse must continue frequent reassessments throughout the primary and secondary survey and communicate findings and changes in exam [3].

Geriatric Considerations:

Physiologic*:* Normal aging changes decrease baroreceptor response to the release of adrenaline and norepinephrine. Additionally, reduced cardiac reserve limits protective responses to even minor changes in volume status [12].

Comorbidities*:* Heart disease is present in 30% of older adults and the symptom of underlying hypertension is present in 50% of elderly patients [1]. Many of these patients take anti-hypertensive and rate control medications, altering outcomes and normal compensatory responses to shock. Additionally, patients with ischemic heart disease or heart failure are at increased risk of rapid decompensation due to excessive fluid and/or blood loss [8].

Trauma: The healthcare team must consider that preceding the trauma myocardial ischemia or infarction may have occurred; the nurse should communicate any new patient complaints of chest discomfort [8]. Remain aware that pelvic fractures require frequent reassessments for occult bleeding that may be missed on imaging [1]. Finally, *heart rate > 90 beats per minute* and *systolic blood pressure ≤110 mmHg* are associated with increased mortality [13].

Interventions:

- Ensure access—at least *two 18 gauge* peripheral intravenous catheters (fragile skin and torturous veins may limit peripheral access, notify provider if central or intraosseous access is necessary).
- Obtain blood pressure and document vital sign trends remembering a normal blood pressure or heart rate may be present but will not always represent patient stability.
- If able, access past medical chart for baseline blood pressure readings as an outpatient.
- Assist in early lab collection anticipating the need for complete blood count and coagulation studies.
- Ask patient, family, or caregivers about blood pressure medications, anticoagulants, antiplatelet agents, and over the counter medications and herbs, communicating results to the provider [14].
- Assist the provider by ensuring assessment is made for the presence of a pacemaker, recognizing its presence denotes underlying cardiac dysrhythmia and/or disease [1].
- If necessary, assist in controlling bleeding by using direct pressure, elevation, pelvic binders, tourniquets, and appropriate blood pressure management [9].

- Anticipate early administration of packed red blood cells to improve oxygenation and possible administration of vitamin K, fresh frozen plasma, or coagulation factors to reverse prolonged bleeding time [4].
- If fluids are administered assess patient's pulmonary and cardiac status following small boluses, such as 500 ml, before administering additional fluids. Also, check with provider about rate of infusions for patients with heart failure [10].
- Maintain a *high suspicion for bleeding* throughout exam.

Disability or the Neurologic Examination

Altered neurologic status resulting from either acute or chronic injuries or disease processes can obscure standard neurological screening tools. For example, the Glasgow Coma scale if often unreliable, therefore it is crucial to ensure a detailed neurological exam is performed and documented [14]. The nurse can assist in obtaining baseline cognitive function from family or caregivers and must independently perform their own exam for reassessment and hand-off reporting. Physiologic changes such as cerebral atrophy place the older adult at greater risk for subdural hematomas secondary to stretching of the parasagittal veins [14]. This, paired with decreased cerebral mass, allows additional room for accumulation of blood prior to signs of increased intracranial pressure. Thus, when head injury is suspected the emergency nurse should prepare for rapid and early transportation for head computed topography (CT) [15]. Pupillary exams should be performed, however note that cataracts, macular degeneration, and delayed response can impact physical assessment findings normally indicative of uncal herniation. Continue frequent reassessments and consider other neurologic altering causes such as hypoglycemia, hypoxia, hypothermia, or hyperthermia [15].

Exposure and Environmental Temperature Control

The patient will need to be exposed for a full assessment, on a cold stretcher, but the emergency nurse should intervene to ensure warming or cooling measures are in place. Consideration of the location and timing of injury is important for any traumatic patient, especially older adults, as they are more susceptible to environmental exposure. Reduced subcutaneous tissue, a decreased ability to sweat, decreased temperature regulation, and possible underlying vascular or endocrine disease places these patients at risk for hypothermia and hyperthermia [4]. Hypothermia is more commonly seen, and interventions to prevent possible premature ventricular contractions, ventricular tachycardia, or coagulopathies include infusing warm fluid, and the use of warming blankets [3]. Rectal temperature may be necessary to initially assess core temperature, properly lubricate and gently insert as the rectal lining thins in older adults.

Resuscitation Adjuncts

While the "ABC's" of the primary survey are being addressed the nurse is also confirming the resuscitation adjuncts below are performed or delegated.

Full Set of Vital Signs: Obtain a complete set of vital signs upon admission and monitor the patient throughout the survey. Comorbidities may impact baseline pulse pressure and respirations; trends in vital signs and frequent assessment of hemostasis can guide clinical intervention. Maintain oxygen saturation at 94–98%, noting that over-oxygenation is associated with increased rates of morbidity and mortality [13].

Family Presence: The family is an invaluable resource for the geriatric patient. The loud, chaotic environment of the emergency room and common decreases in patient neurosensory function can exacerbate the older adult's confusion, fear, and neurologic exam. A familiar face or voice to calm and orient the elderly can improve care and provide a clearer picture of the patient's baseline cognitive and functional status. Additionally, the family can communicate the older adult's wishes and provide advanced directives to guide healthcare goals.

Laboratory Studies: As described above, it is critical to obtain a complete coagulation panel to assess bleeding time. Critical injuries may require consideration of blood lactate and base deficit values to assess for metabolic acidosis [16]. Cardiac enzymes can assess for myocardial events, and a urine analysis for possible urinary tract infections.

Monitoring: The patient should be attached to a cardiac monitor, pulse oximetry, and blood pressure cuff with recommendations to cycle every 5 min during the primary and secondary survey, and every fifteen minutes for the following first hour, then hourly [8, 9]. Also, a 12-lead electrocardiogram is often performed to assess for myocardial ischemia or injury.

Pain: Older adults may not be able to accurately describe pain and are often under-medicated [17]. Assess the patient's behavior and use non-verbal cues such as muscle tension or clenched brow to assess discomfort. Do not rely on vital signs such as hypertension and tachycardia for assessment of pain. Make sure medications administered are weight based and "start low, and go slow" [4]. Monitor for respiratory depression and changes in level of consciousness.

Reevaluation: When the primary assessment is complete it is critical for the team to reassess the patient's response to interventions. Anticipate discussion and patient transfer to a trauma center if not already performed. During this time the emergency nurse should prepare for patient transport for imaging, surgery, or to final disposition [9].

Secondary Survey

Goal: The goal of the secondary survey is to identify less severe injuries, prevent further injury, and obtain a more detailed event and patient history [14]. Central to this survey is the detailed head-to-toe examination.

Patient History

Assist the provider in obtaining the history from the patient, designated liaison, or family. The clinician will need further information about the initial event report, patient's allergies, medications, previous medical and surgical history, and last meal [14].

Medications often impacting geriatric care include [8]:

- Antihypertensives
- Anticoagulants
- Antiplatelet agents—Aspirin/Plavix
- Diabetes medications
- Analgesics
- Nitroglycerin

Comorbidities associated with increased mortality in trauma [2]:

- Cirrhosis
- Coagulopathies
- Ischemic heart disease
- COPD
- Diabetes mellitus
- Malignancy
- Renal failure

Head-to-toe Exam

A more comprehensive physical exam is indicated following the primary survey (see Table 44.2 for specific assessment recommendations). As the nurse for the geriatric patient an individual exam should be performed and documented in addition to the clinician. It is critical to inspect the patient's posterior surface and remove spine board as only 30 to 45 minutes on a hard surface can result in skin breakdown. Reassess for subtle changes, document detailed skin assessments, and use this time to screen for elder maltreatment, reporting suspected abuse per hospital protocol. Signs of potential maltreatment include changes in personality in front of abuser, caregiver's inability to leave patient alone, history of multi-emergency room visits, and dementia mimicking symptoms from the older adult [4].

Table 44.2 *Geriatric Considerations in the Secondary Survey Physical Exam* Common traumatic injuries seen in the older adult are broken into physical exam systems and nursing considerations for the head-to-toe exam are included

Geriatric considerations in the head-to-toe exam	
System & Traumatic injuries seen	Nursing consideration
Head, Eyes, Ears, Nose, Throat (HEENT) • Traumatic Brain Injury • Subdural Hematoma • Intraparenchymal hematomas • Craniofacial fractures • Cervical Spine fractures	• *Screen for anticoagulant medication use rapidly and anticipate reversal factors* • Inspect the head and neck for lacerations • Breakdown instructions and information, speaking slowly and clearly to the patient. • Attempt to provide information in more than one way (verbal and visual for example) • Consider acute or chronic disability and drug or alcohol abuse as cause of altered neurologic exam [15] • Early subdural bleeds may demonstrate subtle signs of confusion or lethargy [15] • The Glasgow Coma Scale may be unreliable in the older adult, consider confusion, agitation, or somnolence to guide changes in mental status • Suspect cervical injury even with minor blunt trauma [8] • Communicate any small changes immediately as repeat head imaging is recommended for any small changes in neurological status [15] • Avoid use of restraints if able, as they may increase agitation
Chest • Pneumothorax • Hemothorax • Pulmonary contusions • Rib fractures • Aortic injury • Pericardial tamponade • Esophageal perforation • Clavicle fracture	• If the patient is alert begin pulmonary hygiene exercises immediately as this population is at increased risk for pneumonia [4] • Facilitate positioning to allow maximum ventilation • Ensure adequate pain control to assist in lung expansion • Monitor blood pressure and heart rate every 5 min for the initial primary and secondary survey [9] • Assess for other causes of abnormal cardiac function such as hypoxia or electrolyte imbalances [8] • Troponin levels >1.2 mcg/L indicate myocardial injury [10]

Abdomen
• Blunt abdominal trauma (contusion or laceration):
  – Spleen
  – Liver
• Penetrating abdominal trauma
• Bowel perforation
• Mesenteric Ischemia
	• Similar mechanisms and grades of solid organ injuries are used for geriatric and younger patients [18]
	• Patient has less abdominal organ protection; assess for early abdominal bruising, palpate for tenderness, guarding, distension, and rigidity [19]
	• Decreased pain sensation reduces sensitivity of abdominal exam; facilitate early imaging such as the FAST exam or CT-abdomen to assess injury [19]

Pelvis and Perineum • Pelvic Fracture (major trauma) • Pubic rami, sacral ala, acetabular fractures (minor trauma) (#89-UTD) • Blunt genitourinary trauma	• Assess femoral pulse and distal vascular perfusion • If fracture is diagnosed assess the joints above and below the area for injury [3] • Assist in pelvic stabilization if necessary • Prepare patient for angiography if FAST exam demonstrates retroperitoneal bleeding [19] • Check the urinary meatus for blood [9] • Avoid the use of urinary catheters as older women have the highest rate of catheter associated urinary tract infections. If catheter is needed, use appropriate lubrication for catheter placement and secure device [8] • Prepare to send urinalysis
Extremities • Distal extremity fractures • Long bone fracture	• Assess for obvious deformities, abrasions, and ecchymosis • Control active bleeding • Assist with plain films and splinting of extremities as necessary • Inspect the posterior surface of the patient and remove rigid spine board as patient is at risk for skin breakdown after only 30–45 min of immobility [9] • Check for compartment syndrome in fractured extremities, assessing the five "P's": pain, pallor, paresthesia, pulselessness, and paralysis [11] • Continue frequent neurovascular checks

Definitive Care or Transport

The goal of the emergency resuscitation is to identify and treat immediate life-threatening injuries and to stabilize the patient, expediting transfer to definitive care [9]. Definitive care may be in another unit in your hospital (operating room, angiography suite, intensive care unit), or it might mean a transfer to a facility with greater resources. As the primary caregiver it is important for the emergency nurse to have a broad, but detailed understanding of the geriatric patient's injuries and potential complications. Facilitate early transfer and effectively communicate verbal report to the transferring staff. Make sure all belonging are with the patient, or family. Finally, although aggressive resuscitation aids in successful rehabilitation of the older adult, patient comorbidities, injury, or directives may limit extension of life. Consider resources such as a chaplain if appropriate, and support those present, allowing time and privacy to grieve.

Summary

The geriatric trauma patient presents a unique challenge in the recognition and management of their injuries. Normal physiologic changes that occur during aging must be recognized during the initial evaluation, and the common presence of comorbidities complicates the clinical care priorities. Additionally, the elderly are more likely to sustain injury in response to low energy blunt forces, such as falls, low-speed motor vehicle crashes, and any pedestrian-related collisions. The role of the emergency nurse in the comprehensive care of the injured geriatric adult involves pivotal assessment skills specific to this population while acting as an effective liaison for the patient, family and healthcare team. Continued education and training for the emergency staff is crucial, and it will guide the evidenced-based management of the older adult in trauma.

References

1. Keller JM, Sciadini MF, Sinclair E, O'Toole RV. Geriatric trauma: demographics, injuries, and mortality. J Orthop Trauma. 2012;26(9):e161–5.
2. Labib N, Nouh T, Winocour S, et al. Severely injured geriatric population: morbidity, mortality, and risk factors. J Trauma. 2011;71:1908–14.
3. Cutugno CL. The 'graying' of trauma care: addressing traumatic injury in older adults. Amer J Nurs. 2011;111(11):40–8.
4. Jagos C. Special populations: the older adult trauma patient. In: Gurney D, editor. Trauma nursing Core course: provider manual. 7th ed. Des Plaines: Emergency Nurses Association; 2014. p. 259–68.
5. Centers for Disease Control and Prevention (CDC). The state of aging and health in America, vol. 2013. Atlanta, GA: Centers for Disease Control and Prevention, US Department of Health and Human Services; 2013.
6. Calland JF, Ingraham AM, Martin N, Marshall GT, Schulman CI, Stapleton T, Barraco RD. Evaluation and management of geriatric trauma: an eastern Association for the Surgery of trauma practice management guideline. J Trauma Acute Care Surg. 2012;73(5):S345–50.
7. Moyer VA. Screening for intimate partner violence and abuse of elderly and vulnerable adults: US preventive services task force recommendation statement. Ann Intern Med. 2013;158(6):478–86.
8. Yelon JA, Luchette FA, editors. Geriatric trauma and critical care. 1st ed. New York: Springer; 2014.
9. Emergency Nurses Association. Trauma nurse core course. http://www.ena.org/education/ENPC-TNCC/tncc/Pages/aboutcourse.aspx. Accessed 25 Feb 2016.
10. Brock AJ, Jablonski RA. Physiology of aging: impact on critical illness and treatment. In: Foreman MD, et al., editors. Critical care nursing of older adults: best practices. New York: Springer Publishing Company; 2010. p. 241–66.
11. Bonne S, Schuerer DJE. Trauma in the older adult: Epidemiology and evolving geriatric trauma principles. Clin Geriatr Med. 2013;29(1):137–50.
12. Brooks SE, Mukherjee K, Gunter OL, Guillamondegui OD, Jenkins JM, Miller RS, May AK. Do models incorporating comorbidities outperform those incorporating vital signs and injury pattern for predicting mortality in geriatric trauma. J Am Coll of Surg. 2014;219(5):1020–7.
13. Heffernan DS, Thakkar RK, Monaghan SF, Ravindran R, Adams CA Jr, Kozloff MS, Gregg SC, Connolly MD, Machan JT, Cioffi WG. Normal presenting vital signs are unreliable in geriatric blunt trauma victims. J Trauma Acute Care Surg. 2010;69(4):813–20.
14. Secondary Survey for Trauma [Internet]. Adhb.govt.nz.2016 [cited 1 March 2016]. http://www.ahdb.govt.nz/trauma/T_guidelines/secondary_survey.html. Accessed 30 Feb 2016.

15. Kehoe A, Rennie S, Smith JE. Glasgow Coma scale is unreliable for the prediction of severe head injury in elderly trauma patients. Emerg Med J. 2015;32(8):613–5.
16. Callaway DW, Shapiro NI, Donnino MW, Baker C, Rosen CL. Serum lactate and base deficit as predictors of mortality in normotensive elderly blunt trauma patients. J Trauma Acute Care Surg. 2009;66(4):1040–4.
17. Quattromani E, Normansell D, Storkan M, Gerdelman G, Krits S, Pennix C, Sprowls D, Armbrecht E, Dalawari P. Oligoanalgesia in blunt geriatric trauma. J Emerg Med. 2015;48(6):653–9.
18. American College of Surgeons (ACS). Trauma quality improvement program. https://www.facs.org/quality-programs/trauma/tqip. Accessed 10 Feb 2016.
19. Mangram AJ, Mitchell CD, Shifflette VK, Lorenzo M, Truitt MS, Goel A, Lyons MA, Nichols DJ, Dunn EL. Geriatric trauma service: a one-year experience. J Trauma Acute Care Surg. 2012;72(1):119–22.

45 Nursing Care of the TBI Patient

Jami Zipf

Traumatic brain injury can be devastating to the patient as well as the family, resulting in lifelong physical and mental disabilities. It is important for the nurse to minimize complications to insure the best outcomes for these patients. Hypotension and hypoxia are directly related to increased morbidity and mortality in the severe TBI patient and must be avoided.

Careful assessment of patients with traumatic brain injuries is imperative as most of these patients are unable to communicate. A basic neurological assessment begins by assessing level of consciousness, movement and muscle tone, pupil size and reactivity, reflexes, posturing, response to pain, and respiratory patterns. The Glasgow Coma Scale (GCS) is used to assess three components (eye, verbal, and motor) based on scores of 3–15. Scores of 8 or less indicate a severe head injury with a greater possibility of permanent disability. GCS should be monitored frequently and any changes called to physicians.

Blood pressure should be monitored as hypotension is to be avoided. An arterial catheter allows for accurate monitoring in the acute phase of injury. Intravenous access allows for fluids to maintain adequate BP as well as drug administration. Central venous catheters are often used but should be removed as soon as the patient stabilizes to minimize risk of bloodstream infections.

A urinary catheter is used to assess renal function and perfusion. Accurate I&O is to be monitored on an hourly basis as the kidney is one of the first organs to demonstrate impaired organ perfusion. A preventative bowel regimen should be established to prevent constipation due to limited mobility and fluid restrictions. Hydrogen ion blockers may be used as TBI patients are at risk for developing stress ulcers.

Monitoring devices are inserted into the skull for the purpose of evaluating intracranial pressure and is indicated for patients with GCS ≤ 8 if CT imaging shows evidence of structural brain damage. Devices such as ventriculostomy allow for drainage of intraventricular fluids, and PbtO2 monitors that measure brain oxygenation may also be used. Goal is to maintain ICP < 20 mmHg and maintain CPP at 50–70 mmHg. Tips in maintaining ICP < 20 mmHg and CPP at 50–70 mmHg include: elevation of HOB 30°; providing sedation; loosen cervical collar; draining CSF; administering mannitol prn; initiating insulin therapy; and promoting normothermia. Remember to follow aseptic technique when caring for these devices. Assess the characteristics of the CSF looking for cloudiness and volume changes. Secure the devices and restrict changes in HOB elevation to prevent dislodgement.

J. Zipf, R.N., B.S.N.
Conemaugh Health System,
Johnstown, PA 15905, USA
e-mail: jzipf@conemaugh.org

A. Rodriguez et al. (eds.), *Geriatric Trauma and Acute Care Surgery*,
https://doi.org/10.1007/978-3-319-57403-5_45

Hypoxia is to be avoided at all costs. Systemic oxygen levels are not always indicative of the brain's oxygen level. A special device may be inserted directly into the brain or jugular vein to adequately assess the brain tissue oxygenation. TBI patients often require prolonged mechanical ventilation and may have a tracheotomy performed. By performing this procedure, the risk of ventilator-associated pneumonia may be decreased. Suctioning of the secretions above the tracheostomy cuff, along with good oral care, should be performed every 4 h.

The patient with TBI may need to have surgical intervention to evacuate clots, stop the bleeding, or create more room in the skull as the brain swells. A large hematoma should be evacuated immediately to prevent neurological deterioration. A decompressive craniectomy may be performed on those patients whose ICP continues to rise despite interventions. In this procedure, a bone in the skull is removed to allow the brain to swell without restriction in the cranium.

Some anesthetic and sedative agents such as propofol and fentanyl may be used. Dosages are decreased to perform a more accurate neurological assessment. As patient improves, doses are reduced. Pentobarbital coma may be induced for patients who don't respond to other therapies used to control ICP.

Lab values such as CO_2 levels and osmolality should also be monitored. CO_2 levels should be maintained at a low-normal range as a very low CO_2 level can decrease cerebral blood flow from vasoconstriction. Osmolality should be increased to help pull excess fluids from the brain tissues. Hypertonic saline may be used to promote this effect. Serum sodium levels should be monitored and hyponatremia should be avoided as this causes cerebral edema to occur.

A damaged brain is susceptible to increased temperature; therefore it is necessary to maintain the patient in normothermic conditions with a core body temperature of $<38\ °C$. Cool water circulated through body wraps or cooling catheters may be used to maintain normal temperature.

VTE prophylaxis is necessary as patients with TBI are at higher risk for developing DVT and PE. Pneumatic compression devices are most often used as well as anti-embolic stockings. Once the risk of bleeding is reduced, low molecular weight heparin is often used prophylactically.

Nutrition should be started as soon as tolerated as the metabolic demands are higher in patients with TBI. A small feeding tube may be placed into the small intestine to deliver nutrition. Goal is to begin adequate nutrition within 72 h of admission with full caloric intake by post injury day 7. It is also important to maintain a normal glucose level; insulin protocols may be used to achieve the desired levels.

TBI patients have an increased risk at developing seizures. Seizures can arise early as a result of the initial trauma but can also develop 2 weeks or later due to damage to the structure of the brain. Seizures increase the metabolic demands on the brain and can cause further damage; therefore it is important to minimize the risk of seizure by starting anti-seizure medications. These medications may be continued for the first 7 days. An EEG may also be used to identify patients at risk for developing seizure.

Positioning of the patient with increased ICP levels may not be possible but the HOB should be at least 30 degrees to promote venous drainage of the brain. Loosening the cervical collar, while maintaining neutral alignment, may help alleviate pain and discomfort which can cause ICP to elevate.

Minimize environmental stimulation as the injured brain cannot process information normally. Increased stimulation may lead to increased ICP, agitation, and restlessness. Keep light low in the patient's room. Minimize conversation and noise.

Rehabilitation consults are made early to start range of motion exercises and splinting to prevent contractures.

Care for patient's family is just as important as caring for the patient. The nurse should prepare the family by explaining the patient's progress and it may be slow with good days and bad days. Encourage the family to seek out support from other family members, clergy, and friends. Consult social services and case management who may assist families with resources. Family meetings should be held frequently with the multidisciplinary team to discuss patient's progress and family needs.

Bibliography

1. ACS TQIP. Best practices in the management of traumatic brain injury; January 2015.
2. Caring for patients with traumatic brain injuries: are you up to the challenges?; October 2009; Https://americannursetoday.com
3. Guidelines for the management of severe trauma brain injury, 3rd ed. 2007.
4. Nursing Management of Adults with severe traumatic brain injury; December 2009. AANN.
5. Trauma nursing: trauma brain injury. www.modernmedicine.com

46 Geriatric Trauma: Spinal Injury Nursing Care

Kai Bortz

Spinal injuries in the elderly can be devastating. Osteoporosis and degenerative joint disease increase the risk of a spine injury in the older adult patient [1]. In addition, decreased muscle mass and ligament strength further increases the older adults risk of a spinal injury following a traumatic event. Odontoid fractures are the most common spinal fracture, accounting for 11% of all traumatic cervical spine injuries, of which 40–60% are Type II odontoid fractures [2]. Spinal injuries often occur as the result of a low velocity fall [2]. A cervical collar must be maintained until a fracture can be ruled out [1].

In the older adult population, spinal injury is often seen without neurological damage [2]. Older adults often have more complications as a result of multiple comorbidities as well as the result of treatment, including nonunion, morbidity, and mortality [2]. Currently, there is no clear consensus on treatment for spinal injuries [2]. Treatment decisions remain inconsistent between trauma centers worldwide [3]. Management is complicated by the presence of multiple medical conditions, including cardiopulmonary compromise, and diminished potential for osseous union [4].

Older adults typically have less functional reserve, which limits treatment options for cervical spine fractures [5]. Management associated with prolonged bed rest is not tolerated well in the elderly [5]. Studies have shown that respiratory failure is the primary cause of death in older adults with spinal injuries, attributable to atelectasis and pneumonia [5]. Despite the treatment provided for a spinal injury, nursing care must focus on preventing complications associated with immobilization, pain, comorbidity exacerbation, and consideration of physiological changes that occur with aging that increase the older adult's risk of complications following a spinal injury.

Central Cord Syndrome is the most common type of spinal cord injury seen in the geriatric population. Central cord treatment is based on severity of initial neurologic injury, degree of spinal canal stenosis, age of patient, and presence of medical comorbidities [3]. Depression screening should be initiated in older adults with a spinal injury resulting in neurologic deficit or any motor function loss. Emotional support and encouragement should be provided as well as involvement of pastoral care and psychiatry as indicated. Nursing care should focus on prevention of further loss of function.

K. Bortz, M.S.N., R.N.-B.C., C.M.S.R.N., C.N.L., T.C.R.N
Transitional Trauma Unit, Lehigh Valley Health Network, 1200 South Cedar Crest Blvd, Allentown, PA 18103, USA
e-mail: Kai_L.Bortz@lvhn.org

A. Rodriguez et al. (eds.), *Geriatric Trauma and Acute Care Surgery*,
https://doi.org/10.1007/978-3-319-57403-5_46

Respiratory Issues

Lower respiratory infections are of great concern following cervical spine immobilization, secondary to dysphagia, delirium, and decreased mobility [10]. Aspiration pneumonia has been linked to death after cervical spine fractures [10]. This could be related to decreased vital capacity and delirium, which may increase the risk of aspiration [10].

A number of physiological changes occur with aging that increases the risk of pulmonary complications in the older adult with a spinal injury. Respiratory function begins to decline and deteriorates with age. Respiratory muscle strength decreases and the chest wall stiffens which decreases chest wall compliance [18, 19]. In addition, immobilization, comorbid conditions, and concomitant injuries in the older adult increases the risk of complications further. Early clearance for head of bed elevation is key to maintaining a patent airway. Nursing care must focus on maintaining a patent airway through upright positioning/repositioning and suctioning. Oxygen should be provided as needed to maintain adequate oxygenation. Incentive spirometry, cough and deep breathe, and mobilization should be encouraged for mobilization of secretions. Incentive spirometry volumes should be monitored for trends in volume, recorded, and followed by the trauma team. Consultation to respiratory therapy should be considered, which may be especially beneficial for cognitively impaired patients who are immobile and unable to participate in incentive spirometry.

Neurological Assessment

The neurological exam in the older adult can be challenging. Normal age-associated changes that occur include a decrease in neurons and neurotransmitters, slower speed of cognitive processing, decrease in general muscle strength, deep tendon reflexes, sensation of touch, pain, and vibration, and nerve conduction velocity [6, 7]. These changes result in slowed coordinated movements and increased response time to stimuli [8]. Thorough neurological assessments should be completed on a routine basis. Baseline cognition should be determined, as well as any motor or sensory deficits prior to their injury. Cognitive impairment prior to injury must be considered during the neurological assessment. Preexisting injuries or medical conditions may limit the patient's mobility or sensory function, which must be considered during assessment of the patient's baseline. The patient must be monitored for changes from this baseline assessment. Family involvement may be necessary to assist in cognitive assessment and activities of daily living assessment, especially in cognitively impaired or mechanically ventilated patients.

Hospitalized older adults have an increased risk of developing delirium. Interventions to prevent delirium should be implemented, and any avoidable precipitating risk factors should be eliminated. In addition, older adults have an increased risk of sleep disorders [9]. Sleep interruptions during hospitalization are common, but should be reduced to prevent delirium. Routine assessments for delirium should be completed by the nurse, and the physician notified with a positive screen for delirium.

Pain

Acute pain control in the older adult patient can be challenging. However, adequate and appropriate pain control in the geriatric trauma patient is essential to the patients' recovery. Pain assessments must be completed frequently using an appropriate pain scale. Cognitively impaired patients are at highest risk of uncontrolled pain [13]. Nonverbal pain scales should be used when necessary to assess for pain [13]. Barriers to adequate pain control include cognitive impairment, fear of addiction, side effects, sensory impairment, and under-reporting of pain [14, 15]. Uncontrolled pain can lead to delirium, decreased mobility, decreased participation in activities of daily living (ADL's), and respiratory compromise. It is important to treat pain in the older adult as soon as pain is identified [16].

Assessment of chronic pain and previous pain interventions should be completed prior to treatment of acute pain. The doses of pain medications need to be lower than the normal dose given to younger patients, as the "start low and go slow but go" motto is often used [16]. Doses should be titrated upwards until the patient reaches their pain level goal [16]. Non-pharmacological pain interventions should be included as an adjunct to pharmacological pain interventions, which assists in avoiding undesired medication side effects in the older adult population. In addition, a bowel regimen should be initiated for all patients receiving opioids and decreased mobility to prevent constipation.

Mobilization

Despite the treatment chosen for treatment of a spine injury, there should be great focus on early mobilization. Patients requiring surgical intervention should be considered for early operative treatment. Older adults with a spinal injury have an increased risk for activities of daily living assistance and gait aid for safe mobilization [10]. Studies have shown that those requiring immobilization were more likely to be functionally impaired, and require supportive care following discharge [10]. Studies have shown decreased function in older adults following the use of external orthotic devices [10]. Older adults may be unable to tolerate the extra weight and decreased range of motion associated with immobilization [10]. Patients requiring orthotic devices should have fall precaution interventions implemented to prevent falls associated with limitations related to orthotic devices. Mortality and complication rates are low when the rigid cervical collar is combined with early patient mobilization [11].

Due to a number of preexisting medical conditions, the older adult patient's functional status must be determined. The patient's functional status is their ability to perform basic self-care activities. Prolonged bed rest in the older adult patient can lead to poor outcomes and should be prevented or reduced whenever possible [12]. Overall mobilization during hospitalization in older adults has shown to be poor. Due to the mobility restrictions associated with spinal injury, it is expected that mobilization in this population may be even worse than the general medical/surgical population. Early physical and occupational therapy consultation should be initiated to assist in expediting mobilization and participation in activities of daily living. Physical activity should be encouraged with health education and goal setting to maintain function.

Nutrition

Nutrition plays an important part in the overall health and recovery of the older adult trauma patient. Preexisting medical conditions and physiological changes that occur with aging that affect appetite as well as malnutrition prior to their trauma may increase the patient's risk of poor outcomes and delayed healing following a traumatic injury [17]. Older adult patients may have difficulty swallowing following a cervical spine injury. As a result, a dysphagia screening should be completed prior to start of oral feedings. Collars and braces, inadequate pain control, and bed rest may decrease oral intake [17]. If possible, the patient should be placed in an upright position and out of bed when eating. Weight, body mass index (BMI), dietary intake, and fluid balance should be monitored closely in the older adult with a spinal injury. Nutrition consultation should be considered for patients at high risk of malnutrition. Dietary supplements may aid in providing nutritional needs for healing and recovery.

Urinary Retention

The immobilized older adult with a spinal injury may have an increased risk of urinary retention. A bladder scan protocol should be followed for appropriate emptying of the bladder. Post void residuals may also need to be monitored to assure complete emptying of the bladder.

Gastrointestinal Issues

Older adult patients with a spinal injury have an increased risk of constipation due to immobilization and medication side effects. Nursing strategies include early mobilization, hydration, assessment of normal bowel frequency and home regimen related to bowel function, and providing stool softeners and/or laxatives as indicated.

Skin

Pressure ulcers/devices—Patients with cervical spine immobilization have an increased risk of developing pressure ulcers. All patients with orthotic devices to prevent spinal mobilization require close monitoring due to the risk of developing pressure ulcers as well as the overall management of the medical condition [20].

References

1. Weber J, Jablonski R, Penrod J. Missed opportunities: under-detection of trauma in elderly adults involved in motor vehicle crashes. J Emerg Nurs. 2010;36:6–9.
2. Fehlings M, Arun R, Vaccaro A, Arnold P, Chapman J, Kopjar B. Predictors of treatment outcomes in geriatric patients with odontoid fractures. Spine. 2013;38(11):881–6.
3. Fehlings M, Wilson J, Dvorak M, Vaccaro A, Fisher C. The challenges of managing spine and spinal cord injuries. Spine. 2010;35(21):161–5.
4. Sander A, Saman A, Delfosse P, Wutzler S, Meier S, Marzi I, Laurer H. Cervical spine fractures in the elderly: morbidity and mortality after operative treatment. Eur J Trauma Emerg Surg. 2013;39:469–76.
5. Damadi A, Saxe A, Fath J, Apelgren K. Cervical spine fractures in patients 65 years or older: a 3-year experience at a level I trauma center. J Trauma. 2006;64(3):745–8.
6. Mattson M. Cellular and neurochemical aspects of the aging human brain. In: Halter JB, Ouslander JG, Tineeti ME, Studenski S, High KP, Asthana S, editors. Hazzard's geriatric medicine and gerontology. 6th ed. New York: McGraw-Hill; 2009. p. 739–50.
7. Hall KE. Aging and neural control of the GI tract. II. Neural control of the aging gut: can an old dog learn new tricks? Am J Physiol Gastrointest Liver Physiol. 2002;283(4):G827–32.
8. Matsumura BA, Ambrose AF. Balance in the elderly. Clin Geriatr Med. 2006;22(2):395–412.
9. Espiritu JR. Aging-related sleep changes. Clin Geriatr Med. 2008;24(1):1–14.
10. Moran C, Kipen E, Chan P, Niggenmeyer L, Simon S, Hunter P, Fitzgerald M, Gruen R. Understanding post-hospital morbidity associated with immobilization of cervical spine fractures in older people using geriatric medicine assessment techniques: a pilot study. Injury. 2013;44(12):1838–42.
11. Molinari R, Khera O, Gruhn W, McAssey R. Rigid cervical collar treatment for geriatric type II odontoid fractures. Eur Spine J. 2012;21:855–62.
12. Padula C, Hughes C, Baumhover L. Impact of a nurse-driven mobility protocol on functional decline in hospitalized older adults. J Nurs Care Qual. 2009;24(4):325–31.
13. Horgas AL, Elliott AF. Pain assessment and management in persons with dementia: relationship between self-report and behavioral observation. J Am Geriatr Soc. 2009;57(1):126–32.
14. American Geriatrics Society Panel on Persistent Pain in Older Persons. The management of persistent pain in older persons. J Am Geriatr Soc. 2002;50:S205–24.
15. Gordon DB, Pellino TA, Miaskowski C, McNeill JA, Paice JA, Laferriere D, Bookbinder M. A 10-year review of quality improvement monitoring in pain management: recommendations for standardized outcome measures. Pain Manag Nurs. 2002;3(4):116–30.
16. Boltz M, Capequti E, Fulmer T, Zwicker D. Evidence-based geriatric nursing protocols for best practice. 4th ed. New York: Springer Publishing Company; 2012.
17. Campbell J, Degolia P, Fallon W, Rader E. In harm's way: moving the older trauma patient toward a better outcome. Geriatrics. 2009;64(1):8–13.
18. Buchman AS, Boyle PA, Wilson RS, Gu L, Bienias JL, Bennett DA. Pulmonary function, muscle strength and mortality in old age. Mech Ageing Dev. 2008;129(11):625–31.
19. Imperato J, Sanchez LD. Pulmonary emergencies in the elderly. Emerg Med Clin North Am. 2006;24(2):317–38.
20. Walker J. Pressure ulcers in cervical spine immobilization: a retrospective analysis. J Wound Care. 2012;21(7):323–7.

47 Cardiothoracic Geriatric Trauma: Nursing Considerations

Matthew Mowry

Thoracic trauma is a serious injury at any age, where patients can quickly succumb to massive exsanguination or injuries from obstructive shock. Thoracic injury is related to 20% of all trauma-related deaths [1]. In the geriatric trauma population, 60% suffer thoracic injuries as opposed to 10% in their younger counterparts [2]. Physiologic changes and preexisting conditions can predispose the elderly to injuries, as well as complicating their recovery.

Trauma centers across the country have been seeing an increase in geriatric trauma for the past few decades. Through medical advances, adults are living longer with chronic medical conditions and at a higher quality life. At Allegheny General Hospital, a Level I trauma center in Pittsburgh, PA, Trauma Registry data confirms such high rates of geriatric thoracic trauma. From 2011 to 2015, there has been a 10% increase in geriatric patients admitted to the Trauma Service, reaching 40% in 2015. The primarily mechanism is falls and motor vehicle crashes (MVCs), with 24% having chest injuries. Sixty percent had major chest trauma, categorized as an Abbreviated Injury Score (AIS) chest score 3 or higher. Of all the geriatric patients with chest trauma, over half of those patients were admitted to the ICU. Mortality rates with chest trauma were a third higher than the general geriatric mortality rate. The most common injuries were rib fractures.

As noted earlier, falls are the leading cause of geriatric trauma. Falls may be a result of a dysrhythmia, hypoxia, anemia, polypharmacy, or mechanical in nature [3]. Mortality rates are often higher for falls than from MVCs, as the fall is often a sign of an underlying cognitive decline or undiagnosed medical condition. Eighty-two percent of all older adults have a chronic medical condition. Those with a medical history of lung disease greatly contributes to their mortality [2].

When managing a geriatric trauma patient, the same standards established for adult are to be used. However, considerations are to be made to adjust for the physiologic changes not only during assessment but also treatment and recovery. The first step in ensuring improved outcomes is appropriate triage. While geriatric trauma is typically defined as 65 and older, studies have shown there is a precipitous decline in outcomes after the age of 70 [2]. Trauma activation guidelines should be tailored to meet those needs, as those under triaged have a four times higher mortality rate [4]. Geriatric trauma patients have a 30% higher rate of admission and 25% higher mortality rate [2]. Once admitted, it is the nurse's primary role to facilitate a positive outcome. Proactive in early ambulation, use of incentive spirometer, and adherence to infection control

M. Mowry, R.N., M.S.N., C.E.N.
Trauma Performance Improvement
Coordinator, Level 1 Adult Trauma Center,
Allegheny General Hospital, Pittsburgh, PA, USA
e-mail: mattmowry@msn.com

A. Rodriguez et al. (eds.), *Geriatric Trauma and Acute Care Surgery*,
https://doi.org/10.1007/978-3-319-57403-5_47

protocols will achieve the goals of reducing nosocomial infections. It has also been noted that over 30% of preventable complications occur in geriatric trauma patient deaths [4].

Once an elderly trauma patient arrives, begin by assessing the patient according to Advanced Trauma Life Support (ATLS) protocols. While the nurses involved in the resuscitation may be working to treat emergent conditions, care should also be taken to provide explanations and comfort to the patient. Patients with baseline cognitive impairment including dementia or hearing loss may show increased compliance with their care when the extra time is taken. Though it may be difficult to obtain details from a patient's living will in the acute phase, efforts should be taken to address goals of care with the patient or power of attorney. Determining code status and interventions early on is ultimately in the best interest for the patient and family.

Assessment of the thorax begins with the upper airway. The airway should be assessed for obstruction, hypoxia, stridor, or air hunger. Geriatric considerations include the potential for mechanical obstruction as a result of loose teeth or dentures, but most often, it is from the tongue. The airway may be occluded from secretions due to a progressively weak gag and cough reflex. Suction should be used as needed but kept to a minimum if at all possible. Attention to duration and intensity, as suction can remove needed oxygen as well as damaging frail skin [4]. Provide oxygen as needed and anticipate intubation, as aggressive and early intervention may be indicated. If intubated, evaluate the position and patency of the endotracheal tube. Airway obstructions may be also due to mandibular fractures, direct laryngeal and tracheal trauma, and expanding neck hematomas [5]. The latter should be a concern for those taking anticoagulants, as intervention and reversal are key components to their management.

When assessing the pulmonary system, several physiologic factors need to be taken in consideration. Ventilatory capacity declines due to a decrease in muscle strength and endurance. Rib cartilage becomes weak and calcified, and the rigid chest wall limits compliance. Vessels throughout the body, including the chest, become atherosclerotic. Therefore, when an elderly patient is involved in a low energy mechanism, such as a ground level fall, they are at risk for rib fractures, as well as pneumothorax, hemothorax, and pulmonary contusion.

The physical exam of the pulmonary system includes inspecting the chest wall for equal expansion, as well as any other deformities or discolorations. Palpate the chest for crepitance, subcutaneous air, and pain. If feasible, place both hands on the two hemithoraces to assess symmetry of the chest wall motion. Additional challenges can occur when assessing an elderly patient with kyphosis or a "barrel chest" from COPD (chronic obstructive pulmonary disease). Auscultate both lung fields for the presences of breath sounds. Ambient noise during resuscitation may make auscultation and percussion difficult [1]. A chest X-ray may be performed initially followed by a more sensitive CT scan for definitive diagnosis.

The most common chest injury in the elderly is rib fractures. Rib calcification can be a setup for fractures, and the decreased chest wall compliance and muscle loss is a predisposition for complications after the injury. Those with COPD and cardiac disease are at particular risk. Falls are the primary mechanism but can also occur from seat belt injuries during MVCs. When assessing patients for rib fractures, evaluate for respiratory distress, including respiratory rate > 35, SpO2 below 90, and a pCO2 > 55 [5]. The decreased alveolar surface area also makes it difficult to oxygenate these patients. Particular concern is for flailed segments; where two or more ribs are fractured in two more or places leading to paradoxical motion. Pain associated with flailed segments lead to increased work of breathing, which can have a spiraling effect of short ineffective breaths and quickly tiring out the patient. This ineffective breathing can lead to atelectasis and respiratory failure, even though oxygen levels are normal.

Pulmonary contusion may accompany rib fractures or flailed segments. These patient will see an event greater challenge avoiding hypoxemia. Treatment is supportive care, maintaining oxygen saturation, aggressive pulmonary toilet, and analgesia. Mechanical ventilation with PEEP (positive end-expiratory pressure) may be needed for the more severe contusions.

A pneumothorax occurs when air enters the pleural space from either an injury to the lung parenchyma or through the chest wall. As the pressure increases and air is unable to escape, a tension pneumothorax develops. The patient will have respiratory distress, unilateral breath sounds, and hemodynamic instability. Deviated trachea and jugular vein distention (JVD) may be a late finding. The goal is to quickly decompress the chest with a needle followed with tube thoracostomy. Once converted to a simple pneumothorax, the chest tube will be connected to an underwater seal device and apply 20 cm water suction. If the patient is intubated and on positive pressure ventilation, monitor the patient for an increase in their pneumothorax.

A hemothorax is when the pleural space is filled with blood instead of air, or there could be both. Typically, this is from injuries to major arteries or damage to the intercostal vessels due to rib fractures. The neck veins may be flat due to exsanguination into the hemothorax, which each can hold up to 3 liters. Or, JVD may be present due to the obstructive effects of the intrathoracic blood. Lungs sounds may be dull to percuss and chest X-ray showing a "whited out" or opacified lung field. If tube thoracostomy is indicated, monitor output in the underwater seal device, as greater than 1500 mL initially or >200 mL/h over 4 h will necessitate operative intervention [5].

In the event the patient decompensates during resuscitation to the point where vital signs are lost, the physician may proceed to open the left chest with an anterolateral thoracotomy. This maneuver allows for control of massive hemorrhage in the chest, release cardiac tamponade, or cross clamp the aorta to improve central perfusion. If the heart is fibrillating, the patient will need to be defibrillated with internal cardiac paddles at 20 J, followed by 30 J as needed. If the heart is not beating, cardiac massage will need to be initiated. This procedure may be considered based on mechanism of injury, as penetrating has a higher success rate than blunt mechanisms. Elderly patients do not do as well as their younger counterparts, as patients who require this procedure already have a high mortality rate.

As for all patients with pulmonary injuries, the priority is to maintain and monitor oxygenation through the SpO2 and serial arterial blood gases. Nursing Diagnoses Impaired Gas Exchange and Ineffective Breathing Pattern apply to these patients [6]. ABGs are helpful in monitoring oxygen levels as well as for CO_2 narcosis and base deficit. Monitor the patient's ability to clear secretions. Maintain adequate hydration and air humidification [7]. If the patient needs pain control due to rib fractures or other chest wall trauma, the Acute Pain Service or Anesthesia may be consulted to place an epidural or paravertebral catheter. Pain may also be controlled with multimodal therapy, including a Patient Controlled Analgesia (PCA) device. If not contraindicated, keep the head of the bed elevated at least 30° [7]. It is also important to obtain a good medical history, including pulmonary disease such as emphysema and COPD, smoking, and environmental or occupational exposures, that would negatively impact their lungs [7].

Along with supportive therapy that includes oxygenation and pain control, encourage the patient in proper breathing techniques. Pursed lip breathing and abdominal breathing exercises will aid in their ability to keep their lungs fully expanded. Assess ongoing pulmonary function with the incentive spirometer. The acceptable range is 15 mL/kg. For every 10% increase in vital capacity in the first 48 h, it was associated with a 36% decrease in pulmonary complications. Rib Fracture Pathways have been shown to decrease unplanned return to the ICU for respiratory issues, decrease length of stay, and improve disposition. Initially presented by York Hospital at the national TQIP Conference in 2014, a PIC (Pain, Inspiration, and Cough) Protocol validated those results. Their targeted approach was to improve mobility, coughing, deep breathing, and pain control to decrease complications. With formal protocols and education with nursing, respiratory therapy, patients and families alike, their results have inspired other trauma centers across to the country to implement similar programs.

The cardiovascular system also goes through a series of physiologic changes as we age. The heart's walls become thickened, thereby slowing the conduction system. There is also a decreased sensitivity to catecholamine, which effects the body's fight or flight response [2]. Coronary arteries become stiff as well as decreased vessel compliance and greater systemic vascular resistance [7]. As a result of these cardiovascular changes, it can be even more challenging to evaluate patients from a hemodynamic standpoint. Heart rates above 90 and systolic blood pressures below 110 mmHg have been considered triage set points for the elderly in trauma activations [8]. Typically, an adult will have signs and symptoms after 30% blood loss [1]. The elderly have a poor physiologic reserve and require more time for diastolic filling and systolic emptying. These patients are at risk for the Nursing Diagnosis of Impaired Tissue Perfusion [6]. Patients who are on Beta Blocker or have a pacemaker can further complicate the initial assessment, as it can prevent an increase in their cardiac output [2].

EAST's Geriatric Trauma Guidelines have stated early and aggressive resuscitation should be initiated in the geriatric population. Begin by inserting two large bore IVs, followed by 1–2 L of normal saline or lactated ringers, with consideration of blood products [4]. Due to the thickened heart wall and sclerosing atrial and mitral valves, this dysfunction leaves patients at risk for developing heart failure during resuscitation. Judicious fluid administration must be balanced with an adequate resuscitation. This should also be considered in patients who required reversal for coagulopathy. Medications such as Prothrombin Complex Concentrate (PCC) have dramatically reduced the large volume of fresh frozen plasma associated with reversing the effects of warfarin in elderly head injuries. For patients on Direct Thrombin and Xa inhibitors, these once nonreversible medication have newly developed antidotes.

Cardiac tamponade is a life-threating condition where a physical obstruction is in the heart and great vessels. Often due but not exclusive to penetrating trauma, 75–100 mL of blood in the pericardial sac can lead to patients presenting in shock. Though not to be confused with dementia, these patients can present with combativeness and anxiousness. Additional challenges are those with a history of congestive heart failure. These patients can present with JVD and muffled heart tones, similar to those with tamponade. Additional signs and symptoms include hypotension, acidosis, and a base deficit. The diagnosis may also be suspected with a mediastinal hematoma or hemothorax on chest X-ray. The tamponade may also be seen on ultrasound during the FAST (Focused Assessment with Sonography for Trauma). These patients need immediate action, either with a temporizing intervention of pericardiocentesis or by definitive action in releasing the clot with a pericardial window or anterolateral thoracotomy [5].

A direct blow to the chest can result in a Blunt Cardiac Injury. The results can vary from a minor contusion to the heart, heart failure, or even cardiac rupture [5]. Dysrhythmias are a common symptom, ranging from tachycardia, premature beats, bundle branch blocks, and atrial fibrillation. Blunt Cardiac Injury can put the elderly further at risk for developing lethal dysthymias if they have underlying heart disease, which impacts 1 in 3 adults over the age of 60 [7]. These patients need supportive therapy for their dysrhythmias per ACLS protocol and admission to a telemetry floor. If signs of heart failure are identified, often by visualizing hypokinetic heart motion on an echocardiogram, they may need invasive monitoring in the ICU [5].

Traumatic rupture of the thoracic aorta is a tear in the vessel's wall and contained by the adventitia or pleural space. In the elderly, this is often due to MVCs, particularly severe lateral impacts. Age-associated stiffness inhibits the aorta's mobility, further putting the elderly at risk for these deceleration-related injuries. Overall, 80% of all ruptured thoracic aortas die at the scene, as a free rupture is often rapidly fatal [5]. Patients may complain of chest pain but 50% have no signs of injury. Widened pulse pressures and a wide mediastinum will be present on chest XR. The gold standard for diagnosis has been Aortography but CT is now the most common diagnostic modality. Initial treatment is to control hypertension and stress on the systolic wall of the aorta. Esmolol is commonly started at 500 mcg/kg bolus followed by a 50 mcg/kg/min drip. The goal is keep heart rate and blood pressure below 100. Unstable patients will go directly to the OR for definitive repair, most often with an endovascular aortic stent graft.

Ongoing assessment includes maintaining pulmonary function as well as optimizing cardiac function. Other concerns include monitoring hydration and nutritional status. In aging, blood pressure may be affected during positioning due to impaired baroreceptors. Careful attention to those at risk for orthostatic hypotension, as it can prevent further falls and injury. In the event your patient develops heart failure during resuscitation or an exacerbation of chronic disease, assess for JVD, bibasilar crackles, pitting edema, and monitor B-type natriuretic peptide (BNP). Diuretics may be needed to remove excess sodium and water [7]. Capillary refill may take longer than the normal 2–3 s if there is a history of vascular or pulmonary disease. Those who are immobile or have contraindications for thromboprophylaxis are at risk for pulmonary embolism. Assess the patient for confusion, dyspnea, slight fever, or pneumonitis [6].

In summary, the geriatric population has several unique factors that make their assessment and treatment more challenging than the typical adult. However, it is important to follow the established national standards and institutional protocols. Because of these challenges, it takes an astute clinician to identify these variations and adjust treatment modalities. There may be times where the treatment and intervention needs to be weighed with the patient's wishes and pre-injury quality of life. The nurse must use a multifaceted approach for the geriatric trauma patient, through injury-specific management needs, education, prevention, and rehabilitation. This full spectrum of geriatric trauma care can be applied to all patients regardless of the injury system.

References

1. McQuillan K, et al. Trauma nursing: from resuscitation through rehabilitation. 4th ed. St. Louis: Saunders Elsevier; 2009.
2. Hawk M, et al. Blunt thoracic injury in older adults: application of Haddon's phase-factor matrix model. J Gerontol Nurs. 2012;38(2):14–27.
3. Campbell J, et al. In harm's way: moving the older trauma patient toward a better outcome. Geriatrics. 2009;64(1):8–13.
4. Cutugno C. The 'graying' of trauma care: addressing traumatic injury in older adults. Am J Nurs. 2011;111(11):40–8.
5. Peitzman A, et al. The trauma manual: trauma and acute care surgery. 4th ed. Philadelphia: Lippincott Williams & Wilkins; 2013.
6. Eliopoulos C. Gerontological Nursing. 7th ed. Philadelphia: Lippincott Williams & Wilkins; 2010.
7. Boltz M, et al. Evidence-based geriatric nursing protocols for best practice. 4th ed. New York City: Springer Publishing Company; 2012.
8. Hefferan D, et al. Normal presenting vital signs are unreliable in geriatric blunt trauma victims. J Trauma. 2010;69(4):813–20.

Nursing Care of the Client with Abdominal Trauma

48

Elizabeth D. Katrancha

Nursing care of the patient with blunt abdominal trauma begins with an assessment of the abdomen. The abdominal assessment is often less than effective due to the often subtle signs and symptoms and the other distracting injuries a patient may have. Observe the abdomen for contusions, abrasions and distension or penetrating wounds. Consider that wounds above the umbilicus could have thoracic implications. Auscultate for bowel sounds and bruits. Absent bowels sounds should be considered in conjunction with other assessment data. Bruits may indicate injury to a great vessel, liver or spleen. Assess for guarding or rigidity, keeping in mind the older adult often has more subtle signs of peritoneal irritation than their younger counterparts.

Most trauma centers now use ultrasound for the focused assessment with sonography for trauma (FAST) examination. The FAST examination can determine the presence of free fluid in the abdomen which would indicate bleeding. If the FAST examination is positive and the patient is hemodynamically unstable, the nurse should begin to prepare for rapid intervention.

The hemodynamically stable blunt abdominal trauma patient will usually undergo a computed tomography (CT) of the abdomen and pelvis to evaluate solid organ injury. The nurse should consider renal function and medications that have potential interactions with contrast dye.

The nurse should be monitoring for changes in mental status, changes in vital signs such as hypotension, tachycardia and oliguria as signs of hypoperfusion. Consider intra-abdominal bleeding as a possible cause. Keep in mind older adults on beta-blockers may not demonstrate tachycardia.

The older adult with penetrating abdominal injuries may be managed operatively. The nurse should assess the patient, keep families informed of the prognosis and prepare for possible emergent surgery. The nurse should anticipate a damage control method of surgical care in unstable patients, meaning the immediate surgical operations will control immediate life-threatening injuries, followed by ongoing resuscitation efforts in the intensive care unit (ICU). The patient will then be taken to the OR later for final surgical repairs. In the ICU, the care will focus on keeping the patient normothermic, monitoring and correcting coagulopathies and maintaining adequate perfusion. The nurse must be continually assessing the geriatric client being observant for subtle changes in assessment and monitoring parameters. The client may return to the ICU from the OR with an open abdominal wall. The nurse may be required to maintain sterile dressings, negative pressure dressing systems or some

E.D. Katrancha, DNP, CCNS, RN, CNE, CSN
Department of Nursing, University of Pittsburgh, Johnstown, PA, USA
e-mail: ekatrancha@pitt.edu

A. Rodriguez et al. (eds.), *Geriatric Trauma and Acute Care Surgery*,
https://doi.org/10.1007/978-3-319-57403-5_48

variation of temporary closure. Using careful aseptic technique is imperative.

The nurse should expect to start enteral feedings in the client with abdominal trauma. This is usually achieved through some form of gastric tube such as a nasally inserted small bore feeding tube or percutaneous endoscopic gastrostomy (PEG) depending on the patient injuries and status. Early feeding has been shown to decrease morbidity and mortality. The nurse will monitor bowel sounds, patient tolerance of the feeding and institute measures to decrease aspiration.

Lastly, the nurse and care team should be in communication with the family and begin discharge planning early.

49 Nursing Considerations for Traumatic Geriatric Orthopedic Injuries

Elizabeth L. Price, Rajesh R. Gandhi, and Therese M. Duane

Nursing care for patients with traumatic orthopedic injuries should focus on preoperative optimization and on decreasing postoperative complications. Preoperative nursing care should include a thorough history and physical, cognitive screening, cardiac and pulmonary evaluations, frailty assessment, nutritional status, medication history, pain control and ensuring the patient has been adequately resuscitated. Postoperatively, the most important nursing considerations should circle around decreasing postoperative complications, including decreasing risks of delirium, deep vein thrombosis, infection, bed decubitus, poor nutrition, depression, and muscle wasting. Nonoperative management of elderly orthopedic fractures such as rib fractures, pelvic fractures, and patients with poor physiological status where surgery is more of a risk than benefit should have nursing care that includes pain control, aggressive pulmonary toilet, early ambulation, adequate nutrition and hydration, and prevention of infection to expedite discharge and to increase the likelihood of best functional outcome.

Preoperative Nursing Considerations

The preoperative period begins once the patient arrives in the emergency department and should not exceed 48 h. Geriatric patients who have prolonged preoperative times, greater than 48 h, have increased 30-day all-cause mortality rates of 41% and a 1-year all-cause mortality of 32% [1]. Patients should be medically optimized for the operating room, if possible, within 12 h of admission and undergo operative fixation within 48 h of admission. A thorough history including past medical history, past surgical history, social history, and medication list should be performed on all patients. Medical history should include all comorbidities and name of primary care physician. Contacting the pharmacy where the patient fills their prescriptions is also helpful as they can offer a current prescription list with strength and frequency if the patient is unable to provide that at the time of admission. Frequency of falls should be questioned especially if the patient is arriving to the emergency department as a result of a fall. Typically, patients who have had more than one fall in the last year experience a decline in functionality or have fall hazards in their

E.L. Price, R.N., M.S.N., A.C.N.S.-B.C. (✉)
Department of Trauma Services, John Peter Smith Health Network, Fort Worth, TX 76104, USA
e-mail: eprice@jpshealth.org

R.R. Gandhi, M.D., Ph.D.
T.M. Duane, M.D., M.B.A
Department of Surgery, John Peter Smith Health Network, Fort Worth, TX 76104, USA
e-mail: rgandhi@jpshealth.org; tduane@jpshealth.org

A. Rodriguez et al. (eds.), *Geriatric Trauma and Acute Care Surgery*,
https://doi.org/10.1007/978-3-319-57403-5_49

current living environment that can be corrected before discharge to prevent subsequent falls. A past medical and surgical history can also help to identify any other comorbidities that the patient may have not identified. The social history should include alcohol, tobacco, and illicit drug use and also include their living environment and support system at home.

While performing the history, be aware of any cognitive impairment that can provide insight into underlying dementia or mental health disease. Patients should undergo a quick assessment for cognitive ability in the emergency department to assess any underlying cognitive deficits that could complicate their hospital stay, such as inability to consent for procedures, postoperative delirium, and pain control challenges. The Six Item Screener (SIS) or Mini-Cog are quick and easy tools to assess for cognitive defects. If cognitive impairments are either known or discovered during the assessment, understand that the patient is at risk for postoperative delirium and nursing measures should be taken to prevent delirium postoperatively. Patients who develop postoperative delirium are at higher risk of complications resulting in higher rates of mortality, poorer functional recovery, and higher hospital costs because of increased lengths of stay [2].

Pulmonary and cardiac assessments start with baseline pulmonary function tests, electrocardiogram (EKG) and chest X-ray or CT of the thorax. The patient's functional capacity should be included in this assessment as patients with low functional capacity are at higher risk for perioperative cardiac adverse events. If the patient's baseline EKG is normal or appropriate to the patient's history, no further cardiac testing should be performed unless it will change the course of management. For example, if your patient arrives to the emergency room in atrial fibrillation with rate control and has a known history, an echocardiogram or cardiac enzymes are not indicated unless there is accompanying chest pain or acute coronary symptoms. If an echocardiogram is indicated, ensure that the test is done quickly and anesthesia is notified since this is a common reason why surgeries are postponed. Baseline pulmonary function tests should be performed on patients with chest trauma, history of chronic obstructive pulmonary disease (COPD), congestive heart failure, obstructive sleep apnea, tobacco use, poor nutrition, or frail by definition. The pulmonary function tests should be trended, with at least three tests over 8 h, as postoperative pulmonary complications occur in the elderly population with the above risk factors 15% of the time (Chow et al. 2009). Patients who have poor pulmonary status or chest trauma should have aggressive pulmonary toilet to prevent atelectasis and pneumonia. Aggressive pulmonary toilet includes scheduled positive expiratory pressure (PEP) every 4 h with chest percussion therapy (CPT), as tolerated, to encourage coughing and deep breathing. Nurses should assess the patient's ability to use the incentive spirometer several times a shift to ensure adequate pulmonary function.

Adequate resuscitation is imperative to preventing complications, increased mortality and ensuring that operative fixation is performed in a timely fashion. Upon arrival to the emergency department, even patients with minor injuries from low mechanisms should be assessed for adequate hydration and occult hypoperfusion. Elderly patients presenting with "normal" vital signs may be in a state of hypoperfusion due to beta blocker use, baseline organ dysfunction, and hypertension. The best indicator for occult hypoperfusion is an elevated lactate and base deficit. If the patient has a lactate greater than 2.5 mM or a base deficit less than −2, the patient is considered to have poor tissue perfusion and should be volume resuscitated. Cardiac monitoring that includes cardiac output, cardiac index, and stroke volume variance should be assessed with invasive monitoring. High mortality rates have been directly linked to undiagnosed occult hypoperfusion and the patient's inability to clear lactate. Salottolo et al. assessed a large population of geriatric trauma patients and found that occult hypoperfusion was common in this population and associated with a twofold increase in mortality [3]. Calloway et al. performed a retrospective study and looked at normotensive geriatric patients, admission lactate levels, and base deficit. Patients with elevated serum lactate and base deficit had a mortality rate of 60%. If lactate levels were normalized within 24 h, mortality risks decreased; but if lactate levels stayed elevated past 48 h, the risk of mortality was 86% [4]. Therefore, patients have significantly better outcomes when lactate levels are corrected within 24 h of admission. However, resuscitation of geriatric patients, especially those with cardiac dysfunction, should be done conservatively and started with boluses of 250–500 mL to prevent volume overload. Baseline renal function should also be assessed with random urine creatinine, urine electrolytes, urine osmolarity, and urinalysis. Any identification of urinary tract infections should be treated appropriately with antibiotics.

The final stages of the preoperative period include assessment for frailty, nutritional status, and treatment goals. There are several definition measures for frailty available. Frailty has been shown to independently predict higher postoperative complications, longer lengths of stay, and higher likelihood of patients to be discharged to an inpatient facility including skilled nursing or assisted-living facilities. Nutritional status should be assessed with consultation to a nutritionist if the patient's serum albumin is less than 3 g/dL with a BMI less than 18.5 kg/m^2 or unintentional weight loss over the last 6 months of more than 10% [5]. Ensuring that patients are getting enough calories is important during the preoperative period and essential postoperatively for proper healing and preventing muscle wasting. Treatment goals should be discussed with all patients but especially with geriatric trauma patients within 24 h of admission. Do Not Resuscitate and Living Wills should be discussed with the patient to help guide appropriate care within the patient's own desires to achieve the best quality of life. Discharge disposition that is realistic for the individual patient should be discussed with the patient's support system present whether that be home with assistance, inpatient rehabilitation, or skilled nursing facility. Keeping clear communication between the surgeon, nursing, the patient, and their family is essential in patient satisfaction and a timely discharge.

Finally, but not any less important, pain control is essential to preventing complications both preoperatively and postoperatively. If available, patients should undergo peripheral nerve blocks to prevent high intravenous or oral narcotic use. Nerve blocks not only offer sufficient pain control but also help with decreasing the incidence of delirium [6]. Examples of nerve blocks include femoral nerve blocks and fascia iliaca compartment blocks for hip or proximal femur fractures. Patients can benefit from paravertebral or serratus anterior plane blocks for rib fractures. If nerve blocks are not an option, an epidural catheter can be placed for many cases of rib fractures. Not all patients are candidates for nerve blocks or epidurals, and, therefore, should be given scheduled Tylenol or introduction of opiates to adequately control their pain. Elderly patients with inadequate pain control have higher rates of complications including delirium, depression, poor functional status, and poor nutritional status at discharge, if not properly treated. Non-steroidal anti-inflammatory drugs (NSAIDs) can be considered, but renal function should be assessed prior to use, especially with Toradol. Muscle relaxants also serve as great adjunctive therapy and should be considered.

Postoperative Nursing Considerations

The postoperative period begins at the completion of operative intervention and ends at discharge. Nursing considerations should focus on pain management and prevention of complications, such as decreasing risks of delirium, deep vein thrombosis, infection, bed decubitus, poor nutrition, and muscle wasting. Patients should be seen by physical and occupational therapy within 12 h of their surgery and be out of bed to chair with every meal. In the instance that the patient is not able to stand postoperatively, sitting on the side of the bed can be effective if able. Baseline functionality should be considered when performing physical therapy. If a patient was ambulating with a walker prior to surgery, then expecting them to walk without assistive devices would not be realistic. The goal of therapy is to regain the patient's individual functionality prior to injury. Early ambulation, especially in the elderly population, has many benefits including prevention of delirium, deep vein thrombosis, muscle wasting, bed decubitus, and depression. During a time when patients may fear a change in quality of life due to pain or decreased mobility, early ambulation can give them hope and a goal to work toward.

Prior to ambulation, it is important to ensure the patient's pain is under control. Whether patients have a postoperative nerve block or oral medications, severe pain during mobilization can cause depression, poor nutritional intake, and an unwillingness to cooperate. Uncontrolled pain can also increase the incidence of postoperative delirium. Patients with fascia iliaca compartment blocks (FICBs) can ambulate with the block in place as long as quad weakness is not present. Physical therapy and nursing staff should have the patient raise their hips off the bed prior to getting out of bed to ensure the patient is not experiencing quad weakness that could potentially cause a fall. Scheduled Tylenol can be very effective in the elderly population and should be tried before opiate introduction. However, if initiation of opiates is necessary to control pain, dosing should start at the lowest dose available and slowly increase, especially in opiate naive individuals.

Elderly patients, especially patients with baseline cognitive impairment, low functionality, are underweight (BMI < 20 kg/m^2) or frail by definition have an increased risk of postoperative delirium. In a prospective cohort study conducted in Norway, elderly patients were evaluated for risk factors of preoperative and postoperative delirium. The study screened patients daily, utilizing the Confusion Assessment Method (CAM) and found that patients who developed postoperative delirium had a body mass index (BMI) less than 20 or had an indoor injury. Low BMI was the most important independent risk factor in predicting postoperative delirium and was associated with a threefold increase in postoperative delirium [7]. Patients who develop inpatient delirium, whether it be preoperative or postoperative, have increased morbidity and mortality, longer lengths of stay, and utilize more resources, ultimately increasing the cost of care compared to those patients who do not experience delirium [7]. Nursing measures to prevent delirium include adequate pain control, frequent reorientation, early ambulation, adequate nutrition and hydration, and facilitating normal sleep and wake cycles. In a study performed on two surgical floors of patients 70 years of age or older, nursing interventions were implemented to decrease the risk factors of postoperative delirium and compared to patients who did not receive any interventions. The nursing interventions included early ambulation, adequate fluid and nutritional intake, non-drug sleep improvement, and improved sensory stimulation which were provided by nurses with training in management and identification of delirium. Patients who received nursing interventions to prevent delirium had a 4.9% incidence of delirium compared to 20.2% in patients without interventions [8]. It is important to prevent inpatient delirium, the first step being nursing interventions at the bedside.

Prevention of infection postoperatively includes removing unnecessary invasive lines, most commonly a Foley catheter. Unless the patient requires catheterization for a medical reason, remove all Foleys postop day one. Patients who are incontinent of urine may have pads weighed for measurement of output. Studies have shown that catheter dwell time is the most important factor in preventing catheter-associated urinary tract infections (CAUTIs). Therefore, early removal of catheters is key to preventing preventable infections. Central lines and peripherally inserted central catheters (PICC) should be removed when no longer needed and a peripheral intravenous (IV) catheter should be placed.

Nonoperative Nursing Considerations

In patients with fractures that are considered nonoperative, the same geriatric assessment that is acquired in the preoperative timeframe should be performed. This includes a thorough medical/surgical/social history and cognitive evaluation, baseline EKG, baseline pulmonary function, nutrition, frailty and functionality, and lactate to ensure proper resuscitation. Patients with fractures that impair mobility, such as nonoperative pelvic fractures, should have early mobilization and pain control. In nonoperative fractures, pain control and adequate mobility to prevent complications are the main focus.

Fall Prevention

The risk of falling increases with each decade in life, especially in females. Many falls in the elderly are preventable with proper assessment by healthcare professionals, medication management, and involving the patient and families in community resources. The Centers for Disease Control and Prevention (CDC) provides fall prevention tips including exercise, proper medication administration, monitoring of patient vision, and eliminating hazards in the patient's home environment. There are many exercise programs available for elderly patients that not only offer education and exercise but also increase confidence in patients that fear falling again. Vellas et al. performed a prospective study assessing patient's feelings of fear of recurrent falls and the effect on health status following a recent fall. Patients who had a fear of falling again had more balance and gait disorders than those who did not experience fear [9]. Therefore, building confidence and providing security during mobilization is important to prevent functional decline and recurrent falls. Another aspect of prevention of recurrent fractures is treatment of osteoporosis for patients with fragility fractures. Treatment should begin before hospital discharge and continue with outpatient treatment with their primary care physician.

References

1. Shiga T, Wajima Z, Ohe Y. Is operative delay associated with increase mortality of hip fracture patients? Systematic review, meta-analysis, and meta-regression. Can J Anesth. 2008;55(3):146–54. https://doi.org/10.1007/BF03016088.
2. Chow WC, Ko CY, Rosenthal RA, Esnaola NF. American College of Surgeons NSQIP/ American Geriatrics Society best practice Guidelines: Optimal Preoperative Assessment of the Geriatric Surgical Patient. American College of Surgeons. 2009; 1–52. Retrieved from. https://www.facs.org/~/media/files/quality%20programs/nsqip/acsnsqipagsgeriatric2012guidelines.ashx.
3. Salottolo KM, et al. A retrospective analysis of geriatric trauma patients: venous lactate is a better predictor of mortality than traditional vital signs. Scand J Trauma Resusc Emerg Med. 2013;14(21):7. https://doi.org/10.1186/1757-7241-32-7.
4. Callaway DW, et al. Serum lactate and base deficit as predictors of mortality in normotensive elderly blunt trauma patients. J Trauma. 2009;66:1040–4.
5. Chow WB, Ko CY, Rosenthal RA, Esnaola NF. Optimal preoperative assessment of the geriatric surgical patient: a best practice guideline from the American college of surgeons national surgical quality improvement program and the American Geriatrics Society. J Am Coll Surg. 2012;215(4):453–66.
6. American Academy of Orthopedic Surgeons. Management of hip fractures in the elderly: evidence-based clinical practice guidelines. 2014.
7. Juliebo V, Bjoro K, Krogseth M, et al. Risk factors for preoperative and postoperative delirium in elderly patients with hip fracture. J Am Geriatr Soc. 2009;57(8):1354–61. https://doi.org/10.1111/j.1532-5415.2009.02377.x.
8. Kratz T, Heinrich M, Schlaub E, Diefenbacher A. Preventing postoperative delirium. Dtsch Arztebl Int. 2015;112(17):289–96. https://doi.org/10.3238/arztebl.2015.0289.
9. Vellas B, Wayne S, Romero L, et al. Fear of falling and restriction of mobility in elderly falls. Age and Aging. 1997;26:189–93.

50 Geriatric Peripheral Vascular Injuries: Nursing Implications

Elizabeth Seislove

Epidemiology

Trauma in the elderly is the fifth leading cause of death in patients greater than 65 years of age. Often the elderly have a lower mechanism of injury but display an increased severity of injury due to frailty and pre-morbid conditions [1]. We often under-triage this patient population due to lack of pre-hospital triage guidelines along with trauma center geriatric triage criteria. The elderly often present to our trauma centers "looking good" which places many practitioners in a false sense of security. Geriatric patients have little reserve so with swift identification and appreciation of an injured geriatric patient will lead to efficient assessment and treatment.

Comorbidities

As noted in previous chapters regarding changes as we age, many of those changes will directly impact the vascular system and impact the severity of injury. Changes such as a decline in cognition, decreased peripheral vision and proprioception, decreased cervical mobility causing slower reaction times, decreased hearing, and mobility including agility all contribute to increased injury [1]. Medication intake will also cause varied changes in patient functionality and ability to adapt to injury. As a nurse, the knowledge of these changes will be essential to provide skilled geriatric care.

Other comorbidities include cardiovascular compromise with decreased circulation, HTN, CHF, A-fib and CAD, diabetes, stroke, renal insufficiency, and COPD, to name a few. Many of these aforementioned comorbidities cause a decrease in circulation increasing the potential for vascular injury in the elderly more than in the younger patient.

Resuscitation

Resuscitation efforts will follow ATLS principles along with an acute awareness of geriatric issues including fluid resuscitation, medication administration, and diagnostics. During the resuscitation efforts, the judicious use of fluids will be important. Fluids will be required and the importance surrounds the timely administration and the volume infused. The cardiovascular system is not as resilient as it is in the younger population; vessels are more rigid and inflexible leading to potential overload. Assessing circulation will include hard and soft signs for arterial vascular injuries. Hard signs include absent distal pulses, palpable thrill or

E. Seislove, M.S.N., R.N., A.V.P.
Trauma Services, Hospital Corporation of America (HCA), Nashville, TN, USA
e-mail: Betsy.seislove@hcahealthcare.com

A. Rodriguez et al. (eds.), *Geriatric Trauma and Acute Care Surgery*,
https://doi.org/10.1007/978-3-319-57403-5_50

audible bruit, actively expanding hematoma, and active pulsatile bleeding. Soft signs include diminished distal pulse, history of significant hemorrhage, neurologic deficit, and proximity of a wound to a named vessel. Upon the identification of one of these signs, preparation for definitive treatment will be required. The patient may necessitate an angiography to either rule out an injury or use as a treatment. Surgical intervention may be an option; preoperative preparation will be required [2].

The importance of knowing current medications the patient may have been taking will be essential: anticoagulation, ASA, beta blockers, ACE inhibitors, steroids, narcotics, will be imperative to assist in resuscitation efforts and aid in definitive treatment such as reversal of anticoagulation therapy.

Continued monitoring of lab values such as lactic acid or base deficit, and those that reflect coagulation (PT/PTT/INR or Thrombelastogram (TEG)), renal function (BUN, CR, GFR), blood alcohol/tox screen, and serum electrolytes will be obtained. The timely identification of abnormalities will enable rapid management of any abnormalities.

Secondary survey is designed to reveal any other injures not discovered during the primary survey, facilitating the appropriate consults and post Emergency Department needs, supporting the overall timely and efficient plan of care.

Injury Patterns

The elderly are most prone to falls followed by MVCs. The most common patterns of injury are fractures [3]. As health care practitioners, we often underestimate the impact of a ground level fall where the elderly may have an increase in injury severity due to the patient's comorbidities. The importance in following ATLS protocol for resuscitation, the timely identification and appreciation of injuries will be important.

Since arteries lose elasticity in the geriatric population the increased possibility of vascular injuries exists. Most commonly injured vessels are the large vessels such as the thoracic aorta, innominate and subclavian arteries [2]. Injuries to these major vessels lead to a high mortality rate. Many patients including the geriatric population who suffer from one of these major vessel injuries will expire at the scene. With advancement in prehospital care, if they survive the scene to arrive at the hospital, surgical intervention may be required, rapid assessment of the injury is imperative along with timely notification to the appropriate specialist for definitive care. Some of these injuries may be treated non-operatively but will require intense hemodynamic monitoring and specific medications for treatment.

Assessment

Nursing assessment will be essential to assure the rapid identification of injured vessels, allowing sufficient circulation and permitting adequate tissue oxygenation. If circulation is compromised due to the lack of blood supply due to an injured vessel, adverse events such as delayed wound healing, loss of tissue, loss of limb, and potential death could occur if circulation is not restored [4].

Circulation is part of the primary survey, being the time for early recognition of life-threatening injuries, and the delivery of rapid treatment is accomplished. If a vascular injury is found during the primary survey, the team must be prepared to assist with hemorrhage control and possible vessel repair and preparation for operative procedures if necessary. Constant reassessment will be required to assure that treatment modalities provided have worked and no further injuries have been found.

Nursing assessment will include evaluation of the peripheral pulses: what do they feel like; are they bounding, thready, equivalent? Is it more pronounced on one side than the other? What is the capillary refill time? What is the skin's color, temperature, and tone? All of the subsequent assessments will assist the nurse in assuring that circulation is adequately restored or maintained. At any time that the patient's vascular assessment changes, it must be approached with a keen sense of why this may have occurred and prompt notification of the trauma attending is necessary to ensure further evaluation is completed [4].

Diagnosis

Several diagnostic tools can be used to diagnose vascular injuries: CXR is the first test performed in the trauma bay and it can be a rough identifier of potential vessel injuries such as the aorta and subclavian arteries. A CT angiogram will be a more definitive diagnostic test. In many cases, an angiogram is the gold standard. An MRI/MRA may also be used in the appropriate circumstance.

Treatment

Once the diagnostic phase is completed and definitive diagnosis have been made, treatment will be based upon the severity of injury.

If a named vessel is noted to be torn, sheared, or have active extravasation, immediate intervention is required. Interventional radiology or endovascular intervention may be utilized for stenting or embolization of the injured vessel. Nursing care for the patient who has received angiographic intervention will require frequent pulse checks on the side of the embolization as well as assessment at the insertion site. Infrequently the entry site may develop a hematoma or pseudoaneurysm causing decrease in circulation on the affected side, and early recognition and follow-up care will be significant.

Depending on the nature of the injury, operative treatment may be required. If circulation has been compromised for a significant period of time, fasciotomies may be conducted, requiring standard wound care along with assessment of muscle, tissue, and skin integrity and scheduled dressing changes [2]. Continued assessment post-operatively of perfusion and pulses is essential.

Some injuries may only require medical treatments such as anticoagulants (low molecular weight heparin or one of the novel anticoagulants) and antihypertensives such as beta blockers to keep the patient's heart rate and blood pressure within acceptable ranges to reduce shear forces on the vessels. If the patient will be treated with medications, understanding the treatment modality of each medication including interactions with other medications, the impact on existing comorbidities and understanding the plan of care and expected outcome are critical for good result [1]. Informing the patient of medications that will be required is a nursing intervention and is our obligation to keep our patients and family informed.

Outcomes

Once a vascular injury has been identified and treatment has been implemented, the care provided thereafter is to sustain the circulation and to prevent secondary injury. Continued assessment of the injured area as well as assessment of peripheral circulation, hemodynamics including heart rate, blood pressure, and oxygenation, medication regimen, and skin integrity will lead to positive outcomes and lead to a healthy recovery [4].

Summary

This chapter identified the importance of understanding the epidemiology of the geriatric patient by considering comorbidities along with mechanisms of injury, injury patterns and physical appearance of the patient will assist the trauma team to identify injuries that may be life-threatening or may lead to further injury.

The identification of a vascular injury occurs during the primary survey and assuring continuous assessment and reassessment after intervention, along with constant hemodynamic monitoring, and vascular and skin checks all will be essential to lead to a healthy recovery and discharge plan.

References

1. American College of Surgeons (ACS). Trauma quality improvement program. https://www.facs.org/quality-programs/trauma/tqip. Accessed 10 Feb 2016.
2. Gregory L. Monet. Year book of vascular surgery. 2012. p. 273–86.
3. Konstantinidis A, Inaba K, Dubose J, Barmparas G, Lam L, Plurad D, Branco BC, Demetriades D. Vascular trauma in geriatric patients: a National Trauma Databank Review. J Trauma Inj Infect Crit Care. 2011;71(4):909–16.
4. McQuillan K, et al. Trauma nursing: from resuscitation through rehabilitation. 4th ed. St. Louis: Saunders Elsevier; 2009.

51 Geriatric Trauma Book: Urologic Trauma

Kai Bortz

Minimal research has been done on urologic injuries in the geriatric trauma population. A number of preexisting conditions may be seen and should be considered in the care of the older adult patient with urologic trauma. With aging, there is a loss of functional glomeruli and tubules as well as a reduction in blood flow, due to the decrease in mass of the kidney [1]. This impacts the ability of the kidneys to excrete medications that rely on renal clearance, therefore increasing the risk of adverse drug reactions [2]. Decreased functional reserve in the older adult also increases the risk of renal failure [3]. Nursing care must include a thorough physical assessment that incorporates the location of pain, assessment for patterns of bruising or lacerations, as well as consideration for associated injury [4]. Hematuria, flank pain/bruising, and abdominal pain have all been associated with assessment of renal injury [4]. There should be a high suspicion of renal injury with rib fractures or spinal process fractures [4]. Hemodynamic stabilization of the patient and treatment of concomitant injuries are critical components of immediate nursing care [4]. Many older adults are currently taking anticoagulants, which can profoundly impact the care of older adult patients with a renal injury. It is critical to complete a thorough review of medications and preexisting comorbidities on admission.

Initial management of most renal injuries includes fluid resuscitation, bed rest, serial vital signs, and serial hemoglobin levels. Urology consultation should be obtained promptly. Renal function should be assessed. Nephrotoxic medications and renally cleared drugs should be avoided to prevent further injury and complications [2]. Fluid balance should be maintained throughout hospitalization.

Ureteral Injury

Ureteral injuries are typically seen in penetrating trauma, not blunt trauma and are therefore uncommon in the elderly population.

Bladder Injury

In the lower urinary tract, there is reduced bladder elasticity and innervation, which leads to decreased urine flow rate, voided volume, and increased postvoid residual in the older adult. In the older adult male, benign prostatic hyperplasia (BPH) can result in urinary urgency, hesitancy,

K. Bortz, M.S.N., R.N.-B.C., C.M.S.R.N., C.N.L., T.C.R.N
Transitional Trauma Unit, Lehigh Valley Health Network, 1200 South Cedar Crest Blvd, Allentown, PA 18103, USA
e-mail: Kai_L.Bortz@lvhn.org

A. Rodriguez et al. (eds.), *Geriatric Trauma and Acute Care Surgery*,
https://doi.org/10.1007/978-3-319-57403-5_51

and frequency [1]. Bladder injuries are often managed with an indwelling urinary catheter, even in younger trauma patients [4]. Urinary catheter insertion should only be attempted after appropriate evaluation for a urethral injury [4]. In general, urinary catheters in the older adult patient should only be used when absolutely necessary and should be avoided whenever possible. Assessment for urinary tract infection should be considered prior to insertion of an indwelling urinary catheter. Daily review of urinary catheters should be performed to prompt early removal of the catheter or removal of the catheter when no longer necessary, to prevent Catheter Associated Urinary Tract Infections.

Due to difficulties with voiding, the older adult patient should be encouraged to get out of bed to void when possible. A bladder scan protocol should be followed for appropriate emptying of the bladder. Post void residuals may also need to be monitored to assure complete emptying of the bladder. Medications that increase urinary retention should be avoided.

References

1. Boltz M, Capequti E, Fulmer T, Zwicker D. Evidence-based geriatric nursing protocols for best practice. 4th ed. New York: Springer Publishing Company; 2012.
2. Beyth RJ, Shorr RI. Principles of drug therapy in older patients: rational drug prescribing. Clin Geriatr Med. 2002;18(3):577–92.
3. Lerma EV. Anatomic and physiologic changes of the aging kidney. Clin Geriatr Med. 2009;25(3):325–9.
4. Tonkin J, Tisdale B, Jordan G. Assessment and initial management of urologic trauma. Med Clin North Am. 2011;95:245–51.

52 Geriatric Trauma Book: Skin

Kai Bortz

There are a number of physiological changes that occur with aging that make the older adult more susceptible to traumatic wounds, as well as pressure ulcers following a traumatic injury. Nursing care of wounds in the older adult trauma patient should include control of comorbidities, particularly those that may inhibit wound healing. Additional risk factors for the older adult that can impair the wound-healing process include dehydration, malnutrition, unresolved pressure/shear and friction, excessive skin moisture, pruritus and dry skin, increased levels of wound exudate, and inappropriate management of wound exudate [1].

Wound Management

A thorough assessment of all wounds should be completed by the nurse and treatment modalities discussed with the trauma team. Nurses must complete routine assessments of the wound, assess for wound type, as well as exudate volume, consistency, color, odor, and the wound-dressing saturation. Treatment modalities will be based on wound type, location, and exudate. The patient should be monitored for signs and symptoms of infection.

If not appropriately managed, wound exudate can have a destructive action on the surrounding, periwound skin [1]. Exudate is a natural component of the wound-healing process and will transport essential nutrients, white blood cells (WBCs), and growth factors to the wound bed [1]. Wound exudate contains waste products that can breakdown the surrounding healthy skin, causing irritation, excoriation, and maceration [1]. In the elderly, this breakdown of the periwound can lead to further damage and prolonged healing time.

Atypical Presentation of Infection

Traumatic wounds can lead to infection. Signs and symptoms of infection in the older adult are often subtle, and may present with nonspecific decline in function, cognitive status, malnutrition, incontinence, falls, or exacerbation of chronic illness [2]. In addition, fever is often blunted or absent with increased age [3]. Temperature should be assessed routinely and a lower threshold for fever should be considered [3]. Nursing care should have increased awareness focused on atypical presentation of infection for older adults and monitor closely in patients with wounds.

K. Bortz, M.S.N., R.N.-B.C., C.M.S.R.N., C.N.L., T.C.R.N
Transitional Trauma Unit, Lehigh Valley Health Network, 1200 South Cedar Crest Blvd, Allentown, PA 18103, USA
e-mail: Kai_L.Bortz@lvhn.org

A. Rodriguez et al. (eds.), *Geriatric Trauma and Acute Care Surgery*,
https://doi.org/10.1007/978-3-319-57403-5_52

Fluid Balance

The older adult with traumatic wounds should be closely monitored for fluid and electrolyte balance [4]. Chronic illnesses as well as side effects of fever or medication may cause fluid and electrolyte imbalances [4]. Fluid and electrolyte imbalances should be corrected. The older adult is at increased risk of dehydration and should be monitored closely for signs and symptoms associated with dehydration, particularly in cognitively impaired patients. When possible, oral fluids should be initiated and encouraged frequently to prompt oral intake.

Nutrition

Malnutrition is more common among the elderly compared with younger patients and is associated with poor outcomes [5]. Hospitalized elders are at a higher risk of developing malnutrition than in the community setting [5]. Many older adults present to the hospital malnourished at the time of injury and should be monitored closely. All patients should be screened for malnutrition at the point of admission and appropriate interventions put in place. Additional focus and interventions to prevent malnutrition and assist with wound healing and overall recovery may need to be implemented for the older adult patient. In patients with traumatic injuries, early and adequate feeding has been linked to improved outcomes [5].

Interruptions to meals and/or tube feedings should be minimized and prevented whenever possible. Many trauma patients require repeated surgeries, making adequate delivery of nutrition during periods of nothing by mouth and surgery difficult to achieve [5]. Weight, body mass index (BMI), dietary intake, and fluid balance should be monitored closely in the older adult [4]. Nutrition consultation should be considered for patients at high risk of malnutrition. Dietary supplements may aid in providing nutritional needs for healing and recovery.

Pressure Ulcers

Nursing care must focus on pressure ulcer prevention in the older adult trauma patient, regardless of the injury type. Immobilization should be minimized to prevent pressure ulcer development. In addition, studies have shown an increase in pressure ulcer development in patients with longer surgery waiting times [6] and longer operating room times [7]. Patients must be assessed for pressure ulcers from the time of admission, as some elderly patients may present to the hospital with pressure ulcers on admission. Nursing care should include routine screening for pressure ulcer risk, skin assessment, and prevention interventions initiated during hospitalization following a traumatic injury. Nursing care of the older adult trauma patient should focus on pressure ulcer prevention, including skin care, maintenance of orthotic devices, appropriate fitting of orthotic devices, protection from moisture associated damage, prevention of friction and shearing, repositioning, and nutrition.

Immobilized patients and the use of immobilization devices exacerbate the risk of pressure ulcer development [8]. Pressure ulcers can cause significant problems for patients with spinal injuries, leading to additional pain, prolonged recovery periods, and additional dependence on healthcare staff. Duration of time in cervical collar was noted to be significant predictor of skin breakdown [8]. Particular attention should be focused on the occipital area, as the occipital pressure ulcers are often being the most serious and frequently detected later [8].

Many factors are associated with an increased risk of developing pressure ulcers in spinal immobilization, such as reduced mobility, application of medical devices, malnutrition, hypoperfusion, and the presence of other comorbidities [8]. While pressure ulcers are usually preventable by repositioning regularly to alleviate pressure, this may not always be possible in the patient with a spinal injury due to spinal instability [8].

Admission to the intensive care unit, mechanical ventilation, and time to cervical spine clearance have shown to be predictors of collar-related pressure ulcers [8]. The risk of pressure ulcer development associated with immobilization devices increases every day the patient is treated with the device [8]. The multidisciplinary team should be aware of the high risk of pressure ulcer development in any patient with an orthotic device, especially if the patient is not able to relieve the pressure or verbalize any discomfort felt [8].

As the risk of collar-related pressure ulcers increases in correlation to time spent in the collar, it is recommended that any patients with a cervical orthosis have skin integrity assessed on a regular basis [8]. Anatomical areas of great concern for skin integrity include the occiput, chin, and mandible [8]. The ears, shoulders, laryngeal prominence, suprascapular region, and sternum should also be considered as areas at risk of developing pressure ulcers [8]. Nursing care should focus on appropriate fitting, care, and education related to cervical collars and orthotic devices.

Early mobilization should be encouraged. Studies have found the mobility subscale of the Braden pressure ulcer risk assessment to be highly predictive of skin breakdown and should be taken into consideration in the older adult trauma patient [8]. Once patients are able to mobilize in their collar, it is important that the patient and family are given clear information on how to care for their device following discharge from the hospital and are provided with clear instructions for follow-up care.

References

1. Tickle J. Managing wounds in older people: the risk of skin damage from high-exudate levels. Br J Community Nurs. 2016;21(3):S20–4.
2. Htwe TH, Mushtaq A, Robinson SB, Rosher RB, Khardori N. Infection in the elderly. Infect Dis Clin North Am. 2007;21(3):711–43.
3. High KP. Infection in the elderly. In: Halter JB, Ouslander JG, Tinetti ME, Studenski S, High KP, Asthana, editors. Hazzard's geriatric medicine and gerontology. 6th ed. New York: McGraw-Hill; 2009. p. 1507–15.
4. Boltz M, Capequti E, Fulmer T, Zwicker D. Evidence-based geriatric nursing protocols for best practice. 4th ed. New York: Springer Publishing Company; 2012.
5. Wade C, Kozar R, Dyer C, Bulger E, Mourtzakis M, Heyland D. Evaluation of nutrition deficits in adult and elderly trauma patients. J Parenter Enteral Nutr. 2015;39(4):449–55.
6. Baumgarten M, Margolis DJ, Berlin JA, Strom BL, Garino J, Kagan SH, Carson JL. Risk factors for pressure ulcers among older hip fracture patients. Wound Repair Regen. 2003;11(2):96–103.
7. Houwing RH, Rozendaal M, Wouters-Wesseling W, Beulens JW, Buskens E, Haalboom JR. A randomized, double-blind assessment of the effect of nutritional supplementation on the prevention of pressure ulcers in hip-fracture patients. Clin Nutr. 2003;22(4):401–5.
8. Walker J. Pressure ulcers in cervical spine immobilization: a retrospective analysis. J Wound Care. 2012;21(7):323–7.

53 Nursing Considerations in the Care of Elderly Burn Patients

Jason Sheaffer

Introduction

Nurses play a pivotal role in the management of burn patients; this role is of particular importance in the care of geriatric burn patients. Considerations for this population begin with the observation of a fundamental relationship between age, burn size, and outcomes. According to the National Burn Repository data for 2016 [1], there continues to be a demonstrable correlation between increasing age and increasing burn size with regard to Burn Mortality. For example, a 60 year old (yo) patient with greater than 40–50% TBSA burn is associated with greater than 50% mortality. A patient in the 60–70 yo age group will carry >50% risk of mortality for the smaller burn size group of 30–40% and a patient in 80–90 yo category will carry a greater than 50% risk of mortality in the 20–30% burn size group. This correlation between managing age and associated comorbidities against the burn size of a patient provides the foundation for understanding the nursing considerations and care of the patient.

J. Sheaffer, R.N., M.S.N.
Blocker Burn Unit, University of Texas Medical Branch at Galveston, Galveston, TX 77550, USA
e-mail: jlsheaff@utmb.edu

Risk Factors

As patients age, they typically accrue comorbidities that play a role in outcomes. The aging patient will potentially present with a variety of risk factors [2]. Such factors can include:

- Underlying cardiac anomalies
- Underlying chronic health concerns, i.e., diabetes and heart disease
- A general trend towards less lean body mass, which predisposes the patient towards further muscle wasting and cachexia.
- Age-related skin changes: Changes in the composition of the aged's epidermis and dermal layers decrease wound healing and increase recovery time of damaged tissues. In general, there is a strong correlation between increased time to heal and increased risk of secondary complications such as infection.

Nursing Considerations

Nursing considerations for this patient population can best be described according to the phase of care that the burn patient is undergoing. The initial phase of care for significant burn injury can be defined as an acute or resuscitative phase lasting 24–48 h. The subsequent post-resuscitation period

A. Rodriguez et al. (eds.), *Geriatric Trauma and Acute Care Surgery*,
https://doi.org/10.1007/978-3-319-57403-5_53

can extend from days to months depending on the size of the initial burn. The post-acute and reconstructive phases can ultimately last for the rest of a patient's life.

Resuscitative Phases

The identification of a significant burn injury (generally 20% or greater) in a patient should prompt initiation of a well-conceived resuscitation plan. There is debate as to what constitutes adequate resuscitation, but generally, the use of well-described formulae is followed. The Parkland formula (4 mL/kg/%tbsaBurned, ½ administered in first 8 h and subsequent volume in remaining 16 h) is often cited as a means for guiding burn patient resuscitation. Recent modifications to the Parkland formula include the modified Brooke formula which calls for a range of 2–4 mL/kg/%tbsa (1/2 given in the first 8 h, subsequent half in the next 16 h) burned as a means gauging fluid needs. Ideal outcomes are predicated more on identifying an endpoint that indicates successful resuscitation [3, p. 115–124]. As a general rule, a satisfactory endpoint would be a urine output of 30–50 cm^3/h for nonelectrical thermal injury [3, p. 115–124]. The geriatric patient, however, represents a significant challenge in resuscitation because they often have both cardiac and renal comorbidities that can complicate successful resuscitation [4, p. 415–420]. For example, a patient with renal insufficiency may not be capable of producing 30–50 cm^3/h, an over-resuscitated geriatric patient will likely experience a higher incidence of congestive heart failure (CHF)-like complication leading to pulmonary edema, acute respiratory failure and contributing ultimately to mortality. This relationship between a patient's underlying comorbidity and presenting burn size underscores the need for careful goal-directed therapies in which the nurse often acts as the implementing agent.

Assessment in Acute Resuscitative Phase

Nursing assessments include assisting with obtaining the information necessary to manage the patient. On presentation to the burn nurse, an accurate weight, height, and complete set of vital signs are essential. The patient should be cleaned so that an exact determination of burn size, as well as any preexisting sores/wounds or skin-related phenomena, can be assessed. Once weight, BSA burned, and vital signs are known, the resuscitation strategy can be implemented. Regardless of which formula or technology is used during resuscitation, nursing staff should be well educated and versed in carrying out the plan.

Physical assessment. Initial physical assessment of the patient should proceed along normal lines, monitoring the ABC's (airway, breathing, and circulation) with notation of inhalation injury, and any circumferential injuries to the trunk and or extremities. These findings should be promptly communicated to the provider so that a determination of the need for emergent procedures (intubation or escharotomy/fasciotomy) can be made. Assessment should proceed along conventional means from that point on.

Nursing Diagnosis

Fluid volume deficit: Burn patients have fluid volume deficits owing to massive insensible loss from open burn wounds as well as increased capillary permeability in the first 24 h as a result of inflammatory mediators released after burn injury. These two factors combine to form the basis for burn resuscitation formulas [5].

Hypothermia: The larger the burn size of the patient, the more significant the likelihood of encountering hypothermia. As a general rule, the burn patient with significant injury should be maintained at a core temp of 37.5–38.5 Celsius [5].

Pain: The presence of pain in the burn setting is inevitable and will be the chief complaint of any patient presenting with first- or second-degree burns unless the patient has underlying neuropathy or deeper burns owing to underlying nerve damage. Pain can be a useful assessment tool for helping to ascertain burn depth. Treatment of acute burn pain is done with judicious use of narcotics. The patient ideally can complete a competent neurological exam and tolerate care with sedation [5].

Planning and Implementation in the Acute Resuscitative Phase

The nurse caring for the burn patient is responsible for administering the IV fluids as directed through appropriate intravenous (IV) access. The use of two large bore IVs is appropriate, and central line access is often attempted and obtained during the resuscitation phase. The nurse administers pain medications and assesses the effect of the medication on the patient as pertains to sensorium, pain levels, and impact on vital signs, especially blood pressure. The nurse(s) will also have likely cleaned the burn wound so that a plan can be formulated to address the burn injury needs. A nurse can anticipate a plan to treat/dress a burn wound with topical and or synthetic dressing, or participate in progressively more advanced burn care procedures including the performance of escharotomies or fasciotomies depending on hospital practice and policy and procedure.

Key factor: The providing nurse must realize that burned skin, whether the second or third degree, will not allow tape or occlusive dressing to adhere when securing IV catheters. IV or central line(s) placed through burn wounds must be sutured in place such that dislodgement will not occur.

Evaluation

Nurses evaluating the burn patient in the resuscitation phase are focused on the patient's response to resuscitation, frequently by monitoring an established appropriate endpoint of resuscitation. The production of 30–50 mL/h of urine (usually) indicates adequacy of resuscitation [3, p. 115–124], but in older patients with comorbid conditions, other endpoints for resuscitation may need to be identified. The bedside nurse should be familiar with the accepted norms and be prepared to communicate parameters that fall outside established normative values promptly. Possible other parameters could include mean arterial pressure (MAP), lactic acid levels, serum bicarbonate, base deficit, and hematocrit depending on the provider's protocols for managing resuscitation. Other evaluation criteria during resuscitation will include the patient's physiologic response to resuscitation. It is entirely likely that the patient will develop edema requiring elevation of extremities and evaluation for development of compartment syndrome. The development of adventitious breath sounds can indicate that pulmonary edema is developing particularly if O_2 saturation and PaO_2 begin to trend downwards. This pattern can indicate over-resuscitation. It can also indicate a comorbid phenomenon (CHF) requiring medical management with inotropic support [4, p. 415–424]. In any case, the bedside nurse is positioned to identify and respond to the trend proactively.

Other Nursing Consideration in the Acute Resuscitative Phase

Psycho-Social: The patient should be interviewed and queried as to their wishes in regard to management. Older clients may have pre-injury instruction such as Do Not Resuscitate/Do Not Intubate that preclude lifesaving interventions. Any family associated with the patient should be identified and brought to the bedside as soon as possible so that clear communication between staff, family, and patient are established. The nurse is often a facilitator of these discussions [6].

Ethical: Ethical considerations in the management of elderly acute burn patients often revolve around the issue of futility [6]. Assigning futility in burn cases is a complicated decision due in part to significant advances made in the care of burn patients in the last 30 years [6]. The survivability of burns has increased dramatically across all age and burn size groups. The family and/or patient should be made aware of the realistic chance of survival as well as the plan of care being considered to heal the burn injury. A family should be encouraged to make careful consideration and consider all options. The nurse has a duty to act as a patient advocate. Therefore it is essential that staff nurses thoroughly understand the patient wishes, rights under self-determination, underlying (patient) cultural and ethnic norms regarding the end of life and death and ensure that the plan of care conforms to the reasonable requests of the patient or the patient's designate. In the context of direct management, the patient's physiologic support (resuscitation) is usually in progress as these issues are identified and evaluated. Changing course from full treatment to palliative/comfort measures can be indicated for even relatively small burns in older patients [6]. Thus, the patient and patient's family should be central in such discussions.

Post Resuscitation-Acute Phase

Once fluid resuscitation is complete and increased capillary permeability third spacing resolves, the patient considerations will focus on wound closure and management during the acute healing process. Nationwide the accepted 1 day length of stay per percent open area burned can be used as a guide [1] with the understanding that underlying comorbidities and considerations of care must be carefully and methodically addressed in the geriatric population. The nurse is the primary provider of treatment, medication, nutrition, pain relief, and usually first responder in the event of sudden deterioration of the patient. The nurse's responsibility at this point is to implement the plan of care and *protect the patient from the hospital environment.*

Assessment

A thorough head to toe nursing assessment is done at least every shift on burn patients, (frequency dependent on hospital policy) as well as upon a noted change in status. The patient assessment should include a thorough review of systems, a detailed inspection of the equipment in use and validation of infusions of medications and an inspection of the safety apparatus in use at the bedside. In the burn patient, there are very specific reasons for stressing these seemingly obvious interventions. For example, a burn patient with facial burns requiring intubation may sustain a significant amount of facial edema in the resuscitation phase, during the post-acute phases the edema can and often does resolve very quickly. If the patient requires continued intubation during this period, it may be necessary to resecure the endotracheal tube multiple times. The previously mentioned considerations centered on maintaining IV patency and central lines should be sutured and secured whenever placed through burned skin.

Airway and Inhalation Injury

Airway edema resulting from inhalation of hot gas and smoke typically forms immediately after exposure. This edema can persist for several days thus necessitating the placement of an artificial airway to maintain airway patency. The key assessments are focused upon the patency of artificial airways (presence of breath sounds), lessening of airway edema (presence of an auscultated air leak), and management of secretions [7]. The bedside nurse will, often in conjunction with respiratory therapists, be responsible for the suctioning and pulmonary toileting of intubated patients. A key consideration in the management of burn patients and particularly elderly burn patients is the threat posed by mucus plugs, i.e., airway obstruction. In the face of inhaled smoke, gas, and heat, inhalation injury can manifest. As the days progress and management of the injury continues, it is common for sloughing of casts, tissue, and mucus to proceed, followed by mucus plug formation which can be a viable threat, especially during the first 3–5 days post injury. These casts can be thick enough to obstruct an endotracheal tube quickly and grossly impair oxygenation/ventilation [8]. The bedside nurse should be trained to observe and intervene when a mucus plug is suspected. Adding to the complication of this scenario is the tendency for a rapid progression from respiratory failure to cardiac failure, which can divert attention from the underlying complication. The mnemonic of Airway, Breathing, and Circulation (ABC) is the accepted means of combatting this complication. When responding to sudden deterioration of the burn patient with inhalation, the confirmation of a patent airway should always be the first action. The evacuation of a mucus plug and prompt restoration of oxygenation can avert a cardiac event many times [8]. In the elderly patient, the threshold for tolerating a plug will be lower, and the progression from plug to the cardiac event may be very quick, necessitating prompt identification and treatment. It should also be noted that pulmonary toileting in the inhalation burn may require near constant attention and reassessment to prevent mucus plugging [11, p. 257]. Proper assessment, toileting, and management of respiratory needs for these patients as well as extubation at the earliest, safest convenience are essential for the prevention of pneumonia which is a well-known complication in the care of the burn patient [1]. Patients who are extubated and "fail" due to coexisting respiratory or pre-morbid issue may need to undergo tracheostomy for long term care. The use of tracheostomy and frequency/conditions for placement vary widely from burn unit to burn unit. Generally the consensus is that optimal outcome is achieved by the patient managing their secretions without artificial airway at the earliest outset.

Cardiac Considerations

Elderly burn patients will require telemetry and monitoring with an underlying evaluation of the electrocardiogram (EKG). The baseline assessment should include the notation of background cardiac history, i.e., afib and CHF, and the presence of any cardiac assistive device (pacemaker). This thorough need to understand the current cardiac health of the patient cannot be overstated. Patients might require sophisticated monitoring to match therapy to symptoms particularly if their underlying cardiac health is compromised. The use and placement of Swan–Ganz catheter or similar technology varies from institution to institution. The presence of a Do Not Resuscitate (DNR) order must be clearly noted, understood, and displayed so that all responding staff is aware of the patient's wishes.

Renal/GU Considerations

Urine output and strict intake and output recording are the primary responsibility of the burn nurse. The administration of nephrotoxic agents should be discussed and evaluated with the bedside nurse participating. The collection of labs and review of values should occur and be communicated from nurse to nurse. Hypotension and ensuing renal insult should be avoided at all costs so as to protect against Acute Kidney Injury (AKI). Burn nurses should be able to assess for AKI and alert med staff so that quick adjustments to the plan of care can be made. In the face of older patients with pre-morbid renal problems, this vigilance is heightened. In the face of kidney failure, therapy considerations include the potential use of dialysis via Continuous Renal Replacement Therapy (CRRT) or via conventional hemodialysis. If CRRT is the chosen modality, the bedside nurse should be prepared to respond to complications involving equipment and catheter maintenance. Acute renal failure (AKI) is a grave development in the treatment of an elderly burn patient [4] and the negative impact on prognosis and care implications should be made clear to the family.

The Foley catheter is the method for monitoring urine output on an hourly basis. However, upon discontinuation of the need for hourly monitoring, indwelling urinary catheters should be removed as soon as is feasible. The 2016 NBR demonstrates UTI as a highly likely complication of care for the elderly patient [1].

GI/Nutrition Considerations

GI and nutritional considerations revolve around the following concepts. Elderly patients, like all trauma patients, are under considerable stress and may present with pre-morbid conditions such as GERD or peptic ulcers. The prompt initiation of ulcer prophylaxis is warranted, the use of proton-pump inhibitors (PPI) as opposed to H_2 blockers is under debate as to best outcomes and guided by institutional preference, the development of GI ulcer is a feared complication that is preventable. The nurse should recognize the need for this therapy and ensure that its presence is in the plan of care.

Constipation is another GI complication of care in burn patient commonly attributable to or aggravated by the use of large quantities of narcotics. Bowel attention and regimen is a standard issue in the geriatric population and should be treated as a serious consideration. Bowel regimen should and often does include the use of stool softeners, probiotics, and food strategies (high fiber) designed to promote regular bowel health. The bedside clinician should assess, identify, and note the presence of constipation, obtain orders to address, and ensure the patient has regular bowel movements. Failure to address these issues places the patient at high risk for impaction and obstruction. In some cases, this can lead to further complications.

The possibility of diarrhea in the care of these patients is present as well. The definition of symptomatic diarrhea can vary widely from provider to provider. Patients experiencing more than 1 L of watery stool per day can be anticipated to experience electrolyte derangement and some degree of dehydration. Hypokalemia and or hypernatremia are common assessments in this scenario. The bedside nurse is often the first to note the presence of diarrhea, particularly in the context of vital signs and lab changes, and should promptly address with a provider to formulate an appropriate plan.

The burn patient's underlying nutritional considerations are a prime factor. There are different formulas used to ascertain the caloric needs of the burn patient; regardless of a method for determining need, the administration of a patient-specific, caloric goal based nutritional plan is the best practice for the nurse [9]. The nurse should expect to place enteral tubes when indicated, quantify dietary intake, and be able to make a basic assessment as to nutritional health. These can be as easy as understanding the weight trend of the patient and describing the physical appearance, especially noting the loss of lean body mass. The use of pictures throughout the course of care helps to capture this phenomenon.

Skin/Wound Care Considerations

Skin care concerns in this population fall into two nursing focuses. The cleansing and provision of wound care with the goal of rapid/early wound closure and the prevention of a hospital-acquired wound.

Acute wound care: Hospitals may have different processes for the delivery of wound care and varying degrees of resources/technology available. The essential premise however generally remains the same. Burn wound care involves the cleaning/preparation of a wound bed followed by removal of devitalized tissue usually in a hydrotherapy setting. The removal of necrotic elements on a regular basis is essential to the prevention of infection and wound health. The administration of a topical medication and/or medication impregnated dressing follows cleaning and is designed to limit bacterial overgrowth and possibly further aid in debridement upon removal. Finally, the dressed wound bed is covered with an outer dressing meant to prevent desiccation of the wound as well as to apply pressure via elastic bandage (Ace wraps) for the purpose of promoting venous return and limiting dependent edema. The specific processes vary from facility to facility but are meant to accomplish the goals above.

Prevention of hospital-acquired wounds. Due to changes in the skin characteristics of the older client coupled with wounds from burn injury, the elderly patient presents as high-risk for acquiring pressure sores. The assessment and management of these patients include a detailed initial skin survey designed to identify preexisting injury and the development of a plan to address concerns. It should be noted that while the use of pressure relieving surfaces, mattresses and similar devices may be indicated and useful, they do not replace offloading of pressure points. The standard of care for prevention of pressure ulcers remains to turn patients off of bony prominences including offloading of the heel. The bedside nurse should also be wary of the possibility for device induced wound(s). Intubated patients or patients with various indwelling tubes/catheters may be at risk of developing pressure sores and or skin breakdown from these devices, particularly if these devices are in contact with compromised skin. Finally, the threat posed by the formation of incontinence dermatitis and breakdown from fecal incontinence cannot be understated. The burn patient must be kept clean and dry, the use of moisture trapping dressings or diapers is often contraindicated making quality peri-care complicated and challenging. Adding to the difficulty is the high preponderance of documented UTI as complications in the management of elderly burn patients [1].

Infection Control/Management

As the bedside nurse, the nurse is uniquely positioned to manage and prevent infection in the burn patients. Patients are often colonized by bacteria upon injury, and due to loss of skin integrity, the colonization may progress towards infection. The nurse assessment should include the noting of physical signs of infection including the presence of odor, cellulitis, purulent drainage, fever, increased or unusual pain, and changes in mental status. Laboratory assessments would include monitoring of white blood cell counts, changes in platelet count (thrombocytopenia), development of insulin resistance (hyperglycemia), and lactic acidosis. Vital sign assessments could include temperature, changes in blood pressure, and tachycardia. Advanced hemodynamic monitoring signs of sepsis would likely include a drop in measured systemic vascular resistance. A sharp increase in the cardiac index is a typical sign of compensation for healthy individuals in the face of sepsis. In the elderly or comorbid populations, compensatory mechanisms may be compromised leading to profound hypotension.

Nurses can and do play a prominent role in infection prevention. Meticulous hand hygiene and use of contact isolation for burn patients are indicated [10]. Further, the nurse should actively advocate for the patient by teaching family and visitors to comply with infection control measures and ensure that all members including visiting and consulting staff comply with the hand washing and isolation. The use of the proper sterile technique is a must when aseptic techniques are indicated, and the bedside nurse plays a role in both assisting with and identifying breakdowns in technique. Advocating for prompt removal of central lines and Foley catheters are other opportunities for nursing staff to support and protect their patients from hospital-acquired infections. Another opportunity for nurses to impact hospital-acquired infection is through the administration of adequate oral care/suctioning, which can reduce ventilator-associated pneumonia. This simple stratagem can have a significant impact not just on patient health but hospital reimbursement, as insurers increasingly seek to avoid paying for hospital-acquired conditions.

Other Considerations

The mobilization and ambulation of the patient are typically a rehabilitation responsibility. However, the nurse often plays a role in assisting or encouraging the safe mobilization of their patients. Patients who spend significant amounts of time in bed avoiding weight bearing are predisposed to developing pneumonia, developing pressure sores, encountering loss of lean body mass, development of deep vein thrombosis, and ultimately impaired wound healing. The simple act of getting a patient out of bed and into the chair, progressing to a weight bearing status at the earliest opportunity, and continuously stressing exercise at least every day can have a dramatic impact on patient outcome. The bedside nursing staff, including support staff, plays a significant role in this by assisting rehab services and encouraging their patients to participate to their fullest ability.

Psycho-Social

Pain management will continue to be a focus throughout the acute course of care, with the patient requiring some degree of narcotic support. The presence of pneumonia as a predominant complication in this population underscores the need to minimize sedation as much as possible. Patients must be able to clear secretions (cough and deep breathe) and ideally move and ambulate to mitigate the risk of secretions. Overuse of narcotic can reduce particiapation in therapy and also impact bowel health. The balance between the appropriate and safe use of narcotics in this setting can be the source of considerable stress for family members, and of course for the patient. In the setting of geriatric burn care, the degree of pain encountered can be a consideration in trying to arrange for best outcomes. Many families cannot fathom allowing their elder loved ones to suffer through a painful post-recovery course. This dilemma is especially evident in the face of patients with preexisting neurologic derangements or delirium who may not fully be aware of what is happening. Constant communication with family and honest appraisal of progress are essential. Assessment of the patient's ongoing psychological health should be ongoing throughout the course with vigilance for delirium. Early on in the course of care, if not upon admission, discharge planning should be addressed. This plan begins with an understanding of the family resources available, the financial resources available, and a history of the incident as pertains to safety. Elder abuse is a known phenomenon and can be malicious, i.e., intentionally perpetrated by a family member or caregiver, or a result of negligence, inadequate resources, or unsafe living conditions. As caregivers, we have a duty to ensure that patients are safely discharged upon recovery. If abuse is suspected or reported, the nurse or whoever receives the information should alert the multidisciplinary team and ultimately the authorities.

Patient Safety

As with all patients, necessary patient safety assessment should include risk for fall, pressure sore risk, and presence, use of, and need for safety equipment (side rails up, beds low to the ground, Ambu bags at the bedside).

Nursing Diagnoses (Not All Inclusive)

- Altered gas exchange (inhalation injury)
- Ineffective airway clearance (mucus plug)
- Decreased cardiac output
- Acute pain
- Constipation
- Diarrhea
- Caregiver role strain
- Patient safety
- Infection risk/actual

Planning/Implementation

The identification of care plans triggered by assessment should lead to the safe care of the elderly client undergoing burn care. The emphasis on safety and prevention of injury or acquired condition decreases the length of stay and ultimately leads to better outcomes. The prompt initiation and maintenance of enteral support for large thermal injuries rely on nursing and medical staff communication. *Whenever possible, maximal nutritional support should be delivered with preference given to enteral as opposed to parenteral delivery.*

Evaluation

Evaluation of the plan will focus on wound healing, presence (or absence) of infection, and continuous monitoring of the patient's mental and physical response to care. The patient family input should be solicited and considered with the plan of care monitored and adjusted daily if necessary in a multidisciplinary fashion.

Post-Acute Reconstructive/ Rehabilitative Phases

The elderly burn patient who survives significant burn injury will likely require a significant amount of assistance upon discharge. They will grapple with limitations in mobility requiring preparation, chronic pain, and lingering wounds requiring some degree of wound care. The disposition of this patient often requires coordination of resources and location of assistance appropriate to the location of family. Discharge planning, therefore, begins with admission and continues throughout care. The bedside nurse participates in this continuum and often has significant interactions with patients for many years afterward.

Nursing Considerations in Post-Acute Care Planning

Assessment

Assessment of the post-acute burn needs focuses primarily on meeting the needs of the patient safely upon discharge and ensuring that a proper follow-up plan has been formulated. Consideration includes the home environment, family dynamic, and equipment needs. In many cases, the assistance that an elderly client will require regarding activities of daily living may require placement into a Skilled Nursing Facility (SNF), Long Term Acute Care (LTAC) facility or rehab facility. The financial possibilities or limitations should be well understood long before attempting to make arrangements before discharge. If a patient is discharged home, training of the family and consideration as to the availability of dressings and home care equipment will have to be addressed.

Functional assessments include the safety of the patient in regard to performing, activities of daily living, fall risk, and monitoring for the development of burn-related complications such as burn scar contractures that can impede range of motion in the future.

Planning/Implementation

Burn discharge planning begins on admission. In the care of the elderly burn patient, having family participate in learning care that will be performed at home is paramount. Having a comprehensive follow-up plan in place is important both to ensure that the patient continues to recover from their burns, but also to ensure they do not develop secondary complications such as pneumonia or other infection in the outpatient setting. Ensuring that a patient has reliable transportation and that family understands the plan of care is essential for successful post-acute outcomes.

Evaluation

The goal of transitioning from inpatient setting to outpatient is for the patient to resume as much of their previous functionality as possible. This functionality will be determined based on the extent of remaining wounds, limitations in range of motion and thus mobility caused by scar formation, pain in healed or healing wounds, and overall health of the client.

Summary

The nursing care of the elderly burn client requires consideration of all burn phenomena typically encountered in burn injury. Additional factors include an emphasis on early family involvement with open and honest dialogue between health care providers and relatives regarding outcomes and needs. The nurse caring for this patient must be especially vigilant against the development of burn-related complications due to the likely presence of significant comorbidity in the client.

References

1. National Burn Repository (NBR). 2016. https://ameriburn.org.site-ym.com/store/default.aspx? (Available for purchase).
2. NANDA-I. Nursing diagnoses: definitions & classification, 2015–2016. 10th ed. Philadelphia: NANDA International; 2015.
3. Herndon DN. Fluid resuscitation and early management. In: Total burn care. 4th ed. Edinburgh: Saunders Elsevier; 2012. p. 115–24.

4. Herndon DN. Care of geriatric patients. In: Total burn care. 4th ed. Edinburgh: Saunders Elsevier; 2012. p. 415–20.
5. Herndon DN. Care of geriatric patients. In: Total burn care. 3rd ed. Edinburgh: Saunders Elsevier; 2012. p. 496–501.
6. Herndon DN. The ethical dimension of burn care. In: Total burn care. 4th ed. Edinburgh: Saunders Elsevier; 2012. p. 687–9.
7. Herndon DN. Anesthesia for burned patients. In: Total burn care. 4th ed. Edinburgh: Saunders Elsevier; 2012. p. 180–4.
8. Herndon DN. Respiratory care. In: Total burn care. 4th ed. Edinburgh: Saunder Elsevier; 2012. p. 239–48.
9. Herndon DN. Care of geritatric patients. In: Total burn care. 4th ed. Edinburgh: Saunders Elsevier; 2012. p. 417.
10. Herndon DN. Treatment of infection in burns. In: Total burn care. 4th ed. Edinburgh: Saunders Elsevier; 2012. p. 137.
11. Herndon DN. Total burn care. 4th ed. Edinburgh: Saunders Elsevier; 2012. p. 257.

54 Perioperative Nursing Considerations

Elizabeth D. Katrancha

Many older adults must undergo surgery after a traumatic injury. The nurse must consider many factors that complicate surgical procedures in the older adult, including comorbidities, decreased physiological reserve, and a more limited functional capacity. It is often the nurse who must compile the whole of the patient information and ensure review by the attending surgeon prior to a procedure. Of course, emergent situations will differ.

Preoperative

Nursing is responsible for ensuring a complete history and physical is recorded, laboratory examination results are reviewed, and assessment of risks is completed prior to a surgical procedure, when possible. Informed consent should be obtained and witnessed by the nurse, taking into consideration the patient's decision-making capacity. If the patient is unable to make decisions, the care team will need to confer with family or legal documentation regarding surrogate decision-making rights.

The history and physical examination should include nutritional status. Many older adults are nutritionally deficient, which can lead to postoperative complications. There are some laboratory values that are helpful in determining nutritional status. Albumin levels of less than 3.2 g/dL, cholesterol levels of less than 160 mg/dL, or a body mass index of less than 20 kg/m^2 have been shown to be predictive of mortality. On physical exam the skin, tongue, and oral mucous membranes help with the evaluation of nutritional and hydration status. Consider nutritional supplementation before and after surgery where appropriate. An early consultation with a registered dietician is recommended.

Patient and family teaching should begin in the preoperative phase. The nurse should be prepared to provide information on the procedure and expectations following the procedure. Consider discharge planning and destination in these early discussions. After a traumatic injury, patients and families need time to process what has occurred and often need guidance and reassurance.

Intraoperative

The care team is responsible for all recommended surgical site infection prevention measures recommended by the Centers for Disease Control and Prevention (CDC) and the Joint Commission's

E.D. Katrancha, D.N.P., C.C.N.S., R.N., C.N.E., C.S.N.
Department of Nursing, University of Pittsburgh at Johnstown, Johnstown, PA 15904, USA
e-mail: ekatrancha@pitt.edu

A. Rodriguez et al. (eds.), *Geriatric Trauma and Acute Care Surgery*,
https://doi.org/10.1007/978-3-319-57403-5_54

core measures in the Surgical Care Improvement Project (SCIP). These include prophylactic antibiotics, blood glucose control, early removal of urinary catheters postoperatively, temperature management, continuation of beta blockers, and venous thromboembolism prophylaxis [1, 2].

The intraoperative nurse must validate all pertinent information and be attentive to detail and ensure all usual safety measures are in place. Patient handoff communication between the preoperative nurse and intraoperative nurse is important. The nurses should review the patient history and physical and review laboratory results. It is also important to check for assistive devices such as hearing aid and dentures. Examine the skin for breakdown. During the surgical procedure, the OR nurse must be mindful of patient positioning and the increased risk for pressure ulcer development, which can happen quickly in the older adult with decreased subcutaneous tissue over bony prominences.

Temperature regulation in the older adult is less effective than younger patients, requiring close monitoring and intervention to maintain a normal body temperature. Blood glucose levels should also be monitored at regular intervals to prevent hyper- or hypoglycemia. Hypertension is a very common comorbidity in the older adult and many patients are managed with beta-blocker therapy which must be continued intraoperatively.

Postoperative

The immediate postoperative period should be focused on recovering the older adult from anesthesia, making airway and breathing the focus. In addition, pain control is one of the most pressing issues in the postoperative phase. The nurse must complete a thorough pain assessment including the pain control goals of the patient. Consideration should be made to both pharmacologic and nonpharmacologic treatments. Consult with the pharmacist and attending physician to develop a routine pain control schedule with allowances for breakthrough pain. Consider and monitor for the adverse effects of opioids on the geriatric client. If patient controlled analgesia (PCA) is to be utilized, the nurse must ensure the patient comprehends how to use the device and is physically able to operate the machine. The nurse should carefully document the effect of the pain control modalities and alert the team to adverse reactions, unwanted side effects, or uncontrolled pain.

Early mobilization is important to prevent complications in all surgical clients. Complications such as atelectasis, pneumonia, deep vein thrombosis, and delirium are consequences of prolonged immobility. The nurse should determine the client's previous functional status and make any necessary assistive devices are available and functioning. Early consultation with physical and occupational therapy is important. The nurse must also ensure that mobilization occurs during the off shifts and weekends. The nurse should continue to reevaluate the discharge plan and progress being made toward the goal.

References

1. The Joint Commission. Surgical Care Improvement Project. 2016. http://www.jointcommission.org/surgical_care_improvement_project/
2. The Centers for Disease Prevention and Control (CDC). Surgical Site Infection. 2016. http://www.cdc.gov/HAI/ssi/ssi.html

Index

A. Rodriguez et al. (eds.), *Geriatric Trauma and Acute Care Surgery*,
https://doi.org/10.1007/978-3-319-57403-5

O

P

R

S

MIX
Papier aus verantwortungsvollen Quellen
Paper from responsible sources
FSC® C105338

If you have any concerns about our products,
you can contact us on
ProductSafety@springernature.com

In case Publisher is established outside the EU,
the EU authorized representative is:
Springer Nature Customer Service Center GmbH
Europaplatz 3, 69115 Heidelberg, Germany

Printed by Libri Plureos GmbH
in Hamburg, Germany